# Cancer of the Testis

M. Pilar Laguna • Peter Albers
Carsten Bokemeyer • Jerome P. Richie
Editors

# Cancer of the Testis

Springer

M. Pilar Laguna, MD PhD
Associate Professor Department of Urology
Academic Medical Center
University of Amsterdam
Amsterdam
The Netherlands

Peter Albers, MD
Professor of Urology
Chairman Department of Urology
Düsseldorf University
Düsseldorf
Germany

Carsten Bokemeyer, MD
Director Department of Oncology and
Hematology with section Pneumology
Hubertus Wald Tumorzentrum
University Medical Center Hamburg
Eppendorf, Hamburg
Germany

Jerome P. Richie, MD
Elliott C. Cutler
Professor of Urologic Surgery
Harvard Medical School
Chief of Urology
Brigham and Women's Hospital
Boston
USA

ISBN: 978-1-4471-5729-8 ISBN: 978-1-84800-370-5 (eBook)

DOI: 10.1007/978-1-84800-370-5

A catalogue record for this book is available from the British Library


Softcover re-print of the Hardcover 1st edition 2011


Printed on acid-free paper

Springer Science+Business Media (www.springer.com)

*Before this book saw the light, one of the authors Dr. John P. Stein passed away. Because of his multiple contributions to the profession, recognized value, and dedication to his patients, it is the wish of the editors and co-authors to dedicate this book in his memory.*

# Foreword

Testis cancer is a relatively uncommon tumor but it is the most common cause of cancer in men between the ages of 20 and 40 and for this reason is looked on with great importance by urologists and medical and radiation oncologists worldwide. As it is well known that it was associated with a very poor prognosis in the past, but the advent of an aggressive approach to surgical removal of lymph node metastases and the lymphatic drainage in general, along with huge improvements in imaging and chemotherapy, has completely turned the tables. Testis cancer is now associated with significant cure rates and an overall improvement in cancer-specific survival.

Closer links have been formed between the urologists and physicians who treat the condition. Every case now involves a discussion with those treating testis cancer as well as those involved in imaging and histopathological assessment. All of this has contributed to the excellent results now achievable and which we can offer to our patients. In addition, the division of opinion that existed between urologists in different countries about the best way to treat early stage testis cancer has also been addressed by roundtable discussions and interaction at conferences between the various interested parties.

This excellent book is an attempt to bridge the various gaps that may have existed and represents a significant transatlantic cooperation. Many of the chapters consist of collaboration between authors in Europe and in the United States. There is also antipodean contribution which adds a further width to the book. Every aspect of testis cancer is covered and I believe that this will become the reference text book for this condition. I would like to congratulate the editors of the book in getting together a very eminent group of authors, all leaders in their field.

John Fitzpatrick
Dublin, Ireland

# Preface

Although the incidence of testis tumors is the lowest among the urological malignancies, the conditions surrounding its diagnosis are more dramatic, if possible, than those concerning other cancers. It appears in adolescents or young adults, most of them still without children, and when metastatic, a multidisciplinary approach including various medical and surgical specialists is often required.

The introduction of cisplatin-based chemotherapy in the early 70s was the turning point in the history of this cancer. Long remission rates were achieved and patients were almost uniformly cured. Together with the modern radiotherapy schemas, chemotherapy has been the corner point in the most curable urological cancer to date.

With the increasing knowledge of this cancer came the population awareness and the possibility of early diagnosis, minimizing treatment toxicity and long-term effects. In parallel, quality of life has always been a capital issue in young groups of patients who want and deserve an active full social and personal life.

More recently, a new spectrum is increasingly depicted in the population with testis tumors. Those are subfertile or infertile patients in whom the diagnosis of tumor accompanies the efforts for fathering children. Inguinal orchidectomy, the classical treatment in the presence of a contralateral nontumoral testis, is no longer the gold standard for these serendipitous tumors. Two reasons justify a partial approach in this special group: the need for preserving sperm producing tubules and the high incidence of benign tumors among those incidentally diagnosed tumors.

Current efforts focus on defining the environmental and genetic factors that might determine the development of a testis cancer and exclusively identifying those malignancies that may ultimately respond to less intensive chemotherapy or radiotherapy schedules.

However, a number of patients are still diagnosed in an advanced stage. For those patients, cure is achieved at the cost of multiple different treatment modalities and under a strict surveillance, both conditions best served in centers of reference.

But the work is not yet accomplished. Although the incidence seems to have reached a plateau and the rate of Stage I cancers is higher than ever, some points deserve the full attention of the medical community. Some alarming reports point out the lack of tumor marker documentation at diagnosis and the treatment deviations. While good quality randomized controlled trials determined the landmarks in the treatment of testis cancer, clinical variability in follow-up is still a weak point in the protocols. Whether the clinical variation in follow-up is prompted by the different treatment options in early stages, or by country or worldwide policies, this variation calls for research, well designed studies, and cooperation among the different specialties involved in the treatment of this disease.

The present book, a Euro-American collaboration, is the result and an example of such cooperation. Not all the authors who have made a significant contribution to the history of this disease are present, but all those who are present have contributed in different forms and grades to the modern approach of testicular cancer.

M. Pilar Laguna
Peter Albers
Carsten Bokemeyer
Jerome P. Richie

# Acknowledgment

Acknowledgements to: Talal Akhter, Judy Crable, and Robin Osborn, DO for their valuable assistance. We also like to acknowledge our families for their patience and support. A special thanks to Dr. Mubin Syed's wife, Afshan Syed and father, Ibrahim Syed.

# Contents

# Part I

# Classification and Risk Factors

# Histological Classification and Pathology of Testicular Tumors

# 1

Ferran Algaba and Isabell A. Sesterhenn

Any testicular tissue can develop into a tumor. Tumors that grow from nonspecialized testicular stroma have the same pathological aspects as those that develop in other anatomical regions; however, tumors from the germ cell, sex cord, and gonadal stroma are completely different. The object of this chapter is to describe these peculiar tumors.

## 1.1 Pathological Expression of the Germ Cell Testicular Tumors and Their Biology

The characteristics of testicular germ cell tumors (TGCTs) are complex, mainly because of the peculiarities of each of the morphological variants and their heterogeneous mixture forming different patterns. Pathological reports present very intricate information for the urologist, so it is sufficient to consider morphological data alone. The goal of this chapter is to expose the basic morphological aspects of the TGCT and the best application of this information in the clinical–pathological correlation.

After a long search for an accurate classification, currently the most widely used system is the *WHO histological classification* (Eble et al. 2004a) (Box 1), which organizes TGCTs in two large groups according to their histological patterns depending on whether they are pure or mixed.

**Box 1 WHO Histological Classification of Germ Cell Testicular Tumors**

Intratubular germ cell neoplasia, unclassified.
Other types
Tumors of one histological type (pure forms)
Seminoma
Seminoma with syncytiotrophoblastic cells
Spermatocitic seminoma
Spermatocitic seminoma with sarcoma
Embryonal carcinoma
Yola sac tumor
Poliembrioma
Trophoblastic tumors
Choriocarcinoma
Trophoblastic neoplasm other than choriocarcinoma
Monophasic choriocarcinoma
Placental site trophoblastic tumor
Teratoma
Dermoid cyst
Monodermal teratoma
Teratoma with somatic-type malignancies
Tumors of more than one histological type (mixed forms)
Mixed embrional carcinoma and teratoma
Mixed teratoma and seminomas
Choriocarcinoma and teratoma/embryonal carcinoma
Others

It is believed that different types of TGCTs are derived from cells belonging to the germ cell lineage with characteristics of fetal germ cell differentiation (loss of OCT3/4-*transcription factor* and increased staining for VASA – a germ cell line-specific protein) (Honecker et al. 2006; Zeeman et al. 2002); variants

F. Algaba (✉)
Pathology Department, Fundacio Puigvert Universitat Autonoma de Barcelona, Calle Cartagena 340-350, Barcelona 08025, Spain
e-mail: falgaba@fundacio-puigvert.es

M.P. Laguna et al. (eds.), *Cancer of the Testis*,
DOI: 10.1007/978-1-84800-370-5_1, 

can be derived from a common cell after passing through the seminoma form (Ferreiro 1994).

Three observations (intratubular germ cell neoplasia, aneuploidy, and isochromosome 12p) sustain the idea that the majority of germ cell tumors originate from an undifferentiated transformed germ cell (that of the intratubular neoplasia of the germ cells), which acquires a morphological appearance when infiltrated, and that seminomas (the most frequent and pure form) can occasionally be constituted in the process of forming into non-seminoma variants (Srigley et al. 1987), Hittmair.

The most well-known findings on the histogenesis of the TGCT seem to demonstrate that there is a close relationship between the *intratubular germ cell neoplasia* and the invasive components of the TGCT that mimic embryogenesis (de Jong et al. 1990; van Echten et al. 1995; Soosay et al. 1991; Giwercman et al. 1990).

*Aneuploidy* is one of the characteristics of the TGCT (Suster et al. 1998; El Naggar et al. 1992; Oosterhuis et al. 1989), although this is not the same for all the variants. It is observed that the average DNA index is similar in intratubular germinal neoplasias and the seminomas, and the value of the latter is higher than that of non-seminoma tumors (Suster et al. 1998), which suggests that some morphological forms can transform into others through the loss of DNA.

The *isochromosome 12p – i(12p)* – is the most frequent chromosomal disorder, and is present in 80% of thecases of established tumors (van Kessel Geurts et al. 1993) and in 50% of intratubular neoplasias of germ cells (de Jong et al. 1997). It has even been found that seminomas have a lesser number of copies of i(12p) than non-seminomas, suggesting that this is the expression of a progression from seminoma to non-seminoma tumors through an increment of copies of this isochromosome.

For the description of the principal morphological characteristics of the different varieties, the above-mentioned WHO histological classification will be followed.

## 1.1.1 Intratubular germ cell neoplasia, unclassified

The presence of neoplastic germ cells in the seminiferous tubules is considered as the preinvasive form of the TGCT. After several publications and meetings, its nomenclature was fixed, advising against the term of carcinoma "in situ," as the intratubular neoplastic cells lack epithelial characteristics. The term intratubular germ cell neoplasia, unclassified (ITGCNU) (Reuter 2005), was suggested and accepted by the WHO (Eble et al. 2004a).

### 1.1.1.1 Morphological Features with Clinical Implications

A TGCT is characterized by the presence of enlarged and atypical cells of clear cytoplasm, with irregular nuclei and multiple prominent nucleoli. They are located immediately above the basal membrane, isolated or in a single row. There is no active spermatogenesis and at times only occasional Sertoli cells displaced toward the light by the neoplastic cells are recognized. The tubules are reduced in diameter and the tubular walls are thicker than normal (Fig. 1.1) (Reuter 2005; Rorth et al. 2000). These morphological characteristics must be strictly used in order not to diagnose the intratubular growth as ITGCNU with complete filling of the tubules in some cases of TGCT (from 7% to 19%) that occasionally can be secondary to an intratubular spread of the TGCT (Lau et al. 2007a).

A subject of discussion is the relation of the ITGCNU with testicular microlithiasis. Although it is true that microlithiasis is more frequent in tubules with ITGCNU (39%), they are also present in 2% of normal testicles (Ganem et al. 1999), and no definitive relation has been established between both lesions (Peterson et al. 2001).

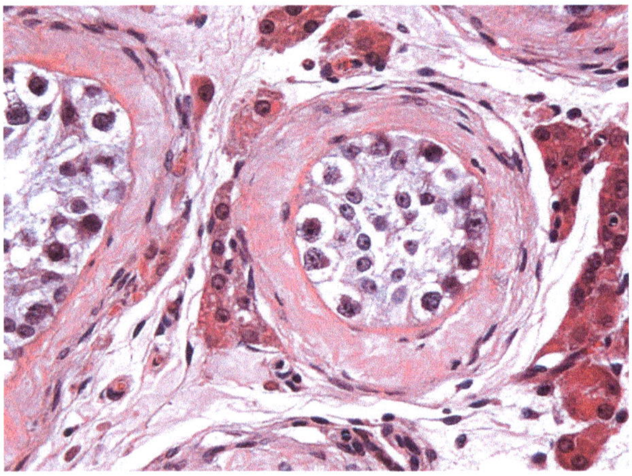

**Fig. 1.1** Intratubular germ cell tumor. Small tubules with fibrosis of the wall

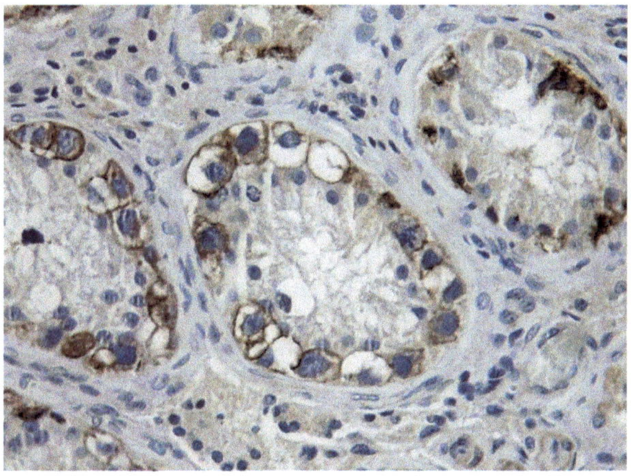

**Fig. 1.2** c.kit expression of the intratubular germ cell tumor

Usually ITGCNU is extensive and a single biopsy is sufficient to make the diagnosis; nevertheless, it has been demonstrated that the diagnostic yield increases as a higher number of biopsies is taken (from 3–5% to 7.8%) (Kliesch et al. 2003).

The immunophenotype is characterized by the expression of placental alkaline-like phosphatase (PLAP) in membrane or cytoplasm pattern (Burke and Mostofi 1988), c-kit (CD117) (Jorgensen et al. 1995) and OCT3/4 (Cheng et al. 2007) (Fig. 1.2).

#### 1.1.1.2 Clinical Features

It can be found in an isolated form in 1% of the biopsies for infertility.

As an odd detail, it may be highlighted that in some cases a decrease in testicular size has been observed, which can be explained by tubular fibrosis and a reduction in the diameter of the seminiferous tubules (Trias et al. 1991).

A 2–8% incidence rate has been observed in cryptorchidic testicles (von der Maase et al. 1986); however, the finding of ITGCNU in children is strongly debated. The majority of the literature is against it, but others are in favor in yolk-sac tumors (Hu et al. 1992), with certain differences in the expression of the PLAP (Soosay et al. 1991; Renedo and Trainer 1994).

ITGCNU is concomitant in nearly all testicular tumors (88%) (Lau et al. 2007a), except in cases of spermatocytic seminoma (Reuter 2005). This finding in a patient with a TGCT does not worsen prognosis.

The clinical bearing of cases with ITGCNU in the contralateral testicle on TGCT is strongly debated. The incidence of this situation varies according to geographic areas, ranging from 5% in countries with a high incidence of TGCT (von der Maase et al. 1986) to 1.2% in those with low incidence (Tabernero et al. 2004), which evidences the different approaches in systematically performing a contralateral testicular biopsy on a TGCT.

#### 1.1.1.3 Evolution

As stated previously, the majority of the ITGCNU have cytological and nonspecific immunohistochemical characteristics (similar to the seminomas) and are associated with any type of TGCT, for which reason they are considered undifferentiated cells; however, some authors have defended the possibility of intratubular differentiation (Berney et al. 2004, 2005) although the differential diagnosis always approaches the intratubular extension of a macroscopically nearby TGCT (Ulbright 1993).

Between 8% and 43% of TGCTs show areas of microinvasive germ cell tumor around the ITGCNU (von Eyben et al. 2004), and rete testis pagetoid extension can be observed (Reuter 2005). In isolated ITGCNU, transformations to microinvasive forms or TGCT have been referenced at 50% (Reuter 2005) to 98% (von Eyben et al. 2005), which leads to the consideration that it must be treated in order to avoid the progression to TGCT (von Eyben et al. 2005).

### *1.1.2 Seminoma*

In its pure form it represents 40–50%, approximately, of the testicular tumors between 25 and 55 years of age, and additionally 15% of seminomas are combined with other morphological variants.

#### 1.1.2.1 Morphological Features

The gross appearance of this neoplasia is usually a tumoration with 5 cm average diameter, lobed, well marked, without capsule, of a whitish color and homogeneous appearance. Occasionally fibrous areas

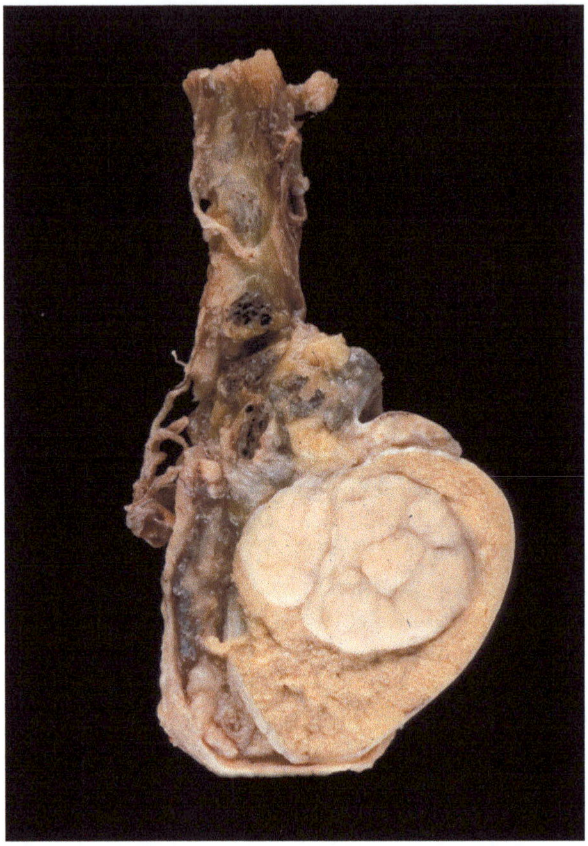

Fig. 1.3 Seminoma. Well-outlined tumor with lobular aspect

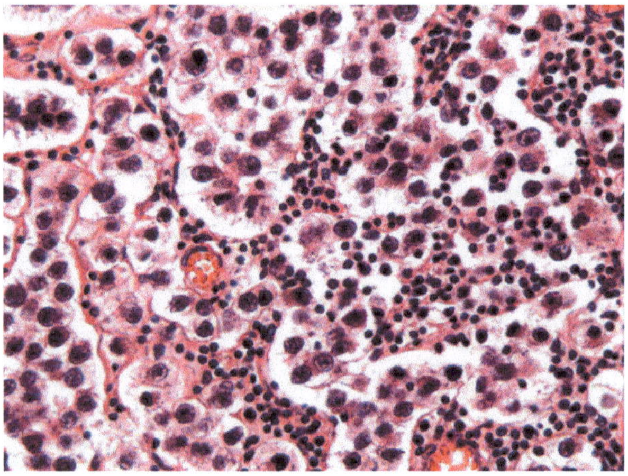

Fig. 1.4 Seminoma with lymphocytes in the stroma

are recognized and in larger tumors necrosis can be observed (Fig. 1.3).

Typically the cells of the seminoma are of clear cytoplasm, with a large-sized, single central nucleus of irregular chromatin and with nucleoli. They are distributed in solid or cord-like aggregates with a thin connective tissue characteristically occupied by T-lymphocytes and macrophages/dendritic cells with occasional granulomas with Langhans cells and foreign body appearance which, if distributed, can have a cytotoxic action on the tumor (Fig. 1.4) (Talerman 1980; Cope et al. 1999).

Its immunophenotype (Table 1.1) is characterized by a membranous expression of PLAP in 87% of the cases (Niehans et al. 1988), of c-kit (CD117) in 77% of the cases (Leroy et al. 2002), and of nuclear expression of the OCT3/4 in all the cases (Hattab et al. 2005). In 20% of seminomas, cytokeratins are expressed (CAM5.2) (Suster et al. 1998), and 10–20% have mononuclear or multinucleated trophoblast cells with secretion of hCG, which must not be interpreted as areas of choriocarcinoma (Ulbright 1993) (Fig. 1.5).

To this classic pattern we must add a series of morphological variations that, although without clinical significance, are important to know, especially for the pathologist, in order to avoid a mistaken diagnosis. These have been described as follows:

- Cases with *exclusive intertubular growth* (Henley et al. 2004) without tumoration that can even go unnoticed in macroscopic observation and that possibly evolve to no more than a microinvasive ITGCNU.
- *Microcystic* pattern that causes confusion with yolk-sac tumor (Ulbright and Young 2005).
- *Tubular growth* that mimics a Sertoli cell neoplasm (Ulbright and Young 2005).
- Cases with marked eosinophilia of the cytoplasm of the seminoma cells that imitate a plasmacytoma (Ulbright 2005)

Other pathological differential diagnoses are: malignant lymphomas (if there is a huge quantity of lymphocytes in the stroma), rete testis carcinoma (in case of rete testis pagetoid extension of the seminoma cells), and granulomatous orchitis when a granulomatous stroma is very prominent. In all these circumstances the demonstration of cells with the typical immunophenotype is of great utility.

#### 1.1.2.2 Clinical Features

From the oncological viewpoint, distinguishing between seminoma and non-seminoma is fundamental for the treatment because of the great significance that the pathological differential diagnosis has.

**Table 1.1** Immunophenotype of the germ cell tumors

| Antibody | Seminoma | Spermatocytic seminoma | Embryonal carcinoma | Yolk-sac tumor | Chorio carcinoma |
|---|---|---|---|---|---|
| OCT3/4 | 90% | – | 90% | – | – |
| PLAP | 87% | – | 86% | 53% | 54% |
| CD30 | <10% | – | 100% | <10% | – |
| AFP | – | – | 33% | 74% | – |
| β-hCG | Trophoblast | – | Trophoblast | Trophoblast | 100% |
| c-kit (CD117) | 85–100% | Dot-like | – | 70–100% | |
| CK | 10% | | 95% | 100% | 100% |
| EMA | – | | 2% | 5% | 46% |
| Vimentin | 30% | – | 19% | 16% | 4% |
| CEA | – | | – | 11% | 25% |

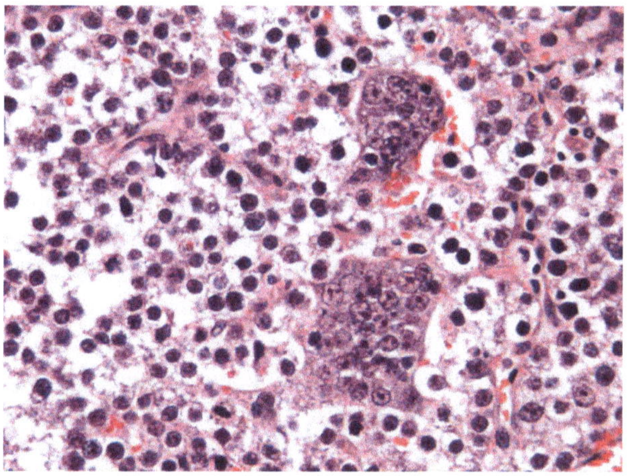

**Fig. 1.5** Seminoma with isolated syncytiotrophoblast cell

The average age of presentation is around 40 years. The majority of the patients consult for local symptoms, but around 2.5% have symptoms related to the metastasis.

As observed, the seminoma lacks serum markers, except for the small group of those that produce hCG. Current therapy achieves a high success rate in initial tumors (Albers 2007) and overall survival rate of around 95% in all the seminoma cases (Steele et al. 1999). However, for those cases with more aggressive evolution than expected, besides the clinical stage there are no morphological data that allow for a recognition of aggressiveness. Despite the fact that some authors give some prognostic value to the atypical nuclear and proliferative index (Tickoo et al. 2002), it has no therapeutic consequence (Ulbright 2005).

#### 1.1.2.3 Evolution

The significance of a seminoma with elevated serum AFP is a widely debated subject in the literature. One possibility is that it is a seminoma with a hidden area of yolk-sac or embryonal carcinoma; however, there are a series of data that reinforce the idea that a tumor is capable of being somatically differentiated between embryonal carcinoma and choriocarcinoma (Suster et al. 1998), such as: scattered single-cell expression of CD30 (2%) (Tickoo et al. 2002), cytokeratin expression in 10% (Niehans et al. 1988), p53 overexpression in 77%, K-ras mutation in 40% (Suster et al. 1998), demonstration in a group of seminomas with a protein molecular profile similar to embryonal carcinoma (Hofer et al. 2005), and demonstration of the presence of mRNA AFP in 60% of pure seminomas that showed neither immunohistochemical expression nor elevation of serum AFP (Yuasa et al. 1999).

Even so, there is no evidence that cases with anomalous expression of cytokeratins or with isolated trophoblast cells have a worse prognosis (Ulbright 1993; Talerman 1980).

### 1.1.3 Spermatocytic Seminoma

There is no relation to the described seminoma, without changes in chromosome 12 and characteristic gains in chromosome 9.

It represents 1–2% of TGCTs (Ulbright 1993). The average age of clinical presentation is 53.6 years, although cases have been reported in the third and fourth decades as well (Chung et al. 2004). It has not been found in children or adolescents.

No mixed cases have been described; nor is it found in the ovaries or in extratesticular locations.

#### 1.1.3.1 Morphological Features

Grossly it is a tumor measuring an average diameter of 7 cm with a gelatinous appearance because of an edematous interstitial component.

The three typical cells are (Fig. 1.6): small cells – *diploid*, resembling lymphocytes; medium-sized cells – *aneuploid*, which are the most frequent with round nuclei and a fine granular chromatin pattern surrounded by a rim of dense eosinophilic cytoplasm; and giant cells – *polyploid*, which are large uninucleated or multinucleated cells with granular or long spireme filaments (Eble 1994). The stroma, with few lymphocytes, has the characteristic edema fluid that forms small cystic spaces or large pools. No cases have been demonstrated with ITGCNU in the non-tumoral parenchyma and the intratubular involvement is related to the extension of the tumor (Eble 1994). Some cases have been published with marked anaplasia but apparently this fact does not have any bearing on its biology (Albores-Saavedra et al. 1996). Around 5% (Eble 1994) of the cases have areas of sarcoma, generally nonspecific, and some are of the rhabdomyosarcoma type (Burke and Mostofi 1993).

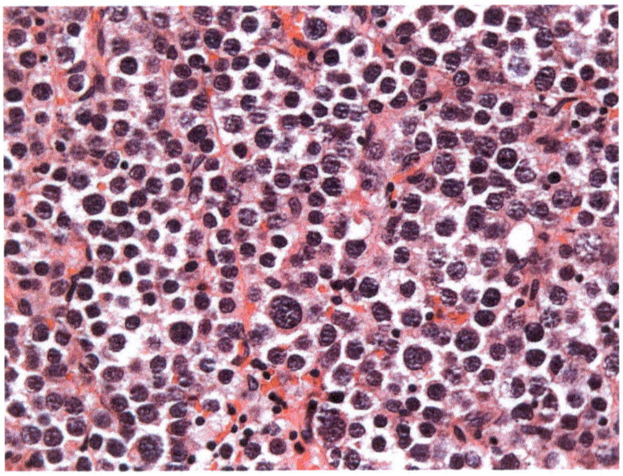

**Fig. 1.6** Spermatocytic seminoma with different types of cell and spirema in some of them

The lack of expression of PLAP, OCT3/4, AFP, and CD30, the occasional dot-like perinuclear reaction for low-molecular-weight cytokeratins, and the expression in 40% of cases of c-kit (CD117) (Cummings et al. 1994; Looijenga et al. 2003) are immunophenotype characteristics. Recently the expression of VASA has been demonstrated (Zeeman et al. 2002).

#### 1.1.3.2 Clinical Features and Evolution

The presence of this tumor is exceptional in maldescended testicles (Stevens et al. 1993).

Its origin is still unknown since its description in 1946 by Pierre Masson. Its germ cell origin is confirmed with the expression of VASA (Zeeman et al. 2002). Because of the filamentous-*spireme* appearance of the nucleus of intermediate and large cells, it is assumed that it could be related to spermatocytes; however, the lectins that it expresses are not those of the post-meiotic cells (Lee et al. 1985). The immunohistochemical expression pattern of Chk2, p53, p19INK4d, and MAGE-A4 is highly consistent with the origin of spermatocytic seminoma from a premeiotic germ cell, which has lost embryonic traits and has committed to spermatogenic lineage but has not yet passed the meiotic checkpoint (Rajpert-De Meyts et al. 2003).

Except for two cases with metastasis (Matoska et al. 1988; Steiner et al. 2006) all the pure spermatocytic seminomas published are in stage I, without being aggressive, and are unlikely to need any treatment beyond orchidectomy, but surveillance is still required because of limited published data (Chung et al. 2004).

In patients with spermatocytic seminoma associated with sarcoma, this element can be metastatic and the approach must be completely different (Floyd et al. 1988; True et al. 1988).

### 1.1.4 Embryonal Carcinoma

In the pure form it presents in 3–10% of the cases, but in the mixed form it accounts for more than 40% of TGCTs (Ulbright 1993, 2005). The age of presentation varies between 25 and 35 years.

#### 1.1.4.1 Morphological Features

Pure embryonal carcinoma is usually a small tumor, with an average diameter of 4 cm, frequently associated with hemorrhage and necrosis. In mixed cases, the gross appearance depends on the other components (Fig. 1.7).

The tumor is made up of cells with little differentiation in the epithelial appearance, rather undefined cellular edges, atypical nuclei and macronuleoli, and abundant mitosis distributed in solid, glandular, and papillar masses (Fig. 1.8). Like in the seminomas, there may be isolated cells of syncytiotrophoblasts in 85%, and intermediate trophoblast in 35% of the cases (Manivel et al. 1987a) (Fig. 1.9).

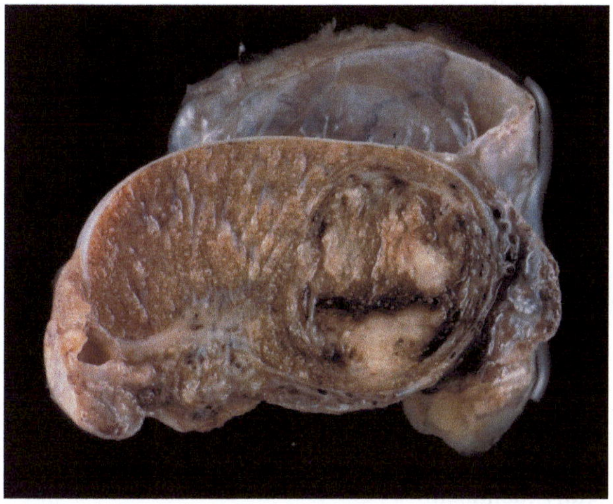

Fig. 1.7 Embryonal cell carcinoma with a heterogeneous aspect

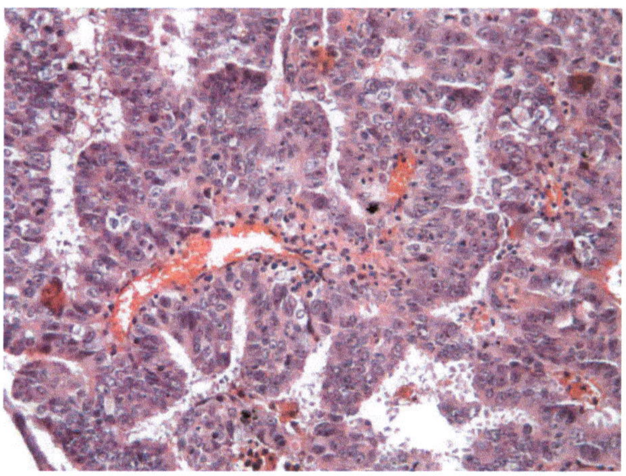

Fig. 1.8 Embryonal cell carcinoma. Atypical cells epithelial-like aspect

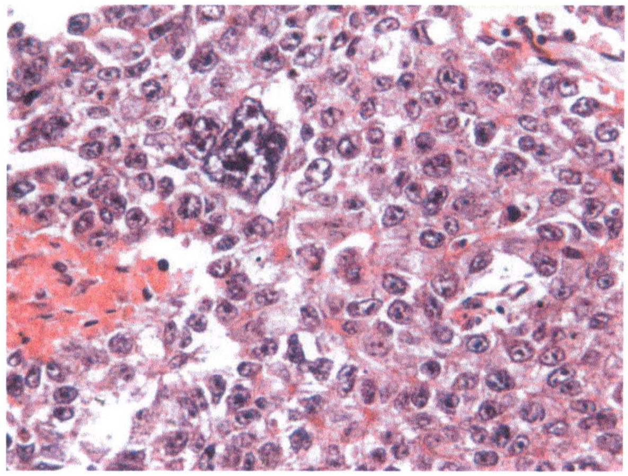

Fig. 1.9 Embryonal cell carcinoma with isolated syncytiotrophoblastic cells

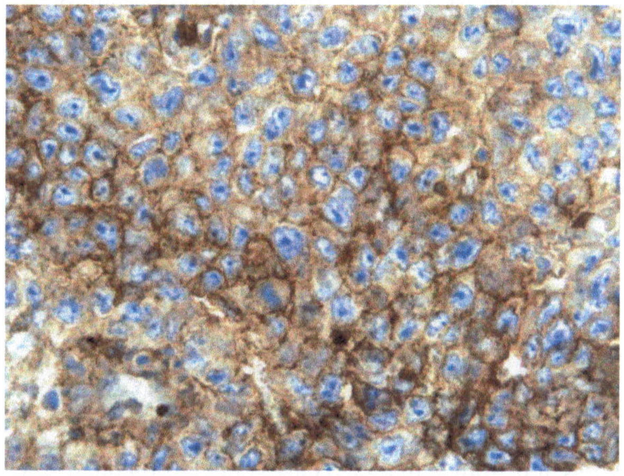

Fig. 1.10 Embryonal cell carcinoma with CD30 expression

With the immunohistochemical method, (Table 1.1) one can demonstrate that the expression of cytokeratins is found in 95%, PLAP in 86%, CD30 in 93% (Fig. 1.10), that the c-kit (CD117) is negative, EMA is practically negative, and AFP is seen in isolated cells in 33% of the cases (Niehans et al. 1988; Lau et al. 2007b).

#### 1.1.4.2 Clinical Features and Evolution

The majority of the patients consult for tumoral mass, and because they have a faster growth speed than seminomas, they present with greater frequency of local pain. Around 10% of the metastasis expresses the initial symptomatology.

Given the scant evidence of AFP production it is very rare that people with very high AFP serum have pure forms of embryonal carcinoma (Mostofi et al. 1988), for which reason one must search for a concomitant yolk-sac tumor. As with seminomas, elevations of hCG can be found because of the occasional isolated trophoblast.

From a therapeutic viewpoint, embryonal carcinoma is included in the group of non-seminomatous TGCTs, and the protocols that are applied depend to a great extent on the extension of the disease.

### *1.1.5 Yolk-Sac Tumor*

This tumor is also known as endodermal sinus tumor or orchioblastoma in the British classification.

In its pure form it is the most common variant (82%) observed in testicles of infants and young children of an average age of 17 months (Kaplan et al. 1988).

In adults, it appears between 17 and 40 years (Talerman 1975). It is practically never pure and is found in 40–50% of adult TGCTs (Ulbright 1993).

#### 1.1.5.1 Morphological Features

The pure yolk-sac tumor is usually a tumoration of 2–6 cm, poorly delimited, with a gray-white infiltrating appearance, and is occasionally microcystic. The gross appearance in mixed cases depends on the different combinations of tumors.

The major pathological–anatomical problem of this tumor is its great diversity of patterns – of which up to 12 varieties have been described (Box 2) – that represent variations of the epithelial component of the reticular yolk-sac. These subtypes do not seem to have any clinical bearing, and are almost always mixed, as there are very rare cases of a single pattern (Jacobsen 1986), but they must be taken into account by the pathologist to avoid diagnostic errors; therefore the aspects of clinical–biological interest of these varieties are described below.

The *microcystic or reticular pattern* is the most frequent (67%) (Jacobsen 1986), comprising small, widely vacuolated cytoplasm cells as if it were adiposity (Fig. 11). Probably, the coalescence of the microcystic pattern is what constructs the *macrocystic pattern* (44%) (Jacobsen 1986) and could even acquire the appearance of a *polyvesicular pattern* (Fig. 1.12).

**Box 2 Histological Subtypes of the Yolk-Sac Tumor**

- Microcystic or reticular
- Macrocystic
- Solid
- Glandular–alveolar
- Endodermal
- Papillary
- Myxomatous
- Polyvesicular
- Hepatoid
- Enteric
- Parietal
- Spindle cell

**Clinical Features**

Around 90% of the cases have AFP serum elevation. At presentation, 10% to 20% are metastatic, and there is a great prevalence of hematogenous dissemination.

The absence of ITGCNU in infantile yolk-sac tumor (Manivel et al. 1988), the practical inexistence of pure forms in the adult, and the genetic differences (Eble et al. 2004a) suggest that there are differences in the yolk-sac tumors according to the age of apparition, although they are morphologically identical.

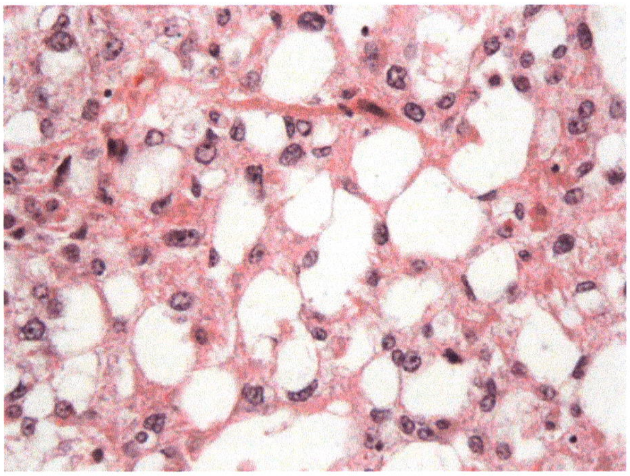

**Fig. 1.11** Yolk-sac tumor microcystic pattern

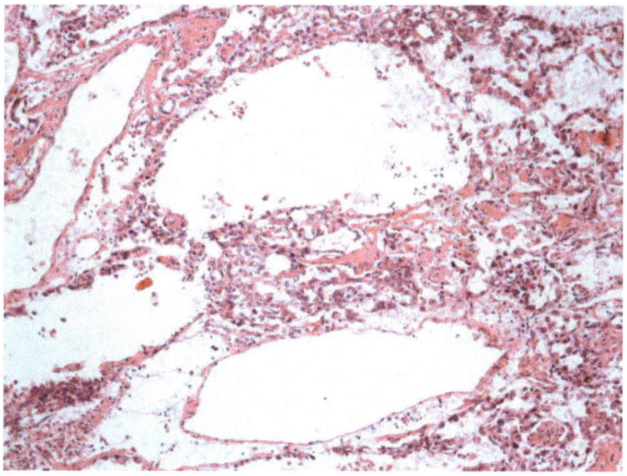

Fig. 1.12 Yolk-sac tumor polivesicular pattern

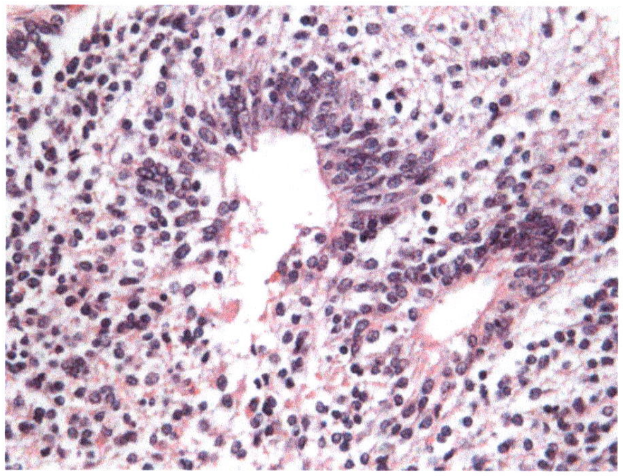

Fig. 1.14 Yolk-sac tumor glandular pattern

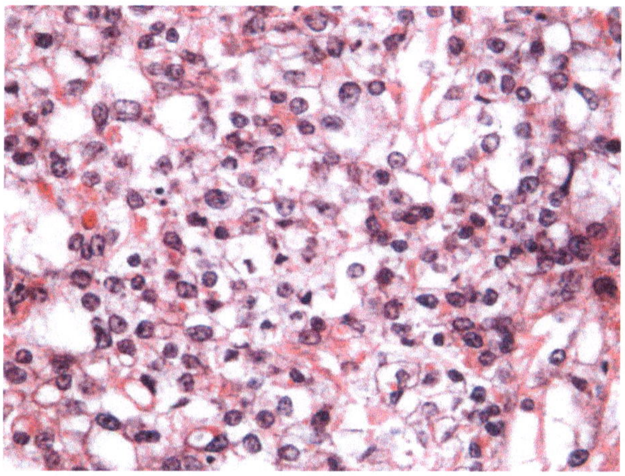

Fig. 1.13 Yolk-sac tumor solid pattern

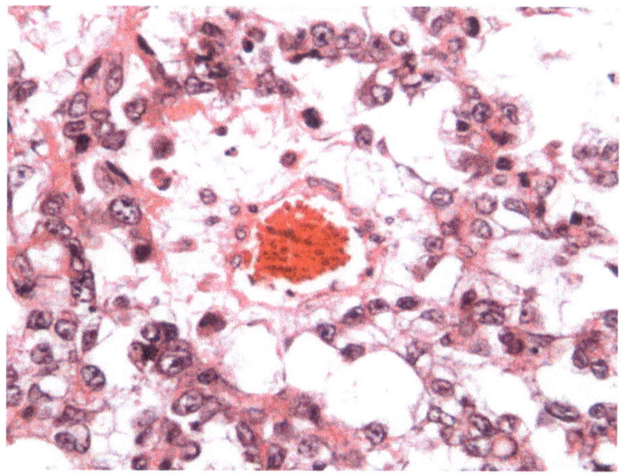

Fig. 1.15 Yolk-sac tumor. Schiller–Duval body

The *solid pattern* (Fig. 1.13) can be found in many cases (27%) (Jacobsen 1986), and according to the extension, it is the one that can most easily lead to an error because of its resemblance to a seminoma; however, the nuclear atypia, the vascular network, and the immunophenotype can help in the differential diagnosis (Ulbright 2005; Ulbright et al. 1999a).

The *glandular–alveolar pattern* (Fig. 1.14) shows glandular structures whose resurfacing cells can range from very flat to cuboid with clear cytoplasm that can imitate an endometrioid carcinoma and is more frequent in the ovary than in the testicle.

The *endodermal pattern* (Fig. 1.15) presents in 9% of cases (Jacobsen 1986) and is comprised of the typical Schiller–Duval bodies with a capillary center and a ring of cuboidal cells of clear cytoplasm and an atypical nucleus with the presence of PAS positive globules. The *papillary pattern* (Fig. 1.16) is constituted when the central capillary pattern with surrounding cells is lengthened.

The *parietal pattern* (Fig. 1.17) is recognized by the presence of eosinophilic bands of basement membrane material that in small areas are found in up to 92% of the cases but are exceptional in large areas of pseudo-sclerotic change (Ulbright et al. 1999a).

Some morphological variants of great interest are those that are characterized by the appearance of somatic tissue which can be assessed as teratomas (see below) when in reality they result from the transformation of the yolk-sac tumor. These variants are the *hepatoid* cell, which focally can be found in 20% of cases (Ulbright et al. 1999a); the *enteric* cell (Fig. 1.18), with a formation

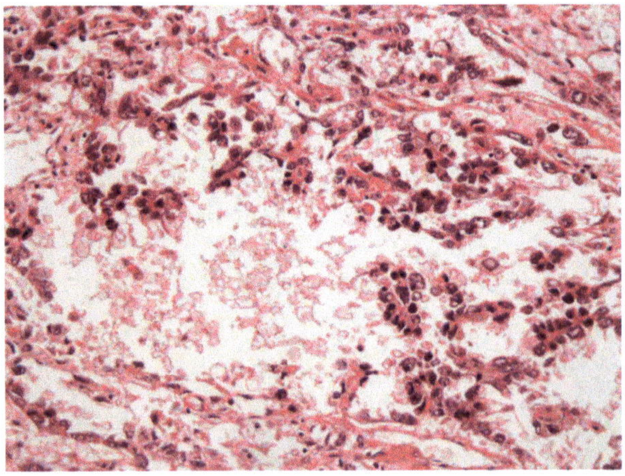

Fig. 1.16 Yolk-sac tumor papillary pattern

of isolated glands that resembles the intestine; the *mixoid* (with angioblastic appearance) and *spindle cell*, which it was believed recapitulated the extraembryonic mesenchyma or magma reticularis with a pluripotential capacity to evolve from non-differentiated spindle proliferation to skeletal muscle and cartilage (Fig. 1.19) (Michael et al. 1989). The isolated presence of these tissues, surrounded by the unquestionable yolk-sac tumor, together with the expression of cytokeratin and AFP, are data that permit distinguishing these variants from teratomas.

The immunohistochemical methods (Table 1.1) show AFP expression (Fig. 1.20) (remember that the yolk-sac tumor is the principal origin of serum AFP) as well as PLAP and cytokeratins, with the OCT3/4 being negative (Looijenga et al. 2003) and expression in 10% of cases of c-kit, EMA, vimentin, and CEA (Niehans et al. 1988).

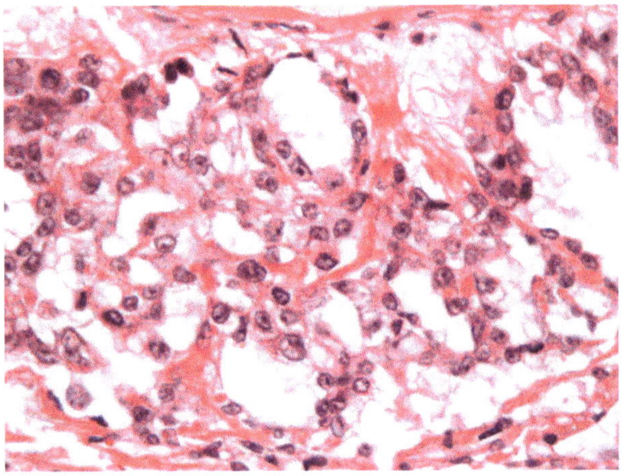

Fig. 1.17 Yolk-sac tumor parietal pattern

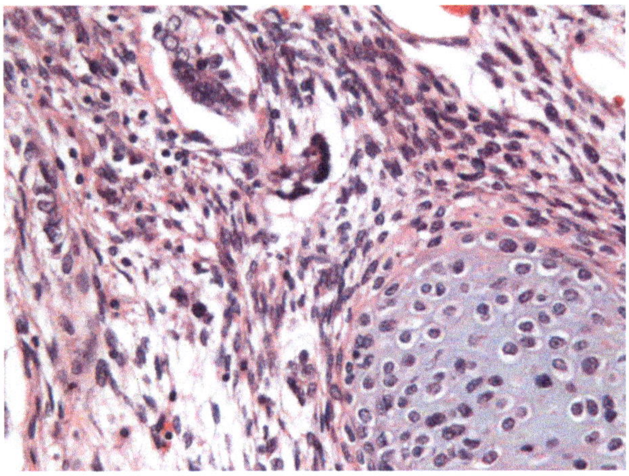

Fig. 1.19 Yolk-sac tumor with stromal (cartilagenous) differentiation

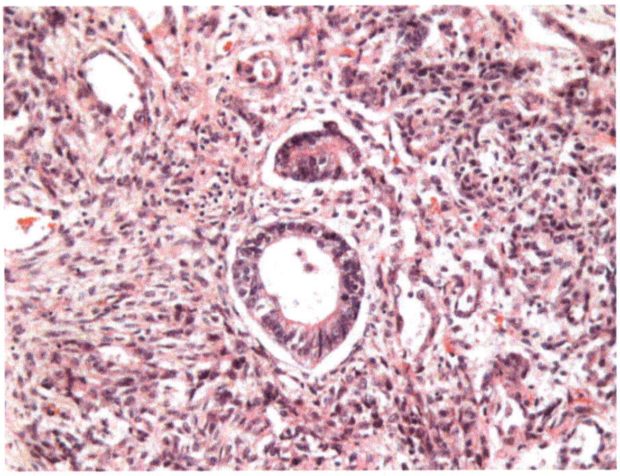

Fig. 1.18 Yolk-sac tumor with intestinal differentiation

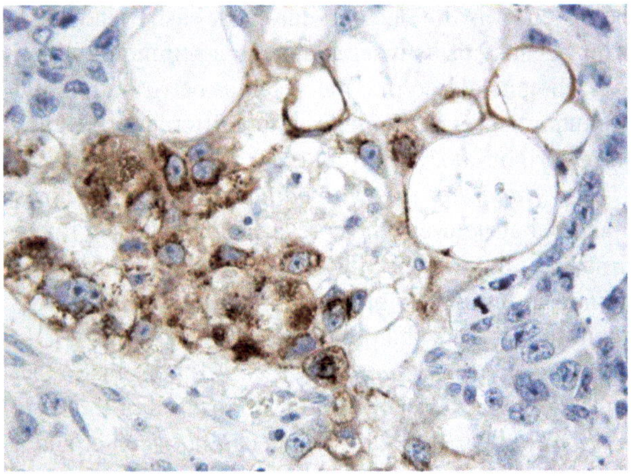

Fig. 1.20 Alfa-1 fetoprotein expression in yolk-sac tumor

## 1.1.6 Choriocarcinoma and Other Trophoblastic Tumors

Choriocarcinoma is the most classic form of a trophoblastic tumor.

In the pure form, it is exceptional (0.3%) and infrequent in the mixed forms (7%) (Ulbright 1993) because, as mentioned above, the presence of isolated trophoblastic cells should not be considered as choriocarcinoma, although they elevate the serum hCG.

### 1.1.6.1 Morphological Features

Generally, hemorrhage is the most typical component.

In order to define a choriocarcinoma, multinucleated syncytiotrophoblastic and mononucleated cytotrophoblastic (with water-clear cytoplasm) as well as intermediate trophoblastic cells (with eosinophilic cytoplasm) are needed (Eble et al. 2004a) (Fig. 1.21) generally in a hemorrhagic and necrotic background. Occasionally, the syncytiotrophoblastic cells surround the aggregates of the other trophoblastic cells, simulating placental villi.

All the cells express (Table 1.1) cytokeratins and PLAP in a focused form in 54% (Ulbright et al. 1999a). The syncytiotrophoblast express strong β-hCG (Fig. 1.22), EMA, and α-inhibin, but the cytotrophoblast is weakly positive. The intermediate trophoblasts express human placental lactogen (Manivel et al. 1987b). EMA (46%), CEA (25%), and vimentin (4%) can also be found (Ulbright et al. 1999a).

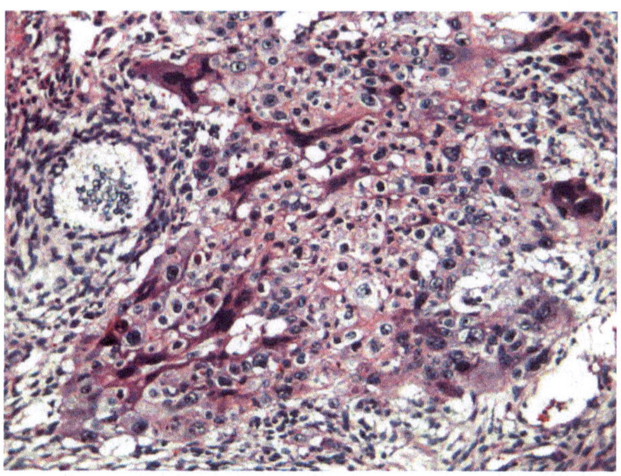

**Fig. 1.21** Choriocarcinoma. Cytotrophoblast and syncytiotrophoblast

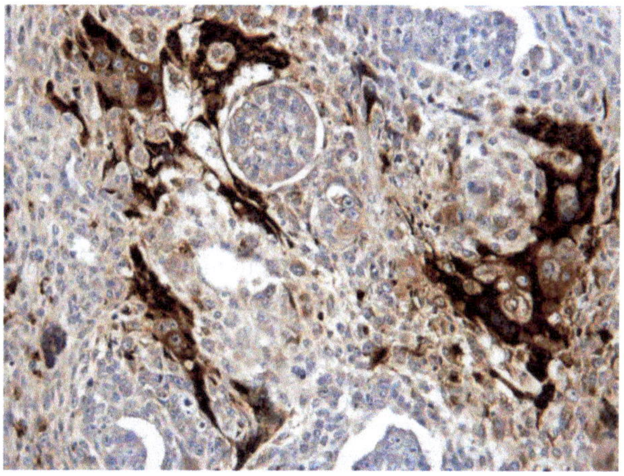

**Fig. 1.22** Choriocarcinoma. β-hCG expression

Cases of trophoblastic tumor have been described without the classic pattern; they are preferably named *monophasic choriocarcinoma* if they are composed only of cytotrophoblasts without syncytiotrophoblasts, and *placental site trophoblastic tumor* if the intermediate trophoblastic cells are the component of the tumor. In these cases, the pathologist must make the differential diagnosis considering the seminoma, the solid variety of the yolk-sac tumor, and even the Leydig tumor cells, especially when there are eosinophil cytoplasm cells (Ulbright et al. 1997).

### 1.1.6.2 Clinical Features

The occasional pure cases are usually metastatic at the time of diagnosis and 10% present with gynecomastia (Ulbright et al. 1999a).

In mixed germ cell tumors, hCG levels over 100,000 IU/L are indicative of choriocarcinoma. It is therefore possible to differentiate these cases, which are highly frequent, from isolated trophoblastic cells.

As expected, the component of choriocarcioma is that which marks the prognosis in the mixed forms.

## 1.1.7 Teratoma

The tumor consisting tissue from the three germ cell layers (endoderm, ectoderm, and mesoderm) is considered a teratoma. Different terms have been used to refer to the mature and immature (fetal-like) appearance of the tissue or its atypia, but attention has always been focused on the biological, and therefore clinical, differences of the teratomas according to the age at appearance and the gonad affected (ovary or testicle).

It is the most frequent TGCT in children, following the yolk-sac tumor, but in adults, it mainly presents as another component of the other varieties, appearing in 22% of the cases (Ulbright 1993).

All these observations have culminated in a different approach to the histogenesis of the different types of gonad teratoma.

#### 1.1.7.1 Histogenetic Hypothesis of the Different Types of Teratoma

In the comparative study of pure infantile teratomas (prepubertal teratomas) and adult teratomas (post-pubertal teratomas), it is observed that the prepubertal teratomas are dyploid and the post-pubertal are hyperdyploid to hypotriploid with 12p amplification [i(12p)] in parallel allelic changes as the other components of the tumor (Ulbright 2005; Mostert et al. 2000). These findings suggest that the prepubertal teratoma comes from a normal germ cell, which through a parthenogenetic-like pathogenesis is transformed into a teratoma, while the postpubertal teratoma is a transformation through an ITGCNU.

#### 1.1.7.2 Morphological Features

The characteristic macroscopic appearance is cystic although large solid areas can be found, both in combination with other cellular types and by itself.

Following the proposed scheme, we can microscopically observe two distinct types (Ulbright 2005; Manivel et al. 1989):

*Prepubertal teratoma* (Fig. 1.23), which has an organoid distribution imitating anatomic structures. There is no cytological atypia, no mitosis, and no concomitant ITGCNU.

*Post-pubertal teratoma* (Fig. 1.24), in which the tissues are distributed in an irregular manner. There is cytological atypia with mitosis and in 90% of the cases concomitant ITGCNU is evidenced.

From the descriptive point of view, mature or immature tissues can be observed. The presence of immature tissues does not have any clinical bearing, except for the proportion of the neuroepithelial component, especially in prepubertal teratomas.

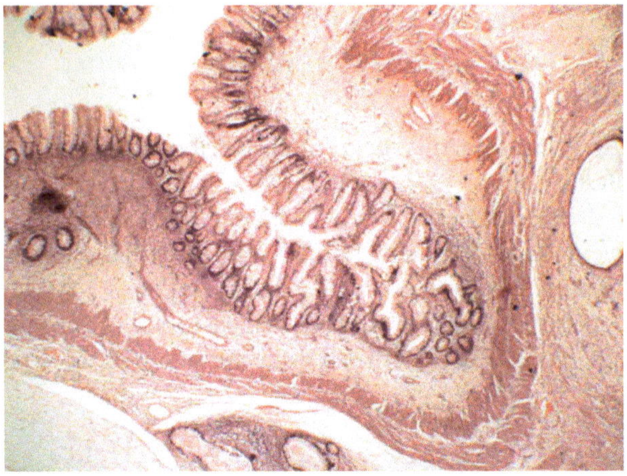

Fig. 1.23 Prepubertal teratoma. All the tissues are in order. The same as in anatomical arrangement

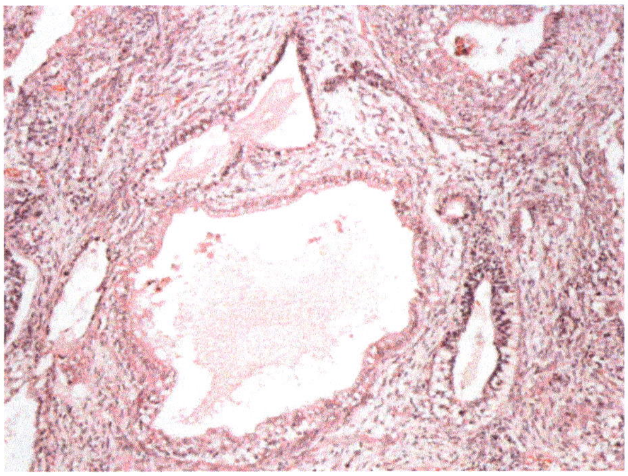

Fig. 1.24 Post-pubertal teratoma. All the components are in irregular arrangement

There are certain special variants such as the *dermoid cyst* (Fig. 1.25), characterized by one or more cysts with predominance of scaly epithelium with skin appendages, benign behavior, and which must be distinguished from the epidermoid cyst (without skin appendages). Other much more infrequent *monodermal teratomas* are those comprising cartilage.

*Teratomas with somatic malignancies* have special interest when any of the tissues have an outstanding growth or an invasive pattern. The quantification of malignant biological significance is arbitrary, although for some authors a fill field of 4× suffices to recognize

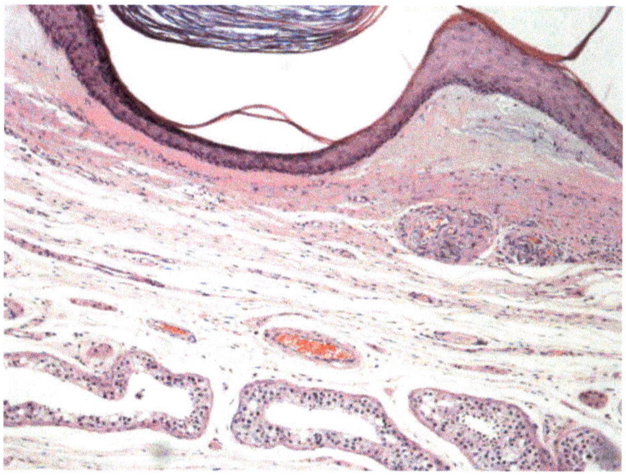

**Fig. 1.25** Dermoid cyst

an initial malignant transformation (Eble et al. 2004a). Most of the time the malignant component is of the sarcoma type, but it seems that only the *intratesticular rhabdomyosarcoma* is the one with a bad prognosis (Ulbright et al. 1984). The other malignant variants, both mesenchymal and epithelial, only seem to negatively influence the evolution when they are located in the metastasis (Michael et al. 1997, 1998).

The immunohistochemical profile depends on the tissues that comprise it. It can be highlighted that the intestinal components can express AFP, and that chromogranin A can be found in these same areas (Pichmann et al. 1993).

## 1.1.8 Tumors of More than One Histological Type

Any mixture is possible although those that do not include seminomas are predominant.

The presence of embryoid bodies that represent embryonal carcinoma and yolk-sac tumors is frequent in many TGCTs. Some authors call the cases with a predominance of embryoid bodies *polyembryoma* (Nakashima et al. 1988). On the other hand, this same combination of embryonal carcinoma and yolk-sac tumor in similar proportions and with a certain ribbon and circular pattern is called *diffuse embryoma* (de Almeida PC and Scully 1983) by other authors.

## 1.1.9 Pathological Prognostic Factors of TGCT

As in all malignant neoplasias, the evolution of TGCT is marked by the stage. The primary objective of the pathologists is to search for prognostic factors of utmost importance in stage I (pT1-4, N0, M0).

The first prognostic factor is the *cellular type*, which in a simplified form has been subdivided into seminoma tumors and non-seminoma tumors.

### 1.1.9.1 Prognostic Factors in Stage I Seminomas

At diagnostic, between 15% and 20% of clinical Stage I seminomas have sub-clinical metastasis and can recur after the orchiectomy (Stenberg 1998). The factors that may call on a possible recurrence are the *size of the tumor* (over 4 cm) and the *invasion of the rete testis* (Jacobsen et al. 1995; Warde et al. 1998). Vascular invasion (Jacobsen et al. 1995) does not seem to have as much significance. The greater number of recurrences appears within 4 years after orchiectomy (Warde and Jewett 1998).

### 1.1.9.2 Prognostic Factors in the Non-seminoma Stage I Tumors

If we exclude the cases with persistence of postorchiectomy elevated markers, 30% of non-seminomas may have affected retroperitoneal nodes. Among those with a negative lymphadenectomy, 7–15% will recur later (Lashley and Lowe 1998). The *vascular invasion* is the most important factor of bad prognosis (50% recurrence among those that have vascular invasion and only 15–20% in those that do not have it) (Klepp et al. 1997).

For positive lymph nodes patients under clinical control alone, tumoral recurrence occurs in 10–50% and is generally extra-abdominal if extensive retroperitoneal surgery has been performed. The risk of this second occurrence is in relation to the *volume of the tumor previously excised* (Pizzocaro 1984). Eighty percent of the recurrences take place during the first year, 12% during the second, 6% during the third, and 1% from the fourth year onward (Freedman et al. 1987; Read et al. 1992).

#### 1.1.9.3 Future Prognostic Markers of Stage I Tumors

Although the factors with the greatest prognostic value are still the classic ones, this has not been an obstacle in going ahead with the research of molecular markers, which are so much in fashion at the present time, and so certain observations need to be made such as the following:

The expression of *collagenase* (metalloprotein of 72 kDA that fragments to the type IV collagen) is more intense in the embryonal carcinoma, the yolk-sac tumor, and the choriocarcinoma than in the seminoma or the teratoma (Boag 1996), and hence it can be related with the tumor's aggressivity although all of them can express it.

The loss of certain *molecules of cellular adherence*, such as the E-cadherins and the alpha-3-integrins, is associated with the progression of the tumors (Hou et al. 1996; Timmes et al. 1994).

The high expression of the *cellular proliferation markers,* specifically the Ki67 (MIB-1), seems to be related to the aggressivity of the embryonal carcinoma and of the yolk-sac tumor (Albers et al. 1997).

However, the expression of the p53 is equivocal, because a large amount is probably expressed in the native form (not mutated) (Boag 1996).

Therefore, and without losing certain expectations from the new prognostic factors, we must continue using the classic factors for daily practice.

### 1.1.10 Evolution of the Post-Chemotherapy Retroperitoneal Masses

In a broad series of post-chemotherapy retroperitoneal masses (Sonneveld et al. 1998), 45.1% of cases were diagnosed as teratoma, 8.8% as germ cell tumor, 43.4% as necrosis and fibrosis, and in 2.7% the tumoral mass was not confirmed surgically. Among patients with teratoma alone, 17.6% of the cases have a postsurgical recurrence, the majority in the form of "*growing syndrome*," with the non-germ cell malignant transformation being rare.

The incomplete resection of the mass or the presence of any form of non-teratoma mature or immature germ cell tumor signifies a risk of progression of the disease (Stenning and Parkinson 1998).

## 1.2 Sex Cord/Gonadal Stromal Tumors

Sex-cord/gonadal stromal tumors account for 3–6% of testicular tumors in adults and 20–30% in prepubertal children (Mostofi and Price 1973; Lawrence et al. 1986; Young and Talerman 1987; Young and Scully 1990; Ulbright et al. 1999b; Young 2005; Eble et al. 2004b). Unlike germ cell tumors they are equally common in patients of different race. The histology of these tumors recapitulates the appearance of Leydig, Sertoli, granulosa, and theca cells, as well as nonspecific stromal cells of the immature and mature testis. The tumors may consist of only one cell type (pure form) or of admixtures of cell types or undifferentiated cells. In addition to the microscopic appearance, immunohistochemistry is helpful. The most common markers are inhibin-α (McCluggage et al. 1998; Iczkowski et al. 1998; Zheng et al. 2003) and calretinin (McCluggage and Maxwell 2001; Cao et al. 2001; Augusto et al. 2002), although the absence of these markers does not exclude the diagnosis of a stromal tumor (Iczkowski et al. 1998; Zheng et al. 2003). Occasionally inhibin can be seen in germ cell tumors and other neoplasms (Cobellis et al. 2001). Other markers include cytokeratins (Düe et al. 1989), desmin (McCluggage et al. 1998), S100 protein, MelanA (Ulbright et al. 2002), CD99 (Comperat et al. 2004), chromogranin, and synaptophysin (Iczkowski et al. 1998).

The classification of these tumors is similar to their counterparts in the ovary and is listed in Box 3 (Eble et al. 2004b). The behavior of sex cord/stromal tumors is difficult to predict as tumors with bland histological features can metastasize. However, tumors exhibiting necrosis, nuclear anaplasia, frequent and abnormal mitoses, irregular borders and large size (greater than 5 cm), extension into paratesticular tissue, and vascular invasion are more likely to progress (Mostofi and Price1973; Lawrence et al. 1986; Young and Talerman 1987; Young and Scully 1990; McCluggage and Maxwell 2001).

### 1.2.1 Pure Forms

Included in this category are Leydig cell tumors, Sertoli cell tumors, granulosa cell tumors, and tumors of the thecoma/fibroma group.

### Box 3 Classification of Stromal Tumors

Sex Cord/Gonadal Stromal Tumors
Leydig cell tumor
Malignant Leydig cell tumor
Sertoli cell tumor
Sertoli cell tumor lipid-rich variant
Sclerosing Sertoli cell tumor
Large cell calcifying Sertoli cell tumor
Others
Malignant Sertoli cell tumor
Granulosa cell tumor
Adult-type granulosa cell tumor
Juvenile-type granulosa cell tumor
Tumors of the thecoma/fibroma group
Thecoma
Fibroma
Sex cord/gonadal stromal tumors, incompletely differentiated
Sex cord/gonadal stromal tumors, mixed forms
Malignant sex cord/gonadal stromal tumors
Tumors containing both germ cell and sex cord/gonadal stromal elements
Gonadoblastoma
Germ cell–sex cord/gonadal stromal tumor, unclassified

#### 1.2.1.1 Leydig Cell Tumor

Leydig cell tumors are the most common stromal tumors and account for about 3% of adult testis tumors, while in prepubertal children they represent about 15% of testis tumors. Bilateral tumors are rare. Prepubertal children present invariably with precocious puberty and macrogenitosomia. The physical changes may be associated with behavioral aberrations (Mostofi and Price 1973; Young and Scully 1990; Ulbright et al. 1999b). About 30% of adults have gynecomastia or decreased libido. Most patients present with painless testicular enlargement. The clinical symptoms depend on the type of hormones produced by the tumor cells, mainly testosterone in prepubertal children and estrogen in adults.

Macroscopically, the tumor appears circumscribed, even encapsulated, homogeneous, bulging, and yellowish or mahogany brown. Histologically, it is composed of elements recapitulating normal development and evolution of Leydig cells (Mostofi and Price 1973; Young and Scully 1990; Ulbright et al. 1999b; Mostofi et al. 1959). The most common appearance is that of medium-sized cells with distinct cell borders, eosinophilic cytoplasm and a round or oval vesicular and rarely grooved nucleus, frequently containing a prominent nucleolus. The cells may be larger with finely or coarsely vacuolated cytoplasm containing lipids, while others consist of elongated, spindle-shaped cells with granular eosinophilic cytoplasm. The nuclei may vary from small to large, round to oval, or vesicular to pyknotic. Occasional cells may be binucleated. The Reinke crystals are helpful in the identification of a Leydig cell tumor, but they are detectable in only about 40% of the cases (Fig. 1.26). Lipofuscin pigment is often present. The cells appear in sheets, columns, cords, and trabeculae (Mostofi et al. 1959; Kim et al. 1985). Rare tumors are microcystic (Billings et al. 1999; Loyd and Boorjian 2006). By immunohistochemistry, most tumors are positive for inhibin-α and calretinin. Rarely, MelanA and other proteins have been observed. About 10% of Leydig cell tumors are malignant. Criteria for the diagnosis of malignancy are anaplasia of the cells, individual cell necrosis, large areas of tumor necrosis, extension to the tunica or epididymis, frequent mitoses, vascular invasion, and tumor size of 5 cm or more (Kim et al. 1985; Cheville et al. 1998; Grem et al. 1986) (Fig. 1.27). However, in rare cases, the tumor may show none of these features but still metastasize. In such cases, the metastases are usually delayed by five years or more.

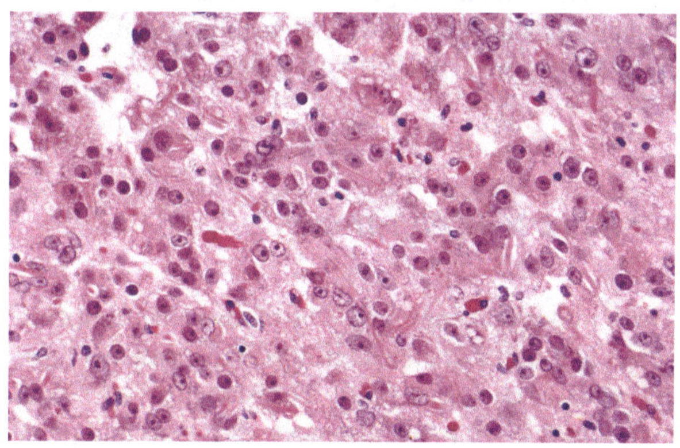

**Fig. 1.26** Leydig cell tumor. Note Reinke crystals

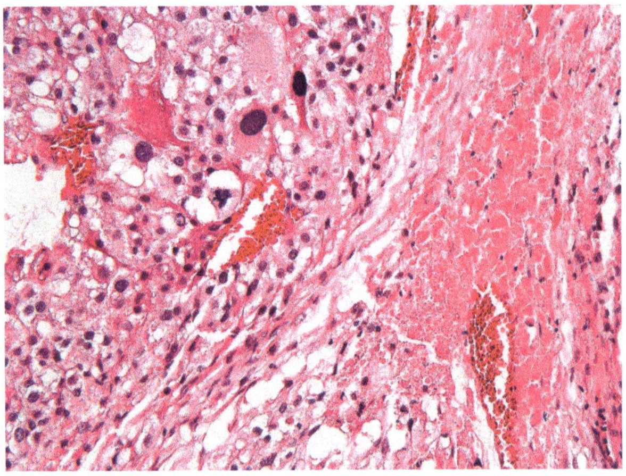

**Fig. 1.27** Malignant Leydig cell tumor. Nuclear anaplasia, abnormal mitosis, and necrosis are present

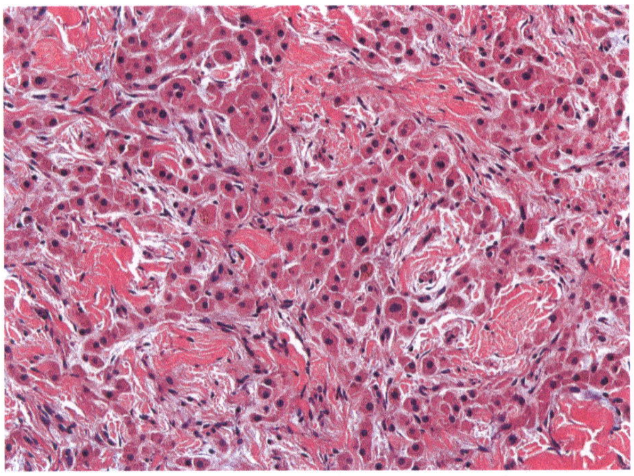

**Fig. 1.28** "Tumor" of adrenal genital syndrome. Large pink cells in hyalinized stroma

Leydig cell tumors have to be distinguished from nodules of Leydig cell hyperplasia found in the testes of persons with atrophy, cryptorchidism, Klinefelter syndrome, or Klinefelter-like syndrome. In such cases, the testes are small and the seminiferous tubules are also small and often sclerotic. Hyperplasia differs from neoplasia in that the tubules are entrapped in the former but not in the latter although a few entrapped tubules may be seen in the periphery of a tumor. Leydig cell tumors and hyperplasia can be distinguished from similar changes in the androgen insensitivity (Kommoss et al. 2000) and the adrenogenital syndromes by the absence of clinical symptoms or laboratory evidence of those syndromes. In patients with adrenogenital syndrome (congenital adrenal hyperplasia), tumorous proliferations of cells resembling both hyperplastic adrenal cortical and Leydig cells occur associated with variable amounts of fibrous tissue. The cells are large, show nuclear variation, and contain abundant lipofuscin. The nodules are often bilateral (Rutgers et al. 1988) (Fig. 1.28).

## 1.2.2 Sertoli Cell Tumor

These tumors account for 1–2% of testicular tumors in adults and occur in all age groups. Most patients present with a testicular mass, occasionally (4%) with gynecomastia. In a few instances, estrogens and pregnanediol are elevated. Bilaterality is unusual (Mostofi and Price 1973; Young and Scully 1990; Ulbright et al. 1999b; Eble et al. 2004b; Collins and Symington 1964; Young et al. 1998).

Macroscopically, the tumors are rather firm, grayish-white or yellow and appear encapsulated. Histologically, the cells range in shape from oval to columnar. They have a small or medium-sized, round or oval vesicular nucleus with a fine chromatin network and a solitary, small basophilic nucleolus. The cytoplasm may be scanty or abundant with multiple small lipid vacuoles or a single large one. The cells form tubules with a more or less distinct lumen which may contain basement membrane-like material, or the tubules appear solid as in the prepubertal testis (Collins and Symington 1964; Young et al. 1998) (Fig. 1.29). The tumor may occur in sheets with only occasional tubule formation. The stroma can be scanty or composed of abundant, sometimes hyalinized, fibrous tissue. A tumor with extensive hyalinization is known as the "sclerosing Sertoli cell tumor" (Zukerberg et al. 1991). About 10% of Sertoli cell tumors are malignant, and terminal patients usually die within 1 year (Henley et al. 2002; Jacobsen 1993) (Fig. 1.30).

Sertoli cell tumors must be distinguished from the small nodules of coiled tubules lined by immature Sertoli cells found in over 20% of cryptorchids and occasionally in descended testes. Such nodules are sometimes mislabeled Sertoli cell or tubular adenoma. Occasionally, scattered spermatogonia are found within the tubules of the Sertoli cell nodules.

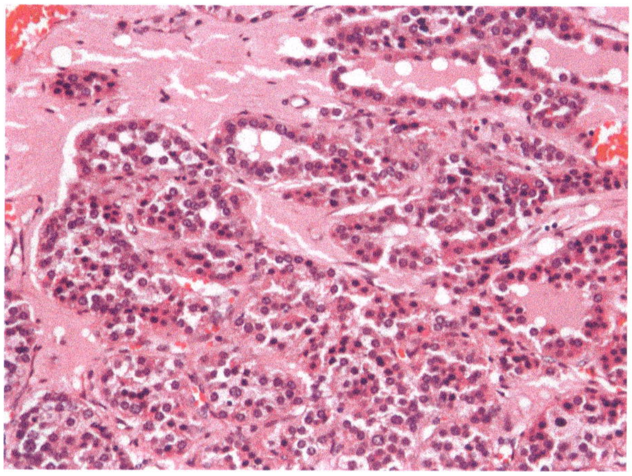

**Fig. 1.29** Sertoli cell tumor. The tumor forms open and closed tubules

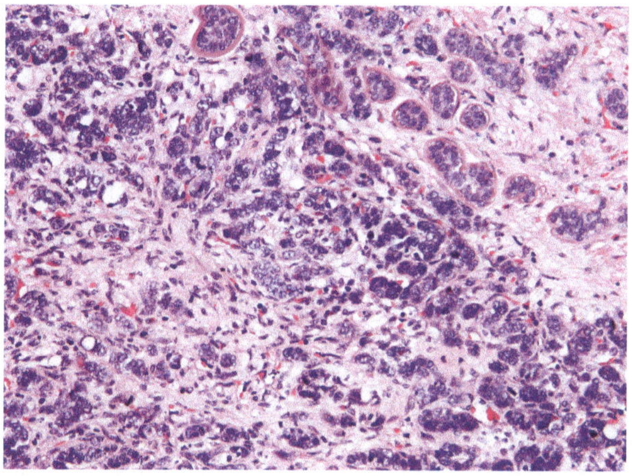

**Fig. 1.30** Malignant Sertoli cell tumor. Most of the tumor cells show nuclear anaplasia

### 1.2.3 Large Cell Calcifying Sertoli Cell Tumor

The large cell calcifying Sertoli cell tumor (Proppe and Scully 1980, 1982) is most common in children and is often associated with Carney syndrome. Twenty percent are bilateral and most of these are associated with Carney syndrome manifested by hyperplasia and neoplasia of other endocrine organs, bilateral primary adrenocortical hyperplasia and pituitary adenomas, spotty mucocutaneous pigmentation, and cardiac myxomas (Carney et al. 1985). Clinical associations include sexual precocity, acromegaly, pituitary gigantism, hypercortisolemia, and sudden death.

On gross examination, the tumors are tan to yellow, often multifocal, and firm. The cells are large, cuboidal, hexagonal, columnar, or spindle-shaped. The cytoplasm is abundant, finely granular, and eosinophilic, but may be amphophilic and slightly vacuolated, and contain abundant lipid in fine droplets or large vacuoles. The nuclei are round, oval, or elongated with one or two small nucleoli. Mitoses are generally absent or rare. The neoplastic cells often form tubules or cords, clusters, trabeculae, or solid sheets. The stroma may be loose, myxoid, or densely collagenous with varying degrees of calcification (Fig. 1.31). Calcifications appear as large, wavy, laminated nodules or massive deposits; sometimes it is sparse. In the absence of prominent tubule formation and minimal calcification, the tumor may simulate a Leydig cell tumor, especially in a child with precocious puberty (Proppe and Scully 1980; Kratzer et al. 1997). In adult patients, rare cases develop metastases (Kratzer et al. 1997). Histologically, they show similar features as other malignant stromal tumors.

### 1.2.4 Testicular Tumors in Peutz–Jeghers Syndrome

Stromal "tumors" in Peutz–Jeghers syndrome resemble the sex-cord stromal tumor with annular tubules or the large cell calcifying Sertoli cell tumor. Most of the

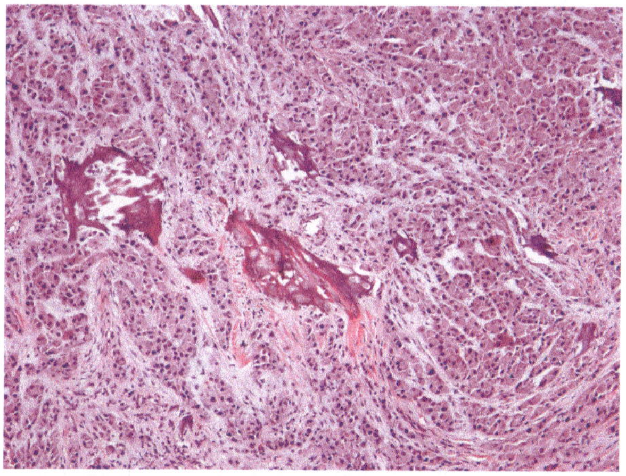

**Fig. 1.31** Large cell calcifying Sertoli cell tumor. Cords of pink tumor cells and scattered calcifications

tumors have a prominent intratubular growth of Sertoli cells with abundant cytoplasm and deposition of basement membrane-like material. Calcifications are uncommon (Cantu et al. 1980; Young et al. 1995). Ulbright et al. (2007; Venara et al. 2001) reported eight children with this syndrome. All had gynecomastia and bilateral testicular lesions.

### 1.2.5 Granulosa Cell Tumors

Two types are recognized: the adult and the juvenile. Both display the same histologic patterns as their ovarian counterparts.

### 1.2.6 Granulosa Cell Tumor, Adult Type

Only 27 cases were reported in the literature. The patients range in age from 10 to 80 years with most in the third to sixth decades. The symptoms are usually a mass, and in 25% of patients gynecomastia (Mostofi et al. 1959; Nistal et al. 1992a; Jimenez-Quintero et al. 1993; Wang et al. 2002). Five patients developed metastases.

The gross appearance is grayish-white or yellow, and homogeneous or lobulated. The nuclei are vesicular and grooved, but they may be large, round, and hyperchromatic. The cells are small, round, or hexagonal; the cytoplasm is generally scant. The tumor may have a diffuse or micro-follicular pattern with Call–Exner bodies (Fig. 1.32).

### 1.2.7 Granulosa Cell Tumor, Juvenile Type

This tumor is almost always encountered before the age of 2 years (Crump 1983; Lawrence et al. 1985; Goswitz et al. 1996; Fagin et al. 2003). It is the most common testicular tumor of the newborn, and indeed it is possible to detect these prenatally by ultrasound (Peterson and Skoog 2008). A few cases have been reported in undescended testes with intersex disorders (Young et al. 1985).

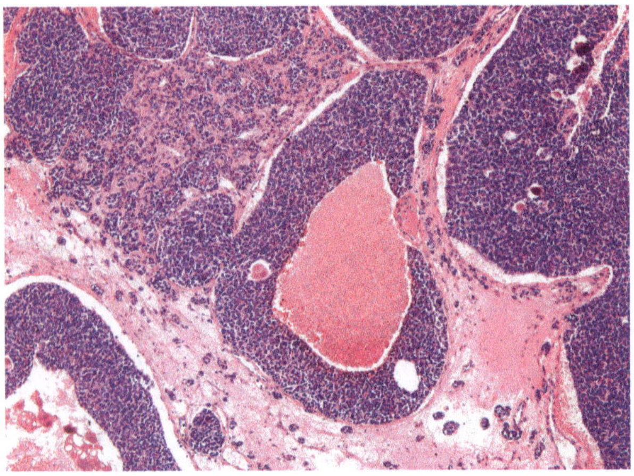

**Fig. 1.32** Granulosa cell tumor, adult type. Follicles in addition to large and small aggregates of tumor cells

Macroscopically, they are lobulated, often with a cystic component. Microscopically, the cells are polyhedral or round and contain abundant pale to eosinophilic cytoplasm. The nuclei are round or oval and hyperchromatic with occasional nucleoli. There may be many mitoses. Histologically, the tumor is usually cystic but may be follicular or have solid areas (Fig. 1.33). The follicles are usually large and may contain mucoid material. By immunohistochemistry, these and Sertoli cell tumors are positive not only for vimentin but also for cytokeratins and actin Harms 1997. Similarly, granulosa cell and Sertoli cell tumors express to a variable degree the anti-Müllerian

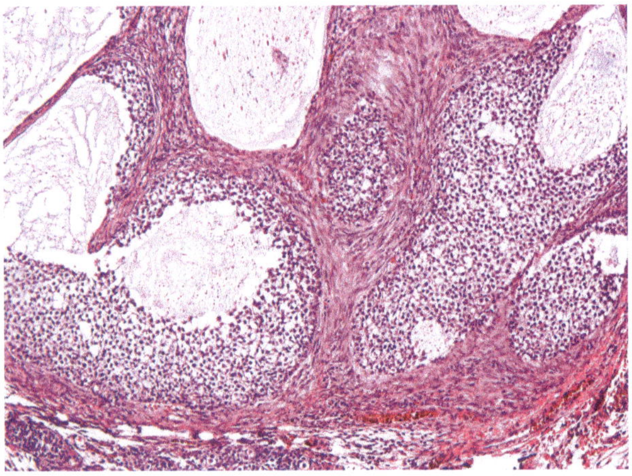

**Fig. 1.33** Granulosa cell tumor, juvenile type. Cystic spaces are partially obliterated by small granulosa cells

hormone, in contrast to Leydig and theca cell tumors (Rey et al. 2000). Kalfa and colleagues (Kalfa et al. 2008) identified FOXL2, a marker of ovarian differentiation, in the nuclei of juvenile granulosa cell tumors, whereas SOX9, a marker of testicular differentiation, was absent. This finding is indicative of the multipotential nature of Sertoli cells.

## 1.2.8 Tumors of the Thecoma/Fibroma Group

These rare tumors are predominantly encountered in young men, who present with a slowly enlarging mass. To date none of these has metastasized. They have a number of synonyms and are now considered to be fibromas with the histologic features of their ovarian counterparts (Allen et al. 1990; Nistal et al. 1992b). Macroscopically, they are white-yellow and firm. They consist of spindle cells with varying fibrosis. By immunohistochemistry they are positive for smooth muscle actin, desmin, vimentin, and S100 protein (Miettinen et al. 1986; Nistal et al. 1996; Renshaw et al. 1997).

## 1.2.9 Sex Cord/Gonadal Stromal Tumors, Unclassified

These tumors consist of nonspecific spindle cells, which are identifiable as stromal tumors by the occasional presence of Leydig, Sertoli, or granulosa cells (Ulbright et al. 1999b; Eble et al. 2004b).

## 1.2.10 Tumors Showing Both Germ Cell and Gonadal Stromal Elements

### 1.2.10.1 Gonadoblastoma

Gonadoblastomas arise almost exclusively in patients with rudimentary or streak gonads, most of whom are phenotypic females, and almost all of whom are X-chromatin-negative and have a Y-chromosome.

Macroscopically, the tumor is multinodular with a yellowish gritty cut surface. The nodules are composed of two principal cell types: large germ cells and small cells resembling immature Sertoli and granulosa cells; elements resembling Leydig and lutein cells may also be present. The two cells (germ cell and sex cord/gonadal stromal elements) are usually in irregular or rounded discrete nests presenting one or more of three patterns. Most often the sex cord cells surround rounded hyaline nodules of basement membrane substance, which merges with the surrounding basement membrane. The germ cells are interspersed between the Sertoli cells. The second pattern consists of nests composed of large germ cells surrounded by many smaller Sertoli cells (Fig. 1.34). In the third growth pattern, the Sertoli cells form a ring of single cells at the periphery of a central nest of germ cells. Focal calcification may consist of fibrous tissue. Large polyhedral cells resembling Leydig cells but without Reinke crystals may be present after puberty (Scully 1970). By immunohistochemistry, the germ cells are positive for VASA, p53, and other germ cell markers. They can also be positive for PLAP and c-kit. The stromal cells are positive for inhibin, Müllerian-inhibiting substance, and WT-1 (Hussong et al. 1997).

Sometimes, the germ cells of a gonadoblastoma transgress the margins of the nests and grow as a seminoma or embryonal carcinoma with only small foci of gonadoblastoma within them or at their margins. The type of germ cell tumor should be specified.

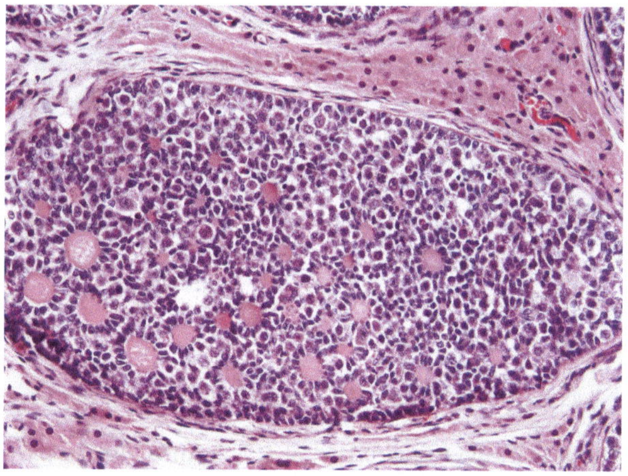

**Fig. 1.34** Gonadoblastoma. Nest of Sertoli cells admixed with germ cells and eosinophilic basement membrane-like material

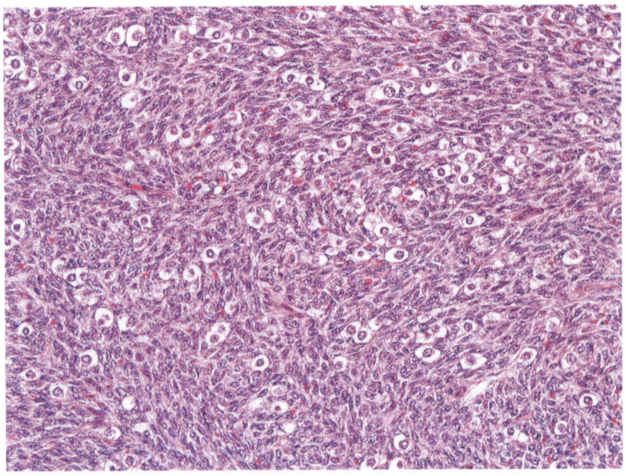

**Fig. 1.35** Mixed germ cell–sex cord/gonadal stromal tumor, unclassified. Germ cells scattered throughout unclassified stromal cells

### 1.2.11 Mixed Germ Cell–Sex Cord/ Gonadal Stromal Tumors, Unclassified

Adult patients between 30 and 60 years of age presenting with a testicular mass may have a tumor consisting of closely admixed germ cells and sex/cord gonadal stromal cells. The germ cells resemble spermatogonia with ample cytoplasm and varying amounts of glycogen. The nuclei are round and may have nucleoli. The germ cells are seen either as single cells or in small groups and grow in association with cells resembling Sertoli, granulosa, and/or Leydig cells (Fig. 1.35). The proportions of the constituent cells vary. Mitotic activity can occur, but the tumor appears to be benign. The germ cells are probably entrapped and not neoplastic (Talerman 1972; Bolen 1981; Ulbright et al. 2000) In contrast to gonadoblastomas, these tumors occur in testes of normal males.

These tumors should not be equated with unclassified stromal tumors containing malignant germ cells indistinguishable from seminoma or unclassified intratubular germ cell neoplasia.

## References


Albers P (2007) Management of stage I testis cancer. Eur Urol 51:34–43

Albers P, Bierhoff E, Neu D et al (1997) MIB-1 immunohistochemistry in clinical stage I nonseminomatous testicular germ cell tumors predicts patients at low risk for metastasis. Cancer 79:1710–1716

Albores-Saavedra J, Huffman H, Alvarado-Cabrero I, Ayala AG (1996) Anaplastic variant of spermatocytic seminoma. Hum Pathol 27:650–655

Allen PR, King AR, Sago MD et al (1990) A benign gonadal stromal tumor of the testis of spindled fibroblastic type. Pathology 22:227–229

Augusto D, Leteurtre E, De La Taille A et al (2002) Calretinin a valuable marker of normal and neoplastic Leydig cells of the testis. Appl Immunohistochem Mol Morphol 10:159–162

Berney DM, Lee A, Randle SJ, Jordan S, Shamash J, Oliver RT (2004) The frequency of intratubular embryonal carcinoma: implications for the pathogenesis of germ cell tumours. Histopathology 45:155–161

Berney DM, Lee A, Shamash J, Oliver RT (2005) The frequency and distribution of intratubular trophoblast in association with germ cell tumors of the testis. Am J Surg Pathol 29:1300–1303

Billings SD, Roth LM, Ulbright TM (1999) Microcystic Leydig cell tumors mimicking yolk sac tumor: a report of four cases. Am J Surg Pathol 23:546–551

Boag AH (1996) Type collagenase expression in testicular germ cell neoplasia. J Urol Pathol 4:147–154

Bolen JW (1981) Mixed germ cell-sex cord stromal tumor: a gonadal tumor distinct from gonadoblastoma. Am J Clin Pathol 75:565–573

Burke AP, Mostofi FK (1988) Placental alkaline phosphatase immunohistochemistry of intratubular malignant germ cells and associated testicular germ cell tumors. Hum Pathol 19:663–670

Burke AP, Mostofi FK (1993) Spermatocytic seminoma. A clinicopathologic study of 79 cases. J Urol Pathol 1:21–32

Cantu JM, Rivera H, Ocampo-Campos R et al (1980) Peutz–Jeghers syndrome with feminizing Sertoli cell tumor. Cancer 46:223–228

Cao QJ, Jones JG, Li M (2001) Expression of calretinin in human ovary, testis, and ovarian sex cord-stromal tumors. Int J Gynecol Pathol 20:346–352

Carney JA, Gordon H, Carpenter PC et al (1985) The complex of myxomas, spotty pigmentation, and endocrine overactivity. Medicine 64:270–283

Cheng L, Sung MT, Cossu-Rocca P, Jones TD, MacLennan GT, De Jong J, Lopez-Beltran A, Montironi R, Looijenga LH (2007) OCT4: biological functions and clinical applications as a marker of germ cell neoplasia. J Pathol 211:1–9

Cheville JC, Sebo TJ, Lager DJ, Bostwick DG et al (1998) Leydig cell tumor of the testis: a clinicopathologic, DNA content, and MIB-1 comparison of nonmetastasizing and metastasizing. Am J Surg Pathol 22:1361–1367

Chung PW, Bayley AJ, Sweet J, Jewett MA, Tew-George B, Gospodarowicz MK, Warde PR (2004) Spermatocytic seminoma: a review. Eur Urol 45:495–498

Cobellis L, Cataldi P, Reis FM et al (2001) Gonadal malignant germ cell tumors express immunoreactive inhibin/activin subunits. Eur J Endocrinol 145:779–784

Collins DH, Symington T (1964) Sertoli-cell tumour. Br J Urol 25(Suppl):52–61

Comperat E, Tissier F, Boye K, De Pinieux G, Vieillefond A (2004) Non-Leydig sex-cord tumors of the testis. The place of immunohistochemistry in diagnosis and prognosis. A study of twenty cases. Virchows Arch 444:567–571

Cope NJ, McCullagh P, Sarsfield PTL (1999) Tumour responding accessory cells in testicular seminoma: an immunohistochemical study. Histopathology 34:510–516

Crump WD (1983) Juvenile granulosa cell (sex cord-stromal) tumor of fetal testis. Urology 129:1057–1058
Cummings OW, Ulbright TM, Eble JN, Roth LM (1994) Spermatocytic seminoma: an immunohistochemical study. Hum Pathol 25:54–59
de Almeida Cardoso PC, Scully RE (1983) Diffuse embryoma of the testis. A distinctive form of mixed germ cell tumor. Am J Surg Pathol 7:633–642
de Jong B, Oosterhuis JW, Castedo SM, Vos A, te Meerman GJ (1990) Pathogenesis of adult testicular germ cell tumors: a cytogenetic model. Cancer Genet Cytogenet 48:143–167
de Jong B, van Echten J, Looijenga LHJ et al (1997) Cytogenetics of the progression of adult testicular germ cell tumors. Cancer Genet Cytogenet 95:88–95
Düe W, Dieckmann KP, Loy V et al (1989) Immunohistological determination of oestrogen receptor, progesterone receptor, and inflammation filaments in Leydig cell tumours. Leydig cell hyperplasia, and normal Leydig cells of the human testis. J Pathol 157:225–234
Eble JN (1994) Spermatocytic seminoma. Hum Pathol 25: 1035–1042
Eble JN, Sauter G, Epstein JI, Sesterhenn IA (eds) (2004a) World Health Organization classification of tumours. Pathology and genetics tumours of the urinary system and male genital organs. IARC Press, Lyon
Eble J, Sauter G, Epstein J, Sesterhenn I (2004b) Pathology and genetics of tumours of the urinary system and male genital organs. IARC Press, Lyon, France
El Naggar AK, Ro JY, McLemore D et al (1992) DNA ploidy in testicular germ cell neoplasms. Histogenetic and clinical implications. Am J Surg Pathol 16:611–618
Fagin R, Berbescu E, Landis S et al (2003) Juvenile granulosa cell tumor of the testis. Urology 62:351
Ferreiro JA (1994) Ber.H2 expression in testicular germ cell tumors. Hum Pathol 25:522–524
Floyd C, Ayala AG, Logothetis CJ, Silva EG (1988) Spermatocytic seminoma with associated sarcoma of the testis. Cancer 61: 409–414
Freedman LS, Parkinson MC, Jones WG et al (1987) Histopathology in the prediction of relapse of patients with stage I testicular teratoma treated by orchiectomy alone. Lancet 2(8554):294–298
Ganem JP, Workman KR, Shaban SF (1999) Testicular microlithiasis is associated with testicular pathology. Urology 53:209–213
Giwercman A, Lindenberg S, Kimber SJ et al (1990) Monoclonal antibody 43-9F as a sensitive immunohistochemical marker of carcinoma in situ of human testis. Cancer 65:1135–1142
Goswitz JJ, Pettinato G, Manivel JC (1996) Testicular sex cord-stromal tumors in children: clinicopathologic study of sixteen children with review of literature. Pediatr Pathol Lab Med 16:451–470
Grem JL, Robins HI, Wilson KS, Gilchrist K, Trump DL (1986) Metastatic Leydig cell tumor of the testis. Report of three cases and review of the literature. Cancer 58:2116–2119
Harms D, Kock LR (1997) Testicular juvenile granulosa cell and Sertoli cell tumours: a clinicopathologic study of 29 cases from the Kiel Paediatric Tumour Registry. Virchow Arch 430:301–309
Hattab EM, Tu PH, Wilson JD, Cheng L (2005) OCT4 immunohistochemistry is superior to placental alkaline phosphatase (PLAP) in the diagnosis of central nervous system germinoma. Am J Surg Pathol 29:368–371
Henley JD, Young RH, Ulbright TM (2002) Malignant Sertoli cell tumors of the testis. A study of 13 examples of a neoplasm frequently misinterpreted as seminoma. Am J Surg Pathol 26:541–550
Henley JD, Young RH, Wade CL, Ulbright TM (2004) Seminomas with exclusive intertubular growth: a report of 12 clinically and grossly inconspicuous tumors. Am J Surg Pathol 28:1163–1168
Hittmair A, Rogastsch H, Hobisch A et al (1996) CD30 expression in seminoma. Hum Pathol 27:1166–1171
Hofer MD, Browne TJ, He L, Skotheim RI, Lothe RA, Rubin MA (2005) Identification of two molecular groups of seminomas by using expression and tissue microarrays. Clin Cancer Res 11:5722–5729
Honecker F, Stoop H, Mayer F, Bokemeyer C, Castrillon DH, Lau YF, Looijenga LH, Oosterhuis JW (2006) Germ cell lineage differentiation in non-seminomatous germ cell tumours. J Pathol 208:395–400
Hou J, Kallaburg BVS, Bui HX et al (1996) E-Cadherin and p53 expression in pure testicular seminoma. J Urol Pathol 5: 109–118
Hu LM, Phillipson J, Barsky SH (1992) Germ cell neoplasia in infantile yolk sac tumor. Verification by tandem repeat sequence in situ hybridization. Diagn Mol Pathol 1:118–128
Hussong J, Crussi FG, Chou PM (1997) Gonadoblastoma: immunohistochemical localization of Muellerian –inhibiting substance, inhibin, WT-1 and p53. Mod Pathol 10:1101–1105
Iczkowski KA, Bostwick DG, Roche PC et al (1998) Inhibin A is a sensitive and specific marker for testicular sex cord-stromal tumors. Mod Pathol 11:774–779
Jacobsen GK (1986) Histogenetic considerations concerning germ cell tumours. Morphological and immunohistochemical comparative investigation of the human embryo and testicular germ cell tumours. Virchows Arch A Pathol Anat Histopathol 408:509–525
Jacobsen GK (1993) Malignant Sertoli cell tumor of the testis. J Urol Pathol 1:233–255
Jacobsen GK, von der Maase H, Specht L et al (1995) Histopathological features in stage I seminoma treated with orchidectomy only. J Urol Pathol 3:85–94
Jimenez-Quintero LP, Ro JY, Zavala-Pompa A et al (1993) Granulosa cell tumor of the adult testis: a clinicopathologic study of seven cases and a review of the literature. Hum Pathol 24:1120–1126
Jorgensen N, Rajpert-De Meyts E, Graem N, Muller J, Giwercman A, Skakkebaek NE (1995) Expression of immunohistochemical markers for testicular carcinoma in situ by normal human fetal germ cells. Lab Invest 72: 223–231
Kalfa N, Fellous M, Boizet-Bonhoure B et al (2008) Aberrant expression of ovary determining gene FOXL2 in the testis and juvenile granulosa cell tumor in children. J Urol 180 (4 Suppl):1810–1813, Epub 2008 Aug 21
Kaplan GW, Cromie WC, Kelalis PP, Silber I, Tank ES Jr (1988) Prepubertal yolk sac testicular tumors – report of the testicular tumor registry. J Urol 140:1109–1112
Kim I, Young RH, Scully RE (1985) Leydig cell tumors of the testis. A clinicopathological analysis of 40 cases and review of the literature. Am J Surg Pathol 9:177–192

Klepp O, Dahl O, Flodgren P et al (1997) Risk-adapted treatment of clinical stage I non-seminoma testis cancer. Eur J Cancer 33:1038–1044

Kliesch S, Thomaidis T, Schutte B, Puhse G, Kater B, Roth S, Bergmann M (2003) Update on the diagnostic safety for detection of testicular intraepithelialneoplasia (TIN). APMIS 111:70–74

Kommoss F, Oliva E, Bittinger F et al (2000) Inhibin-alpha CD99, HEA125, PLAP, and chromogranin immunoreactivity in testicular neoplasms and the androgen insensitivity syndrome. Hum Pathol 31:1055–1061

Kratzer SS, Ulbright TM, Talerman A et al (1997) Large cell calcifying Sertoli cell tumor of the testis: a study of six malignant and six benign cases and a review of the literature. Am J Surg Pathol 21:1271–1280

Lashley DB, Lowe BA (1998) A rational approach to managing stage I nonseminomatous germ cell cancer. Urol Clin North Am 25:405–423

Lau SK, Weiss LM, Chu PG (2007a) Association of intratubular seminoma and intratubular embryonal carcinoma with invasive testicular germ cell tumors. Am J Surg Pathol 31: 1045–1049

Lau SK, Weiss LM, Chu PG (2007b) D2-40 immunohistochemistry in the differential diagnosis of seminoma and embryonal carcinoma: a comparative immunohistochemical study with KIT (CD117) and CD30. Mod Pathol 20:320–325

Lawrence WD, Young RH, Scully RE (1985) Juvenile granulosa cell tumor of the infantile testis. A report of fourteen cases. Am J Surg Pathol 9:87–94

Lawrence WD, Young RH, Scully RE (1986) Sex cord-stromal tumors. In: Talerman A, Roth LM (eds) Pathology of the testis and its adnexa. Churchill Livingstone, New York

Lee MC, Talerman A, Oosterhuis JW et al (1985) Lectin histochemistry of classic and spermatocytic seminoma. Arch Opathol Lab Med 109:938–942

Leroy X, Augusto D, Leteurtre E, Gosselin B (2002) CD30 and CD117 (c-kit) used in combination are useful for distinguishing embryonal arcinoma from seminoma. J Histochem Cytochem 50:283–285

Looijenga LH, Stoop H, de Leeuw HP, de Gouveia Brazao CA, Gillis AJ, van Roozendaal KE, van Zoelen EJ, Weber RF, Wolffenbuttel KP, van Dekken H, Honecker F, Bokemeyer C, Perlman EJ, Schneider DT, Kononen J, Sauter G, Oosterhuis JW (2003) POU5F1 (OCT3/4) identifies cells with pluripotent potential in human germ cell tumors. Cancer Res 63:2244–2250

Loyd E, Boorjian S (2006) A painless testicular mass in a 50-year-old man. Leydig cell tumor of the testis, microcystic variant. Arch Pathol Lab Med 3:39

Manivel JC, Niehans G, Wick MR, Dehner LP (1987) Intermediate trophoblast in germ cell neoplasms. Am J Surg Pathol 11:693–701

Manivel JC, Simonton S, Wold LE, Dehner LP (1988) Absence of intratubular germ cell neoplasia in testicular yolk sac tumors in children. A histochemical and immunohistochemical study. Arch Pathol Lab Med 112:641–645

Manivel JC, Reinberg Y, Niehans GA, Fraley EE (1989) Intratubular germ cell neoplasia in testicular teratomas and epidermoid cysts. Correlation with prognosis and possible biologic significance. Cancer 64:715–720

Matoska J, Ondrus D, Hornak M (1988) Metastatic spermatocytic seminoma. A case report with light microscopic, ultrastructural, and immunohistochemical findings. Cancer 62:1197–1201

McCluggage WG, Maxwell P (2001) Immunohistochemical staining for calretinin is useful in the diagnosis of ovarian sex cord-stromal tumors. Histopathology 38:403–408

McCluggage WG, Shanks JH, Whiteside C, Maxwell P et al (1998) Immunohistochemical study of testicular sex cord - stromal tumors, including staining with anti-inhibin antibody. Am J Surg Pathol 22:615–619

Michael H, Ulbright TM, Brodhecker CA (1989) The pluripotential nature of the mesenchyme-like component of yolk sac tumor. Arch Pathol Lab Med 113:1115–1119

Michael H, Hull MT, Ulbright TM et al (1997) Primitive neuroectodermal tumors arising in testicular germ cell neoplasms. Am J Surg Pathol 21:896–904

Michael H, Hull MT, Foster RS et al (1998) Nephroblastoma-like tumors in patients with testicular germ cell tumors. Am J Surg Pathol 22:1107–1114

Miettinen M, Salo J, Virtanen I (1986) Testicular stromal tumour. Ultrastructural, immunohistochemical, and gel electrophoretic evidence of epitelial differentiation. Ultrastruct Pathol 10:515–528

Mostert M, Rosenberg C, Stoop H, Schuyer M, Timmer A, Oosterhuis W, Looijenga L (2000) Comparative genomic and in situ hybridization of germ cell tumors of the infantile testis. Lab Invest 80:1055–1064

Mostofi FK, Price EB Jr (1973) Tumors of the male genital system. In: Atlas of tumor pathology, second Series, fascicle 8. Armed Forces Institute of Pathology, Washington, DC

Mostofi FK, Theiss EA, Ashley DJB (1959) Tumors of specialized gonadal stroma in human male subjects. Cancer 12: 944–957

Mostofi FK, Sesterhenn IA, Davis CJ Jr (1988) Developments in histopathology of testicular germ cell tumors. Semin Urol 6:171–188

Nakashima N, Murakami S, Fukatsu T, Nagasaka T, Fukata S, Ohiwa N, Nara Y, Sobue M, Takeuchi J (1988) Characteristics of "embryoid body" in human gonadal germ cell tumors. Hum Pathol 19:1144–1154

Niehans GA, Manivel JC, Copland GT et al (1988) Immunohistochemistry of germ cell and trophoblastic neoplasms. Cancer 62:1113–1123

Nistal M, Lazaro R, Garcia J et al (1992a) Testicular granulosa cell tumor of the adult type. Arch Pathol Lab Med 116: 284–287

Nistal M, Martinez-Garcia C, Paniagua R (1992b) Testicular fibroma. J Urol 147:1617–1619

Nistal M, Puras A, Perna C et al (1996) Fusocellular gonadal stromal tumour of the testis with epithelial and myoid differentiation. Histopathology 29:259–264

Oosterhuis JW, Castedo SM, de Jong B et al (1989) Ploidy of primary germ cell tumors of the testis. Lab Invest 60:14–21

Peterson C, Skoog S (2008) Prenatal diagnosis of juvenile granulose cell tumor of the testis. J Pediatr Urol 4:472–474

Peterson AC, Bauman JM, Light DE, McMann LP, Costabile RA (2001) The prevalence of testicular microlithiasis in an asymptomatic population of men 18 to 35 years old. J Urol 166:2061–2064

Pichmann S, Mikuz G, Schmid KW (1993) Chromogranin A and B in nonseminomatous testicular tumors. An immunohistochemical study. J Urol Pathol 1:43–54

Pizzocaro G (1984) Monfardini S No adjuvant chemotherapy in selected patients with pathological stage II nonseminomatous germ cell tumors of the testis. J Urol 131(4):677–680

Proppe KH, Scully RE (1980) Large-cell calcifying Sertoli cell tumor of the testis. Am J Clin Pathol 74:607–619

Proppe KH, Scully RE (1982) Large cell calcifying Sertoli cell tumor of the testis: light microscopic and ultrastructural study. Hum Pathol 13:1109–1114

Rajpert-De Meyts E, Jacobsen GK, Bartkova J, Aubry F, Samson M, Bartek J, Skakkebaek NE (2003) The immunohistochemical expression pattern of Chk2, p53, p19INK4d, MAGE-A4 and other selected antigens provides new evidence for the premeioticoriginofspermatocyticseminoma. Histopathology 42:217–226

Read G, Stenning SP, Cullen MH et al (1992) Medical research council prospective study of surveillance for stage I testicular teratoma. J Clin Oncol 10:1762–1768

Renedo DE, Trainer TD (1994) Intratubular germ cell neoplasia (ITGCN) with p53 and PCNA expresssion and adjacent mature teratoma in a infant testis. An immunohistochemical and morphologic study with a review of the literature. Am J Surg Pathol 18:947–952

Renshaw AA, Gordon M, Corless CL (1997) Immunohistochemistry of unclassified sex cord-stromal tumors of the testis with a predominance of spindle cells. Mod Pathol 10:693–700

Reuter VE (2005) Origins and molecular biology of testicular germ cell tumors. Mod Pathol 18(Suppl 2):S51–S60

Rey R, Sabourin JC, Venara M et al (2000) Anti-Müllerian hormone is a specific marker of Sertoli- and granulosa-cell origin in gonadal tumors. Hum Pathol 31:1202–1208

Rorth M, Rajpert-De Meyts E, Andersson L, Dieckmann KP, Fossa SD, Grigor KM, Hendry WF, Herr HW, Looijenga LH, Oosterhuis JW, Skakkebaek NE (2000) Carcinoma in situ in the testis. Scand J Urol Nephrol Suppl (205): 166–186

Rutgers JL, Young RH, Scully RE (1988) The testicular "tumor" of the adrenogenital syndrome: a report of six cases and review of the literature on testicular masses in patients with adrenocortical disorders. Am J Surg Pathol 12:503–513

Scully RE (1970) Gonadoblastoma: A review of 74 cases. Cancer 25:1340–1356

Sonneveld DJA, Sleijfer DT, Koops HS et al (1998) Mature teratoma identified after postchemotherapy surgery in patients with disseminated nonseminomatous testicular germ cell tumors. A plea for an aggressive surgical approach. Cancer 82:1343–1351

Soosay GN, Bobrow L, Happerfield L et al (1991) Morphology and immunohistochemistry of carcinoma in situ adjecent to testicular germ cell tumours in adults and children: implications for histogenersis. Histopathology 19:537–544

Srigley JR, Toth P, Edwards V (1987) Diagnostic electron microscopy of male genital tumors. Clin Lab Med 7: 91–115

Steele GS, Richie JP, Stewart AK, Menck HR (1999) Fort on patterns of care for testicular carcinoma, 1985–1996. Cancer 86:2171–2183

Steiner H, Gozzi C, Verdorfer I, Mikuz G, Bartsch G, Hobisch A (2006) Metastatic spermatocytic seminoma – an extremely rare disease. Eur Urol 49:183–186

Stenberg CN (1998) The management of stage I testis cancer. Urol Clin North Am 25:435–449

Stenning SP, Parkinson MC (1998) Postchemotherapy residual masses in germ cell tumor patients. Content, clinical features, and prognosis. Cancer 83:1409–1419

Stevens MJ, Gildersleve J, Jameson CF, Horwich A (1993) Spermatocytic seminoma in a maldescended testis. Br J Urol 72:657–659

Suster S, Moran CA, Dominguez-Malagón H et al (1998) Germ cell tumors of the mediastinum and testis: a comparative immunohistochemical study of 120 cases. Hum Pathol 29:737–742

Tabernero J, Paz-Ares L, Salazar R, Lianes P, Guerra J, Borras J, Villavicencio H, Leiva O, Cortes-Funes H (2004) Incidence of contralateral germ cell testicular tumors in South Europe: report of the experience at 2 Spanish university hospitals and review of the literature. J Urol 171:164–167

Talerman A (1972) A distinctive gonadal neoplasm related to gonadoblastoma. Cancer 30:1219–1224

Talerman A (1975) The incidence of yolk sac tumor (endodermal sinus tumor) elements in germ cell tumors of the testis in adults. Cancer 36:211–215

Talerman A (1980) Germ cell tumors of the testis. Prog Surg Pathol 1:175–204

Tickoo SK, Hutchinson B, Bacik J, Mazumdar M, Motzer RJ, Bajorin DF, Bosl GJ, Reuter VE (2002) Testicular seminoma: a clinicopathologic and immunohistochemical study of 105 cases with special reference to seminomas with atypical features. Int J Surg Pathol 10:23–32

Timmes A, Oosterhuis JW, Koops HS et al (1994) The tumor microenviroenment: possible role of integrins and the extracellular matrix in tumor biological behaviour of intratubular germ cell neoplasia and testicular seminomas. Am J Pathol 44:1035–1044

Trias I, Algaba F, Hocsman H (1991) Intratubular germ cell tumor. Relation with "burned-out" tumor and testicular germinal neoplasia. Eur Urol 19:81–84

True LD, Otis CN, Delprado W, Scully RE, Rosai J (1988) Spermatocytic seminoma of testis with sarcomatous transformation: a report of five cases. Am J Surg Pathol 12:75–82

Ulbright TM (1993) Germ cell neoplasms of the testis. Am J Surg Pathol 17:1075–1091

Ulbright TM (2005) Germ cell tumors of the gonads: a selective review emphasizing problems in differential diagnosis, newly appreciated, and controversial issues. Mod Pathol 18(Suppl 2):S61–S79

Ulbright TM, Young RH (2005) Seminoma with tubular, microcystic, and related patterns: a study of 28 cases of unusual morphologic variants that often cause confusion with yolk sac tumor. Am J Surg Pathol 29:500–505

Ulbright TM, Loehrer PJ, Roth LM (1984) The development of non-germ cell malignancies within germ cell tumors. A clinicopathologic study of 11 cases. Cancer 54:1824–1833

Ulbright TM, Young RH, Scully RE (1997) Trophoblastic tumors of the testis other than classic chriocarcinoma: "Monophasic" choriocarcinoma and placental site trophoblastic tumor: a report of two cases. Am J Surg Pathol 21:282–288

Ulbright TM, Amin MB, Young RH (1999a) Tumors of the testis, adnexa, spermatic cord, and scrotum. Atlas of tumor pathology. AFIP, Washington
Ulbright TM, Amin MB, Young RH (1999) Tumors of the testis, adnexa, spermatic cord and scrotum. In: Atlas of tumor pathology, third Series, No. 25. Armed Forces Institute of Pathology, Washington, DC
Ulbright TM, Srigley JR, Reuter VE et al (2000) Sex cord-stromal tumor of the testis with entrapped germ cells. A lesion mimicking unclassified mixed germ cell sex cord-stromal tumors. Am J Surg Pathol 24:535–542
Ulbright TM, Srigley JR, Hatzianastassiou DK et al (2002) Leydig cell tumors of the testis with unusual features: adipose differentiation, calcification with ossification, and spindle-shaped tumor cells. Am J Surg Pathol 26:1424–1433
Ulbright TM, Amin MB, Young RH (2007) Intratubular large cell hyalinizing sertoli cell neoplasia of the testis: a report of 8 cases of a distinctive lesion of the Peutz–Jeghers syndrome. Am J Surg Pathol 6:827–835
van Echten J, van Gurp RJHLM, Stoepker M et al (1995) Cytogenetic evidence that carcinoma in situ is the precursor lesion for invasive testicular germ cell tumors. Cancer Genet Cytogenet 85:133–137
van Kessel Geurts A, Suijkerbuijk RF, Sinke Rj et al (1993) Molecular cytogenetics of human germ cell tumours: i(12p) and related chromosomal anomalies. Eur Urol 23:23–29
Venara M, Rey R, Bergada I et al (2001) Sertoli cell proliferations of the infantile testis. An intratubular form of Sertoli cell tumor? Am J Surg Pathol 25:1237–1244
von der Maase H, Rorth M, Walbom-Jorgensen S, Sorensen BL, Christophersen IS, Hald T, Jacobsen GK, Berthelsen JG, Skakkebaek NE (1986) Carcinoma in situ of contralateral testis in patients with testicular germ cell cancer: study of 27 cases in 500 patients. Br Med J (Clin Res Ed) 293: 1398–1401
von Eyben FE, Jacobsen GK, Rorth M, Von Der Maase H (2004) Microinvasive germ cell tumour (MGCT) adjacent to testicular germ cell tumours. Histopathology 44:547–554
von Eyben FE, Jacobsen GK, Skotheim RI (2005) Microinvasive germ cell tumor of the testis. Virchows Arch 447:610–625
Wang BY, Rabinowitz DS, Granato RC Sr et al (2002) Gonadal tumor with granulosa cell tumor features in an adult testis. Ann Diagn Pathol 6:56–60
Warde P, Jewett MAS (1998) Surveillance for stage I testicular seminoma. Is it good option? Urol Clin North Am 25: 425–433
Warde P, von der Maase H, Horwich A (1998) Prognostic factors for relapse in stage I seminoma managed by surveillance (Abstract 1188). Proc Am Soc Clin Oncol 17:1188
Young RH (2005) Sex cord-stromal tumors of the ovary and testis: their similarities and differences with consideration of selected problems. Mod Pathol 18:S81–S98
Young RH, Scully RE (1990) *Testicular Tumors*. ASCP Press, Chicago, pp 101–136
Young RH, Talerman A (1987) Testicular tumors other than germ cell tumors. Semin Diagn Pathol 4:342–360
Young RH, Lawrence WD, Scully RE (1985) Juvenile granulosa cell tumor-another neoplasm associated with abnormal chromosomes and ambiguous genitalia. A report of three cases. Am J Surg Pathol 9:737–743
Young S, Gooneratne S, Straus FH et al (1995) Feminizing Sertoli cell tumors in boys with Peutz–Jeghers syndrome. Am J Surg Pathol 19:50–58
Young RH, Koelliker DD, Scully RE (1998) Sertoli cell tumors of the testis, not otherwise specified. A clinicopathologic analysis of 60 cases. Am J Surg Pathol 22:709–721
Yuasa T, Yoshiki T, Ogawa O, Tanaka T, Isono T, Mishina M, Higuchi K, Okada Y, Yoshida O (1999) Detection of alpha-fetoprotein mRNA in seminoma. J Androl 20:336–340
Zeeman AM, Stoop H, Boter M, Gillis AJ, Castrillon DH, Oosterhuis JW, Looijenga LH (2002) VASA is a specific marker for both normal and malignant human germ cells. Lab Invest 82:159–166
Zheng W, Senturk BZ, Parkash V (2003) Inhibin immunohistochemical staining: a practical approach for the surgical pathologist in the diagnoses of ovarian sex cord-stromal tumors. Adv Anat Pathol 10:27–38
Zukerberg LR, Young RH, Scully RE (1991) Sclerosing Sertoli cell tumor of the testis: a report of 10 cases. Am J Surg Pathol 15:829–834

# Risk Factors and Genetical Characterization

## 2

Leendert H.J. Looijenga

## Abbreviations

| | |
|---|---|
| AFP | Alpha feta protein |
| CTA | Cancer testis antigens |
| CIS | Carcinoma in situ |
| CAIS | Complete androgen insensitivity |
| c- and a-CGH | Chromosomal- as well as array-comparative genomic hybridization |
| DSD | Disorders of sex development |
| GBY | Gonadoblastoma region of the Y chromosome |
| hCG | Human chorionic gonadotropin |
| GCTs | Human germ cell tumors |
| HDAC | Histone deacetylase |
| ISH | In situ hybridization (ISH) |
| IGCNU | Intratubular germ cell neoplasia unclassified |
| LDH | Lactate dehydrogenase |
| MSI | Microsatellite instability |
| miRNA | MicroRNA |
| PAIS | Partial androgen insensitivity |
| PGC | Primordial germ cell |
| SCF | Stem cell factor |
| SNP | Single nucleotide polymorphism |
| SS | Spermatocytic seminomas |
| TDS | Testicular dysgenesis syndrome |
| TIN | Testicular intratubular neoplasia |
| UGT | Undifferentiated gonadal tissue |
| XIST | X inactive specific transcript |

L.H.J. Looijenga
Josephine Nefkens Institute, Pathology Department, Erasmus MC, Rotterdam, The Netherlands

## 2.1 Introduction

The testis is a highly specialized male specific organ with in principle two main functions: generation of germ cells by a process called spermatogenesis, and formation of hormones crucial for normal male phenotypic development as well as initiation and maintenance of spermatogenesis (Grootegoed et al. 2000; Loveland et al. 2005). The final goal of the germ cells is transmitting genetic information to the next generation (Donovan 1998; McLaren 2001). Therefore, they have to be able to become pluripotent, i.e. capable of forming all differentiation lineages, both embryonal and extraembryonal upon fertilization (Cinalli et al. 2008). This requires a unique mechanism involving proliferation and maturation of germ cells as well as a germ cell-specific manner of division known as meiosis (Hunt and Hassold 2002). This results finally in generation of a haploid DNA content in highly specialized cells, called spermatozoa, able to penetrate the zona pellucida of the mature egg. The proper formation of these cells requires a delicate temporal and spatial process during embryogenesis resulting in testis formation (Wilhelm et al. 2007), as well as during and after puberty, being dependent on the interaction of many cell types, which are organized within and around the seminiferous tubules, being the functional units wherein spermatogenesis occurs (Grootegoed et al. 2000). The cell of origin of the germ cell lineage is referred to as a primordial germ cell (PGC) (Donovan 1998; McLaren 1992, 2003 Wylie 1993; Kato et al. 1999). These cells originate outside the soma and migrate to the genital ridge. Within the genital ridge they are referred to as gonocytes (to be discussed below). This system of gonadal development and gametogenesis can be disturbed in various ways, both

M.P. Laguna et al. (eds.), *Cancer of the Testis*,
DOI: 10.1007/978-1-84800-370-5_2, 

during early development as well in adult life. In principle, every cell type present within the testis can undergo malignant transformation, and result in cancer, like Sertoli cell tumors, Leydig cell tumors, lymphoma's, sarcomas, etc (Woodward et al. 2004). These types of cancer will not be discussed here. This chapter will be restricted to the various human germ cell tumors (GCTs), which can occur in the human testis. When relevant, the GCTs occurring at other anatomical localizations will be referred to.

## 2.2 General Concept and Perspectives

The last few years, a wealth of information has become available on solid cancers, including human GCTs. This boost is due to the availability of various techniques able to generate high throughput data on (epi) genetics as well as expression profiling (both protein-encoding and noncoding genes, including microRNAs (miRNAs)). These data sets on their own are significant for the elucidation of the pathogenetic steps involved in the formation of the cancer under investigation. An integrated approach will provide an even higher level of understanding of the biology of the systems. When linked to patient characteristics, the data have been shown to be highly relevant for patient management (Swanton and Downward 2008). This approach has resulted in novel insights in the pathobiological pathways, new methods for diagnosis, prognosis, response prediction, and molecular therapies. This will benefit quality of life of the individual patient. In addition, it will allow generation of informative in vitro and in vivo models of disease. There is no doubt that patients already benefit from this endeavor in terms of increasing survival (Joensuu et al. 2001; Druker et al. 2001).

## 2.3 Human Germ Cell Tumors: Introduction

Human GCTs are different from other solid cancers of adults in a number of aspects, related to both biology and clinical behavior (Oosterhuis and Looijenga 2005). This is likely due to their embryonic origin, in spite of their clinical presentation in adult life as observed in most cases (to be discussed below). It is proposed that the origin of GCTs also explains their overall sensitivity to DNA damaging agents (i.e., irradiation and cisplatin-based chemotherapy) (Hong and Stambrook 2004), supported by the fact that this is influenced by the histological composition of the tumor: loss of embryonic features results in induction of treatment resistance (Masters and Koberle 2003). The recent findings on embryonic and adult stem cells in general, and cancer stem cells specifically (Zaehres and Scholer 2007; Rossant 2008; Morrison and Spradling 2008; Knoblich 2008; Jaenisch and Young 2008), are of relevance in the context of the origin and pathobiology of human GCTs (Pera 2008). The following paragraphs will focus on risk factors and genetical characterization of the various types of these tumors. Understanding the impact of these observations is also dependent on knowledge of the pathogenesis of these tumors, which requires information on normal gonadal and germ cell development. Therefore, these aspects will also be discussed where appropriate. In addition, if relevant, clinical data will be integrated in the discussion.

## 2.4 Classification of Human GCTs

Traditionally GCTs are classified on the basis of their histological appearance, as judged by the pathologist (Scully 1978; Mostofi and Sesterhenn 1985; Mostofi et al. 1987; Donohue 1990). Although, without any restriction this approach is relevant and informative, it underestimates the biological diversity of this type of cancer, as discussed extensively elsewhere (Oosterhuis and Looijenga 2005; Reuter 2005). More specifically, taking a different view on this seemingly heterogeneous group of cancers will likely identify novel patterns, making the pathogenesis of these cancers easier to understand, both from a developmental as well as clinical point of view. For this specific purpose, an alternative classification system was proposed in 2005, in which site of presentation of the primary tumor, age of the patient at diagnosis, histological composition, and chromosomal constitution are informative parameters. On the basis of these criteria, five categories (I–V) of GCTs are identified (Oosterhuis and Looijenga

**Table 2.1** Summary of the most differentiating parameters for the type I, II, and III germ cell tumors

| Parameters: | Type I | Type II | Type III |
|---|---|---|---|
| Histology | Teratoma/yolk sac tumor | (Non)Seminoma | Sperm. seminoma |
| Age | Neonates/infants | Adolescents/young adults | Elderly |
| Cell of origin | Embryonic germ cell | Prim. germ cell/gonocyte | Prim. spermatocyte |
| Genomic imprinting | Partial erased | Erased | Partial paternal |
| Genotype | Diploid/gain 1,12p(13),20q, Loss 1p,4,6q | Aneuploid, gain X,7,8,12p,21 Loss 1p,11,13,18 | Aneuploid, gain 9 |
| Risk factors | Unknown | Multiple related to delay germ cell maturation | Unknown |
| Animal model | Mouse teratocarcinomas | Unknown | Canine seminoma |

2005). This has already proven to allow a more straightforward understanding of their origin, histological diversity, as well as clinical behavior. Because of the fact that within the testis predominantly the type I, II, and III GCTs are diagnosed, they will form the topic of this chapter. On the basis of the incidence as well as pathobiological and clinical aspects, emphasis will be on the type II GCTs. The different characteristics relevant to identify the major groups of GCTs of the testis, i.e., type I, II, and III, are summarized in Table 2.1. A more detailed discussion on the other types of GCTs has been made elsewhere (Oosterhuis and Looijenga 2003, 2005; Looijenga and Oosterhuis 1999; Looijenga et al. 1999).

## 2.5 Origin of GCTs of the Testis

To understand the nature of risk factors for the development of human GCTs, especially those of the testis, it is of relevance to have insight into normal gonadal development and the origin of GCTs. The morphological characteristics and expression profiles (see below) of the type II and III GCTs support their germ cell lineage origin (Sperger et al. 2003; Kraggerud et al. 2002; Skotheim et al. 2002; Looijenga et al. 2003a, 2006; Korkola et al. 2005; Hofer et al. 2005; Biermann et al. 2007a, b; Gashaw et al. 2007). However, this is not directly obvious for the type I GCTs, i.e., they show no characteristics mimicking germ cells in any stage of development. In this context, investigation of their pattern of genomic imprinting, defined as the germ cell-specific functional difference between a haploid set of chromosomes depending on the parental origin, is informative (Surani et al. 1990; Tycko 1994; Surani 1994). The partial erasement of the pattern of genomic imprinting supports the view that the majority of the type I GCTs are also of germ cell origin (Sievers et al. 2005a). Therefore indeed, the type I, II, and III GCTs can all be considered as GCTs truly.

The origin and migration of embryonic germ cells from the yolk sac region (proximal epiblast) to the genital ridge (Hayashi et al. 2007), provide an interesting explanation as to why the type I and II GCTs can also be found outside the gonads, i.e., along the midline of the body. In this context, the current knowledge on suppression of the somatic differentiation pathways during formation and migration of embryonic germ cells is highly relevant (see below). Still, the specific localization of GCTs in the brain is unknown on the basis of this assumption (Scotting 2006; Oosterhuis et al. 2007). However, studies on genomic anomalies support the view that they are indeed GCTs (De Bruin et al. 1994; Motzer et al. 1991; Palmer et al. 2007). Expression profiling of mRNA shows that the intracranial GCTs have a similar pattern of gene expression as those of the gonads, both testis and ovary (Looijenga et al. 2006) and Hersmus et al., submitted for publication. The question remains to be answered whether the germ cells at the extragonadal localizations have a specific function during embryogenesis and possibly later, and whether the final cancer is the result of lack of physiological apoptosis or differentiation later in life. Alternatively, the tumors can be the results of initial aberrant migration and unphysiological survival. The recent observations regarding relevant factors in the migration of PGCs, like SDF1 and its receptors CXCR4 and 7 are relevant in this context (Knaut and Schier 2008; Boldajipour et al. 2008). Although these issues are interesting, they will not be discussed here, because of the focus on GCTs of the testis. In the following two paragraphs, the type I and type III GCTs will be discussed in more detail, with emphasis on identified risk factors and genetic anomalies, including mRNA, miRNA, and protein findings. The remaining final part of the chapter will be dedicated to the type II GCTs.

## 2.5.1 Type I GCTs

### 2.5.1.1 Epidemiology and Histological Composition

The type I GCTs of the adult testis are rare (Schneider et al. 2004), and predominantly found in neonates and infants, although exceptions do occur (see below). A higher incidence in industrialized countries has been suggested, without an ethnic preference. Independent of the anatomical localization (see Table 2.1), all proven type I GCTs are composed of teratoma and/or yolk sac tumor. The teratoma can contain both immature and mature elements, possibly mixed, of all differentiation lineages, i.e., endoderm, mesoderm, and ectoderm. Overall, these tumors are clinically benign (Huddart et al. 2003). If however, other histological components are found, like seminoma, embryonal carcinoma, or choriocarcinoma, it is by definition a type II GCT (see below). Visa versa, if a tumor is composed of only a teratoma or a yolk sac tumor, or a mixture of both, diagnosed in a dysgenetic testis (see below) or in a testis after puberty, it must be demonstrated that it is not a variant of a type II GCT. This can be done on the basis of the identification of the precursor lesion or the presence of specific chromosomal anomalies (see below).

### 2.5.1.2 Cell of Origin

No obvious precursor cell for the type I GCTs based on morphological or immunohistochemical characteristics is identified so far. However, on analysis of mouse models, as well as determination of the pattern of genomic imprinting (see above), the cell of origin is found to be a germ cell in the majority of cases (Walt et al. 1993). A somatic origin of the (limited number of) human type I GCTs with a biparental pattern of genomic imprinting so far cannot be excluded. In general, the type I GCTs show a partial pattern of erasement, reflecting the origin of an early embryonic germ cell (Sievers et al. 2005a). Experimental data on migrating (fluorescently labeled) PGCs in Bax-deficient mice, which are therefore apoptosis disturbed, indicate that a specific subpopulation of PGCs migrate along a different route ending in the sacral region, instead of in the genital ridge (Runyan et al. 2008). This sacrococcygeal region is indeed another predominant anatomical site where type I GCTs can be found. Interestingly, this specific PGC population is larger in a female mouse compared to that in a male mouse, possibly reflecting the preferential occurrence of these tumors in baby girls compared to baby boys (Schneider et al. 2004). Although this is an interesting observation, elucidation of the cell of origin and the pathogenetic pathways involved in human type I GCTs still requires much effort. The Wnt pathway has been proposed to be involved, but mainly upon specific differentiation lineages within the tumor, and not in the initiation of the tumor itself (Fritsch et al. 2006). This is of interest because of the significant role of Wnt in stem cell biology (Walsh and Andrews 2003; Constantinescu 2003; Suda and Arai 2008) (see also below).

### 2.5.1.3 Risk Factors and Genetic Changes

No risk factors for type I GCTs have been identified so far (Malogolowkin et al. 1990); this supports an independent origin and pathogenesis from the type II GCTs (see below). A slowly increasing incidence has been noted. Interesting is the observation that teratomas are frequently observed in mice in which the function of a specific gene is disrupted in the germ cell lineage, including kras2, pten, and dnd (Looijenga et al. 2007a). So far, no indications are available that one of these genes is involved in the pathogenesis of the human type I GCTs. Dnd is of specific interest, because of its role in the function of miRNAs (see below). In the mouse, absence of this gene results in a disturbed germ cell development, resulting in infertility as well as bilateral teratomas (Youngren et al. 2005). No studies have been published on the association of a type I GCT and fertility. A rare DNA variant within the DND gene has been identified in a single type II GCT (see below) (Linger et al. 2008). Using an additional series of

18 proven type I GCTs, either teratomas or yolk sac tumors, this specific variant was not found (Looijenga, unpublished observations), and it is therefore unlikely to be a relevant pathogenetic factor. Moreover, a number of inbred mouse strains show development of testicular teratomas, which is to a certain level dependent of the genetic background used. The high tendency to form of teratomas from the germ cell lineage in these strains has been explained assuming that it reflects a rescue mechanism preventing transmission of the affected gene to the next generation (Looijenga et al. 2007a, b). The direct switch from a germ cell to a somatic cell (the stem cell of the teratoma) will generate a relatively benign tumor. Although of interest, no experimental data are available to support it yet, but the heterogeneity in function of genes of which disruption results in the phenomenon is intriguing. The heterogeneity of genes leading to mouse teratoma formation is of interest in the context of the required suppression of the somatic differentiation program in PGCs (to be discussed below). It suggests that this can be disturbed in many different ways, offering a model to study this so-called process of activation to pluripotency, also referred to as reprogramming (Silva and Smith 2008; Surani et al. 2007). This step is also of relevance in the context of type II GCTs, in which reprogramming occurs in about 50% of the tumors during the progression from the precursor lesion to the invasive cancer (see below). However, mice do not show development of type II GCTs, with possibly a single, and highly relevant, exception (to be discussed below).

Because of the lack of proven cell lines derived from type I GCTs, the data on chromosomal constitution are obtained from primary in vivo tumors, which need verification that sufficient numbers of tumor cells are included in the sample under investigation. With this possible restriction, the overall picture is consistent and as follows: no chromosomal changes are identified in teratomas, not even after microdissection, while recurrent genomic imbalances are present in the type I yolk sac tumors (Perlman et al. 1994, 1996; Mostert et al. 2000; Schneider et al. 2001, 2002; Veltman et al. 2003, 2005). These data have been obtained using conventional karyotyping, and more recently also using chromosomal- as well as array-comparative genomic hybridization (c- and a-CGH), as well as (fluorescent) in situ hybridization (ISH). The data from the different approaches are in accordance to each other. The overall pattern is summarized in Table 2.1. On the basis of genetic characteristics, it has been demonstrated that indeed the yolk sac tumor component originates from the teratoma component. This is in line with the observation that upon extensive transplantation it is also observed in mouse embryo-derived teratomas, considered as the animal model for human type I GCTs (Walt et al. 1993; Van Berlo et al. 1990a, b). Of interest is that mouse embryonic stem cells lacking functional Sox2, a regulator of pluripotency (see below), give rise to (polyploid) trophoblastic cells (i.e., reflecting extra-embryonic differentiation) (Li et al. 2007a), in which Cdx2 is a regulatory element (Deb et al. 2006). Indeed, subtle changes in the level of Sox2 regulate differentiation of embryonic stem cells (Boer et al. 2007; Kopp et al. 2008) (see also below). The aneuploidy of the human type I yolk sac tumors also parallels the observation that if mouse embryonic stem cells are tetraploidized, they form trophoblast. This serves as a rescue mechanism to allow embryonic development in gene-disrupted embryonic stem cells which lack the capacity to generate the yolk sac, which is crucial for further development. These data suggest that the processes involved in the progression from teratoma to yolk sac, both in mouse and human tumor cells, might be solely determined by evolutionary retained mechanisms, which are still operational in the type I GCT cells. The intriguing consistency of polyploidy remains unexplained (Otto 2007).

An older age of the patient, beyond the neonatal and infantile period, at clinical diagnosis does not exclude the diagnosis of a type I GCT. This is exemplified by the two Caucasian female patients of respectively 14 and 37 years of age (unpublished observations). They presented with an ovarian tumor histologically composed of pure yolk sac tumor. Because of the rareness of a pure yolk sac tumor at this age, and the knowledge that they are much more frequent at younger age, a-CGH was performed on both tumors, demonstrating the type I characteristic chromosomal imbalances, including loss of 1p, and 4 and 6q, and gain of 1q, 12p(13), and 20q (see Fig. 2.1a). The type II specific chromosomal imbalance (see below), i.e., gain of the short arm of chromosome 12, is absent (see Fig. 2.1b). The second tumor suggests the presence of a teratomatous component based on smooth muscle tissue, but it could not be confirmed. Although of interest from a pathobiological point of view, distinction between

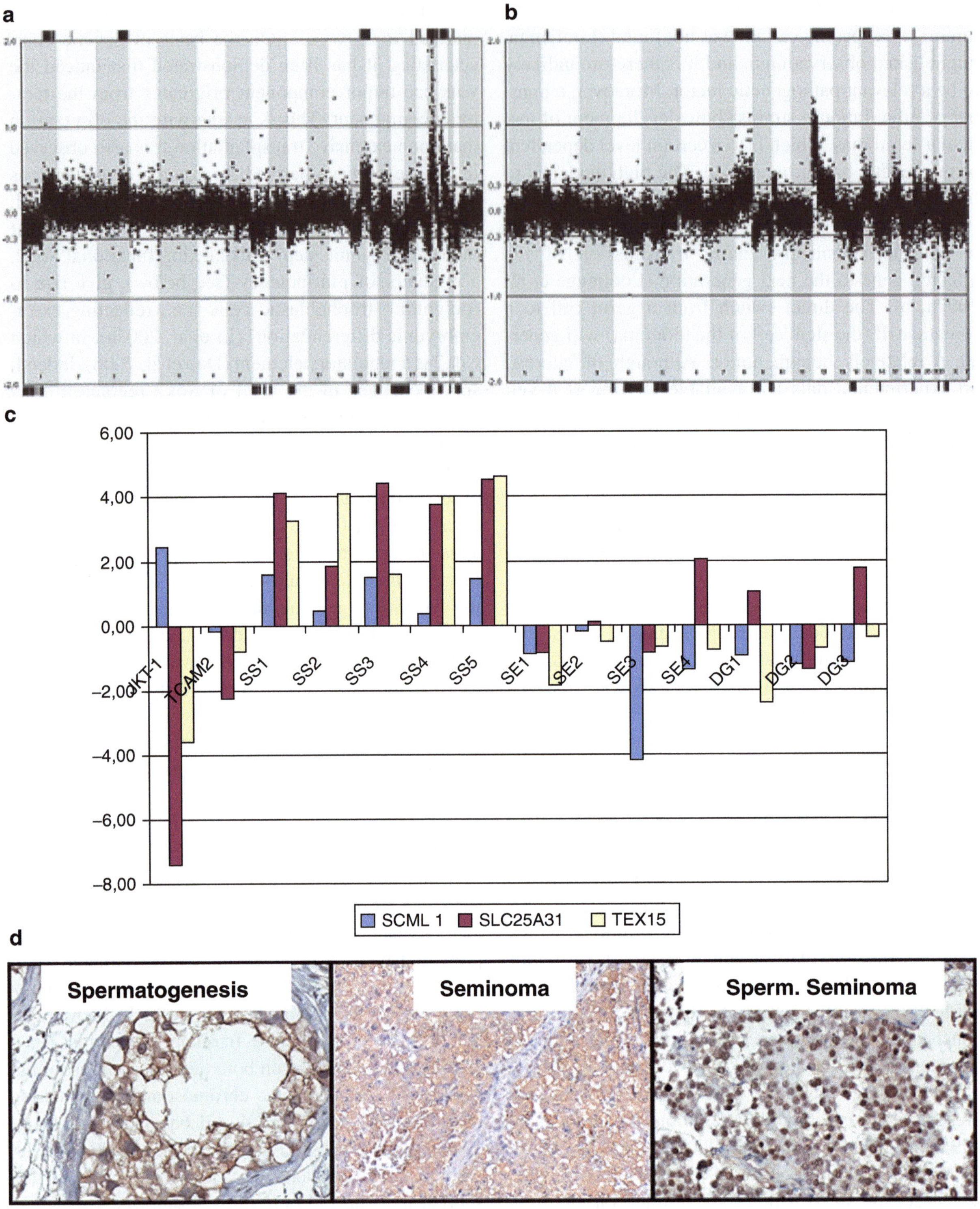


**Fig. 2.1** Example of array-comparative genomic hybridization using DNA of (**a**) a yolk sac tumor of the ovary of a phenotypically normal female patient of 37 years of age. Note the presence of specific chrosomosomal imbalances, but the absence of gain of the short arm of chromosome 12; (**b**) a representative type II testicular GCT, showing the recurrent chromosomal changes, including gain of 12p; (**c**) Expression data based on Affymetrix profiling for SCML1, SLC25A31 (also known as ANT4), and TEX4. Note the specific expression in spermatocytic seminoma (SS) compared to that in seminoma (SE) and dysgerminoma (DG). The seminoma cell line TCam-2 and the nonrelated JKT-1 are included for comparison; (**d**) Represenntative examples of immunohistochemical detection of SCML1 on normal spermatogenesis (*left panel*: positive), seminoma (middle panel: negative), and SS (*right panel*: positive)

a type I and type II yolk sac tumors has no clinical implication as yet.

#### 2.5.1.4 Concluding Points Type I GCTs

No identified risk factors

Histologically composed of either teratoma and/or yolk sac tumor

Predominantly diagnosed in neonates and infants

Early embryonic germ cell is cell of origin

Teratomas show no chromosomal anomalies

Yolk sac tumors show loss of 1p, and 4 and 6q and gain of 1q, 12p(13), and 20q

No representative cell lines available

Various representative animal models identified (i.p. mouse teratocarcinomas)

### 2.5.2 Type III GCTs

#### 2.5.2.1 Epidemiology

Type III GCTs, also known as spermatocytic seminomas (SS), are rare, and preferentially found in elderly males (Muller et al. 1987; Burke and Mostofi 1993). Although they hardly metastasize, up to 30% of the patients will develop bilateral disease (Bergner et al. 1980). Although type II GCTs are significantly less frequently diagnosed in blacks, there seems to be a skewed incidence of SS. This supports the independent origin of both tumor entities (see below). In contrast to the type I and II GCTs, the SS have no counterpart in the ovary or other anatomical localizations. In other words, this tumor is specifically associated with the occurrence of spermatogenesis, which is not the case for the other GCTs, although this has been proposed otherwise (see below). In fact, the type I and II tumors are related to the presence, i.e., retention, of embryonic germ cells, with their specific characteristics (see above and below).

#### 2.5.2.2 Histological Composition

SS have been considered as a variant of seminoma. However, the morphology and histology are in the majority of cases significantly different (Romanenko and Persidskii 1983; Dekker et al. 1992; Cummings et al. 1994; Chung et al. 2004; Talerman 1984). The less experienced pathologists may be misled by the variation of the histological appearance of SS. Generally, SS are characteristically composed of three cell types, with respectively a small, intermediate, and large nucleus, associated with a diploid, tetraploid, and hypertetraploid DNA content. No convincing haploid tumor cells have been identified so far (Looijenga et al. 2007b; Oosterhuis et al. 1989a; Kysela and Matoska 1991; Takahashi 1993). In addition, they usually lack infiltrating lymphocytes, which are characteristic for (classic) seminoma (see below). The precursor lesion is known as intratubular SS, being an accumulation of tumor cells in the luminal space of the seminiferous tubules, suggesting that the tumor cells only proliferate in the luminal compartment of the seminiferous tubule, beyond the tight junctions between the Sertoli cells (Looijenga et al. 2007a, b). This in contrast to the cell of origin of the type II GCTs (see below).

#### 2.5.2.3 Cell of Origin and Markers for Diagnosis

On the basis of the various sizes of the nuclei of the SS tumor cells, it has been hypothesized that these cells undergo meiosis, generating cells with a different DNA content. This was further substantiated using immunohistochemistry for three markers, XPA, SCP1, and SSX2-4, which were indeed able to distinguish SS from (classical) seminoma (Stoop et al. 2001). Subsequently, other markers have been added on the basis of targeted analysis, including P53, CHK2, p16INK4D, and MAGE-4A (Rajpert-De Meyts et al. 2003a), indeed markers of later stages of germ cell development. The pattern of genomic imprinting of SS is highly specific for germ cell developing along the male lineage of spermatogenesis, i.e., it shows a more paternal pattern of genomic imprinting (Sievers et al. 2005a). High throughput mRNA expression profiling shows that these tumors indeed express multiple genes related to spermatogenesis, including cancer testis antigens (CTA), of which MAGE-4A is an example (Looijenga et al. 2006). This study also demonstrated that SS shows expression of genes specific for the prophase of meiosis I, i.e., TCFL5, CLGN, and LDHc. Unpublished results indicate that a number of other genes show a specific pattern of expression in SS compared to other GCTs, including (classic) seminomas. These include SCMH1 (Takada et al. 2007), SLC25A31 (ANT4) (Brower et al. 2007), and TEX15 (Yang et al. 2008) (see Fig. 2.1c). These markers are related to different processes, like germ cell maturation, including regulation of gene expression and meiotic recombination. That the mRNA studies are informative is proven previously (Looijenga et al. 2006). It is here also demonstrated for the specific presence of SCML1 protein in SS and not in seminoma (see Fig. 2.1d, middle vs. right panel; for comparison normal testis is indicated in the left panel). Other markers are less discriminating between SS and seminoma, like PLZF and TAF4B (Dadoune 2007), which are related to spermatogenic stem cell maintenance and renewal (data not shown). Therefore, the summed data suggest that the cell of origin of SS is a later germ cell, most likely a primary spermatocyte. This is, however, difficult to reconcile with the occurrence of bilateral disease in about one-third of the cases (Burke and Mostofi 1993; Bergner et al. 1980; Eble 1994). The explanation could be that the first hit in the pathogenesis of SS in fact occurs in a migrating germ cell before it enters the genital ridge. The affected germ cell is, in spite of the initial hit, able to develop along the male germ cell lineage and the block in maturation becomes only obvious when meiosis is initiated. This hypothesis could be tested experimentally in the various spontaneous and induced animal tumors, like those in *Caenorhabditis elegans* (Subramaniam and Seydoux 2003) and the dog (Looijenga and Oosterhuis 2007; Looijenga et al. 1994). So far, no representative cell lines of SS are available.

### 2.5.2.4 Risk Factors and Genetic Changes

No risk factors for SS are identified yet, although as mentioned, the diagnosis of SS indicates directly that the patient has a significant increase in risk to develop a bilateral cancer. Because SS does not metastasize, orchidectomy is sufficient for cure. It will result in complete castration in some cases because of bilateral disease. The rare progression of SS towards, highly malignant, sarcomatous elements has, however, to be kept in mind (Floyd et al. 1988; True et al. 1988; Matoska and Talerman 1990). The monoclonal origin of the SS and sarcoma element has not been proven so far, for which the identified recurrent chromosomal imbalances might be informative.

Conventional karyotyping, supported by c- and a-CGH revealed that SS have a characteristic pattern of chromosomal anomalies (Looijenga et al. 2006; Oosterhuis et al. 1989a; Kysela and Matoska 1991; Takahashi 1993; Rosenberg et al. 1998; Maiolino et al. 2004; Verdorfer et al. 2004; McIntyre et al. 2007). Overall they lack translocations, duplication, and deletions, but are characterized by additional copies of chromosome 9 (see Table 2.1). Integrated analysis of both chromosomal anomalies and expression profiling demonstrated that DMRT1 is a likely candidate gene/protein to explain the gain of chromosome 9 (Looijenga et al. 2006). Although its mechanistic basis remains to be elucidated, it can be used as an informative diagnostic marker. Interestingly this protein is also found in the testicular seminomas of dogs (Looijenga et al. 2007b), one of the supposed animal models for human SS, and it is recommended to indeed reclassify these canine tumors as SS.

Recent data on expression profiling of miRNA classify SS in the group of more differentiated samples, including normal testis and teratomas (Gillis et al. 2007). Again, this supports the relatively mature stage of differentiation of the tumor cells.

On the basis of these observations, it remains to be decided whether SS are indeed a cancer, or rather a benign tumor. The unsatisfactory explanation of the high incidence of bilaterality of these tumors, often synchronously, prompts another speculation. It is conceivable that these neoplasms originate as a hyperplasia, which is common in hormonally regulated endocrine organs. This thought is supported by the fact that the canine seminomas, in fact SS, are very often multifocal and mixed with gonadal stromal tumors.

### 2.5.2.5 Concluding Points Type III GCTs

No identified risk factors

Histologically composed of small, intermediate, and large germ cells

Predominantly diagnosed in elderly, solely in the testis

Primary spermatocyte likely cell of origin

Gain of chromosome 9 is a recurrent anomaly

DMRT1 is a likely 9p-candidate gene

No representative cell lines available

Various representative animal models identified (*C. elegans* and dog)

Bilateral disease might be explained by early initial genetic change or hyperplasia

## 2.6 Type II GCTs: Introduction

Type II GCTs are the most frequent GCT of the testis, accounting for approximately 1% of all cancers in Caucasian males (Verhoeven et al. 2007; Shah et al. 2007). In contrast to most solid human cancers, type II GCTs have a peak incidence at the adolescent and young adult age, in which group they represent in fact the most frequent solid cancer. The age of presentation can be significantly younger in patients with disorders of sex development (DSD (see below)). In spite of the overall cure rate, they are the second cause of death in young adult Caucasian males (Horwich et al. 2006). In most European countries a significant rise in incidence of these cancers has been reported, although an interesting heterogeneity has been observed (Dieckmann and Pichlmeier 2004; Walsh et al. 2006). This has been linked to both genetic predisposition as well as exposure to environmental compounds, specifically those with estrogen and/or antiandrogen action (see below). A significant lower incidence of type II GCTs of the testis has been reported for other ethnic populations, including Asians and Blacks, which is not influenced by migration (Gajendran et al. 2005; McGlynn et al. 2005).

### 2.6.1 *Histological Composition and Markers of Differentiation*

The type II GCTs are subdivided into seminomas and nonseminomas, both histologically and clinically (Woodward et al. 2004; International Germ Cell Cancer Collaborative 1997). The nonseminomas are further subclassified into embryonal carcinoma, yolk sac tumor, choriocarcinoma, and teratoma (Woodward et al. 2004). In fact, all differentiation lineages as found during normal embryogenesis (both somatic and extra-embryonal) can be represented in these tumors, including the germ cell lineage (Honecker et al. 2006), making these tumors really totipotent. This is in line with the various markers suitable for diagnosis (see below). It must be kept in mind that teratomas and yolk sac tumors can therefore be both part of a type I and type II GCTs, which cannot be distinguished on histological criteria. The markers useful to distinguish the seminoma from the embryonal carcinoma of type II GCTs are summarized in Fig. 2.2a. The list is not meant to include all putative informative markers, but to indicate the overall pattern. It sheds light on the pathobiology of these tumors in general, and identifies putative interesting targets for diagnosis and possibly targeted treatment. These markers have been identified on the basis of either a hypothesis-driven approach, or using high throughput investigations. The markers AFP (for yolk sac tumor), hCG (for choriocarcinoma), and LDH1 (for tumor load) are useful as serum markers in a clinical setting, specifically related to the presence of a yolk sac or choriocarcinoma component, and tumor load, respectively (Horwich et al. 2006). It is interesting to note that most markers suitable to distinguish seminoma and embryonal carcinoma from the more differentiated nonseminoma components, and to specify seminoma from embryonal carcinoma, are known from regulation of pluripotency in (mouse and human) embryonic stem cells, like OCT3/4, NANOG, and SOX2. These and a selection of others will be discussed in more detail, clustered on the basis of their pattern of expression:

#### 2.6.1.1 OCT3/4 (POU5F1) and NANOG

OCT3/4, encoding the POU5F1 protein was the first regulator of pluripotency identified in mouse embryonic stem cells (Nichols et al. 1998). This transcription factor regulates whether the cells will remain undifferentiated or start to differentiate (Hansis et al. 2000; Niwa et al. 2000; Pesce and Scholer 2000, 2001; Donovan 2001). The expression is at least influenced by promoter methylation, both in vivo and in vitro (Hattori et al. 2004; De Jong et al. 2007a) (see also below). On the basis of this observation, the expression of mRNA of OCT3/4 in type II GCTs was initiated. Two specific variants of the protein-encoding OCT3/4 are recognized, of which the A (or I) type is related to pluripotency. The protein is located in the nucleus. The B (or II) variant is localized in the cytoplasm. It is not related to regulation of pluripotency, and will therefore not be discussed here. Detection of OCT3/4 mRNA is not only hampered by the existence of two variants but also by the presence of a number of pseudogenes. This may result in false positive RT-PCR observations (Takeda et al. 1992; Suo et al. 2005; Liedtke et al. 2007; De Jong and Looijenga 2006). A combined approach using PCR amplification of mRNA (after DNAse treatment) and endonuclease digestion

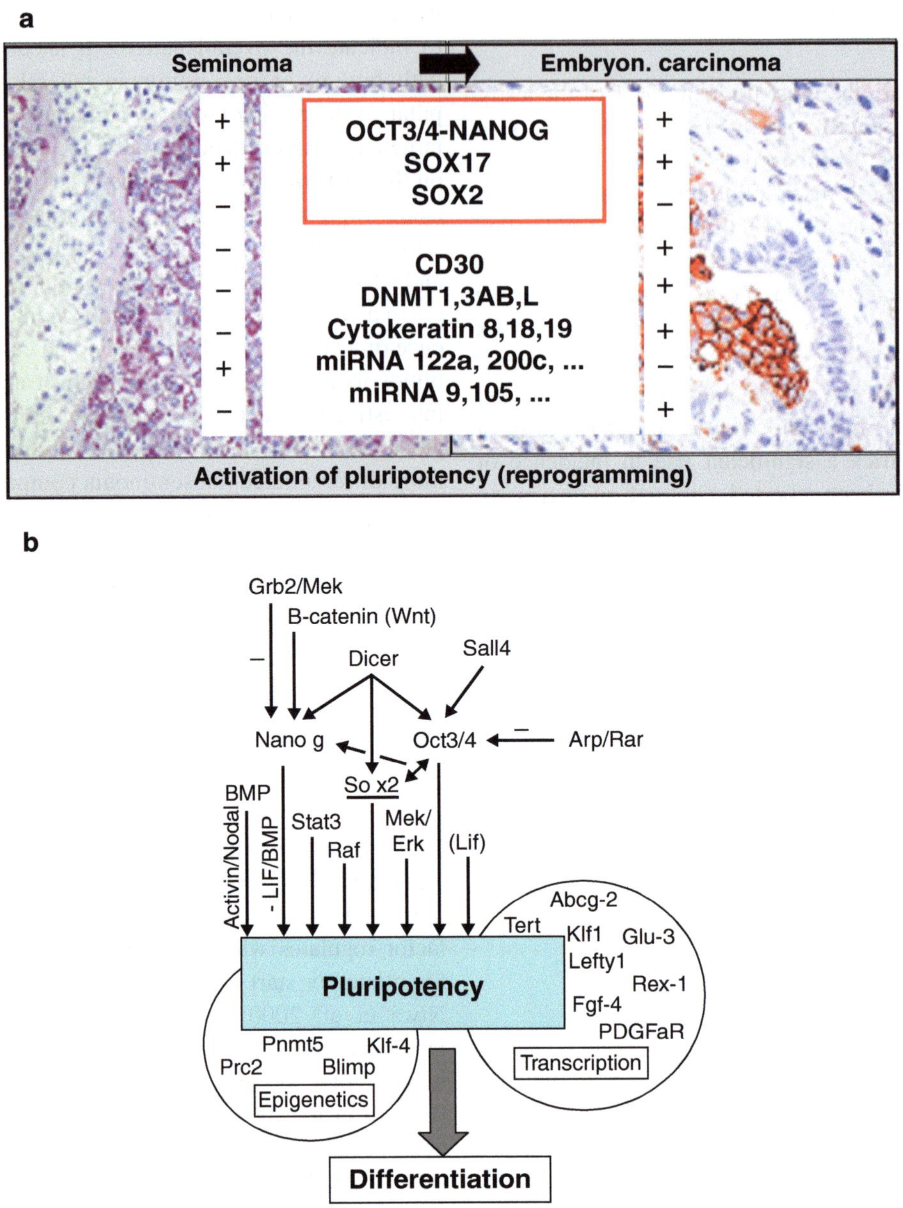


**Fig. 2.2** (**a**) Summary of the different factors involved in the distinction between the human normal and malignant primordial germ cell (seminoma) stage compared to embryonic stem cell (embryonal carcinoma) stage. The *red box* set of genes, i.e., OCT3/4 (NANOG), SOX2/17 is suitable to be used in a clinical setting; (**b**) Various factors and pathways related to the undifferentiated stage of (mouse and human) embryonic stem cells. The genes used to generate pluripotent stem cells from somatic cells are underlined (Oct3/4-SOX2 and Klf-4). The difference between mouse and human embryonic stem cells regarding the need of Lif is illustrated by the use of *brackets*. The effects of these different targets/pathways are on the epigenetic status of the cells as well as their pattern of transcription; (**c**) Affymetrix expression profiling of KLF4 and c-MYC in the same samples is mentioned under Fig. 2.1c, although in addition, embryonal carcinomas (EC) are included; (**d**) Representative example of SOX9 immunohistochemistry on a normal embryonic testis. Note the staining of the Sertoli cells; (**e**) Representative example of FOXL2 immunohistochemistry on a normal adult ovary. Note the staining of the granulosa cells; (**f**) Representative immunohistochemistry for stem cell factor on carcinoma in situ cells (insert is the staining for OCT3/4); (**g**) Affymetrix expression profiling for the various DNA methyl transferases (1, 3A, 3B and 3L) on the samples is described under C; (**h**) Immunohistochemical detection of 5M-cytosine on normal spermatogenesis (positive) and CIS (negative), and the various histological elements of type II GCTs (seminoma is negative, while all nonseminomas are positive). In addition, a chemotherapy resistant seminoma, as well as the seminoma cell line TCam-2 and the embryonal carcinoma cell line (NT2), shows a high level of methylation

c

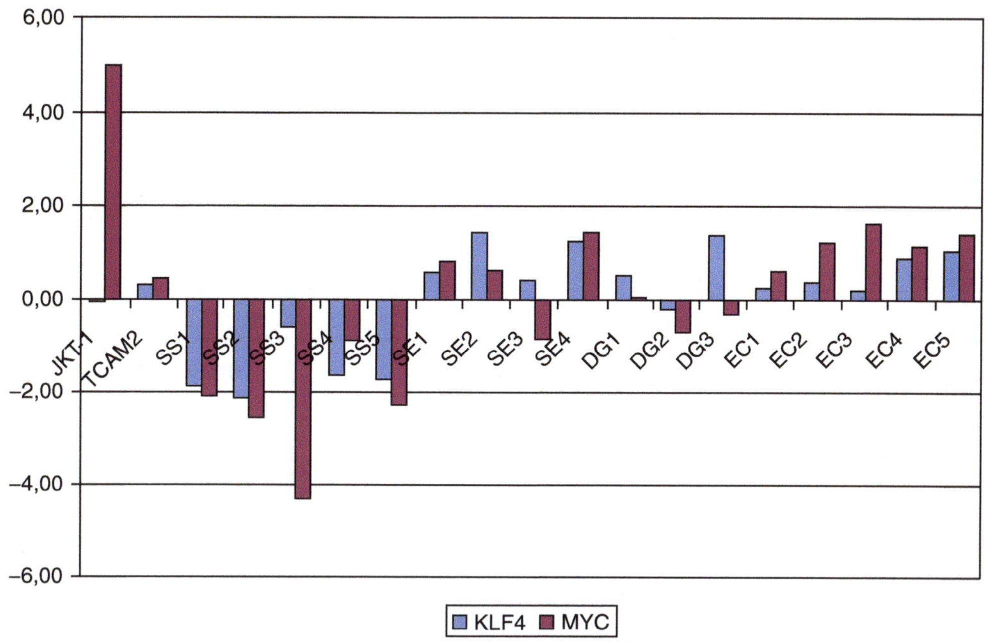


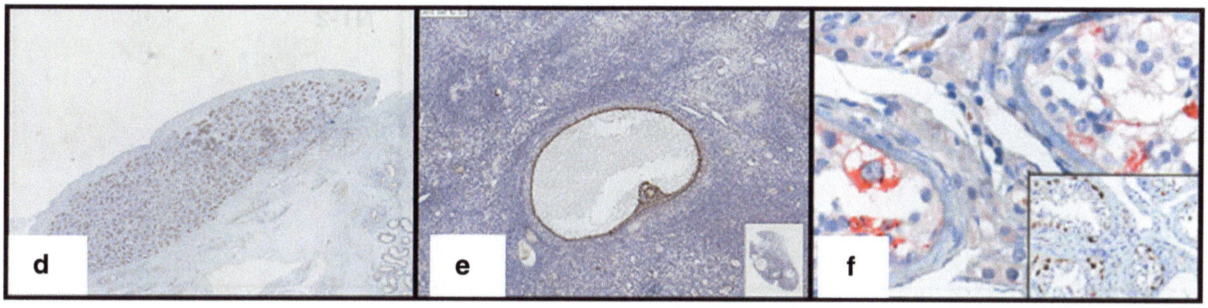


g

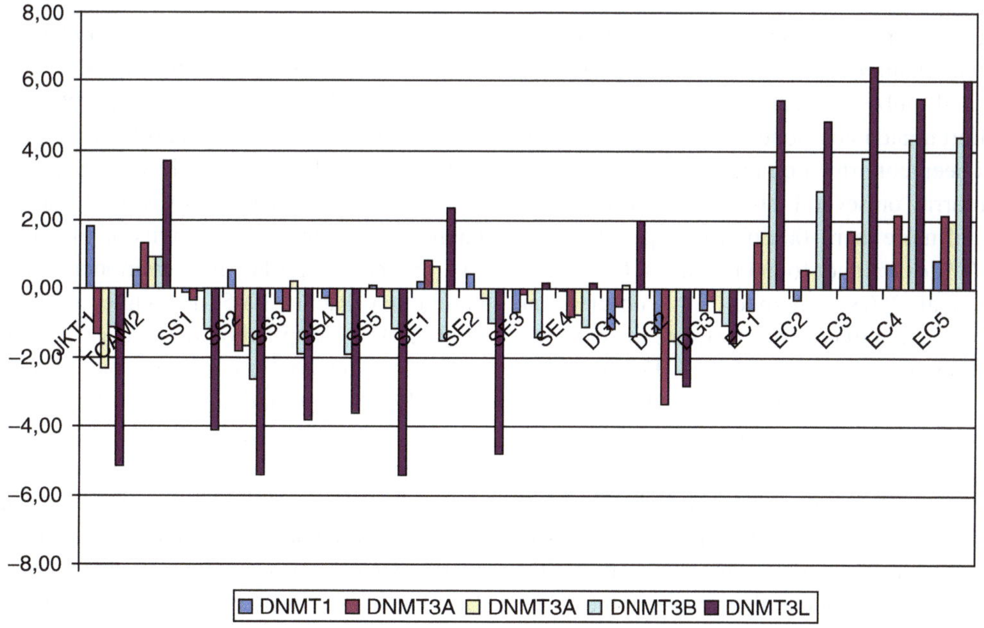


**Fig. 2.2** (continued)

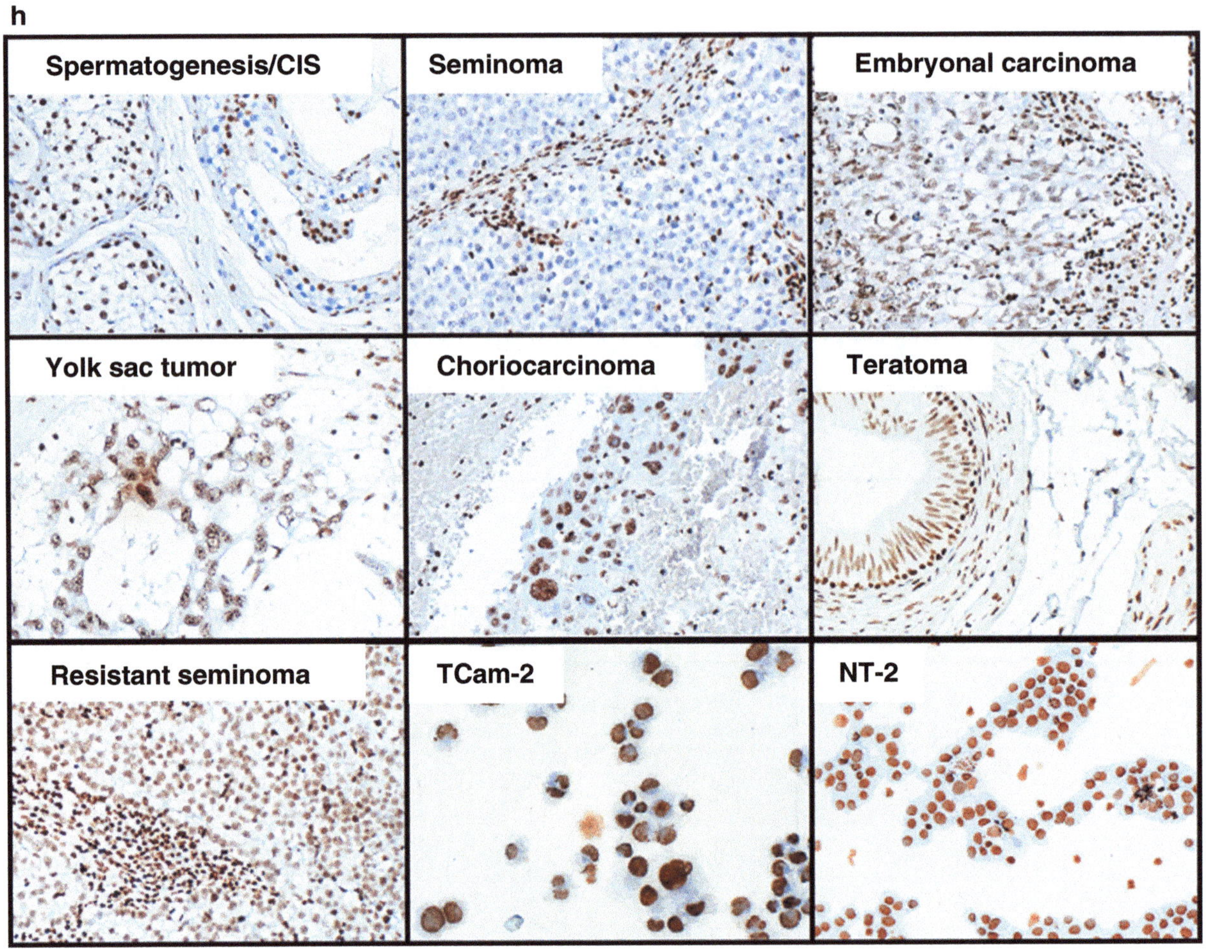


allows investigation of the expression of the POU5F1 encoding gene (Palumbo et al. 2002). It is expressed in seminoma and embryonal carcinoma, and not in the various differentiated components. Subsequently, this pattern has been confirmed on the protein level, using tissue microarray on several thousands of solid cancer specimens, of more than 100 different types. It shows that OCT3/4 is overall not found in other solid cancers (Looijenga et al. 2003a). In spite of this observation, many studies were initiated to investigate the presence of OCT3/4 in nongerm cell cancers (De Jong and Looijenga 2006). Predominantly on the basis of mRNA-based investigation, it has been concluded that this marker was indeed present, which would make it unsuitable as specific marker for type II GCTs. Most of these studies did not include proper protein detection, and indeed it was recently demonstrated that the results were false positive mainly because of the detection of pseudogenes. A specific primer set to detect the mRNA relating to the OCT3/4 protein has been generated, and proven to be specific (Liedtke et al. 2007; de Jong et al. 2008a). Use of this approach, as well as verified antibodies, will exclude false positive (and negative) results. In conclusion, the presence of OCT3/4 protein, detected by verified antibodies and having specificity and sensitivity, is the most informative diagnostic marker for seminoma and embryonal carcinoma (Richie 2005; de Jong et al. 2005a; Cheng et al. 2007). If applied on tissue derived from an adult testis, it is an absolute marker, but overdiagnosis is possible in infants and in the case of germ cell maturation delay (see below for further discussion). This diagnostic value is not limited to the testis, but also shown for other anatomical sites (De Jong et al. 2005b). Moreover, the pattern of staining is not influenced by metastasis or exposure to chemotherapeutic reagents. Besides these invasive components, the precursor lesions, CIS, and gonadoblastoma (see below) are also positive. It remains to be clarified whether OCT3/4 can be considered as an oncogenic driver, as suggested on the basis of experimental data in mouse (Gidekel et al. 2003). No chromosomal anomalies have been identified supporting this model so far. The specificity of OCT3/4 for type II GCTs is in accordance to the observation that absence of this gene is not influencing the adult stem cell properties in mouse (Lengner et al. 2007). Interesting, however, is the block in differentiation and hyperplasia observed in various tissues in case of overexpression of this gene (Hochedlinger et al. 2005). The putative targets under control of regulation by OCT3/4 have been identified, which show a strong specific pattern (Boyer et al. 2005; Loh et al. 2006).

Interestingly, absence of OCT3/4 in mouse PGC does not result in differentiation, as reported in mouse and human embryonic stem cells, but induction of apoptosis (Kehler et al. 2004). This indicates that the function of OCT3/4 is cell dependent, for which so far no explanation has been provided (see also below). Although fewer studies have been published on the other regulator of pluripotency, i.e., NANOG, in type II GCTs, till now it seems that the expression pattern is similar to OCT3/4 (Clark et al. 2004; Ezeh et al. 2005; Hart et al. 2005; Hoei-Hansen et al. 2005; Korkola et al. 2006). It has been suggested that the chromosomal localization of NANOG is of specific interest, being on the short arm of chromosome 12, which is always gained in these tumors (see below). However, it needs to be experimentally verified whether such a relationship exists, because downregulation of NANOG has been reported upon differentiation of embryonal carcinoma towards other lineages (as expected, parallel to OCT3/4), but gain of 12p is still present in differentiated tumors, which indicates that still a positive selection mechanism is involved. In this context, the presence of gain of 12p in human embryonic stem cells upon extensive in vitro growth is also relevant (see below). There are, however, interesting data indicating that upregulation of NANOG is required for induction of apoptosis of mouse embryonic stem cells (Lin et al. 2005). Interestingly, expression of this gene is regulated by Oct3/4 as well as Sox2 (see below) (Loh et al. 2006; Rodda et al. 2005; Masui et al. 2007), and potentiates indeed generation of pluripotency (Silva et al. 2006; Suzuki et al. 2006). This is, among others, influenced by the Wnt pathway, via β-catenin (Takao et al. 2006). Most recently, Rex-1 has been found to distinguish within the Oct3/4 positive mouse embryonic stem cell population. The Rex-1 negative cells are related to primitive ectoderm while the positive cells represent the inner cell mass. These subpopulations are interchangeable, depending on the presence of Leukemia Inhibiting Factor (LIF) (Toyooka et al. 2008). No such subpopulations have been identified so far within type II GCTs (Kristensen et al. 2008). This might be due to the difference in LIF dependence of the mouse and human embryonic stem cells (Ginis et al. 2004). Another interesting finding is that an aberrant Oct3/4 in embryonic stem cells is related to disruption of Dicer expression, which is crucial for normal miRNA function (Cui et al. 2007) (see below).

Finally, although interesting data have been summarized in Fig. 2.2b, still a lot of questions need to be answered. The key question is whether these transcription factors are intrinsic to the cell of origin and therefore consistently present, or whether they play a causative role in the pathogenesis of these tumors.

#### 2.6.1.2 SOX2 and SOX17

Although OCT3/4 and NANOG are valuable markers for the study of tumor biology as well as for diagnostics, they neither distinguish seminoma/CIS from embryonal carcinoma nor PGCs from embryonic stem cells. However, the presence of cytoplasmic as well as nuclear OCT3/4 (A type) staining, especially in combination with the morphological criteria, allows identification of embryonal carcinoma to a certain extent. Of course various other informative markers have been identified for embryonal carcinoma to allow distinction from seminoma, including cytokeratin 8/18/19 and CD30 (see also Figs. 2.2a and 2.3) (Pallesen and Hamilton-Dutoit 1988; Latza et al. 1995; Herszfeld et al. 2006). From a developmental point of view, the observation that SOX2 is positive in embryonal carcinoma and negative in seminoma and CIS is highly interesting. SOX2 is associated with OCT3/4 as a complex in the regulation of gene expression in embryonic stem cells, both mouse and human (Rodda et al. 2005; Masui et al. 2007; Okumura-Nakanishi et al. 2005; Carlin et al. 2006; Nakatake et al. 2006), including NANOG (see Fig. 2.2b for summary). In fact, OCT3/4 levels are regulated by SOX2 (Masui et al. 2007). But, in contrast to OCT3/4 and NANOG, SOX2 is not specific for embryonic stem cells and their malignant counterpart, i.e., embryonal carcinoma. It is found in many different lineages of differentiation, however, always in the absence of OCT3/4 and NANOG (Avilion

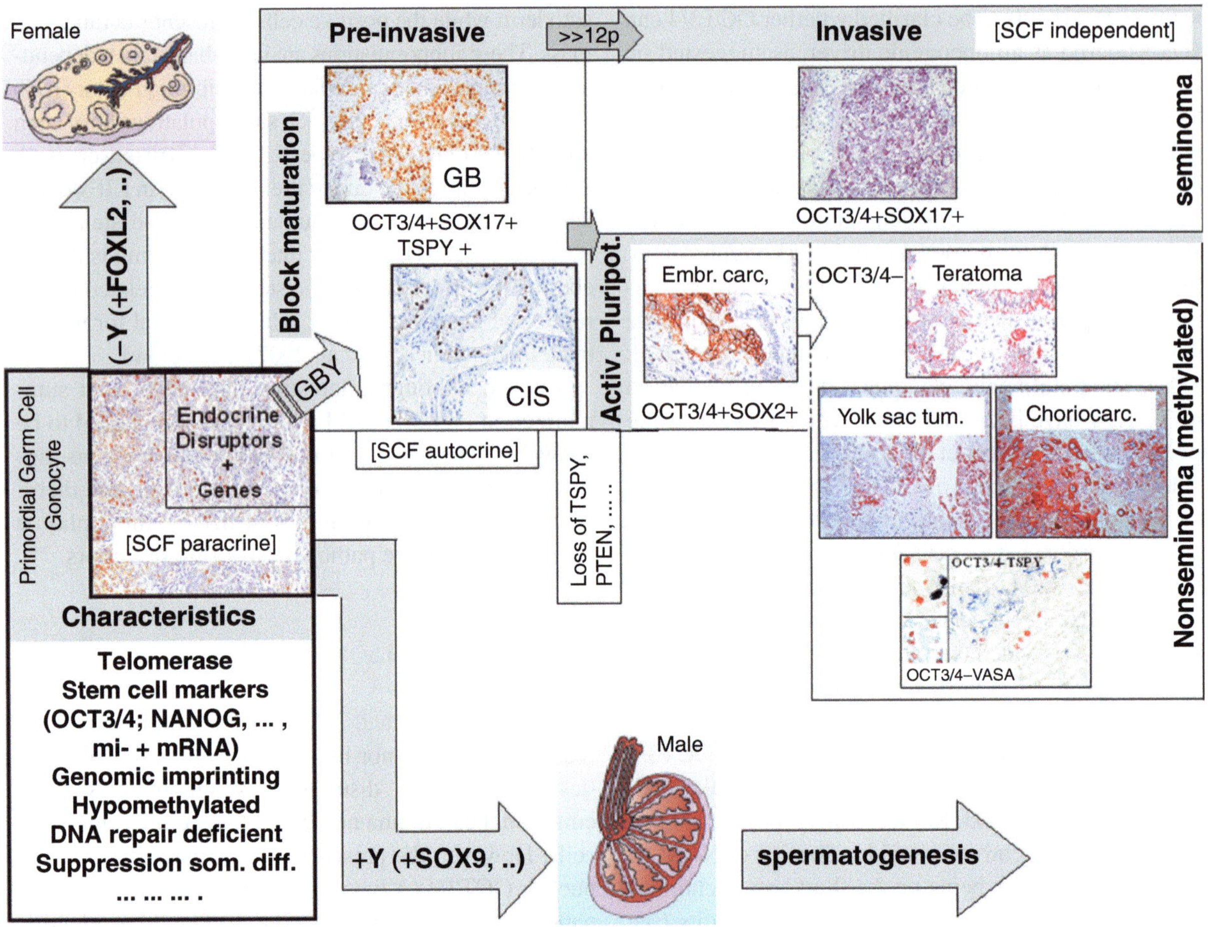


**Fig. 2.3** Pathogenetic model of the initiation and progression of type II GCTs. See text for explanation

et al. 2003; Kelberman et al. 2006). This likely determines the absence of pluripotency of these cells. Interestingly, while SOX2 is found in mouse PGCs, it is absent in the human counterparts, which illustrates species specificities of regulation of pluripotency (Perrett et al. 2008; De Jong et al. 2008b). This is also demonstrated by the presence of Oct3/4 in mouse spermatogonia, in contrast to the human counterparts, which therefore makes it an informative diagnostic marker for CIS. Another intriguing observation is that human Sertoli cells associated with disrupted spermatogenesis or CIS can also show staining for SOX2, but never for OCT3/4 and NANOG. This must be kept in mind to exclude false positive intratubular diagnosis of embryonal carcinoma (De Jong et al. 2008b).

A relevant question is why OCT3/4 has a different function in PGCs and embryonic stem cells, extrapolated to seminoma/CIS and embryonal carcinoma, i.e., regulation of apoptosis vs. differentiation. It might be due to the differential presence of SOX2, which is only positive in embryonal carcinoma (see above). The next question is whether another SOX-member transcription factor is specifically expressed in PGCs, CIS, and seminoma. To get insight into this possibility, a high throughput screening was performed, which showed that SOX17 (and SOX15 to a lesser extent) is indeed specifically expressed in seminoma and CIS, confirmed at the protein level as well as in nonseminoma cell lines. Linking the genetic information to the expression data indicates that seminoma indeed shows specific gain of a region on chromosome 17, in which SOX17 is mapped (Korkola et al. 2008). Interestingly, SOX17 is identified as a regulatory element to distinguish embryonic from adult hematopoietic stem cells (Kim et al. 2007; Jang and Sharkis 2007). This observation opens a new field of experiments linking regulation of gene expression related to pluripotency in type II GCTs, especially on the basis of the use of the various cell lines representative for human type II GCTs.

#### 2.6.1.3 Diagnostic Expression Signature for Seminoma and Embryonal Carcinoma

The cumulated data allow now a rather simple and informative signature for seminoma/CIS and embryonal carcinoma, relevant both for diagnosis as well as investigation of the mechanism of activation of pluripotency, i.e., the transition of a seminomatous (PGC/gonocyte) cell to an embryonal carcinoma (embryonic stem) cell. This is schematically illustrated in Fig. 2.2a (in the red box). In fact, various patterns have been reported, but the most simple and straightforward is seminoma OCT3/4+/SOX17+/SOX2− and embryonal carcinoma OCT3/4+/SOX17−/SOX2+. The power of this rule of thumb is that by definition, besides OCT3/4, a positive differentiating marker is included. This is also true for the nonmalignant counterparts, i.e., human PGC/gonocyte and embryonal stem cell, which has been investigated in several studies (Gashaw et al. 2007; Hoei-Hansen et al. 2005; De Jong et al. 2008b; Rajpert-De Meyts et al. 2004; Stoop et al. 2005; Biermann et al. 2006; Kerr et al. 2008a, b; Honecker et al. 2004). In this context, it is relevant to underline that the PGC/gonocytes are in fact not pluripotent, but are equipped to transmit this capacity to the next generation. In contrast, the embryonal stem cells are capable of showing an intrinsic pluripotency, which will be lost upon derivation of adult stem cells that are committed and thereby have lost pluripotency. This is in line with the absence of OCT3/4 in adult stem cells (Ledford 2007).

#### 2.6.1.4 Generation of Pluripotent Stem Cells Using Defined Set of Genes

It has been shown that pluripotent stem cells can be derived from somatically differentiated cells, both human and mouse, and can be generated by expressing a selected number of genes, i.e., OCT3/4, SOX2, KLF4, and c-MYC. The latter can even be omitted (Zaehres and Scholer 2007; Nakatake et al. 2006; Takahashi and Yamanaka 2006; Meissner et al. 2007; Nakagawa et al. 2007; Okita et al. 2007; Takahashi et al. 2007; Wernig et al. 2007). This however, results in a less efficient approach, and it results in the absence of malignant transformation. Interesting is also that NANOG is not required. So far, no studies specifically on KLF4 in type II GCTs have been performed, but expression profiling analysis demonstrated no differences between seminoma and embryonal carcinoma, like OCT3/4 and NANOG (see above) (Fig. 2.2c). It has been indicated that KLF4 is needed in this specific set of genes to reestablish an embryonic epigenetic pattern of the DNA and histones (see also Fig. 2.2b), which is lost upon physiological differentiation. A similar expression pattern in type II GCTs is found for c-MYC, which is indicated to be needed for proliferation induction (Fig. 2.2c). It must be kept in mind that these data on GCTs are based on mRNA levels, and confirmation on the protein level, including activity status, will be needed to get further insight in the relevance of these proteins. However, it can be concluded so far that embryonal carcinoma (and seminoma, but in the absence of SOX2) seems to express the critical genes of pluripotent stem cells.

The difference between seminoma and embryonal carcinoma might be due to the different expression, among others, of SOX17 and SOX2. In this context, the recent observation that pten and akt are involved in the generation of embryonic stem cells from mouse PGC, i.e., the so-called activation of pluripotency (or reprogramming), is highly relevant (Kimura et al. 2003, 2008). Inactivation of pten in PGCs results in generation of embryonic stem cells, related to activation of Akt. Indeed, PTEN has been found to be inactivated in the transition from CIS to embryonal carcinoma (Di Vizio et al. 2005). Of interest is that suppression of PTEN is required for allowing cellular transformation (including antiapoptotic effects) of activated RAS (Vasudevan et al. 2007) (see below). In the pten/akt mouse model, p53 was found to be a crucial downstream target (see also below). The PTEN/AKT and KRAS2 pathways seem indeed to be active in human embryonic stem cells (Humphrey et al. 2004). KRAS2 is another gene mapped to the short arm of chromosome 12, which makes it a gene of interest in the pathogenesis of type II GCTs (see below), and supportive data are available that it is indeed involved (McIntyre et al. 2008). This interesting model deserves further exploration. Experimental data on the regulatory networks of these transcription factors can be obtained using the available type II GCT cell lines (see below). Interesting is the fact that KRAS2 is also linked to c-KIT targeting, which will be discussed in the next paragraph.

#### 2.6.1.5 c-KIT and KRAS2

c-KIT is a kinase receptor relevant for a number of crucial processes during normal development, including survival and migration of PGCs from the epiblast to the genital ridge (Wylie 1993; Godin et al. 1991; Runyan et al. 2006). Disturbances in the function of the c-KIT pathway, dependent on the ligand stem cell factor (SCF) result in various anomalies, including sub- or infertility (Lennartsson et al. 2005). In normal development of germ cells, c-KIT is downregulated upon arrival of the PGCs in the genital ridge (Wylie 1993; Godin et al. 1991), although it can still be detected at a relatively low level in human spermatogonia (Stoop et al. 2008). In contrast, it remains high in expression in the mouse counterparts, as also reported for Oct3/4 (see above). c-KIT is also present at a high level in CIS and gonadoblastoma, the precursor lesions of type II GCTs (see below) and is overall downregulated upon invasive growth, although still some c-KIT can be found in invasive tumors (Strohmeyer et al. 1991; Izquierdo et al. 1995; De Meyts et al. 1996; Sakuma et al. 2003; Miettinen and Lasota 2005; Nikolaou et al. 2007). Activating mutations, leading to an SCF independent active receptor, have been found predominantly in bilateral type II GCTs. The sensitivity of the mutation detection leads to seemingly conflicting data (Sakuma et al. 2003; Looijenga et al. 2003b; Kemmer et al. 2004; Tate et al. 2005; Biermann et al. 2007c; Rapley et al. 2008). Some studies predominantly find the activating mutations in primary unilateral seminomas. That indeed c-KIT has an important role in the pathogenesis of type II GCTs is also supported by the observation that this gene can be overexpressed because of a highly restricted genomic amplification only including this gene (McIntire et al. 2005). That particular tumor indeed showed a high and consistent staining at the protein level using immunohistochemistry. The c-KIT signaling pathway has been linked to $PI_3K$ (De Miguel et al. 2002; Shivakrupa et al. 2003), both in mouse PGCs as well as type II GCTs. This is of course relevant in the context of the previously described link to PTEN (see above). Moreover, it is of interest because of the observations that activating KRAS2 mutations are also found, in a mutually exclusive manner (Goddard et al. 2007). Activation of a mutated KRAS2 results in an increased in vitro survival of seminoma cells (Olie et al. 1994, 1995a, b), which are normally not able to survive outside the patient, as well as an earlier age at clinical presentation of the tumor.

### 2.6.2 Risk Factors

A number of risk factors have been identified for type II GCTs, including cryptorchidism, in(sub)fertility, familial predisposition, birth weight, and birth order, as well as various forms of DSD (Moller 1993; Skakkebaek et al. 1998; Jacobsen et al. 2000; McGlynn et al. 2003; Pamenter et al. 2003; Raman et al. 2005; Costabile 2007; Sonke et al. 2007; Walsh et al. 2007; Cook et al. 2008). In spite of the overall consistency of the role of these risk factors, various others have been identified, with variable impact. Interestingly, some of them seem to be specific for either seminoma or nonseminoma. In spite of much effort, it has not been possible to identify the gene or genes involved in familial type II GCTs yet (Rapley et al. 2000; Holzik et al. 2004). The link to the long arm of the X chromosome is likely related to the occurrence of cryptorchidism, and thereby indirectly to the development of the cancer. Overall, the genetic predisposition is difficult to investigate because of the small sizes of the affected families, the relationship to subfertility, as well as the possible role of the (micro)environment. Because of their weakness as risk factors, it is often not possible to divide the impact of both parameters within a single family. The likely multigenetic basis of the predisposition makes the identification of genes even more complex (Lutke Holzik et al. 2006). It is noteworthy in this context that immigrants from Finland to Sweden, who have a lower initial risk for type II GCTs, obtain the risk of the Swedish population at the second generation (Hemminki et al. 2002). This demonstrates a significant effect of the environment on the incidence for a limited period of time, and possibly overruling a genetic component, if present. Recent studies of transgenerational effects of exposure to certain chemicals, including endocrine disruptors, are of specific interest (Anway et al. 2005, 2006; Chang et al. 2006; Crews et al. 2007; Skinner 2007a, b). The link to epigenetic regulation is intriguing and might explain for the so-called testicular dysgenesis syndrome (TDS) (see below). It is of interest that the other identified risk factors commonly, in one way or the other, affect the maturation of embryonic germ cells negatively. These factors have been brought together into TDS (Skakkebæk et al. 2001; Fisher et al. 2003; Skakkebaek 2003; Rajpert-De Meyts 2006; Sonne et al. 2008). This model integrates various elements, in which the final outcome will have a negative effect on testicular function, including sub(in)fertility, cryptorchidism, and/or an increased risk for development of a type II GCT. In this model, the role of the supportive element, i.e., the Leydig–Sertoli cells is crucial. Within the subgroup of sub(in)fertility, it has recently been identified that the presence of bilateral microlithiasis is an informative parameter to identify males with a high risk (up to 20%) of CIS (De Gouveia Brazao et al. 2004), which is in line with the observation of a high incidence of these microcalcifications in patients with a unilateral type II testicular GCT, and contralateral CIS (Holm et al. 2003). This finding can be of value for screening purposes (Costabile 2007).

A recent meta-analysis demonstrated that both a low and a high birth weight increase the risk (Michos et al. 2007). In addition, trisomy 21 patients have an increased risk and indeed, a delayed maturation of germ cells has been identified (Cools et al. 2006a). It remains to be elucidated whether the extra chromosome 21 in the germ cells or the supportive cells in the testis results in an increased risk for type II GCTs. Although this was suggested, because of the gain of chromosome 21 in the tumor cells, this seems to be unlikely, because this has not been found for women. Therefore, it is more likely that the suboptimal microenvironment of the testis due to the trisomy status of the individual results in a delayed maturation of germ cells and thereby a higher risk for malignant transformation. In this context, the observation that Klinefelter patients (47,XXY) have no increased risk of type II GCTs of the testis, but rather of the mediastinum, is of interest (Isurugi et al. 1977; Lee and Stephens 1987; Nichols et al. 1987; Hasle et al. 1992, 1995; Volkl et al. 2006). Most recently, such an association has also been suggested for the intracranial GCTs (unpublished observations). The absence of testicular type II GCTs in Klinefelter patients is likely due to induction of apoptosis of germ cells related to an improper microenvironment (Aksglaede et al. 2006). The resulting pituitary/gonadal overstimulation may play a role in the increased risk of mediastinal GCTs. A similar phenomenon has been reported for germ cells in the ovary of Turner syndrome patients (45XO) (Modi et al. 2003), as well as patients with complete androgen insensitivity (CAIS) (Cools et al. 2005) (see below).

The mechanistic basis of the increased risk of the various conditions remains to be elucidated, but the possible role of estrogen and antiandrogen functions, being the basis of the TDS model, is worth investigating in more detail. This hypothesis is supported by multiple observations. The higher level of testosterone in blacks might indeed explain the lower incidence of this type of cancer (Henderson et al. 1988). This is supposedly related to the role of testosterone during embryonal development in pushing the PGCs along their maturation pathway to spermatogonia, which thereby lose their characteristics of PGCs/gonocytes, and therefore their ability to form CIS (see above). The higher risk of the first child in birth order is in line with a role of a higher level of estrogen exposure at early embryonal developmental age (Weir et al. 2000). Although type II GCTs are rather specific for the Caucasian population, the Maori are an interesting exception (Wilkinson et al. 1992). Men of this ethnic group show a similar incidence as Caucasians, possibly again related to an increased level of estrogen. The intrinsically higher level of testesterone in blacks, already during embryonal development, might be related to their lower risk for type II GCTs. This possibly prevents delayed maturation of PGC/gonocytes into the stage of spermatogonia. A number of studies also indicate that polymorphisms in enzymes which increase the level estrogen are related to a higher risk of type II GCTs (Starr et al. 2005). Moreover, the differences between the people of Denmark and Finland are associated with different exposures to chemicals that have estrogen or antiandrogen activity (Toppari et al. 1996; Rajpert-De Meyts et al. 2003b). A counterargument on the role of increased estrogen is that during the early development the level of estrogen is high, but it could be that a critical window is relevant in this context. Of specific interest is that an animal model for disrupted testicular development, used as model for endocrine disruptors in the generation of TDS, indicates the same window (Welsh et al. 2008). The possible role of androgens in the pathogenesis of type II GCTs is also suggested on the basis of the various types of patients with DSD, with a higher or lower risk of a type II GCT. These will be discussed below.

### 2.6.3 Disorders of Sex Development

This group of developmental anomalies, previously referred to intersex, is defined as conditions of incomplete or disordered genital or gonadal development leading to a discordance between genetic sex (i.e., determined by the chromosomal constitution, of the X and Y chromosomes), gonadal sex (the testicular or ovarian development of the gonad), and phenotypic sex (the physical appearance of the individual). Recently, a revised classification system has been proposed, with the aim to reduce uncertainties on description (Hughes et al. 2006). Because of the topic of this review, a number of relevant issues in the context of type II GCTs will be discussed here. Indeed, as expected, these patients have no increased risk for the type I and III GCTs.

#### 2.6.3.1 Parameters Related to Tumor Risk

DSD patients with either hypovirilization or gonadal dysgenesis can show an increased risk for the development of type II GCTs. A number of recent reviews have been published recently (Cools et al. 2006b; Looijenga et al. 2007c). The most important issues will be summarized here. The precursor can indeed be CIS or gonadoblastoma, related to the level of virilization of the gonad. This can nicely be demonstrated by the use of protein detection by immunohistochemistry for SOX9 (indicative for SRY function and Sertoli cell differentiation), and FOXL2 (granulosa cell differentiation) (Hersmus et al. 2008a). In contrast to the link between ovarian differentiation and FOXL2 and that between testicular differentiation and SOX9, the correlation between the presence of the Y chromosome and testicular development is less obvious (Cools et al. 2007). In fact, no correlation between the Y chromosome and testis development has been identified in patients with sex chromosomal mosaicisms, for which no explanation is available so far. It is suggested that in fact CIS and gonadoblastoma are the same type of lesion (Hersmus et al. 2008b), of which the histological context is determined by the level of virilization.

The anatomical position of the gonad also seems to be significantly related to the risk of malignant transformation. This is in line with the fact that cryptorchidism is indeed one of the strongest risk factors for type II GCTs of the testis (Batata et al. 1980; Muller et al. 1984; Giwercman et al. 1987; Abratt et al. 1992). Interestingly, it has been demonstrated that a seminoma is more frequently found in intraabdominal gonads than in gonads localized in the scrotum (Ogunbiyi et al. 1996). This likely also explains the preferential occurrence of dysgerminomas in the ovary, which are always abdominal (Susnerwala et al. 1991; Dietl et al. 1993; Chow et al. 1996; Cusido et al. 1998; Tewari et al. 2000). In addition, it has been shown that an early age of orchiopexy indeed reduces the risk for a type II GCT of the testis (Walsh et al. 2007; Jones et al. 1991; Engeler et al. 2000). This is likely related to the still ongoing maturation of PGC/gonocyte like cells to spermatogonia. Moreover, complete absence or very low level of testosterone also diminishes the risk of a type II GCT. This is nicely illustrated by patients with hypogonadotropic hypogonadism, who always have cryptorchid testis, but never will develop a GCT. In addition, patients with CAIS have a significantly lower risk compared to patients with the partial form of this disorder (Cools et al. 2005, 2006b; Hannema et al. 2006). Most likely this is related to the induction of apoptosis of the germ cells in the testis of CAIS patients, as observed in Klinefelter patients (see above).

Development of type II GCTs in DSD patients seems to be related to formation of specific histological structures. In patients with a certain level of virilization and therefore testis formation, it results in the characteristic lesion of CIS, as also found in men without any sign of DSD, but related possibly to TDS (see above). In contrast, DSD patients lacking such a level of virilization will develop gonadoblastoma, which may in rare cases be combined with seminiferous tubules with CIS. The precursor lesion of gonadoblastoma is known as undifferentiated gonadal tissue (UGT), which allows a better diagnosis at early developmental stages (Cools et al. 2006c). Interestingly, the various genetic anomalies related to an increased risk for type II GCTs indicate that it has a link to the function of Sertoli cells (Hersmus et al. 2008b). This might be the missing link between TDS and DSD (Hutchison et al. 2008). The structures, being the precursors of invasive type II GCTs, contain double positive cells for OCT3/4 and TSPY. The latter is the most interesting candidate gene for the involvement of the Y chromosome, which will be discussed in the next paragraph.

#### 2.6.3.2 Involvement of the Y Chromosome; TSPY as Candidate Gene

The risk of development of a type II GCTs in DSD patients is directly related to presence of a specific part of the Y chromosome, known as the gonadoblastoma region of the Y chromosome (GBY) (Page 1987). This area maps around the centromeric region, and excludes the SRY gene as candidate. This is indeed supported by the clinical observation of patients with a translocation of the SRY gene to an X chromosome or an autosome, resulting in 46,XX men, who have no increased risk of this type of cancer. Although SRY is not the gene of interest in this context, knowledge of its function is relevant. The first downstream target of SRY is the transcription factor SOX9, which in the testis is Sertoli cell specific (see Fig. 2.1d). It has been assumed that simply the absence of this pathway results in formation of an ovary, which has been recently challenged by a number of observations, including identification of FOXL2 (Baron et al. 2005; Uhlenhaut and Treier 2006; Ottolenghi et al. 2007) as the gene required for granulosa cell formation (see Fig. 2.2e). A recent study reports that SOX9 and FOXL2 are indeed highly informative to identify the testicular and ovarian differentiation lineages in gonads of patients with DSD (Hersmus et al. 2008a). The presence of SOX9 is associated with CIS and FOXL2 with gonadoblastoma.

Several candidate genes map within the GBY region, of which TSPY is one of the most interesting ones. It stands for testis specific protein on the Y chromosome, which is in fact a multicopy gene (Vogel and Schmidtke 1998). It has similarities to the DEK/CAN family of proteins; it interacts with cyclin B1 and is therefore supposed to be involved in cell cycle regulation. Various splice variants have been reported, which indeed can be present in type II GCTs. Protein expression analysis demonstrate that the corresponding protein is present in spermatogonia during normal development. The level of protein is increased in CIS and gonadoblastoma, for which the mechanistic basis is unknown so far (Lau 1999; Schnieders et al. 1996; Hildenbrand et al. 1999; Kersemaekers et al. 2005; Delbridge et al. 2004; Li et al. 2007b). The consistent aneuploidy of type II GCTs might be related to this. In fact, the increased level of this protein is used as supportive parameter to distinguish a malignant germ cell from a germ cell showing delayed maturation. Upon invasive growth, expression of the gene is mostly lost, associated with subsequent absence of the protein, although the Y chromosome can still be retained. Therefore, this is due to downregulation of expression. Transfection expression analysis demonstrated that induction of TSPY in human cells lacking this protein results in an increase in proliferation, both in vitro and in vivo. In fact, the cells show a shorter G2 phase of the cell cycle (Oram et al. 2006). Interestingly, a subsequent study shows that a number of the upregulated genes in the TSPY transfected cells map to the short arms of chromosome 12. In fact, a correlation between the level of TSPY and expression of these genes, including KRAS2 and NANOG, was found only in the precursor lesion CIS, and not in the invasive tumors (Li et al. 2007c). This observation nicely fits with the downregulation of TSPY upon progression of the tumor towards invasiveness.

Mice lack TSPY. Transgenic animals containing a human TSPY genomic fragment interestingly show integration in the Y chromosome, in a tandem repeat organization, like the organization in the human genome (Schubert et al. 2003). This is intriguing but unexplained so far. However, no GCTs were identified, not at younger or older age. In other words, the simple overexpression of TSPY in Oct3/4 positive cells is not enough to generate a type II GCT in the mouse.

### 2.6.4 Cell of Origin and Markers of Diagnosis

The presence of the different markers in the precursor cells of type II GCTs of the testis, known as carcinoma in situ (CIS) (Skakkebæk 1972), testicular intratubular neoplasia (TIN) (Loy and Dieckmann 1990), and intratubular germ cell neoplasia unclassified (IGCNU) (Woodward et al. 2004), is supportive to an embryonic origin. As indicated, the counterpart in dysgenetic gonads, with a low level of virilization, is known as gonadoblastoma (Scully 1970). These lesions also contain germ cells showing the same characteristics as CIS cells. The nonmalignant counterpart is most likely a PGC or gonocyte. The difference between these two is only that a gonocyte is a PGC that has arrived in the genital ridge, after migration from the yolk sac region. In other words, they only differ in anatomical localization. The consistent biallelic expression of imprinted genes in invasive type II GCTs, as well as CIS, is in agreement with this origin (Van Gurp et al. 1994; Szabo and Mann 1995; Rachmilewitz et al. 1996; Verkerk et al. 1997; Looijenga et al. 1998; Ross et al. 1999; Sievers et al. 2005b; Kawakami et al. 2006; Lind et al. 2007). Interestingly, induction of erasement of imprinting in mouse embryonic stem cells results in development of a number of hematopoietic and solid cancers, including a single testicular seminoma (Holm et al. 2005). Although this is a single observation, and the histology of the tumor is not confirmed independently, its existence is highly relevant, because it indicates that an animal model can possibly be generated, and that an erased pattern of genomic imprinting is required.

During this migratory and early gonadal stage of germ cell development, the cells are positive for c-KIT, PLAP, OCT3/4, NANOG, etc., the markers of which are also found to be expressed in CIS and gonadoblastoma, as well as seminoma (Oosterhuis and Looijenga 2005; Rajpert-De Meyts 2006). Normally, upon maturation from the gonocytes to spermatogonia, these markers are downregulated, and others, including MAGE-4A, are initiated (Gashaw et al. 2007; Biermann et al. 2006). In addition, high throughput expression profiling shows that CIS cells shows strong overlap with embryonic stem cells regarding expression profile (Almstrup et al. 2005). This supports the model of an embryonic origin of type II GCTs, which is in line with the epidemiological observation of the dip in the incidence of this type of cancer in men who were conceived during World War II (Moller 1993; Moller and Skakkebæk 1996), as well as other risk factors. This clearly distinguishes this population of cells from the adult stem cell identified of the spermatogenetic lineage (Hofmann et al. 2005; Chen et al. 2005; Kanatsu-Shinohara et al. 2006). The alternative model in which type II GCTs originate from a pachytene spermatocyte is in disagreement with these observations (Chaganti and Bosl 1995). Possibly, the most convincing argument against this latter model is the fact that patients with various forms of DSD, most of whom will never develop proper spermatogenesis, not even spermatogonia, have an increased risk for this type of cancer. Therefore, it can be concluded that the cell of origin of type II GCTs is a germ cell blocked in their PGC/gonocyte stage. This also explains why similar tumors can be found in the ovary, as well as extragonadal sites. The occurrence of mediastinal type II GCTs in Klinefelter patients also strongly argues against a pachytene spermatocyte as cell of origin, as these patients have no spermatogenesis.

That indeed OCT3/4 has additional diagnostic value for the detection of CIS is demonstrated by a recent study. This is a retrospective analysis on testicular biopsies of men for fertility related problems. None of these was initially diagnosed as having CIS, although they all in time developed an invasive tumor. Expert pathology review identified in 50% of the cases the malignant cells, which were identified in 70% using immunohistochemistry for OCT3/4 (unpublished observations). The rule of thumb is that every marker showing a specific pattern of expression in embryonic germ cells and which becomes negative upon differentiation will be informative for the diagnosis of CIS and gonadoblastoma, as well as seminoma. This was recently confirmed for newly identified markers. Because of the consistency and specificity of OCT3/4 in staining in the adult testis, there is no need for identification of additional markers from the diagnostic point of view. However, they will be useful in dissecting the biology of these tumors.

There are two exceptions in which OCT3/4 is not as informative as would be needed for the diagnosis of the precursor of type II GCTs. That is in the case of tissue obtained during the first year of life, and in case of gonads showing germ cell maturation delay. Under these conditions, OCT3/4 staining can still be present in germ cells which have not undergone malignant transformation. These cells are also positive for TSPY, as well as SOX17. On the basis of the morphology, as well as additional criteria, supportive arguments can be obtained to diagnose or rule out. These criteria are not easy to apply in routine pathology, and they are not without any restriction (Cools et al. 2005). For this purpose, availability of a more informative marker would be of great clinical diagnostic value in these patients. A possible marker fulfilling these criteria will be discussed in the next paragraph.

### 2.6.5 SCF as Marker for Early Malignant Germ Cells

As mentioned, SCF is the ligand of c-KIT. It is crucial for proper migration and survival of PGCs. Experiments in vitro support this model, and indicate that SCF prevents induction of apoptosis by, among others, activation of the $PI_3K$ pathway (De Miguel et al. 2002; Shivakrupa et al. 2003). Two variants of SCF can be generated by Sertoli cells by alternative exon usage. One is membrane bound and is highly effective in supporting survival of PGCs (Lev et al. 1994; Yan et al. 2000). The soluble form is related to activation of the Leydig cells present in the stromal compartment of the testis. Under normal physiological conditions, both embryonic and adult, no SCF can be identified in human gonads by immunohistochemistry using a specific antibody (Stoop et al. 2008). However, it is consistently present in testis with CIS, but not in case of the presence of germ cells showing delayed maturation. This is in contrast to OCT3/4 (NANOG and c-KIT) being present under all these conditions. Upon invasive growth of the tumor cells, SCF, like c-KIT (Biermann et al. 2006), is predominantly downregulated although it can be present heterogeneously in various histological elements. It could be demonstrated that SCF has a significant additional value to detect the earliest malignant changes in germ cells (see Fig. 2.2f). No specific upregulation of gene expression could be identified using Q-RT-PCR, although mRNA ISH data indicate that the gene is predominantly expressed in CIS cells. This suggests the presence of an autocrine loop, which is in line with the observation of both c-KIT and SCF in a subpopulation of cells of the embryonal carcinoma cell lines, while it is found in all cells of the seminoma cell line TCam-2. Also the effect of inhibition of c-KIT supports an autocrine loop (Goddard et al. 2007). This observation is both biologically and diagnostically relevant. It suggests that during the early stages in the pathogenesis of type II GCTs, a switch occurs between a paracrine to an autocrine loop of the SCF and c-KIT pathway. Upon development of an invasive tumor, either seminoma or nonseminoma, this mechanism is overruled, and not under selective pressure anymore (see Fig. 2.3).

### 2.6.6 Possibilities for Early (Noninvasive Diagnosis)

Various attempts have been undertaken to develop a method for early diagnosis of preferentially the precursor lesions of type II GCTs. This has been on the basis of their aneuploidy (see below), as well as their protein expression profiling (Giwercman et al. 1990a, b; Giwercman 1992; Meng et al. 1998; Hoei-Hansen et al. 2007). Overall, most studies show rather disappointing results. This is likely related to the heterogeneous expression of the markers used, as well as the selection of patients for screening. A recent study shows that if OCT3/4 is used as marker for diagnosis, the majority of patients known to have CIS (80%) can be identified on the basis of the presence of positive cells in semen (Dieckmann 2009; van Casteren et al. 2008). Although various questions have to be answered before this protocol will be applicable in a clinical setting, it was proven that in principle the approach can be informative, using the optimal marker, protocol, and selected patient cohort. This will especially be of interest in populations with an increased risk of development of testicular type II GCTs, such as those with infertility, bilateral microlithiasis, and a previous unilateral tumor. A prospective study will be needed to show the power of the method compared to that of the surgical biopsy, which is considered as the gold standard. In addition, the presence of activating c-KIT mutations in bilateral type II GCTs can also be an interesting target for clinical implementation although, as mentioned, the sensitivity of the detection system might be a limiting factor.

### 2.6.7 Chromosomal Constitution

Many studies have been performed to investigate the chromosomal constitution of type II GCTs, including its precursor lesion (Kraggerud et al. 2002; Oosterhuis et al. 1989a; Castedo et al. 1989; Samaniego et al. 1990; Skotheim et al. 2001; Summersgill et al. 2001; von Eyben 2004). In fact, this started with total DNA content analysis using flow cytometric studies, followed by conventional karyotyping and targeted ISH, and more recently c- and a-CGH as well as single nucleotide polymorphism (SNP) arrays. Overall, the different approaches showed the same results; type II GCTs are highly aneuploid with specific and characteristic changes. The seminomas and CIS are hypertriploid and the nonseminomas hypotriploid. Specific chromosomal gains and losses are identified, some of which are suggested to be histology related. The only recurrent structural imbalance is the gain of the short arm of chromosome 12, mostly as isochromosomes (see Table 2.1). Most studies indicate that gain of 12p is progression related; it occurs when the CIS cells become independent for their interaction with Sertoli cells (Summersgill et al. 2001; Rosenberg et al. 2000). The presence of additional copies of 12p is independent from the histological constitution, as well as anatomical localization. It is interesting that human embryonic stem cells cultured for an extensive period of time also show this anomaly (Draper et al. 2003; Cowan et al. 2004; Li et al. 2006). In spite of many attempts, there is no single 12p-target gene identified. A number of genes have been suggested to be relevant, including KRAS2, NANOG, although the actual proof is lacking so far.

The X chromosome is gained in the majority of tumors, for which a link with familial predisposition has been suggested (see above). The presence of additional X chromosomes is relevant in the context of understanding the biology of type II GCTs, including in the Klinefelter syndrome patients, as well as in patients with various forms of DSD. Moreover, it has a molecular diagnostic value (see below).

SNP analysis in type II GCTs demonstrated the presence of so-called uniparental disomies (Lu et al. 2005). These have been more frequently detected in nonseminomas than in seminomas. The proposed explanation is that the latter originates from fusion of a haploid (postmeiotic) germ cell with a diploid germ cell, also explaining their consistent peritriploid DNA content (Oosterhuis et al. 1989b). This hypothesis is highly unlikely, because these tumors can develop without the presence of spermatogenesis, as discussed before. In addition, this pattern of uniparental disomy has also been found in an ovarian type II GCT (unpublished observations). The most likely explanation is that the tumor cells undergo significant mitotic recombination.

Of interest is that currently an integrated analysis of expression of genes and proteins as well as DNA copy changes is initiated (Skotheim et al. 2002, 2005, 2003a, b; Korkola et al. 2005, 2006, 2008; McIntyre et al. 2004, 2007). Overall, the data suggest a close correlation between the two, in which the expression drives the chromosomal imbalances or vice versa. For example, gain of a specific region of chromosome 17 is found to be overrepresented in seminoma, which includes the SOX17 gene (Korkola et al. 2008), which is characteristic for seminoma (see above). These models are highly relevant to explain the chromosomal changes as observed in solid tumors, which likely will also have clinical impact.

### 2.6.8 Epigenetic Modification

In spite of a wealth of information about the genomic make up of type II GCTs, increasing knowledge on the epigenetic constitution is evolving (Kawakami et al. 2006; Lind et al. 2006, 2007; Peltomäki 1991; Ishii et al. 2007; Zhang et al. 2005; Honorio et al. 2003; Smiraglia et al. 2002; Koul et al. 2002; Okamoto and Kawakami 2007). The role of epigenetics in germ cell development has been reviewed recently (Biermann and Steger 2007). Targeted – as well as genome wide studies demonstrate that overall the seminomas show a hypomethylated DNA status, in contrast to the various histological types of nonseminomas. Interestingly, the supernumerical X chromosomes are inactivated in nonseminomas by methylation (Looijenga et al. 1997). This is, like during normal embryogenesis, the result of the function of the non(protein)-coding XIST gene. This unique phenomenon in men is correlated with hypomethylation of the promoter region, which can be used as molecular target for type II GCTs in men (Kawakami et al. 2003, 2004). The difference in methylation status can indeed be demonstrated using expression profiling for the different forms of the DNA methyltransferases (see Fig. 2.2g). The DNMT1 is required for maintenance of the methylated status during cell division, and previously found to be present in differentiated form of nonseminomas (Omisanjo et al. 2007), while DNMT3A and B are needed for de novo methylation (Karpf and Matsui 2005), as happens during early embryogenesis. DNMT3L has a role in the establishment of the pattern of genomic imprinting (Oakes et al. 2007). Overall, a specific upregulation is observed in the embryonal carcinomas compared to the seminomas. Indeed, this is also reflected by immunohistochemistry using a $^{M}$C-specific antibody. Representative examples are shown in Fig. 2.2g. This pattern of methylation is in accordance to the expected pattern based on observations during embryogenesis, i.e., PGCs are hypomethylated and differentiated derivatives (locally) hypermethylated. In this context, it is relevant to remember that in vitro culturing may induce specific changes in DNA methylation, which may bias the findings made in type II GCT-derived cell lines. Interestingly, indeed, the TCam-2 cell line, representative for seminoma, being hypomethylated, shows a hypermethylated pattern based on immunohistochemistry. Therefore, the observations made in cell lines must always be verified in in vitro tumors.

That possibly the hypermethylated pattern of this seminoma cell might have a biological function is suggested by the hypermethylation of chemotherapy resistant seminomas (see Fig. 2.2h) (unpublished observation). It remains to be investigated whether this relates to specific genetic changes in this cell line (see below). Interestingly, a methylation study was recently done for the promoter region of OCT3/4. In seminoma and embryonal carcinoma, the promoter region is predominantly hypomethylated, in in vitro cell lines as well as in vivo tumors (De Jong et al. 2007a). Microdissection of the embryonal carcinoma cells even demonstrated a complete demethylated pattern. Upon differentiation of the embryonal carcinoma cells, OCT3/4 is downregulated in expression, associated with hypermethylation of the promoter region. Most likely, this pattern is reflecting the situation in most genes related to pluripotency, showing the same pattern of expression as OCT3/4, like NANOG.

Histone modification has also been identified as a significant regulatory element in specification of which genes will be hypermethylated upon differentiation from an undifferentiated stem cell. This is related to the histone H3 methylated at lysine 27 by polycomb proteins, which is a repressive mark, as well as the active mark methylated H3K4 (Ohm et al. 2007). Interestingly, this was indeed found to be the case in cell lines derived from type II GCTs, i.e., embryonal carcinomas, in which two additional repressive marks are identified, being dimethylated H3K9 and trimethylated H3K9, both associated with DNA hypermethylation in adult cancers. This is nicely fitting with the observed pattern of expression of the histone deacetylase (HDAC) in these tumors (Omisanjo et al. 2007). More recently, a related study investigated the expression of BLIMP-1 and PRMT-5 (unpublished observations). These proteins are involved in the suppression of the somatic differentiation program in PGCs/gonocytes, related to dimethylated histone H2A and H4 (Ancelin et al. 2006). Knock out of these genes results in differentiation of mouse PGCs (Hayashi et al. 2007; Ohinata et al. 2005). Indeed, these proteins and epigenetic changes are present in embryonic germ cells, as well as CIS and seminoma, including the representative cell line TCam-2. As expected, upon formation of embryonal carcinoma, these proteins are downregulated, and the dimethylated H2A and H4 are removed. Again, these studies demonstrated the close relationship between normal embryogenesis and type II GCTs.

It remains a challenge to identify which of the mechanisms are reflecting normal development, and which are related to the pathogenetic process. For this purpose, investigation of genetic anomalies affecting genes or pathways might be highly informative. Therefore, the next section will be related to this topic.

### 2.6.9 Mutational Status

Various studies with the goal to identity pathogenetic mutations have been performed on type II GCTs. These included a large number of targets, among others, NRAS, KRAS-2, and HRAS (Goddard et al. 2007; Mulder et al. 1989; Ganguly et al. 1990; Ridanpaa et al. 1993; Przygodzki et al. 1996; Oosterhuis et al. 1997), and BCL10 (van Schothorst et al. 1999; Kakinuma et al. 2001). Although mutations have been identified, these seem to be limited in frequency, with the possible exceptions of c-KIT and KRAS-2 (see above), and more recently BRAF. This latter proto-oncogene has been shown to be mutated in a variety of cancers, including melanoma. Interestingly, the affected pathway is the MEK-pathway, in which RAS also act. Activating mutations of KRAS and BRAF are mutually exclusive in type II GCTs. A correlation between BRAF mutation and hypermethylation of the promoter of hMLH1 has been reported (Imai 2007). hMLH1 is involved in mismatch repair, and improper function of this protein. Absence of or mutations in this gene result in microsatellite instability (MSI). Indeed, MSI instability has been reported to be related to treatment resistance (i.p. cisplatin-based) in multiple studies (Mayer et al. 2002; Devouassoux-Shisheboran et al. 2001; Velasco et al. 2004, 2007). However, the exact link between BRAF status, MSI, and treatment sensitivity of type II GCTs has to be clarified. For this approach, the TCam-2 cell line might be a suitable tool.

An overall low mutation frequency is rather exceptional for solid cancers, although it seems to be the rule for type II GCTs. That this is indeed not due to the preselection of genes under investigation, but an overall phenomenon is supported by the results of a high throughput investigation on the mutation status of the kinome (Bignell et al. 2006; Greenman et al. 2007). This might again be related to the embryonic origin of the tumors. In fact, embryonic stem cells have a unique mechanism in which one of the two DNA strands is kept protected against any form of mutations (Hong and Stambrook 2004). This protects the DNA from anomalies to be transmitted to the next generation. The activation of pluripotency of the germ cell after disruption of the integrity of the genome, in type I GCTs (see above), might be related to loss of pluripotency of the immortal strand. Therefore, the power of the mutation status analysis in type II GCTs is limited in elucidating the involvement of various pathogenetic mechanisms and pathways. However, on the basis of the observations made, a number of interesting conclusions can be drawn, especially when different platforms of data are combined. Besides the already mentioned role of KRAS2 and c-KIT, this also accounts for the role of the TP53 in the pathogenesis of type II GCTs.

#### 2.6.9.1 TP53 and MicroRNAs

One of the intriguing observations is that also TP53 is hardly mutated in type II GCTs (Guillou et al. 1996; Moore et al. 2001; Kersemaekers et al. 2002a, b; Mayer et al. 2003; Emanuel et al. 2006). It is however, interesting that TP53 target genes have been found to be frequently hypermethylated in type II GCTs (Christoph et al. 2007). The absence of TP53 mutations has been a matter of much discussion, especially because the observations in the supposed mouse model are counterindicative. The absence of low level of P53 mutations in type II GCTs is a rare phenomenon among solid cancers. The mutations found in TP53 in type II GCTs are predominantly detected in so-called nongerm cell malignancies (Houldsworth et al. 1998). These are somatic cancers formed as a result of progression of a teratomatous element. In fact, these mimic the mutational status of solid cancer in adults, including the mutational status of TP53. The reason for the presence of wild type TP53 remained elusive for a long period of time. The selective pressure on TP53 to be inactivated in many solid cancers is related to its function in overruling cellular senescence upon for example mutation of a protooncogene (Lundberg et al. 2000; Yeager et al. 1998). Thereby the organism is protected from the formation of cancers due to single mutations. The explanation for the wild type TP53 status in type II GCTs was obtained as a result of the expression analysis of certain miRNAs. MiRNAs are a subgroup of nonprotein-encoding RNA, which interacts with mRNAs to block translation (Dalmay and Edwards 2006; Mattick and Makunin 2005; Hall and Russell 2005; Sontheimer and Carthew 2005). A close link between miRNA and genetics (Calin and Croce 2006) and epigenetics (Chuang and Jones 2007) has been indicated. Several thousands of miRNAs are expected to exist within the mammalian genome, which underwent an increase in evolution in the human genome (Wienholds and Plasterk 2005). It is assumed that about one-third of the protein-encoding mRNAs are also regulated by miRNAs. In type II GCTs, a specific pattern of expression of miRNA has been observed using a high throughput approach (Gillis et al. 2007). In fact, the tumors were classified into undifferentiated and differentiated components, which indeed support the model that shows that miRNA are involved in regulation of differentiation. The miRNA cluster 371–373 (mapped to chromosome 19) is specifically expressed in the seminomas and embryonal carcinomas. As expected, this set of miRNAs is also expressed in human embryonic stem cells (Suh et al. 2004). This cluster of miRNAs was previously found to be able to mimic the presence of a mutated TP53 in overruling cellular senescence in a high throughput in vitro model system (Voorhoeve et al. 2006). Using a unique series of type II GCTs and cell lines, a good correlation between the level of expression of these miRNAs and the mutational status of TP53 was identified. The miRNAs interact with the 3′ UTR of the mRNA encoding the tumor suppressor gene protein LATS-2, which is involved in the regulation of G1–S transition in the cell cycle. LATS-2 is indeed a downstream target of TP53, and inactivation of TP53 results in absence of LATS-2 protein, thereby overruling cellular senescence. A role of LATS-2 in polyploidization has also been suggested (Aylon et al. 2006). Intriguingly, DND is recently identified to be a regulatory element is this process. In brief, the miRNAs 371–373 mimic the effect of mutated TP53 regarding the interaction with LATS-2. However, this does not influence the function of TP53 in the DNA damage response. That miRNAs have a significant role in the causation and possibly also in differentiation of type II GCTs is supported by the observation of the discrepancy between mRNA and protein of E2F1, which is regulated by the miRNA 17–92 cluster (Novotny et al. 2007). In addition, two miRNAs (miR-145 and

324-5p) are highly expressed in seminoma and the cell line TCam-2, and not in the other histologies, including cell lines (De Jong et al. 2008b). These miRNAs are predicted to interact with the mRNA of SOX2, which is indeed specifically expressed in embryonal carcinoma and cell lines but not in seminoma (see above). It is highly interesting to investigate the involvement of these miRNA in the transition of CIS/seminoma to embryonal carcinoma, likely related to the process of activation of pluripotency (reprogramming), which also occurs during normal development (see Figs. 2.2a and 2.3). In addition, it can be related to the mechanism of suppression of the somatic expression program (omnipotency), which is essential for germ cells.

The role of miRNAs in the pathogenesis of type II GCTs opens an exciting area of research, in which indeed the interactive analysis of miRNA and mRNA expression, DNA copy number changes, and protein expression will be highly informative and also useful for understanding treatment sensitivity (Duale et al. 2007). Currently, a number of histological subtype-specific miRNAs have been, besides the above mentioned examples. These miRNA may give insight into the regulatory elements involved in the pluripotency of type II GCTs, and may be of diagnostic and therapeutic relevance. To facilitate the selection of in vitro and/or in vivo models for type II (and also I and III) GCTs, the following paragraph gives an update on the existing models.

### 2.6.10 Available Cell Lines and Models

Till recently, only cell lines representative for nonseminomas, i.p. embryonal carcinomas, were available. These have been proven to be of value for many different studies. The most frequently used cell lines are NT2, Tera-1, 833KE, NCCIT, and 2102Ep. It must be kept in mind that NCCIT originates from a primary extragonadal type II GCT, and lacks a functional P53 (Voorhoeve et al. 2006; Damjanov et al. 1993). The JKT-1 cell line proposed to be representative for seminoma has been proven to be unrelated and therefore not informative in the context of type II GCTs (Jo et al. 1999; Kinugawa et al. 1998; Eckert et al. 2007; de Jong et al. 2007b). Therefore, the data published are not relevant for GCTs. In contrast, the TCam-2 cell line is of interest. This cell line has indeed most characteristics of seminoma (Goddard et al. 2007; Eckert et al. 2007; de Jong et al. 2007b), although some nonseminomatous features also are found (to be published elsewhere). One of the intriguing observations is that this cell line has a mutated BRAF, which is rare in type II GCTs (see above). This probably explains the success in generating this cell line. One of the other type II-derived cell lines, i.e., 833KE, contains a KRAS2 mutation. In spite of this possible limitation, for sure the TCam-2 cell line will be valuable for investigation of pathogenetic mechanisms related to the development of type II GCTs, i.p. transition from a seminomatous to a nonseminomatous phenotype. It has to be kept in mind that cell lines have a high incidence of mutated proto-oncogenes compared to an unselected series of type II GCTs of patients. This might be due to an enhanced in vitro survival caused by these mutations.

### 2.6.11 Pathogenetic Model

On the basis of the different levels of information described, a comprehensive model for the pathogenesis of type II GCTs can be proposed (Fig. 2.3). For sure it does not contain all available information, but it reflects the most interesting observations, and demonstrates the close link with mechanisms involved in normal development.

#### 2.6.11.1 Concluding Points Type II GCTs

- PGC/gonocyte origin
- Various identified risk factors, mostly related to germ cell maturation delay
- Histologically composed of seminoma or nonseminoma
- Nonseminoma are omnipotent
- OCT3/4 is informative diagnostic marker in adult testis
- Seminoma is characterized by OCT3/4+, SOX2−, SOX17 +
- Embryonal carcinoma is characterized by OCT3/4+, SOX2±, SOX17−
- Predominantly diagnosed in adolescent and young adults

Consistently aneuploid with multiple structural anomalies

Gain of short arm of chromosome 12 is characteristic

Mutations are rarely found

TSPY is a candidate gene for the Y-involvement

Multiple representative cell lines available, including a seminoma cell line

Possible model for suppression of somatic differentiation program

No representative animal model identified

## 2.7 Overall Conclusions

Different types of human GCT can be recognized; the subclassification proposed here allows a better understanding of the pathogenesis of this type of cancer, regarding cell of origin as well as mechanisms of progression. Overall, GCTs mimic normal germ cell development to a certain extent, which explains both the biology and clinical behavior of the subtypes. Specific markers for diagnosis for the various histological elements have been identified, on the basis of targeted- as well as high throughput approaches. These give insight into the fundamental mechanisms involved in proliferation, differentiation, and apoptosis, also during normal development. An integrated analysis of the different data sets will allow a high level of understanding of the processes involved. On the basis of these observations, novel approaches are under development, in the field of early (noninvasive) diagnosis, treatment, and generation of informative in vitro and in vivo model systems.

**Acknowledgments** The author would like to thank the following people for their support: Prof. Dr. J.W. Oosterhuis, A.J.M. Gillis, and J. Stoop for critically reading the manuscript and giving helpful suggestions; the pathologists and urologists, and especially the patients, who supported the progress in understanding the intriguing complexity of human germ cell tumors.

## References

Abratt RP, Reddi VB, Sarembock LA (1992) Testicular cancer and cryptorchidism. Br J Urol 70:656–659

Aksglaede L, Wikstrom AM, Rajpert-De Meyts E, Dunkel L, Skakkebaek NE, Juul A (2006) Natural history of seminiferous tubule degeneration in Klinefelter syndrome. Hum Reprod Update 12(1):39–48

Almstrup K, Hoei-Hansen CE, Nielsen JE et al (2005) Genome-wide gene expression profiling of testicular carcinoma in situ progression into overt tumours. Br J Cancer 92(10):1934–1941

Ancelin K, Lange UC, Hajkova P et al (2006) Blimp1 associates with Prmt5 and directs histone arginine methylation in mouse germ cells. Nat Cell Biol 8(6):623–630

Anway MD, Cupp AS, Uzumcu M, Skinner MK (2005) Epigenetic transgenerational actions of endocrine disruptors and male fertility. Science 308(5727):1466–1469

Anway MD, Leathers C, Skinner MK (2006) Endocrine disruptor vinclozolin induced epigenetic transgenerational adult onset disease. Endocrinology 147(12):5515–5523

Avilion AA, Nicolis SK, Pevny LH, Perez L, Vivian N, Lovell-Badge R (2003) Multipotent cell lineages in early mouse development depend on SOX2 function. Genes Dev 17(1):126–140

Aylon Y, Michael D, Shmueli A, Yabuta N, Nojima H, Oren M (2006) A positive feedback loop between the p53 and Lats2 tumor suppressors prevents tetraploidization. Genes Dev 20(19):2687–2700

Baron D, Batista F, Chaffaux S et al (2005) Foxl2 gene and the development of the ovary: a story about goat, mouse, fish and woman. Reprod Nutr Dev 45(3):377–382

Batata MA, Whitmore WF Jr, Chu FCH et al (1980) Cryptorchidism and testicular cancer. J Urol 124:382–387

Bergner DM, Duck GB, Rao M (1980) Bilateral sequential spermatocytic seminoma. J Urol 124:565

Biermann K, Steger K (2007) Epigenetics in male germ cells. J Androl 28(4):466–480

Biermann K, Klingmuller D, Koch A et al (2006) Diagnostic value of markers M2A, OCT3/4, AP-2gamma, PLAP and c-KIT in the detection of extragonadal seminomas. Histopathology 49(3):290–297

Biermann K, Heukamp LC, Steger K et al (2007) Gene expression profiling identifies new biological markers of neoplastic germ cells. Anticancer Res 27(5A):3091–3100

Biermann K, Heukamp LC, Steger K et al (2007b) Genome-wide expression profiling reveals new insights into pathogenesis and progression of testicular germ cell tumors. Cancer Genomics Proteomics 4(5):359–367

Biermann K, Goke F, Nettersheim D et al (2007c) c-KIT is frequently mutated in bilateral germ cell tumours and down-regulated during progression from intratubular germ cell neoplasia to seminoma. J Pathol 213(3):311–318

Bignell G, Smith R, Hunter C et al (2006) Sequence analysis of the protein kinase gene family in human testicular germ-cell tumors of adolescents and adults. Genes Chromosomes Cancer 45(1):42–46

Boer B, Kopp J, Mallanna S et al (2007) Elevating the levels of Sox2 in embryonal carcinoma cells and embryonic stem cells inhibits the expression of Sox2:Oct-3/4 target genes. Nucleic Acids Res 35(6):1773–1786

Boldajipour B, Mahabaleshwar H, Kardash E et al (2008) Control of chemokine-guided cell migration by ligand sequestration. Cell 132(3):463–473

Boyer LA, Lee TI, Cole MF et al (2005) Core transcriptional regulatory circuitry in human embryonic stem cells. Cell 122(6):947–956

Brower JV, Rodic N, Seki T et al (2007) Evolutionarily conserved mammalian adenine nucleotide translocase 4 is essential for spermatogenesis. J Biol Chem 282(40):29658–29666

Burke AP, Mostofi FK (1993) Spermatocytic seminoma. A clinicopathologic study of 79 cases. J Urol Path 1:21–32
Calin GA, Croce CM (2006) MicroRNAs and chromosomal abnormalities in cancer cells. Oncogene 25(46):6202–6210
Carlin R, Davis D, Weiss M, Schultz B, Troyer D (2006) Expression of early transcription factors Oct4, Sox2 and Nanog by porcine umbilical cord (PUC) matrix cells. Reprod Biol Endocrinol 4(1):8
Castedo SM, De Jong B, Oosterhuis JW et al (1989) Chromosomal changes in human primary testicular nonseminomatous germ cell tumors. Cancer Res 49:5696–5701
Chaganti RSK, Bosl GJ (1995) Germ cell tumors: unraveling a biological paradox. Lab Invest 73:593–595
Chang HS, Anway MD, Rekow SS, Skinner MK (2006) Transgenerational epigenetic imprinting of the male germline by endocrine disruptor exposure during gonadal sex determination. Endocrinology 147(12):5524–5541
Chen C, Ouyang W, Grigura V et al (2005) ERM is required for transcriptional control of the spermatogonial stem cell niche. Nature 436(7053):1030–1034
Cheng L, Sung MT, Cossu-Rocca P et al (2007) OCT4: biological functions and clinical applications as a marker of germ cell neoplasia. J Pathol 211(1):1–9
Chow SN, Yang JH, Lin YH et al (1996) Malignant ovarian germ cell tumors. Int J Gynaecol Obstet 53:151–158
Christoph F, Kempkensteffen C, Weikert S et al (2007) Frequent epigenetic inactivation of p53 target genes in seminomatous and nonseminomatous germ cell tumors. Cancer Lett 247(1):137–142
Chuang JC, Jones PA (2007) Epigenetics and microRNAs. Pediatr Res 61(5 Pt 2):24R–29R
Chung PW, Bayley AJ, Sweet J et al (2004) Spermatocytic seminoma: a review. Eur Urol 45(4):495–498
Cinalli RM, Rangan P, Lehmann R (2008) Germ cells are forever. Cell 132(4):559–562
Clark AT, Rodriguez RT, Bodnar MS et al (2004) Human STELLAR, NANOG, and GDF3 genes are expressed in pluripotent cells and map to chromosome 12p13, a hotspot for teratocarcinoma. Stem Cells 22(2):169–179
Constantinescu S (2003) Stemness, fusion and renewal of hematopoietic and embryonic stem cells. J Cell Mol Med 7(2):103–112
Cook MB, Graubard BI, Rubertone MV, Erickson RL, McGlynn KA (2008) Perinatal factors and the risk of testicular germ cell tumors. Int J Cancer 122(11):2600–2606
Cools M, van Aerde K, Kersemaekers AM et al (2005) Morphological and immunohistochemical differences between gonadal maturation delay and early germ cell neoplasia in patients with undervirilization syndromes. J Clin Endocrinol Metab 90(9):5295–5303
Cools M, Honecker F, Stoop H et al (2006a) Maturation delay of germ cells in trisomy 21 fetuses results in increase risk for the development of testicular germ cell tumors. Hum Pathol 37:101–111
Cools M, Drop SL, Wolffenbuttel KP, Oosterhuis JW, Looijenga LH (2006b) Germ cell tumors in the intersex gonad: old paths, new directions, moving frontiers. Endocr Rev 27: 468–484
Cools M, Stoop H, Kersemaekers AM et al (2006c) Gonadoblastoma arising in undifferentiated gonadal tissue within dysgenetic gonads. J Clin Endocrinol Metab 91(6):2404–2413
Cools M, Boter M, van Gurp RJHLM et al (2007) Analysis of Y containing cell lines in the gonads of patients with gonadal dysgenesis: impact on gonadal differentiation patterns and risk for gonadoblastoma formation. Clin Endocr (in press)
Costabile RA (2007) How worrisome is testicular microlithiasis? Curr Opin Urol 17(6):419–423
Cowan CA, Klimanskaya I, McMahon J et al (2004) Derivation of embryonic stem-cell lines from human blastocysts. N Engl J Med 350(13):1353–1356
Crews D, Gore AC, Hsu TS et al (2007) Transgenerational epigenetic imprints on mate preference. Proc Natl Acad Sci USA 104(14):5942–5946
Cui XS, Shen XH, Kim NH (2007) Dicer1 expression in preimplantation mouse embryos: involvement of Oct3/4 transcription at the blastocyst stage. Biochem Biophys Res Commun 352(1):231–236
Cummings OW, Ulbright TM, Eble JN, Roth LM (1994) Spermatocytic seminoma: an immunohistochemical study. Hum Pathol 25:54–59
Cusido MT, Jorda B, Gonzalez J, Garcia A, Xercavins J (1998) Ovarian germ cell tumors. Eur J Gynaecol Oncol 19(2): 130–134
Dadoune JP (2007) New insights into male gametogenesis: what about the spermatogonial stem cell niche? Folia Histochem Cytobiol 45(3):141–147
Dalmay T, Edwards DR (2006) MicroRNAs and the hallmarks of cancer. Oncogene 25(46):6170–6175
Damjanov I, Horvat B, Gibas Z (1993) Retinoic acid-induced differentiation of the developmentally pluripotent human germ cell tumor-derived cell line, NCCIT. Lab Invest 68:220–232
De Bruin TWA, Slater RM, Defferrari R et al (1994) Isochromosome 12p-positive pineal germ cell tumor. Cancer Res 54:1542–1544
De Gouveia Brazao CA, Pierik FH, Oosterhuis JW, Dohle GR, Looijenga LHJ, Weber RFA (2004) Bilateral testicular microlithiasis predicts development of malignant testicular germ cell tumours in subfertile men. J Urol 171:158–160
De Jong J, Looijenga LHJ (2006) Stem cell marker OCT3/4 in tumor biology and germ cell tumor diagnostics: history and future. Crit Rev Oncog 12(3-4):171–203
de Jong J, Stoop H, Dohle GR et al (2005) Diagnostic value of OCT3/4 for pre-invasive and invasive testicular germ cell tumours. J Pathol 206(2):242–249
De Jong J, Weeda S, Gillis AJM, Oosterhuis JW, Looijenga LHJ (2007a) Differential methylation of the OCT3/4 upstream region in primary human testicular germ cell tumors. Oncol Rep 18(1):127–132
de Jong J, Stoop H, Gillis AJ et al (2007b) JKT-1 is not a human seminoma cell line. Int J Androl 30(4):350–365
de Jong J, Stoop H, Gillis AJ et al (2008a) Further characterization of the first seminoma cell line TCam-2. Genes Chromosomes Cancer 47(3):185–196
De Jong J, Stoop J, Gillis AJM et al (2008b) Differential expression of SOX17 and SOX2 in human normal and malignant germ cells and stem cells has biological and clinical implications. J Pathol 215(1):21–30
De Meyts ER, Jorgensen N, Mueller J, Skakkebaek NE (1996) Prolonged expression of the c-kit receptor in germ cells of intersex fetal testes. J Pathol 178:166–169
De Miguel MP, Cheng L, Holland EC, Federspiel MJ, Donovan PJ (2002) Dissection of the c-Kit signaling pathway in

mouse primordial germ cells by retroviral-mediated gene transfer. Proc Natl Acad Sci USA 99(16):10458–10463
Deb K, Sivaguru M, Yong HY, Roberts RM (2006) Cdx2 gene expression and trophectoderm lineage specification in mouse embryos. Science 311(5763):992–996
Dekker I, Rozeboom T, Delemarre J, Dam A, Oosterhuis JW (1992) Placental-like alkaline phosphatase and DNA flow cytometry in spermatocytic seminoma. Cancer 69: 993–996
Delbridge ML, Longepied G, Depetris D et al (2004) TSPY, the candidate gonadoblastoma gene on the human Y chromosome, has a widely expressed homologue on the X - implications for Y chromosome evolution. Chromosome Res 12(4):345–356
Devouassoux-Shisheboran M, Mauduit C, Bouvier R et al (2001) Expression of hMLH1 and hMSH2 and assessment of microsatellite instability in testicular and mediastinal germ cell tumours. Mol Hum Reprod 7(12):1099–1105
Di Vizio D, Cito L, Boccia A et al (2005) Loss of the tumor suppressor gene PTEN marks the transition from intratubular germ cell neoplasias (ITGCN) to invasive germ cell tumors. Oncogene 10:1882–1894
Dieckmann KP (2009) Re: Niels J van Casteren, Hans Stoop, Gert R Dohle, Ronald de Wit, J Wolter Oosterhuis, Leendert HJ Looijenga. Noninvasive detection of testicular carcinoma in situ in semen using OCT3/4. Eur Urol 55(4):e67–e68
Dieckmann KP, Pichlmeier U (2004) Clinical epidemiology of testicular germ cell tumors. World J Urol 22(1):2–14
Dietl J, Horny HP, Ruck P, Kaiserling E (1993) Dysgerminoma of the ovary. An immunohistochemical study of tumor- infiltrating lymphoreticular cells and tumor cells. Cancer 71(8):2562–2568
Donohue JP (1990) The pathology of germ cell tumors of the testis. In: Libertino JA (ed) Testis tumors (International Perspectives in Urology), 7th edn. Lippincott Williams & Wilkins, Baltimore, pp 23–54
Donovan PJ (1998) The germ cell–the mother of all stem cells. Int J Dev Biol 42(7):1043–1050
Donovan PJ (2001) High Oct-ane fuel powers the stem cell. Nat Genet 29(3):246–247
Draper JS, Smith K, Gokhale P et al (2003) Recurrent gain of chromosomes 17q and 12 in cultured human embryonic stem cells. Nat Biotechnol 22:53–54
Druker BJ, Talpaz M, Resta DJ et al (2001) Efficacy and safety of a specific inhibitor of the BCR-ABL tyrosine kinase in chronic myeloid leukemia. N Engl J Med 344(14): 1031–1037
Duale N, Lindeman B, Komada M et al (2007) Molecular portrait of cisplatin induced response in human testis cancer cell lines based on gene expression profiles. Mol Cancer 6:53
Eble JN (1994) Spermatocytic seminoma. Hum Pathol 25(10):1035–1042
Eckert, D. Biermann, K. Nettersheim, D. Gillis, A. J. Steger, K. Jack, H. M. Muller, A. M. Looijenga, L. H. Schorle, H. Expression of BLIMP1/PRMT5 and concurrent histone H2A/H4 arginine 3 dimethylation in fetal germ cells, CIS/IGCNU and germ cell tumors. BMC Dev Biol 8( nov 7): 106.
Eckert D, Nettersheim D, Heukamp LC, Kitazawa S, Biermann K, Schorle H (2007) TCam-2 but not JKT-1 cells resemble seminoma in cell culture. Cell Tissue Res 331(2):529–538
Emanuel PO, Unger PD, Burstein DE (2006) Immunohistochemical detection of p63 in testicular germ cell neoplasia. Ann Diagn Pathol 10(5):269–273
Engeler DS, Hosli PO, John H et al (2000) Early orchiopexy: prepubertal intratubular germ cell neoplasia and fertility outcome. Urology 56(1):144–148
Ezeh UI, Turek PJ, Reijo RA, Clark AT (2005) Human embryonic stem cell genes OCT4, NANOG, STELLAR, and GDF3 are expressed in both seminoma and breast carcinoma. Cancer 104(10):2255–2265
Fisher JS, Macpherson S, Marchetti N, Sharpe RM (2003) Human 'testicular dysgenesis syndrome': a possible model using in-utero exposure of the rat to dibutyl phthalate. Hum Reprod 18(7):1383–1394
Floyd C, Ayala AG, Logothetis CJ, Silva EG (1988) Spermatocytic seminoma with associated sarcoma of the testis. Cancer 61(2):409–414
Fritsch MK, Schneider DT, Schuster AE, Murdoch FE, Perlman EJ (2006) Activation of Wnt/beta-catenin signaling in distinct histologic subtypes of human germ cell tumors. Pediatr Dev Pathol 9(2):115–131
Gajendran VK, Nguyen M, Ellison LM (2005) Testicular cancer patterns in African-American men. Urology 66(3):602–605
Ganguly S, Murty VV, Samaniego F, Reuter VE, Bosl GJ, Chaganti RS (1990) Detection of preferential NRAS mutations in human male germ cell tumors by the polymerase chain reaction. Genes Chromosomes Cancer 1:228–232
Gashaw I, Dushaj O, Behr R et al (2007) Novel germ cell markers characterize testicular seminoma and fetal testis. Mol Hum Reprod 13(10):721–727
Gidekel S, Pizov G, Bergman Y, Pikarsky E (2003) Oct-3/4 is a dose-dependent oncogenic fate determinant. Cancer Cell 4:361–370
Gillis AJ, Stoop HJ, Hersmus R et al (2007) High-throughput microRNAome analysis in human germ cell tumours. J Pathol 213(3):319–328
Ginis I, Luo Y, Miura T et al (2004) Differences between human and mouse embryonic stem cells. Dev Biol 269(2):360–380
Giwercman A (1992) Carcinoma in-situ of the testis: screening and management. Scand J Urol Nephrol 26:1–47
Giwercman A, Grindsted J, Hansen B, Jensen OM, Skakkebaek NE (1987) Testicular cancer risk in boys with maldescended testis: a cohort study. J Urol 138(5):1214–1216
Giwercman A, Lindenberg S, Kimber SJ, Andersson T, Müller J, Skakkebæk NE (1990a) Monoclonal antibody 43-9F as a sensitive immunohistochemical marker of carcinoma *in situ* of human testis. Cancer 65:1135–1142
Giwercman A, Hopman AHN, Ramaekers FCS, Skakkebæk NE (1990b) Carcinoma *in situ* of the testis: detection of malignant germ cells in seminal fluid by means of *in situ* hybridization. Am J Pathol 136:497–502
Goddard NC, McIntyre A, Summersgill B, Gilbert D, Kitazawa S, Shipley J (2007) KIT and RAS signalling pathways in testicular germ cell tumours: new data and a review of the literature. Int J Androl 30(4):337–348; discussion 49
Godin I, Deed R, Cooke J, Zsebo K, Dexter M, Wylie CC (1991) Effects of the steel gene product on mouse primordial germ cells in culture. Nature 352:807–809
Greenman C, Stephens P, Smith R et al (2007) Patterns of somatic mutation in human cancer genomes. Nature 446(7132): 153–158

Grootegoed JA, Siep M, Baarends WM (2000) Molecular and cellular mechanisms in spermatogenesis. Baillieres Best Pract Res Clin Endocrinol Metab 14(3):331–343
Guillou L, Estreicher A, Chaubert P et al (1996) Germ cell tumors of the testis overexpress wild-type p53. Am J Pathol 149:1221–1228
Hall PA, Russell SH (2005) New perspectives on neoplasia and the RNA world. Hematol Oncol 23(2):49–53
Hannema SE, Scott IS, Rajpert-De Meyts E, Skakkebaek NE, Coleman N, Hughes IA (2006) Testicular development in the complete androgen insensitivity syndrome. J Pathol 208(4):518–527
Hansis C, Grifo JA, Krey LC (2000) Oct-4 expression in inner cell mass and trophectoderm of human blastocysts. Mol Hum Reprod 6(11):999–1004
Hart AH, Hartley L, Parker K et al (2005) The pluripotency homeobox gene NANOG is expressed in human germ cell tumors. Cancer 104:2092–2098
Hasle H, Jacobsen BB, Asschenfeldt P, Andersen K (1992) Mediastinal germ cell tumour associated with Klinefelter syndrome. A report of case and review of the literature. Eur J Pediatr 151:735–739
Hasle H, Mellemgaard A, Nielsen J, Hansen J (1995) Cancer incidence in men with Klinefelter syndrome. Br J Cancer 71:416–420
Hattori N, Nishino K, Ko YG, Ohgane J, Tanaka S, Shiota K (2004) Epigenetic control of mouse Oct-4 gene expression in embryonic stem cells and trophoblast stem cells. J Biol Chem 279(17):17063–17069
Hayashi K, de Sousa Lopes SM, Surani MA (2007) Germ cell specification in mice. Science 316(5823):394–396
Hemminki K, Li X, Czene K (2002) Cancer risks in first-generation immigrants to Sweden. Int J Cancer 99(2):218–228
Henderson BE, Bernstein L, Ross RK, Depue RH, Judd HL (1988) The early in utero oestrogen and testosterone environment of blacks and whites: potential effects on male offspring. Br J Cancer 57(2):216–218
Hersmus R, Kalfa N, De Leeuw B et al (2008a) FOXL2 and SOX9 as parameters of female and male gonadal differentiation in patients with various forms of disorders of sex development (DSD). J Pathol 215(1):31–38
Hersmus R, De Leeuw HCGM, Wolffenbuttel KP et al (2008b) New insights into type II germ cell tumor pathogenesis based on the studies of patients with various forms of disorders of sex development (DSD). Mol and Cell Endocrinol 291(1–2):1–10
Herszfeld D, Wolvetang E, Langton-Bunker E et al (2006) CD30 is a survival factor and a biomarker for transformed human pluripotent stem cells. Nat Biotechnol 24(3):351–357
Hildenbrand R, Schroder W, Brude E et al (1999) Detection of TSPY protein in a unilateral microscopic gonadoblastoma of a Turner mosaic patient with a Y-derived marker chromosome. J Pathol 189(4):623–626
Hochedlinger K, Yamada Y, Beard C, Jaenisch R (2005) Ectopic expression of Oct-4 blocks progenitor cell differentiation and causes dysplasia in epithelial tissues. Cell 121: 465–477
Hoei-Hansen CE, Almstrup K, Nielsen JE et al (2005) Stem cell pluripotency factor NANOG is expressed in human fetal gonocytes, testicular carcinoma in situ and germ cell tumours. Histopathology 47(1):48–56
Hoei-Hansen CE, Carlsen E, Jorgensen N, Leffers H, Skakkebaek NE, Rajpert-De Meyts E (2007) Towards a non-invasive method for early detection of testicular neoplasia in semen samples by identification of fetal germ cell-specific markers. Hum Reprod 22(1):167–173
Hofer MD, Browne TJ, He L, Skotheim RI, Lothe RA, Rubin MA (2005) Identification of two molecular groups of seminomas by using expression and tissue microarrays. Clin Cancer Res 11(16):5722–5729
Hofmann MC, Braydich-Stolle L, Dettin L, Johnson E, Dym M (2005) Immortalization of mouse germ line stem cells. Stem Cells 23(2):200–210
Holm M, Hoei-Hansen CE, Rajpert-De Meyts E, Skakkebaek NE (2003) Increased risk of carcinoma in situ in patients with testicular germ cell cancer with ultrasonic microlithiasis in the contralateral testicle. J Urol 170(4):1163–1167
Holm TM, Jackson-Grusby L, Brambrink T, Yamada Y, Rideout WM 3rd, Jaenisch R (2005) Global loss of imprinting leads to widespread tumorigenesis in adult mice. Cancer Cell 8(4):275–285
Holzik MF, Rapley EA, Hoekstra HJ, Sleijfer DT, Nolte IM, Sijmons RH (2004) Genetic predisposition to testicular germ-cell tumours. Lancet Oncol 5(6):363–371
Honecker F, Stoop H, de Krijger RR, Chris Lau YF, Bokemeyer C, Looijenga LH (2004) Pathobiological implications of the expression of markers of testicular carcinoma in situ by fetal germ cells. J Pathol 203(3):849–857
Honecker F, Stoop H, Mayer F et al (2006) Germ cell lineage differentiation in nonseminomatous germ cell tumors. J Pathol 208:395–400
Hong Y, Stambrook PJ (2004) Restoration of an absent G1 arrest and protection from apoptosis in embryonic stem cells after ionizing radiation. Proc Natl Acad Sci USA 101(40): 14443–14448
Honorio S, Agathanggelou A, Wernert N, Rothe M, Maher ER, Latif F (2003) Frequent epigenetic inactivation of the RASSF1A tumour suppressor gene in testicular tumours and distinct methylation profiles of seminoma and nonseminoma testicular germ cell tumours. Oncogene 22(3):461–466
Horwich A, Shipley J, Huddart R (2006) Testicular germ-cell cancer. Lancet 367(9512):754–765
Houldsworth J, Xiao H, Murty VV et al (1998) Human male germ cell tumor resistance to cisplatin is linked to TP53 gene mutation. Oncogene 16(18):2345–2349
Huddart SN, Mann JR, Robinson K et al (2003) Sacrococcygeal teratomas: the UK Children's Cancer Study Group's experience. I. Neonatal. Pediatr Surg Int 19(1–2):47–51
Hughes IA, Houk C, Ahmed SF, Lee PA (2006) Consensus statement on management of intersex disorders. Arch Dis Child 2(3):148–162
Humphrey RK, Beattie GM, Lopez AD et al (2004) Maintenance of pluripotency in human embryonic stem cells is STAT3 independent. Stem Cells 22(4):522–530
Hunt PA, Hassold TJ (2002) Sex matters in meiosis. Science 296(5576):2181–2183
Hutchison GR, Scott HM, Walker M et al (2008) Sertoli cell development and function in an animal model of testicular dysgenesis syndrome. Biol Reprod 78(2):352–360
Imai K, Yamamoto H (2007) Carcinogenesis and microsatellite instability: the interrelationship between genetics and epigenetics. Carcinogenesis 29(4):673–680

International Germ Cell Cancer Collaborative Group (1997) International Germ Cell Consensus Classification: a prognostic factor- based staging system for metastatic germ cell cancers. J Clin Oncol 15(2):594–603

Ishii T, Kohu K, Yamada S et al (2007) Up-regulation of DNA-methyltransferase 3A expression is associated with hypomethylation of intron 25 in human testicular germ cell tumors. Tohoku J Exp Med 212(2):177–190

Isurugi K, Imao S, Hirose K, Aoki H (1977) Seminoma in Klinefelter's syndrome with 47, XXY, 15s+ karyotype. Cancer 39(5):2041–2047

Izquierdo MA, Van der Valk P, Van Ark-Otte J et al (1995) Differential expression of the c-kit proto-oncogene in germ cell tumours. J Pathol 177:253–258

Jacobsen R, Bostofte E, Engholm G et al (2000) Risk of testicular cancer in men with abnormal semen characteristics: cohort study. BMJ 321(7264):789–792

Jaenisch R, Young R (2008) Stem cells, the molecular circuitry of pluripotency and nuclear reprogramming. Cell 132(4): 567–582

Jang YY, Sharkis SJ (2007) Fetal to adult stem cell transition: knocking Sox17 off. Cell 130(3):403–404

Jo Y, Kinugawa K, Matsuki T, Morioka M, Tanaka H (1999) Analysis of the biological properties and use of comparative genomic hybridization to locate chromosomal aberrations in the human testicular seminoma cell line JKT-1 and its highly metastatic cell line JKT-HM. BJU Int 83(4):469–475

Joensuu H, Roberts PJ, Sarlomo-Rikala M et al (2001) Effect of the tyrosine kinase inhibitor STI571 in a patient with a metastatic gastrointestinal stromal tumor. N Engl J Med 344(14):1052–1056

Jones BJ, Thornhill JA, O'Donnell B et al (1991) Influence of prior orchiopexy on stage and prognosis of testicular cancer. Eur Urol 19:201–203

Kakinuma H, Habuchi T, Ito T et al (2001) BCL10 is not a major target for frequent loss of 1p in testicular germ cell tumors. Cancer Genet Cytogenet 126(2):134–138

Kanatsu-Shinohara M, Inoue K, Miki H et al (2006) Clonal origin of germ cell colonies after spermatogonial transplantation in mice. Biol Reprod 75(1):68–74

Karpf AR, Matsui S (2005) Genetic disruption of cytosine DNA methyltransferase enzymes induces chromosomal instability in human cancer cells. Cancer Res 65(19):8635–8639

Kato Y, Rideout WM 3rd, Hilton K, Barton SC, Tsunoda Y, Surani MA (1999) Developmental potential of mouse primordial germ cells. Development 126(9):1823–1832

Kawakami T, Okamoto K, Sugihara H et al (2003) The roles of supernumerical X chromosomes and XIST expression in testicular germ cell tumors. J Urol 169(4):1546–1552

Kawakami T, Okamoto K, Ogawa O, Okada Y (2004) XIST unmethylated DNA fragments in male-derived plasma as a tumour marker for testicular cancer. Lancet 363(9402):40–42

Kawakami T, Zhang C, Okada Y, Okamoto K (2006) Erasure of methylation imprint at the promoter and CTCF-binding site upstream of H19 in human testicular germ cell tumors of adolescents indicate their fetal germ cell origin. Oncogene 25(23):3225–3236

Kehler J, Tolkunova E, Koschorz B et al (2004) Oct4 is required for primordial germ cell survival. EMBO Rep 5(11): 1078–1083

Kelberman D, Rizzoti K, Avilion A et al (2006) Mutations within Sox2/SOX2 are associated with abnormalities in the hypothalamo-pituitary-gonadal axis in mice and humans. J Clin Invest 116(9):2442–2455

Kemmer K, Corless CL, Fletcher JA et al (2004) KIT mutations are common in testicular seminomas. Am J Pathol 164(1): 305–313

Kerr CL, Hill CM, Blumenthal PD, Gearhart JD (2008a) Expression of pluripotent stem cell markers in the human fetal ovary. Hum Reprod 23(3):589–599

Kerr CL, Hill CM, Blumenthal PD, Gearhart JD (2008b) Expression of pluripotent stem cell markers in the human fetal testis. Stem Cells 26(2):412–421

Kersemaekers AMF, Mayer F, Molier M et al (2002a) Role of P53 and MDM2 in treatment response of human germ cell tumors. J Clin Oncol 20:1551–1561

Kersemaekers AM, Mayer F, Molier M, van Weeren PC, Oosterhuis JW, Bokemeyer C, Looijenga LH (2002b) p53 and MDM2 in germ cell cancer treatment response. J Clin Oncol 20(18):1551–1561

Kersemaekers AM, Honecker F, Cools M et al (2005) Identification of germ cells at risk for neoplastic transformation in gonadoblastomas: an immunohistochemical study for OCT3/4 and TSPY. Hum Pathol 36:512–521

Kim I, Saunders TL, Morrison SJ (2007) Sox17 dependence distinguishes the transcriptional regulation of fetal from adult hematopoietic stem cells. Cell 130(3):470–483

Kimura T, Suzuki A, Fujita Y et al (2003) Conditional loss of PTEN leads to testicular teratoma and enhances embryonic germ cell production. Development 130(8):1691–1700

Kimura T, Tomooka M, Yamano N et al (2008) AKT signaling promotes derivation of embryonic germ cells from primordial germ cells. Development 135(5):869–879

Kinugawa K, Hyodo F, Matsuki T et al (1998) Establishment and characterization of a new human testicular seminoma cell line, JKT-1. Int J Urol 5(3):282–287

Knaut H, Schier AF (2008) Clearing the path for germ cells. Cell 132(3):337–339

Knoblich JA (2008) Mechanisms of asymmetric stem cell division. Cell 132(4):583–597

Kopp JL, Ormsbee BD, Desler M, Rizzino A (2008) Small increases in the level of Sox2 trigger the differentiation of mouse embryonic stem cells. Stem Cells 26(4):903–911

Korkola JE, Houldsworth J, Dobrzynski D et al (2005) Gene expression-based classification of nonseminomatous male germ cell tumors. Oncogene 24(32):5101–5107

Korkola JE, Houldsworth J, Chadalavada RS et al (2006) Down-regulation of stem cell genes, including those in a 200-kb gene cluster at 12p13.31, is associated with in vivo differentiation of human male germ cell tumors. Cancer Res 66(2): 820–827

Korkola JE, Heck S, Olshen AB et al (2008) In vivo differentiation and genomic evolution in adult male germ cell tumors. Genes Chromosomes Cancer 47(1):43–55

Koul S, Houldsworth J, Mansukhani MM et al (2002) Characteristic promoter hypermethylation signatures in male germ cell tumors. Mol Cancer 1(1):8

Kraggerud SM, Skotheim RI, Szymanska J et al (2002) Genome profiles of familial/bilateral and sporadic testicular germ cell tumors. Genes Chromosomes Cancer 34(2):168–174

Kristensen DM, Nielsen JE, Skakkebaek NE et al (2008) Presumed pluripotency markers UTF-1 and REX-1 are expressed in human adult testes and germ cell neoplasms. Hum Reprod 23(4):775–782

Kysela B, Matoska J (1991) Flow cytometry analysis of ploidy and proliferation activity in classical and spermatocytic seminoma. Neoplasma 38:3–11

Latza U, Foss H-D, Durkop H et al (1995) CD30 antigen in embryonal carcinoma and embryogenesis and release of the soluble molecule. Am J Pathol 146:463–471

Lau YF (1999) Gonadoblastoma, testicular and prostate cancers, and the TSPY gene. Am J Hum Genet 64(4):921–927

Ledford H (2007) Doubts raised over stem-cell marker. Nature 449(7163):647

Lee MW, Stephens RL (1987) Klinefelter's syndrome and extragonadal germ cell tumors. Cancer 60(5):1053–1055

Lengner CJ, Camargo FD, Hochedlinger K, Welstead GG, Zaidi S, Gokhale S, Scholer HR, Tomilin A, Jaenisch R (2007) *Oct4* expression is not required for mouse somatic stem cell self-renewal. Cell Stem Cell 1:403–415

Lennartsson J, Jelacic T, Linnekin D, Shivakrupa R (2005) Normal and oncogenic forms of the receptor tyrosine kinase kit. Stem Cells 23(1):16–43

Lev S, Blechman JM, Givol D, Yarden Y (1994) Steel factor and c-kit protooncogene: genetic lessons in signal transduction. Crit Rev Oncog 5(2–3):141–168

Li SS, Liu YH, Tseng CN, Chung TL, Lee TY, Singh S (2006) Characterization and gene expression profiling of five new human embryonic stem cell lines derived in Taiwan. Stem Cells Dev 15(4):532–555

Li J, Pan G, Cui K, Liu Y, Xu S, Pei D (2007a) A dominant-negative form of mouse SOX2 induces trophectoderm differentiation and progressive polyploidy in mouse embryonic stem cells. J Biol Chem 282(27):19481–19492

Li Y, Vilain E, Conte F, Rajpert-De Meyts E, Lau YF (2007) Testis-specific protein Y-encoded gene is expressed in early and late stages of gonadoblastoma and testicular carcinoma in situ. Urol Oncol 25(2):141–146

Li Y, Tabatabai ZL, Lee TL et al (2007c) The Y-encoded TSPY protein: a significant marker potentially plays a role in the pathogenesis of testicular germ cell tumors. Hum Pathol 38(10):1470–1481

Liedtke SEJ, Waclawczyk S, Wernet P, Kögler G (2007) *Oct4* and its pseudogenes confuse stem cell research. Cell Stem Cell 1:364–366

Lin T, Chao C, Saito S et al (2005) p53 induces differentiation of mouse embryonic stem cells by suppressing Nanog expression. Nat Cell Biol 7(2):165–171

Lind GE, Skotheim RI, Fraga MF, Abeler VM, Esteller M, Lothe RA (2006) Novel epigenetically deregulated genes in testicular cancer include homeobox genes and SCGB3A1 (HIN-1). J Pathol 210(4):441–449

Lind GE, Skotheim RI, Lothe RA (2007) The epigenome of testicular germ cell tumors. APMIS 115(10):1147–1160

Linger R, Dudakia D, Huddart R et al (2008) Analysis of the DND1 gene in men with sporadic and familial testicular germ cell tumors. Genes Chromosomes Cancer 47(3):247–252

Loh YH, Wu Q, Chew JL et al (2006) The Oct4 and Nanog transcription network regulates pluripotency in mouse embryonic stem cells. Nat Genet 38(4):431–3440

Looijenga LH, Oosterhuis JW (1999) Pathogenesis of testicular germ cell tumours. Rev Reprod 4(2):90–100

Looijenga LH, Oosterhuis JW (2007) Are all testicular seminomas of animals in fact spermatocytic seminomas? Vet Pathol 44(1):126

Looijenga LHJ, Olie RA, Van der Gaag I et al (1994) Seminomas of the canine testis; counterpart of spermatocytic seminoma of men? Lab Invest 71:490–496

Looijenga LH, Gillis AJ, van Gurp RJ, Verkerk AJ, Oosterhuis JW (1997) X inactivation in human testicular tumors. XIST expression and androgen receptor methylation status. Am J Pathol 151(2):581–590

Looijenga LH, Verkerk AJ, Dekker MC, van Gurp RJ, Gillis AJ, Oosterhuis JW (1998) Genomic imprinting in testicular germ cell tumours. APMIS 106(1):187–195; discussion 96–97

Looijenga LH, de Munnik H, Oosterhuis JW (1999) A molecular model for the development of germ cell cancer. Int J Cancer 83(6):809–814

Looijenga LHJ, Stoop H, De Leeuw PJC et al (2003a) POU5F1 (OCT3/4) identifies cells with pluripotent potential in human germ cell tumors. Cancer Res 63:2244–2250

Looijenga LHJ, De Leeuw PJC, Van Oorschot M et al (2003b) Stem cell factor receptor (c-KIT) codon 816 mutations predict development of bilateral testicular germ cell tumors. Cancer Res 63:7674–7678

Looijenga LHJ, Hersmus R, Gillis A et al (2006) Genomic and expression profiling of human spermatocytic seminomas; primary spermatocyte as tumorigenic precursor and DMRT1 as candidate chromosome 9-gene. Cancer Res 66:290–302

Looijenga LHJ, Gillis AJM, Stoop H, Hersmus R, Oosterhuis JW (2007a) Chromosomes and expression in human testicular germ cell tumors: insight it the origin and pathogenesis. Ann NY Acad Science 1120:187–214

Looijenga LH, Stoop H, Hersmus R, Gillis AJ, Wolter Oosterhuis J (2007) Genomic and expression profiling of human spermatocytic seminomas: pathogenetic implications. Int J Androl 30(4):328–335; discussion 35–36

Looijenga LH, Hersmus R, Oosterhuis JW, Cools M, Drop SL, Wolffenbuttel KP (2007c) Tumor risk in disorders of sex development (DSD). Best Pract Res Clin Endocrinol Metab 21(3):480–495

Loveland KL, Hogarth C, Mendis S et al (2005) Drivers of germ cell maturation. Ann NY Acad Sci 1061:173–182

Loy V, Dieckmann K-P (1990) Carcinoma in situ of the testis: intratubular germ cell neoplasia or testicular intraepithelial neoplasia. Hum Pathol 21:457

Lu YJ, Yang J, Noel E et al (2005) Association between large-scale genomic homozygosity without chromosomal loss and nonseminomatous germ cell tumor development. Cancer Res 65(20):9137–9141

Lundberg AS, Hahn WC, Gupta P, Weinberg RA (2000) Genes involved in senescence and immortalization. Curr Opin Cell Biol 12(6):705–709

Lutke Holzik MF, Hoekstra HJ, Sijmons RH et al (2006) Re-analysis of the Xq27-Xq28 region suggests a weak association of an X-linked gene with sporadic testicular germ cell tumour without cryptorchidism. Eur J Cancer 42(12):1869–1874

Moller H (1993) Clues to the aetiology of testicular germ cell tumours from descriptive epidemiology. Eur Urol 23(1):8-13; discussion 4–5

Maiolino P, Restucci B, Papparella S, Paciello O, De Vico G (2004) Correlation of nuclear morphometric features with animal and human World Health Organization International Histological Classifications of canine spontaneous seminomas. Vet Pathol 41(6):608–611

Malogolowkin MH, Mahour GH, Krailo M, Ortega JA (1990) Germ cell tumors in infancy and childhood: a 45-year experience. Pediatr Pathol 10:231–241

Masters JR, Koberle B (2003) Curing metastatic cancer: lessons from testicular germ-cell tumours. Nat Rev Cancer 3(7): 517–525

Masui S, Nakatake Y, Toyooka Y et al (2007) Pluripotency governed by Sox2 via regulation of Oct3/4 expression in mouse embryonic stem cells. Nat Cell Biol 9(6):625–635

Matoska J, Talerman A (1990) Spermatocytic seminoma associated with rhabdomyosarcoma. Am J Clin Pathol 94:89–95

Mattick JS, Makunin IV (2005) Small regulatory RNAs in mammals. Hum Mol Genet 14(Spec no. 1):R121–R132

Mayer F, Gillis AJM, Dinjens W, Oosterhuis JW, Bokemeyer C, Looijenga LHJ (2002) Microsatellite instability of germ cell tumors is associated with resistance to systemic treatment. Cancer Res 62:2758–2760

Mayer F, Stoop H, Scheffer GL et al (2003) Molecular determinants of treatment response in human germ cell tumors. Clin Cancer Res 9(2):767–773

McGlynn KA, Devesa SS, Sigurdson AJ, Brown LM, Tsao L, Tarone RE (2003) Trends in the incidence of testicular germ cell tumors in the United States. Cancer 97(1):63–70

McGlynn KA, Devesa SS, Graubard BI, Castle PE (2005) Increasing incidence of testicular germ cell tumors among black men in the United States. J Clin Oncol 23(24):5757–5761

McIntire KR, Summersgill B, Grygalewicz B et al (2005) Amplification and overexpression of the KIT gene is associated with progression in the seminoma subtype of testicular germ cell tumors of adolescents and adults. Cancer Res 65: 8085–8089

McIntyre A, Summersgill B, Jafer O et al (2004) Defining minimum genomic regions of imbalance involved in testicular germ cell tumors of adolescents and adults through genome wide microarray analysis of cDNA clones. Oncogene 23:9142–9147

McIntyre A, Summersgill B, Lu YJ et al (2007) Genomic copy number and expression patterns in testicular germ cell tumours. Br J Cancer 97(12):1707–1712

McIntyre A, Gilbert D, Goddard N, Looijenga L, Shipley J (2008) Genes, chromosomes and the development of testicular germ cell tumors of adolescents and adults. Genes Chromosomes Cancer: 47(7):547–557

McLaren A (1992) Development of primordial germ cells in the mouse. Andrologia 24:243–247

McLaren A (2001) Mammalian germ cells: birth, sex, and immortality. Cell Struct Funct 26(3):119–122

McLaren A (2003) Primordial germ cells in the mouse. Dev Biol 262(1):1–15

Meissner A, Wernig M, Jaenisch R (2007) Direct reprogramming of genetically unmodified fibroblasts into pluripotent stem cells. Nat Biotechnol 25(10):1177–1181

Meng FJ, Zhou Y, Giwercman A, Skakkebaek NE, Geurts van Kessel AD, Suijkerbuijk RF (1998) Fluorescence in situ hybridization analysis of chromosome 12 anomalies in semen cells from patients with carcinoma in situ of the testis. J Pathol 186(3):235–239

Michos A, Xue F, Michels KB (2007) Birth weight and the risk of testicular cancer: a meta-analysis. Int J Cancer 121(5): 1123–1131

Miettinen M, Lasota J (2005) KIT (CD117): a review on expression in normal and neoplastic tissues, and mutations and their clinicopathologic correlation. Appl Immunohistochem Mol Morphol 13(3):205–220

Modi DN, Sane S, Bhartiya D (2003) Accelerated germ cell apoptosis in sex chromosome aneuploid fetal human gonads. Mol Hum Reprod 9(4):219–225

Moller H, Skakkebæk NE (1996) Risk of testicular cancer and cryptorchidism in relation to socio-economical status and related factors: case-control studies in Denmark. Int J Cancer 66:287–293

Moore BE, Banner BF, Gokden M et al (2001) p53: a good diagnostic marker for intratubular germ cell neoplasia, unclassified. Appl Immunohistochem Mol Morphol 9(3):203–206

Morrison SJ, Spradling AC (2008) Stem cells and niches: mechanisms that promote stem cell maintenance throughout life. Cell 132(4):598–611

Mostert MC, Rosenberg C, Stoop H et al (2000) Comparative genomic and in situ hybridization of germ cell tumors of the infantile testis. Lab Invest 80:1055–1064

Mostofi FK, Sesterhenn IA (1985) Pathology of germ cell tumors of testes. Prog Clin Biol Res 203:1–34

Mostofi FK, Sesterhenn IA, Davis CJJ (1987) Immunopathology of germ cell tumors of the testis. Semin Diagn Pathol 4:320–341

Motzer RJ, Rodriquez E, Reuter VE et al (1991) Genetic analysis as an aid in diagnosis for patients with midline carcinomas of uncertain histologies. J Natl Cancer Inst 83: 341–346

Mulder MP, Keijzer W, Verkerk A et al (1989) Activated *ras* genes in human seminoma: evidence for tumor heterogeneity. Oncogene 4:1345–1351

Muller J, Skakkebaek NE, Nielsen OH, Graem N (1984) Cryptorchidism and testis cancer. Cancer 54:629–634

Muller J, Skakkebaek NE, Parkinson MC (1987) The spermatocytic seminoma: views on pathogenesis. Int J Androl 10(1):147–156

Nakagawa M, Koyanagi M, Tanabe K et al (2007) Generation of induced pluripotent stem cells without Myc from mouse and human fibroblasts. Nat Biotechnol 26(1):101–106

Nakatake Y, Fukui N, Iwamatsu Y et al (2006) Klf4 cooperates with Oct3/4 and Sox2 to activate the Lefty1 core promoter in embryonic stem cells. Mol Cell Biol 26(20):7772–7782

Nichols CR, Heerema NA, Palmer C, Loehrer PJ Sr, Williams SD, Einhorn LH (1987) Klinefelter's syndrome associated with mediastinal germ cell neoplasms. J Clin Oncol 5(8): 1290–1294

Nichols J, Zevnik B, Anastassiadis K et al (1998) Formation of pluripotent stem cells in the mammalian embryo depends in the POU transcription factor Oct4. Cell 95:379–391

Nikolaou M, Valavanis C, Aravantinos G et al (2007) Kit expression in male germ cell tumors. Anticancer Res 27(3B): 1685–1688

Niwa H, Miyazaki J, Smith AG (2000) Quantitative expression of Oct-3/4 defines differentiation, dedifferentiation or self-renewal of ES cells. Nat Genet 24(4):372–376

Novotny GW, Sonne SB, Nielsen JE et al (2007) Translational repression of E2F1 mRNA in carcinoma in situ and normal

testis correlates with expression of the miR-17-92 cluster. Cell Death Differ 14(4):879–882
Oakes CC, La Salle S, Smiraglia DJ, Robaire B, Trasler JM (2007) A unique configuration of genome-wide DNA methylation patterns in the testis. Proc Natl Acad Sci USA 104(1):228–233
Ogunbiyi JO, Shittu OB, Aghadiuno PU, Lawani J (1996) Seminoma arising in cryptorchid testes in Nigerian males. East Afr Med J 73(2):129–132
Ohinata Y, Payer B, O'Carroll D et al (2005) Blimp1 is a critical determinant of the germ cell lineage in mice. Nature 436(7048):207–213
Ohm JE, McGarvey KM, Yu X et al (2007) A stem cell-like chromatin pattern may predispose tumor suppressor genes to DNA hypermethylation and heritable silencing. Nat Genet 39(2):237–242
Okamoto K, Kawakami T (2007) Epigenetic profile of testicular germ cell tumours. Int J Androl 30(4):385–392; discussion 92
Okita K, Ichisaka T, Yamanaka S (2007) Generation of germline-competent induced pluripotent stem cells. Nature 448(7151):313–317
Okumura-Nakanishi S, Saito M, Niwa H, Ishikawa F (2005) Oct-3/4 and Sox2 regulate Oct-3/4 gene in embryonic stem cells. J Biol Chem 280(7):5307–5317
Olie RA, Looijenga LHJ, Dekker MC, De Jong FH, De Rooij DG, Oosterhuis JW (1994) Growth of human seminoma cells on STO feeder depends on phenotype, presence of fetal calf serum and added growth factors. In: Jones WG, Harnden P, Appleyard I (eds) Advances in biosciences. Germ cell tumors III, vol 91. Pergamon, Oxford, pp 95–106
Olie RA, Looijenga LHJ, Boerrigter L et al (1995a) N- and KRAS mutations in human testicular germ cell tumors: incidence and possible biological implications. Genes Chromosomes Cancer 12:110–116
Olie RA, Looijenga LHJ, Dekker MC, De Jong FH, De Rooy DG, Oosterhuis JW (1995b) Heterogeneity in the in vitro survival and proliferation of human seminoma cells. Br J Cancer 71:13–17
Omisanjo OA, Biermann K, Hartmann S et al (2007) DNMT1 and HDAC1 gene expression in impaired spermatogenesis and testicular cancer. Histochem Cell Biol 127(2):175–181
Oosterhuis JW, Looijenga LH (2003) Current views on the pathogenesis of testicular germ cell tumours and perspectives for future research: highlights of the 5th Copenhagen Workshop on Carcinoma in situ and Cancer of the Testis. APMIS 111(1):280–289
Oosterhuis J, Looijenga L (2005) Testicular germ-cell tumours in a broader perspective. Nat Rev Cancer 5(3):210–222
Oosterhuis JW, Castedo SM, de Jong B et al (1989) Ploidy of primary germ cell tumors of the testis. Pathogenetic and clinical relevance. Lab Invest 60(1):14–21
Oosterhuis JW, Gillis AJM, Looijenga LHJ (1997) In vitro survival, RAS mutations, apoptosis and activation of the SAPK-pathway in human seminoma cells. In: Appleyard I (ed) Germ cell tumours IV, 1st edn. John Libbey, London, pp 51–57
Oosterhuis JW, Stoop H, Honecker F, Looijenga LHJ (2007) Why human extragonadal germ cell tumors occur in the midline of the body; old concepts, new perspectives. Int J Androl 30(4):256–263
Oram SW, Liu XX, Lee TL, Chan WY, Lau YF (2006) TSPY potentiates cell proliferation and tumorigenesis by promoting cell cycle progression in HeLa and NIH3T3 cells. BMC Cancer 6:154
Otto SP (2007) The evolutionary consequences of polyploidy. Cell 131(3):452–462
Ottolenghi C, Uda M, Crisponi L et al (2007) Determination and stability of sex. Bioessays 29(1):15–25
Page DC (1987) Hypothesis: a Y-chromosomal gene causes gonadoblastoma in dysgenetic gonads. Development 101 suppl:151–155
Pallesen G, Hamilton-Dutoit SJ (1988) Ki-1 (CD30) antigen is regularly expressed by tumor cells of embryonal carcinoma. Am J Pathol 133(3):446–450
Palmer RD, Foster NA, Vowler SL et al (2007) Malignant germ cell tumours of childhood: new associations of genomic imbalance. Br J Cancer 96(4):667–676
Palumbo C, Van Roozendaal K, Gillis AJM et al (2002) Expression of the PDGF alpha-receptor 1.5 kb transcript, OCT-4 and c-KIT in human normal and malignant tissues. Implications for early diagnosis of testicular germ cell tumors and understanding regulatory mechanisms. J Pathol 196:467–477
Pamenter B, De Bono JS, Brown IL et al (2003) Bilateral testicular cancer: a preventable problem? Experience from a large cancer centre. BJU Int 92(1):43–46
Peltomäki P (1991) DNA methylation changes in human testicular cancer. Biochim Biophys Acta 1096:187–196
Pera MF (2008) Stem cells. A new year and a new era. Nature 451(7175):135–136
Perlman EJ, Cushing B, Hawkins E, Griffin CA (1994) Cytogenetic analysis of childhood endodermal sinus tumors: a Pediatric Oncology Group study. Pediatr Pathol 14:-695–708
Perlman EJ, Valentine MB, Griffin CA, Look AT (1996) Deletion of 1p36 in childhood endodermal sinus tumors by two-color fluorescence in situ hybridization: a pediatric oncology group study. Genes Chromosomes Cancer 16:15–20
Perrett RM, Turnpenny L, Eckert JJ et al (2008) The early human germ cell lineage does not express SOX2 during in vivo development or upon in vitro culture. Biol Reprod 78(5):852–858
Pesce M, Scholer HR (2000) Oct-4: control of totipotency and germline determination. Mol Reprod Dev 55(4):452–457
Pesce M, Scholer HR (2001) Oct-4: gatekeeper in the beginnings of mammalian development. Stem Cells 19(4): 271–278
Przygodzki RM, Moran CA, Suster S et al (1996) Primary mediastinal and testicular seminomas: a comparison of K- ras-2 gene sequence and p53 immunoperoxidase analysis of 26 cases. Hum Pathol 27:975–979
Rachmilewitz J, Elkin M, Looijenga LHJ et al (1996) Characterization of the imprinted IPW gene: allelic expression in normal and tumorigenic human tissues. Oncogene 13:1687–1692
Rajpert-De Meyts E (2006) Developmental model for the pathogenesis of testicular carcinoma in situ: genetic and environmental aspects. Hum Reprod Update 12(3):303–323
Rajpert-De Meyts E, Jacobsen GK, Bartkova J et al (2003) The immunohistochemical expression pattern of Chk2, p53, p19INK4d, MAGE-A4 and other selected antigens provides

new evidence for the premeiotic origin of spermatocytic seminoma. Histopathology 42(3):217–226

Rajpert-De Meyts E, Toppari J, Hoi-Hansen CE, Muller J, Skakkebaek NE (2003) Testicular neoplasia in childhood and adolescence. Endocr Dev 5:110–123

Rajpert-De Meyts E, Hanstein R, Jorgensen N, Graem N, Vogt PH, Skakkebaek NE (2004) Developmental expression of POU5F1 (OCT-3/4) in normal and dysgenetic human gonads. Hum Reprod 19:1338–1344

Raman JD, Nobert CF, Goldstein M (2005) Increased incidence of testicular cancer in men presenting with infertility and abnormal semen analysis. J Urol 174(5):1819–1822; discussion 22

Rapley EA, Crockford GP, Teare D et al (2000) Localization to Xq27 of a susceptibility gene for testicular germ-cell tumours. Nat Genet 24(2):197–200

Rapley EA, Hockley S, Warren W et al (2008) Somatic mutations of KIT in familial testicular germ cell tumours. Genes Chromosomes Cancer 47:34–42

Reuter VE (2005) Origins and molecular biology of testicular germ cell tumors. Mod Pathol 18(suppl 2):S51–S60

Richie JP (2005) OCT4 staining in testicular tumors. A sensitive and specific marker for seminoma and embryonal carcinoma. J Urol 174(2):569–570; discussion 70

Ridanpaa M, Lothe RA, Onfelt A, Fossa S, Borresen AL, Husgafvel-Pursiainen K (1993) K-ras oncogene codon 12 point mutations in testicular cancer. Environ Health Perspect 101(suppl 3):185–187

Rodda DJ, Chew JL, Lim LH et al (2005) Transcriptional regulation of nanog by OCT4 and SOX2. J Biol Chem 280(26):24731–24737

Romanenko AM, Persidskii YV (1983) Ultrastructure and histogenesis of spermatocytic seminoma. Vopr Onkol 19:61–66

Rosenberg C, Mostert MC, Schut TB et al (1998) Chromosomal constitution of human spermatocytic seminomas: comparative genomic hybridization supported by conventional and interphase cytogenetics. Genes Chromosomes Cancer 23: 286–291

Rosenberg C, Van Gurp RJHLM, Geelen E, Oosterhuis JW, Looijenga LHJ (2000) Overrepresentation of the short arm of chromosome 12 is related to invasive growth of human testicular seminomas and nonseminomas. Oncogene 19: 5858–5862

Ross JA, Schmidt PT, Perentesis JP, Davies SM (1999) Genomic imprinting of H19 and insulin-like growth factor-2 in pediatric germ cell tumors. Cancer 85(6):1389–1394

Rossant J (2008) Stem cells and early lineage development. Cell 132(4):527–531

Runyan C, Schaible K, Molyneaux K, Wang Z, Levin L, Wylie C (2006) Steel factor controls midline cell death of primordial germ cells and is essential for their normal proliferation and migration. Development 133(24):4861–4869

Runyan C, Gu Y, Shoemaker A, Looijenga L, Wylie C (2008) The distribution and behavior of extragonadal primordial germ cells in Bax mutant mice suggest a novel origin for sacrococcygeal germ cell tumors. Int J Dev Biol 52(4): 333–344

Sakuma Y, Sakurai S, Oguni S, Hironaka M, Saito K (2003) Alterations of the c-kit gene in testicular germ cell tumors. Cancer Sci 94(6):486–491

Samaniego F, Rodriguez E, Houldsworth J et al (1990) Cytogenetic and molecular analysis of human male germ cell tumors: chromosome 12 abnormalities and gene amplification. Genes Chromosomes Cancer 1:289–300

Schneider DT, Schuster AE, Fritsch MK et al (2001) Genetic analysis of childhood germ cell tumors with comparative genomic hybridization. Klin Padiatr 213(4):204–211

Schneider DT, Schuster AE, Fritsch MK et al (2002) Genetic analysis of mediastinal nonseminomatous germ cell tumors in children and adolescents. Genes Chromosomes Cancer 34(1):115–125

Schneider DT, Calaminus G, Koch S et al (2004) Epidemiologic analysis of 1, 442 children and adolescents registered in the German germ cell tumor protocols. Pediatr Blood Cancer 42(2):169–175

Schnieders F, Dork T, Arnemann J, Vogel T, Werner M, Schmidtke J (1996) Testis-specific protein, Y-encoded (TSPY) expression in testicular tissues. Hum Mol Genet 5(11):1801–1807

Schubert S, Skawran B, Dechend F et al (2003) Generation and characterization of a transgenic mouse with a functional human TSPY. Biol Reprod 69(3):968–975

Scotting PJ (2006) Are cranial germ cell tumours really tumours of germ cells? Neuropathol Appl Neurobiol 32:569–574

Scully RE (1970) Gonadoblastoma. A review of 74 cases. Cancer 25:1340–1356

Scully RE (1978) Germ cell tumors. In: Scully RE (ed) Tumors of the ovary and maldeveloped gonads, 1st edn. Armed Forces of Pathology, Washington, D.C., pp 226–286

Shah MN, Devesa SS, Zhu K, McGlynn KA (2007) Trends in testicular germ cell tumours by ethnic group in the United States. Int J Androl 30(4):206–213; discussion 13–14

Shivakrupa R, Bernstein A, Watring N, Linnekin D (2003) Phosphatidylinositol 3'-kinase is required for growth of mast cells expressing the kit catalytic domain mutant. Cancer Res 63(15):4412–4419

Sievers S, Alemazkour K, Zahn S et al (2005a) IGF2/H19 imprinting analysis of human germ cell tumors (GCTs) using the methylation-sensitive single-nucleotide primer extension method reflects the origin of GCTs in different stages of primordial germ cell development. Genes Chromosomes Cancer 44:256–264

Sievers S, Alemazkour K, Zahn D et al (2005) Analysis of the IGF2/H19 imprinting status with the methylation sensitive single nucleotide primer extension method in human germ cell tumors reflects their origin from different stages of primordial germ cell development. Genes Chromosomes Cancer 44:256–264

Silva J, Smith A (2008) Capturing pluripotency. Cell 132(4): 532–536

Silva J, Chambers I, Pollard S, Smith A (2006) Nanog promotes transfer of pluripotency after cell fusion. Nature 441(7096): 997–1001

Skakkebæk NE (1972) Possible carcinoma-in-situ of the testis. Lancet 2(7776):516–517

Skakkebaek NE (2003) Testicular dysgenesis syndrome. Horm Res 60(suppl 3)49

Skakkebaek NE, Rajpert-De Meyts E, Jorgensen N et al (1998) Germ cell cancer and disorders of spermatogenesis: an environmental connection? APMIS 106(1):3–11; discussion 2

Skakkebæk NE, Rajpert-De Meyts E, Main KM (2001) Testicular dysgenesis syndrome: an increasingly common developmental disorder with environmental aspects. Hum Reprod 16(5):972–978

Skinner MK (2007) Epigenetic transgenerational toxicology and germ cell disease. Int J Androl 30(4):393–396; discussion 6–7

Skinner MK (2007b) Endocrine disruptors and epigenetic transgenerational disease etiology. Pediatr Res 61(5 Pt 2): 48R–50R

Skotheim RI, Kraggerud SM, Fossa SD et al (2001) Familial/bilateral and sporadic testicular germ cell tumors show frequent genetic changes at loci with suggestive linkage evidence. Neoplasia 3(3):196–203

Skotheim RI, Monni O, Mousses S et al (2002) New insights into testicular germ cell tumorigenesis from gene expression profiling. Cancer Res 62(8):2359–2364

Skotheim RI, Korkmaz KS, Klokk TI et al (2003a) NKX3.1 expression is lost in testicular germ cell tumors. Am J Pathol 163(6):2149–2154

Skotheim RI, Abeler VM, Nesland JM et al (2003b) Candidate genes for testicular cancer evaluated by in situ protein expression analyses on tissue microarrays. Neoplasia 5(5):397–404

Skotheim RI, Lind GE, Monni O et al (2005) Differentiation of human embryonal carcinomas in vitro and in vivo reveals expression profiles relevant to normal development. Cancer Res 65(13):5588–5598

Smiraglia DJ, Szymanska J, Kraggerud SM, Lothe RA, Peltomaki P, Plass C (2002) Distinct epigenetic phenotypes in seminomatous and nonseminomatous testicular germ cell tumors. Oncogene 21(24):3909–3916

Sonke GS, Chang S, Strom SS, Sweeney AM, Annegers JF, Sigurdson AJ (2007) Prenatal and perinatal risk factors and testicular cancer: a hospital-based case-control study. Oncol Res 16(8):383–387

Sonne SB, Kristensen DM, Novotny GW et al (2008) Testicular dysgenesis syndrome and the origin of carcinoma in situ testis. Int J Androl 31(2):275–287

Sontheimer EJ, Carthew RW (2005) Silence from within: endogenous siRNAs and miRNAs. Cell 122(1):9–12

Sperger JM, Chen X, Draper JS et al (2003) Gene expression patterns in human embryonic stem cells and human pluripotent germ cell tumors. Proc Natl Acad Sci USA 100:13350–13355

Starr JR, Chen C, Doody DR et al (2005) Risk of testicular germ cell cancer in relation to variation in maternal and offspring cytochrome p450 genes involved in catechol estrogen metabolism. Cancer Epidemiol Biomarkers Prev 14(9): 2183–2190

Stoop H, Van Gurp RHJ, De Krijger R et al (2001) Reactivity of germ cell maturation stage-specific markers in spermatocytic seminoma: diagnostic and etiological implications. Lab Invest 81:919–928

Stoop H, Honecker F, De Krijger R, Bokemeyer C, Looijenga HJ (2005) Differentiation and development of human female germ cells during prenatal gonadogenesis: an immunohistochemical study. Hum Reprod 20:1466–1476

Stoop H, Honecker F, Van de Geijn GJM et al (2008) Stem cell factor as novel diagnostic marker for early malignant germ cells. J Pathol 216(1):43–54

Strohmeyer T, Peter S, Hartmann M et al (1991) Expression of the hst-1 and c-kit protooncogenes in human testicular germ cell tumors. Cancer Res 51:1811–1816

Subramaniam K, Seydoux G (2003) Dedifferentiation of primary spermatocytes into germ cell tumors in *C. elegans* lacking the pumilio-like protein PUF-8. Curr Biol 13(2):134–139

Suda T, Arai F (2008) Wnt signaling in the niche. Cell 132(5):729–730

Suh MR, Lee Y, Kim JY et al (2004) Human embryonic stem cells express a unique set of microRNAs. Dev Biol 270(2): 488–498

Summersgill B, Osin P, Lu YJ, Huddart R, Shipley J (2001) Chromosomal imbalances associated with carcinoma in situ and associated testicular germ cell tumours of adolescents and adults. Br J Cancer 85(2):213–220

Suo G, Han J, Wang X, Zhang J, Zhao Y, Dai J (2005) Oct4 pseudogenes are transcribed in cancers. Biochem Biophys Res Commun 337(4):1047–1051

Surani MA (1994) Genomic imprinting: control of gene expression by epigenetic inheritance. Curr Opin Cell Biol 6: 390–395

Surani MA, Kothary R, Allen ND et al (1990) Genome imprinting and development in the mouse. Dev Suppl 110:89–98

Surani MA, Hayashi K, Hajkova P (2007) Genetic and epigenetic regulators of pluripotency. Cell 128(4):747–762

Susnerwala SS, Pande SC, Shrivastava SK, Dinshaw KA (1991) Dysgerminoma of the ovary: review of 27 cases. J Surg Oncol 46(1):43–47

Suzuki A, Raya A, Kawakami Y et al (2006) Maintenance of embryonic stem cell pluripotency by Nanog-mediated reversal of mesoderm specification. Nat Clin Pract Cardiovasc Med 3(suppl 1):S114–S122

Swanton C, Downward J (2008) Unraveling the complexity of endocrine resistance in breast cancer by functional genomics. Cancer Cell 13(2):83–85

Szabo PE, Mann JR (1995) Biallelic expression of imprinted genes in the mouse germ line: implications for erasure, establishment, and mechanisms of genomic imprinting. Genes Dev 9:1857–1868

Takada Y, Isono K, Shinga J et al (2007) Mammalian Polycomb Scmh1 mediates exclusion of Polycomb complexes from the XY body in the pachytene spermatocytes. Development 134(3):579–590

Takahashi H (1993) Cytometric analysis of testicular seminoma and spermatocytic seminoma. Acta Pathol Jpn 43: 121–129

Takahashi K, Yamanaka S (2006) Induction of pluripotent stem cells from mouse embryonic and adult fibroblast cultures by defined factors. Cell 126(4):663–676

Takahashi K, Tanabe K, Ohnuki M et al (2007) Induction of pluripotent stem cells from adult human fibroblasts by defined factors. Cell 131(5):861–872

Takao Y, Yokota T, Koide H (2006) Beta-catenin up-regulates Nanog expression through interaction with Oct-3/4 in embryonic stem cells. Biochem Biophys Res Commun 353(3):699–705

Takeda J, Seino S, Bell GI (1992) Human Oct3 gene family: cDNA sequences, alternative splicing, gene organization, chromosomal location, and expression at low levels in adult tissues. Nucleic Acids Res 20(17):4613–4620

Talerman A, Fu YS, Okagaki T (1984) Spermatocytic seminoma. Ultrastructural and microspectrophotometric observations. Lab Invest 51(3):343–349

Tate G, Suzuki T, Kishimoto K, Mitsuya T (2005) A c-KIT codon 816 mutation, D816H, in the testicular germ cell tumor: case report of a Japanese patient with bilateral testicular seminomas. Acta Med Okayama 59(1):33–36

Tewari K, Cappuccini F, Disaia PJ, Berman ML, Manetta A, Kohler MF (2000) Malignant germ cell tumors of the ovary. Obstet Gynecol 95(1):128–133

Toppari J, Larsen JC, Christiansen P et al (1996) Male reproductive health and environmental xenoestrogens. Environ Health Perspect 104(suppl 4):741–803

Toyooka Y, Shimosato D, Murakami K, Takahashi K, Niwa H (2008) Identification and characterization of subpopulations in undifferentiated ES cell culture. Development 135(5): 909–918

True LD, Otis CN, Delprado W, Scully RE, Rosai J (1988) Spermatocytic seminoma of testis with sarcomatous transformation. A report of five cases. Am J Surg Pathol 12(2): 75–82

Tycko B (1994) Genomic imprinting: mechanism and role in human pathology. Am J Pathol 144:431–443

Uhlenhaut NH, Treier M (2006) Foxl2 function in ovarian development. Mol Genet Metab 88(3):225–234

Van Berlo RJ, De Jong B, Oosterhuis JW, Dijkhuizen T, Buist J, Dam A (1990a) Cytogenetic analysis of murine embryo-derived tumors. Cancer Res 50:3416–3421

Van Berlo RJ, Oosterhuis JW, Schrijnemakers E, Schoots CJ, de Jong B, Damjanov I (1990b) Yolk-sac carcinoma develops spontaneously as a late occurrence in slow-growing teratoid tumors produced from transplanted 7-day mouse embryos. Int J Cancer 45(1):153–155

van Casteren NJ, Stoop H, Dohle GR, de Wit R, Oosterhuis JW, Looijenga LH (2008) Noninvasive detection of testicular carcinoma in situ in semen using OCT3/4. Eur Urol 54(1):153–158

Van Gurp RJLM, Oosterhuis JW, Kalscheuer V, Mariman ECM, Looijenga LHJ (1994) Human testicular germ cell tumors show biallelic expression of the H19 and IGF2 gene. J Natl Cancer Inst 86:1070–1075

van Schothorst EM, Mohkamsing S, van Gurp RJ, Oosterhuis JW, van der Saag PT, Looijenga LH (1999) Lack of Bcl10 mutations in testicular germ cell tumours and derived cell lines. Br J Cancer 80(10):1571–1574

Vasudevan KM, Burikhanov R, Goswami A, Rangnekar VM (2007) Suppression of PTEN expression is essential for anti-apoptosis and cellular transformation by oncogenic Ras. Cancer Res 67(21):10343–10350

Velasco A, Riquelme E, Schultz M et al (2004) Microsatellite instability and loss of heterozygosity have distinct prognostic value for testicular germ cell tumor recurrence. Cancer Biol Ther 3(11):1152–1158

Velasco A, Corvalan A, Wistuba II et al (2007) Mismatch repair expression in testicular cancer predicts recurrence and survival. Int J Cancer 122(8):1774–1777

Veltman I, Schepens MT, Looijenga LHJ, Strong LC, van Kessel AG (2003) Germ cell tumours in neonates and infants: a distinct subgroup. APMIS 111:152–160

Veltman I, Veltman J, Jeanssen I et al (2005) Identification of recurrent chromosomal aberrations in germ cell tumors of neonates and infants using genome-wide array-based comparative genomic hybridization. Genes Chromosomes Cancer 43:367–376

Verdorfer I, Rogatsch H, Tzankov A, Steiner H, Mikuz G (2004) Molecular cytogenetic analysis of human spermatocytic seminomas. J Pathol 204(3):277–281

Verhoeven RH, Coebergh JW, Kiemeney LA, Koldewijn EL, Houterman S (2007) Testicular cancer: trends in mortality are well explained by changes in treatment and survival in the southern Netherlands since 1970. Eur J Cancer 43(17):2553–2558

Verkerk AJ, Ariel I, Dekker MC et al (1997) Unique expression patterns of H19 in human testicular cancers of different etiology. Oncogene 14(1):95–107

Vogel T, Schmidtke J (1998) Structure and function of TSPY, the Y-chromosome gene coding for the "testis-specific protein". Cytogenet Cell Genet 80(1–4):209–213

Volkl TM, Langer T, Aigner T et al (2006) Klinefelter syndrome and mediastinal germ cell tumors. Am J Med Genet 140(5):471–481

von Eyben FE (2004) Chromosomes, genes, and development of testicular germ cell tumors. Cancer Genet Cytogenet 151(2):93–138

Voorhoeve PM, le Sage C, Schrier M et al (2006) A genetic screen implicates miRNA-372 and miRNA-373 as oncogenes in testicular germ cell tumors. Cell 124(6):1169–1181

Walsh J, Andrews PW (2003) Expression of Wnt and Notch pathway genes in a pluripotent human embryonal carcinoma cell line and embryonic stem cell. APMIS 111(1):197–210; discussion 1

Walsh TJ, Grady RW, Porter MP, Lin DW, Weiss NS (2006) Incidence of testicular germ cell cancers in U.S. children: SEER program experience 1973 to 2000. Urology 68(2):402–405; discussion 5

Walsh TJ, Dall'era MA, Croughan MS, Carroll PR, Turek PJ (2007) Prepubertal orchiopexy for cryptorchidism may be associated with lower risk of testicular cancer. J Urol 178(4):1440–1446

Walt H, Oosterhuis JW, Stevens LC (1993) Experimental testicular germ cell tumorigenesis in mouse strains with and without spontaneous tumours differs from development of germ cell tumours of the adult human testis. Int J Androl 16:267–271

Weir HK, Marrett LD, Kreiger N, Darlington GA, Sugar L (2000) Pre-natal and peri-natal exposures and risk of testicular germ-cell cancer. Int J Cancer 87(3):438–443

Welsh M, Saunders PT, Fisken M et al (2008) Identification in rats of a programming window for reproductive tract masculinization, disruption of which leads to hypospadias and cryptorchidism. J Clin Invest 118(4):1479–1490

Wermann H, Stoop H, Gillis AJM, Honecker F, Van Gurp RJHLM, Ammerpohl O, Richter J, Oosterhuis JW, Bokemeyer C, Looijenga LHJ. Global DNA methylation in fetal human germ cells and germ cell tumors: association with differentiation and cisplatin resistance. Journal of Pathol: in press.

Wernig M, Meissner A, Foreman R et al (2007) In vitro reprogramming of fibroblasts into a pluripotent ES-cell-like state. Nature 448(7151):318–324

Wienholds E, Plasterk RH (2005) MicroRNA function in animal development. FEBS Lett 579(26):5911–5922

Wilhelm D, Palmer S, Koopman P (2007) Sex determination and gonadal development in mammals. Physiol Rev 87(1):1–28

Wilkinson TJ, Colls BM, Schluter PJ (1992) Increased incidence of germ cell testicular cancer in New Zealand Maoris. Br J Cancer 65(5):769–771

Woodward PJ, Heidenreich A, Looijenga LHJ et al (2004) Testicular germ cell tumors. In: Eble JN, Sauter G, Epstein JI, Sesterhann IA (eds) World Health Organization Classification of tumours pathology and genetics of the urinary system and male genital organs. IARC, Lyon, pp 217–278

Wylie CC (1993) The biology of primordial germ cells. Eur Urol 23:62–67

Yan W, Kero J, Huhtaniemi I, Toppari J (2000) Stem cell factor functions as a survival factor for mature Leydig cells and a growth factor for precursor Leydig cells after ethylene dimethane sulfonate treatment: implication of a role of the stem cell factor/c-Kit system in Leydig cell development. Dev Biol 227(1):169–182

Yang F, Eckardt S, Leu NA, McLaughlin KJ, Wang PJ (2008) Mouse TEX15 is essential for DNA double-strand break repair and chromosomal synapsis during male meiosis. J Cell Biol 180(4):673–679

Yeager TR, DeVries S, Jarrard DF et al (1998) Overcoming cellular senescence in human cancer pathogenesis. Genes Dev 12(2):163–174

Youngren KK, Coveney D, Peng X et al (2005) The Ter mutation in the dead end gene causes germ cell loss and testicular germ cell tumours. Nature 435(7040):360–364

Zaehres H, Scholer HR (2007) Induction of pluripotency: from mouse to human. Cell 131(5):834–835

Zhang C, Kawakami T, Okada Y, Okamoto K (2005) Distinctive epigenetic phenotype of cancer testis antigen genes among seminomatous and nonseminomatous testicular germ-cell tumors. Genes Chromosomes Cancer 43(1):104–112

# Part II

# Diagnostic and Staging of Testicular Germ Cell Tumors

# Testicular Tumor Markers

# 3

Nathan Lawrentschuk and Damien M. Bolton

Tumor markers (TM) are usually proteins associated with a malignancy and might be clinically usable in patients with cancer. A TM can be detected in a solid tumor, in circulating tumor cells in peripheral blood, in lymph nodes, in bone marrow, or in other body fluids (ascites, urine, and feces). A TM may be used to define a particular disease entity; it may be used for diagnosis, staging, or population screening. Markers may also be used to detect the presence of occult metastatic disease, to monitor response to treatment, or to detect recurrent disease (Lindblom and Liljegren 2000).

More recently, the term biomarker has become commonplace in oncology. A biomarker is a biological molecule found in blood, other body fluids, or tissues that are a sign of a normal or abnormal process or of a condition or disease. A biomarker may be used to see how well the body responds to a treatment for a disease or condition. As such, biomarkers may overlap with TMs (National Cancer Institute 2009).

Although uncommon, testis cancer serves as a model for solid organ cancer treatment with an expectation of cure in all but very few cases. TMs including human chorionic gonadotropin (HCG), alpha fetoprotein (AFP), and lactate dehydrogenase (LDH) play an important role throughout the management of a disease from diagnosis through treatment response and early detection of relapse (Fleshner and Warde 2002). The importance of TMs in testicular cancer cannot be overemphasized. A clear role for these investigations has been delineated in the American Joint Commission on Cancer staging classification for testis cancer and in standard management algorithms (American Joint Commission on Cancer (AJCC) 2002; National Comprehensive Cancer Network 2009). In this chapter, these markers will be outlined at first in the context of their biology and then their relationship to each type of testicular malignancy. Immunohistochemical TM and future biomarkers will also be briefly outlined.

## 3.1 Tumor Markers in Testicular Cancer

A specific TM is a fusion protein associated with a malignant process in which an oncogene is translocated and fused to an active promoter of another gene. Nonspecific markers include the oncofetal proteins (such as the carcinoembryonic antigen or AFP) expressed by many different types of cancer (Lindblom and Liljegren 2000). It is this second type of TM that is used in testicular cancer. In the European Germ Cell Cancer Consensus group (EGCCCG) guidelines for the diagnosis and staging of germ cell cancer, TM are considered mandatory. This mandates that for seminoma and nonseminoma, AFP and HCG must be done, and to help identify those with metastatic disease LDH also must be done in addition (Table 3.1) (Krege et al. 2008).

AFP and HCG now have highly sensitive radioimmunoassays freely available (Waldmann and McIntire 1974), whereas LDH is an enzyme detected in the serum by catalytic concentration that is now also a routine investigation (Canal et al. 1980; von Eyben 2003). AFP and/or HCG are elevated in up to 80% of patients with nonseminomatous germ cell tumors; HCG is elevated in 15–30% of seminoma patients at the time of diagnosis and LDH is elevated in up to 80% of patients with advanced metastatic seminoma (Carver and Sheinfeld 2005; Trigo et al. 2000). An

N. Lawrentschuk (✉)
Department of Surgery, Urology Unit, Austin Hospital, University of Melbourne, Melbourne, Australia

M.P. Laguna et al. (eds.), *Cancer of the Testis*,
DOI: 10.1007/978-1-84800-370-5_3, 

**Table 3.1** The major serum tumor markers and their relationship to germ cell tumors

| Tumor marker | Seminoma | Nonseminoma |
|---|---|---|
| HCG | Raised in 15–30% (typically <300 IU) | Raised (up to 80%) |
| AFP | – | Raised (up to 80%) |
| LDH | Raised with metastatic disease (up to 80%) | Raised with metastatic disease (up to 80%) |

important point to recognize is that in the follow-up period after initial treatment, a rise in TM may precede the development of radiological or clinical disease (Wylie and Logue 1998). TM should be determined before orchiectomy and thereafter at weekly intervals until normalization.

All of the above mentioned TMs may be present in neoplastic and nonneoplastic conditions, and these are outlined in Table 3.2. It is also important to acknowledge that stable, low increases in serum AFP and HCG may not represent active disease. Careful repeat evaluation determines whether the markers increase. In such instances, if no significant change is noted after appropriate studies have been reviewed by an experienced practitioner, then consideration should be given to managing such cases with close surveillance to avoid unnecessary chemotherapy (Morris and Bosl 2000).

### 3.1.1 Human Chorionic Gonadotropin (HCG)

HCG is mainly used for the detection and monitoring of pregnancy and pregnancy-related disorders, but it is also an extremely sensitive and specific marker for trophoblastic tumors of placental and germ cell origin (Ballieux et al. 2008). HCG is a glycoprotein produced by the syncytiotrophoblasts and is increased in approximately 15% of pure seminomas and in 40% of advanced nonseminomas (Carver and Sheinfeld 2005). The serum half-life of HCG is approximately 24–48 h (Fakouri

**Table 3.2** Neoplastic and nonneoplastic conditions causing raised levels of the major serum tumor markers for germ cell tumors in males

| Elevations (male patients) | Neoplastic | Nonneoplastic | Additional management actions |
|---|---|---|---|
| HCG (Ballieux et al. 2008; Catalona et al. 1979; Fowler et al. 1982; Odell and Griffin 1987; Richie 1992; Wylie and Logue 1998) | Release of entrapped HCG from a tumor mass<br>Irregular forms of HCG produced by malignant tumors, e.g., liver, pancreas, stomach, lung, kidney, and bladder | Assay crossreactivity between the beta subunits of LH and HCG (especially in IgA-deficient patients)<br>Pituitary sources of HCG unrelated to tumor activity<br>Performance enhancing drugs<br>Marijuana<br>Reinfusion of peripheral blood stem cells containing high concentrations of HCG<br>Interference of additives to blood collection tubes | Exclude confounders on history, repeat assay if necessary |
| AFP (Doherty et al. 1997) | Hepatocellular, pancreatic, biliary, and gastric cancers | Processes involving the liver or biliary tree (hepatitis or cirrhosis) | Performance of routine liver function tests and hepatitis studies may be warranted to complement imaging to detect possible recurrent or persistent disease |
| LDH (Flores 2009; Kumar et al. 2003) | Any advanced cancer or high turnover tumor | Any disease causing tissue damage<br>Acute myocardial infarction, liver disease, lung disease, bowel infarction, autoimmune diseases | Exclude other diseases on history and examination ± further investigations |

and Coogan 2003). With complete tumor excision, even markedly elevated serum levels return to normal within 5–7 days (Vugrin et al. 1984) (Table 3.3).

### 3.1.2 Alpha Fetoprotein (AFP)

AFP is a glycoprotein produced primarily in the fetal yolk sac but also in the liver and gastrointestinal tract, and its secretion from germ cell tumors is restricted to nonseminomatous histology. Consequently any patients with histological pure seminomas and an increased serum AFP are classified and treated like those with nonseminomatous germ cell tumor. AFP is increased in approximately 60% of patients with metastatic nonseminoma and 20% of patients with clinical stage I nonseminoma (Carver and Sheinfeld 2005; Leisinger and Donohue 2002). The serum half-life of AFP is approximately 5–7 days (Fakouri and Coogan 2003). With complete tumor excision, elevated serum levels return to normal within 25–30 days (Table 3.3).

**Table 3.3** Typical tumor marker levels in patients being treated for testicular cancer

| * = Abnormal ** = Critical | | | | | | | | | | | |
|---|---|---|---|---|---|---|---|---|---|---|---|
| A. NON SEMINOMA PATIENT | | | | | | | | | | | |
| Date and Time | CEA | PSA | Fr PSA | PSA Ratio | HCG | AFP tu | HCG Tumour | LD | Testostrn | Ca125 |
| 20Aug08 1659 | | | | | | | | 223* | | |
| 20Aug08 1701 | | | | | | 1354* | | | | |
| 20Aug08 2014 | | | | | | | 103* | | | |
| 29Aug08 1249 | | | | | | 345* | 10* | 224* | | |
| 12Sep08 1238 | | | | | | | | 181 | | |
| 7Oct08 1014 | | | | | | 119* | 69* | 209 | | |
| 14Oct08 0949 | | | | | | 75* | 13* | 180 | | |
| 4Nov08 1005 | | | | | | 7* | < 1 | 268* | | |
| 18Nov08 0900 | | | | | | < 5 | < 1 | 251* | | |
| 9Jan09 0923 | | | | | | < 5 | < 1 | 253* | | |
| 9Jan09 1050 | | | | | | < 5 | < 1 | 291* | | |
| B. SEMINOMA PATIENT | | | | | | | | | | |
| Date and Time | CEA | PSA | Fr PSA | PSA Ratio | HCG | AFP tu | HCG Tumour | LD | Testostrn | Ca125 |
| 29Apr05 1008 | | | | | | < 5 | < 2 | 178 | | |
| 21Jun05 1417 | | | | | | < 5 | < 2 | 191* | | |
| 18Aug05 1256 | | | | | | < 5 | < 2 | 201* | | |
| 21Oct05 1134 | | | | | | < 5 | < 2 | 277* | | |
| 22Nov05 1033 | | | | | | < 5 | < 2 | 245* | | |
| 17Feb06 1059 | | | | | | < 5 | < 2 | 181 | | |
| 28Apr06 1021 | | | | | | < 5 | < 2 | 234* | | |
| 7Sep06 0940 | | | | | | < 5 | < 2 | 210* | | |
| 4Jan07 1338 | | | | | | < 5 | | 200* | | |
| 29Jun07 1204 | | | | | | < 5 | < 1 | 166 | | |
| 21Dec07 1141 | | | | | | < 5 | < 1 | 183 | | |
| 23Dec08 1157 | | | | | | < 5 | < 1 | 212 | 212 | 212 |

The nonseminoma patient has a drop as expected after orchiectomy. The seminoma patient had no raised markers but borderline LDH which is not uncommon. *AFP* alpha fetoprotein; *HCG* human chorionic gonadotropin; *LD* lactate dehydrogenase

Pure seminomas never express elevated AFP values. As for beta-HCG, AFP is not specific to testis cancer (Leisinger and Donohue 2002).

### 3.1.3 Lactate Dehydrogenase (LDH)

LDH is a protein enzyme that is known to be a useful marker for cell turnover and is often *raised* in malignancy. The enzyme is especially concentrated in the heart, liver, red blood cells, kidneys, muscles, brain, and lungs. Tissue levels are 500 times greater than those in serum, and thus even a small mass of damaged tissue causes leakage of enzyme and consequently increasing its level in serum significantly (1997; American Joint Commission on Cancer (AJCC) 2002). LDH is generally considered part of routine liver function tests because it is often raised in liver disease. The total LDH can be further separated into five components or fractions labeled by number: LDH-1, LDH-2, LDH-3, LDH-4, and LDH-5. In clinical practice the total LDH value is used for decision making.

Each of these fractions, called isoenzymes, is used mainly by a different set of cells or tissues in the body (Flores 2009). LDH elevation, especially LDH-1 elevation, is noted in patients with large volume disease of all histologic types of germ cell tumors, even in pure seminoma. Increases in serum LDH correlate with tumor burden, growth rate, and cellular proliferation. Elevation of LDH is present in approximately 60% of patients with advanced NSGCT and 80% of patients with metastatic seminoma. Since LDH levels correlate well with the tumor volume, they can be used as a risk factor to assess prognosis (Leisinger and Donohue 2002). The half life of isotype 1 is approximately 3 days (Smith et al. 1987). LDH is valuable as a marker in the surveillance of patients with advanced seminomas, in whom it is an indicator of tumor bulk (Bosl and Chaganti 1994). It can also provide some prognostic information: three multivariate analyses have shown it to be a significant prognostic factor independent of HCG or AFP concentration in both seminomas and teratomas (Birch et al. 1986). Therefore LDH should be measured routinely both preoperatively and in the follow up of patients with testicular germ cell tumors (Hughes and Bishop 1996) (Table 3.3). However, LDH in itself has limited sensitivity, specificity, and positive predictive value for detecting relapse of germ cell tumors; false-positive increases are common and should be interpreted cautiously (Venkitaraman et al. 2007).

## 3.2 Staging and Risk-Stratifying Germ Cell Tumors by Marker

In defining the clinical stage (CS) of a patient with a gonadal germ cell tumor, the American Joint Committee on Cancer (AJCC) has designated it as preferable staging by TNM classification (Table 3.4) (American Joint Commission on Cancer (AJCC)

**Table 3.4** The serum or S section of the AJCC TNM guidelines (American Joint Commission on Cancer (AJCC) 2002)

| S Stage under AJCC guidelines | | Serum tumor markers |
|---|---|---|
| Sx | | Serum marker studies not available or not performed |
| S0 | | Serum marker study levels within normal limits |
| LDH (U/l) HCG (mIU/mL) AFP (ng/mL) | | |
| S1 | | <1.5 × N and <5,000 and <1,000 |
| S2 | | 1.5–10 × N or 5,000–50,000 or 1,000–10,000 |
| S3 | | >10 × N or >50,000 or >10,000 |
| N indicates the upper limit of normal for the LDH assay | | |
| Stage I testicular cancer includes the following substages | | |
| Stage IA | pT1 | N0 M0 S0 |
| Stage IB | pT2, pT3, or pT4 | N0 M0 S0 |
| Stage IC | Any pT/TX | N0 M0 S1–3 |

2002). For verification of CS I disease, markers should be followed after orchiectomy until normalization is achieved. Patients without marker normalization after orchiectomy are defined as stage I S disease (Table 3.4). Patients with metastatic disease are classified according to the classification of the International Germ Cell Cancer Collaborative Group (IGCCCG) (Krege et al. 2008), which includes histology, location of primary tumor, location of metastases, and levels of AFP, b-HCG, and LDH after orchiectomy and before chemotherapy. In this instance markers serve as prognostic markers to categorize patients into "good," Intermediate," and "poor" prognosis groups (Table 3.5) (Krege et al. 2008). The individual treatment strategy is based on both the TNM classification and the IGCCCG classification of prognostic factors.

The TNM classification of GCT includes a separate category, S, for serum TM on top of the usual tumor (T), node (N), and metastasis (M) definitions; such is the importance of the TM (Table 3.3) (American Joint Commission on Cancer (AJCC) 2002).

## 3.3 Seminomatous Germ Cell Tumor

TM is not as important in seminoma because of the simple reason they are rarely raised. Seminoma in the nonmetastatic setting has raised HCG in only 15–30% of cases (markers of a typical seminoma patient are demonstrated in Table 3.3). However, having a raised HCG does not confer a worse prognosis than those HCG negative cases (Suzuki et al. 1998). It has been stated that LDH levels may be even more helpful in patients with seminoma, as only a minority have a raised HCG but half have a raised LDH value (but only usually in the metastatic setting) (Bartlett et al. 1991; Skinner and Scardino 1979).

## 3.4 Nonseminomatous Germ Cell Tumor

The utility of TM in nonseminoma cannot be understated, and they form the basis of risk-adapted strategies as well as the justification for surveillance and

**Table 3.5** IGCCCG prognostic grouping classification (1997)

| Prognosis | 5-year survival (%) | Nonseminoma | Seminoma |
|---|---|---|---|
| Good | 90 | Testis or primary extragonadal retroperitoneal tumor<br>And no nonpulmonary visceral metastases<br>And low markers<br>AFP <1,000 ng/mL<br>And HCG <1,000 ng/mL (<5,000 IU/l)<br>And LDH <1.5× normal level | Any primary localization<br>And no nonpulmonary visceral metastases<br>Any marker level |
| Intermediate | 75 | Testis or primary extragonadal retroperitoneal tumor<br>No presence of<br>Nonpulmonary visceral Metastases<br>And intermediate markers<br>AFP 1,000–10,000 ng/mL<br>And/or HCG 1,000–10,000 ng/mL (5,000–50,000 IU/l)<br>And/or LDH 1.5–10× normal level | Any primary localization<br>Presence of nonpulmonary visceral metastases (liver, CNS, bone, intestinum)<br>Any marker level |
| Poor | 50 | Primary mediastinal germ cell tumor with or without testis or<br>Primary retroperitoneal tumor<br>Presence of nonpulmonary visceral metastases (liver, CNS, bone, intestinum)<br>And/or "high markers"<br>AFP >10,000 ng/mL<br>And/or HCG >10,000 ng/mL (50,000 IU/l)<br>And/ or LDH >10× normal level | — |

early detection of relapse after definitive chemotherapy or surgery. Their role is further enhanced given the fact that up to 80% of patients have one or both HCG and AFP elevated. A raised LDH is noted in a similar percentage of metastatic cases (a typical responding case is outlined in Table 3.3). TM pattern at diagnosis is not a good predictor of the pattern at recurrence in patients with nonseminoma. TM assessment should be included in the follow-up schedule regardless of levels at the time of diagnosis. Early detection of recurrence should not rely only on marker levels, even in patients with elevated levels at presentation (Trigo et al. 2000).

## 3.5 Immunohistiochemical Tumor Markers

While discussing TM, it is also worth considering that immunohistochemical markers play an important role, particularly in the diagnosis of carcinoma in situ (CIS). At present, CIS is only detectable via biopsy. The tissue section needs to be of adequate size and be properly fixed. Evaluation must be supported by at least one solid immunohistochemical marker, such as placental alkaline phosphatase (PLAP), OCT-3/4 or AP-2c (Hoei-Hansen et al. 2007). As an example PLAP is normally produced by primordial germ cells and syncytiotrophoblasts. In testicular cancer, immunohistochemical markers are required only where mixed elements exist or in unusual cases where classic histological features are absent. When required, c-kit and OCT-3/4 are often utilized (Vilar et al. 2006). Oct-3/4 is interesting as it is expressed in all testicular germ cell tumors tested, even in CIS. Additionally, high levels have been suggested potentially to correlate with an increased malignant potential in CIS, but more definitive studies are required in the future (Gidekel et al. 2003).

## 3.6 Appropriate Use of Tumor Markers

With the valid and important role of testicular TM, one may ask if they are indeed used appropriately in practice. Gilbert et al. (Gilbert et al. 2008) in the USA investigated this very question using the SEER cancer registry where there was substantial variation in TM reporting for testis cancer. Approximately 50% of AFP and HCG results were either not performed or unknown, and LDH use was reported for only 21% of cases. In aggregate, all three TM were used in only 16% of patients with testis cancer. When a more liberal definition was applied (minimum of AFP and HCG), around half the cases had documentation of TM use. Because TMs are now an integral part of staging, less than half the patients identified in this SEER cohort would have been staged appropriately using the current AJCC staging classification (American Joint Commission on Cancer (AJCC) 2002). Indeed, it has been proposed that levels of TM assessment are a surrogate for the level of care provided for testis cancer (Bosl and Motzer 1997). This is because information obtained from the use of TMs impacts subsequent treatment and potentially the outcome in patients with testis cancer (Gilbert et al. 2008). Certainly the low rates of use identified within the SEER data set represent a potential quality of care concern that all physicians need to be aware of and address.

## 3.7 Future Biomarkers

The discovery of new biomarkers for both early detection and prognosis of cancer is critical to the hope of better clinical outcomes. Recently there has been an expanding understanding of the underlying molecular etiology of cancer. Consequently molecular targeted therapies for some particularly aggressive cancers such as renal cell carcinoma have been developed. Better understanding of the molecular etiology of cancer and identification of additional therapeutic targets remain important research goals (Tyson and Ornstein 2008).

Tumor biobanks are becoming commonplace and collecting and storing human tissue including blood, urine, and semen are important, particularly for germ cell tumors (Webster 2008). Recently, semen may have uncovered some future biomarkers of CIS (Hoei-Hansen et al. 2007) while seminal expression of NY-ESO-1 and MAGE-A4 are potential markers for testicular cancer (Satie et al. 2009). Studying circulating tumor cells in those patients having already undergone treatment is another target for biomarkers. The CD200 membrane glycoprotein (Moreaux et al. 2008) is one such target. Also, characterization of circulating tumor cell levels using full-length and caspase-cleaved cytokeratin 18 (CK18) is considered a biomarker for chemotherapy-induced cell death and is measured using a combination of the M30 and M65 ELISAs (de Haas et al. 2008). Others such as chemokines and G-protein coupled receptors responsible for the maintenance of adult stem cell niches may have a role in the future (Gilbert et al. 2009).

Over 30 years ago, it was recognized that the clarification of the biology of testicular tumors will provide the basis for future rational therapy (Jewett 1977). Markers have since formed and will continue to form an important part of this process.

## 3.8 Key Points Regarding Testicular Cancer and Tumor Markers

- TMs in testicular cancer have a role in diagnosis and staging to treatment and long-term follow-up.
- No TM is 100% sensitive to testicular tumor or 100% specific to testicular cancer. Imaging and history remain important if undetectable, and other malignant and benign conditions must always be excluded when a TM is raised.
- A rise in TMs may precede the development of radiological or clinical disease.
- The appropriate use of TM in testicular cancer patients may be seen as a surrogate of the level of oncological care being provided.

## References


(1997) International Germ Cell Consensus Classification: a prognostic factor-based staging system for metastatic germ cell cancers. International Germ Cell Cancer Collaborative Group. J Clin Oncol 15:594

American Joint Commission on Cancer (AJCC) (2002) AJCC cancer staging manual, 6th edn. Springer, New York

Ballieux BE, Weijl NI, Gelderblom H et al (2008) False-positive serum human chorionic gonadotropin (HCG) in a male patient with a malignant germ cell tumor of the testis: a case report and review of the literature. Oncologist 13:1149

Bartlett NL, Freiha FS, Torti FM (1991) Serum markers in germ cell neoplasms. Hematol Oncol Clin North Am 5:1245

Birch R, Williams S, Cone A et al (1986) Prognostic factors for favorable outcome in disseminated germ cell tumors. J Clin Oncol 4:400

Bosl GJ, Chaganti RS (1994) The use of tumor markers in germ cell malignancies. Hematol Oncol Clin North Am 8:573

Bosl GJ, Motzer RJ (1997) Testicular germ-cell cancer. N Engl J Med 337:242

Canal P, Bugat R, Soula G et al (1980) The measurement of total lactic dehydrogenase and its isoenzymes in solid tumours. Biomedicine 33:222

Carver BS, Sheinfeld J (2005) Germ cell tumors of the testis. Ann Surg Oncol 12:871

Catalona WJ, Vaitukaitis JL, Fair WR (1979) Falsely positive specific human chorionic gonadotropin assays in patients with testicular tumors: conversion to negative with testosterone administration. J Urol 122:126

de Haas EC, di Pietro A, Simpson KL et al (2008) Clinical evaluation of M30 and M65 ELISA cell death assays as circulating biomarkers in a drug-sensitive tumor, testicular cancer. Neoplasia 10:1041

Doherty AP, Bower M, Christmas TJ (1997) The role of tumour markers in the diagnosis and treatment of testicular germ cell cancers. Br J Urol 79:247

Fakouri B, Coogan C (2003) Testicular tumors. In: Saclarides TJ, Millikan K, Godellas C (eds) Surgical oncology: an algorithmic approach for the general surgeon. Springer, New York

Fleshner N, Warde P (2002) Controversies in the management of testicular seminoma. Semin Urol Oncol 20:227

Flores J (2009) Lactate dehydrogenase isoenzymes test. In: Net B (ed) Encyclopedia of Medicine. http://findarticles.com/p/articles/mi_g2601/is_0008/ai_2601000803 CBS Interactive Inc. Accessed 1 Dec 2009

Fowler JE Jr, Platoff GE, Kubrock CA et al (1982) Commercial radioimmunoassay for beta subunit of human chorionic gonadotropin: falsely positive determinations due to elevated serum luteinizing hormone. Cancer 49:136

Gidekel S, Pizov G, Bergman Y et al (2003) Oct-3/4 is a dose-dependent oncogenic fate determinant. Cancer Cell 4:361

Gilbert DC, Chandler I, McIntyre A et al (2009) Clinical and biological significance of CXCL12 and CXCR4 expression in adult testes and germ cell tumours of adults and adolescents. J Pathol 217:94

Gilbert SM, Daignault S, Weizer AZ et al (2008) The use of tumor markers in testis cancer in the United States: a potential quality issue. Urol Oncol 26:153

Hoei-Hansen CE, Olesen IA, Jorgensen N et al (2007) Current approaches for detection of carcinoma in situ testis. Int J Androl 30:398

Hughes O, Bishop M (1996) Lactate dehydrogenase should be used as marker in testicular tumours. BMJ 313:625

Jewett MA (1977) Biology of testicular tumors. Urol Clin North Am 4:495

Krege S, Beyer J, Souchon R et al (2008) European consensus conference on diagnosis and treatment of germ cell cancer: a report of the second meeting of the European Germ Cell Cancer Consensus group (EGCCCG): part I. Eur Urol 53:478

Kumar U, Sharan A, Kamal S (2003) Raised serum lactate dehydrogenase associated with gangrenous small bowel volvulus: a case report. Indian J Clin Biochem 18:6

Leisinger HJ, Donohue JP (2002) The role of retroperitoneal surgery in testis cancer. Crit Rev Oncol Hematol 44:71

Lindblom A, Liljegren A (2000) Regular review: tumour markers in malignancies. BMJ 320:424

Moreaux J, Veyrune JL, Reme T et al (2008) CD200: a putative therapeutic target in cancer. Biochem Biophys Res Commun 366:117

Morris MJ, Bosl GJ (2000) Recognizing abnormal marker results that do not reflect disease in patients with germ cell tumors. J Urol 163:796

National Cancer Institute (2009) Cancer dictionary, Washington, USA www.cancer.gov/dictionary. Accessed 1 Dec 2009
National Comprehensive Cancer Network (2009) Testicular cancer, Vol. 2. Available at www.nccn.org/professionals/physician_gls/PDF/testicular.pdf. Accessed 26 Mar 2009
Odell WD, Griffin J (1987) Pulsatile secretion of human chorionic gonadotropin in normal adults. N Engl J Med 317:1688
Richie J (1992) Neoplasms of the testis. Saunders, Philadelphia
Satie AP, Auger J, Chevrier C et al (2010) Seminal expression of NY-ESO-1 and MAGE-A4 as markers for the testicular cancer. Int J Androl, Epub
Skinner DG, Scardino PT (1979) Relevance of biochemical tumor markers and lymphadenectomy in management of non-seminomatous testis tumors: current perspective. Trans Am Assoc Genitourin Surg 71:31
Smith DA, Leung FY, Jablonsky G et al (1987) Determination, by radioimmunoassay, of the mass of lactate dehydrogenase isoenzyme 1 in human serum and of its rate of removal from serum after a myocardial infarction. Clin Chem 33:1863
Suzuki K, Nakazato H, Kurokawa K et al (1998) Treatment of stage I seminoma: should beta-HCG positive seminoma be treated aggressively? Int Urol Nephrol 30:593
Trigo JM, Tabernero JM, Paz-Ares L et al (2000) Tumor markers at the time of recurrence in patients with germ cell tumors. Cancer 88:162
Tyson DR, Ornstein DK (2008) Proteomics of cancer of hormone-dependent tissues. Adv Exp Med Biol 630:133
Venkitaraman R, Johnson B, Huddart RA et al (2007) The utility of lactate dehydrogenase in the follow-up of testicular germ cell tumours. BJU Int 100:30
Vilar E, Calvo E, Tabernero J (2006) Molecular biology of testicular germ cell tumors. Clin Transl Oncol 8:846
von Eyben FE (2003) Laboratory markers and germ cell tumors. Crit Rev Clin Lab Sci 40:377
Vugrin D, Friedman A, Whitmore WF Jr (1984) Correlation of serum tumor markers in advanced germ cell tumors with responses to chemotherapy and surgery. Cancer 53:1440
Waldmann T, McIntire K (1974) The use of radioimmunoassay for alpha-fetoprotein in the diagnosis of malignancy. Cancer 34(Suppl 4):1510
Webster P (2008) Biobanks. Canada launches massive study of adult cancer precursors. Science 320:1572
Wylie JP, Logue JP (1998) Pitfalls of hCG monitoring in stage I seminoma. Clin Oncol (R Coll Radiol) 10:131

# Radiographic Diagnosis and Staging

# 4

Maria De Santis, Mark Bachner, Nathan Lawrentschuk, Gregory S. Jack, and Damien M. Bolton

## 4.1 Introduction

This chapter focuses on the standard use of imaging techniques relevant to the diagnosis and staging of testicular carcinoma and highlights the pros and cons of the different imaging tools as well as staging pitfalls.

## 4.2 Diagnostic Imaging of the Testicle

### *4.2.1 Ultrasonography*

Ultrasonography (US) is the recommended imaging modality for the evaluation of testicular pathology (Wittenberg et al. 2006; Nachtsheim et al. 1983; Kim et al. 2007). It is nearly 100% sensitive for the detection of intratesticular tumors (Guthrie and Fowler 1992; Carroll and Gross 1983; Howlett et al. 2000) and it can detect tumors that are nonpalpable and only a few millimeters in size (Horstman et al. 1994; Glazer et al. 1982) (Fig. 4.1). In the setting of a suspected testicular mass, ultrasound should be used to confirm the diagnosis and evaluate the contralateral testis (Sanchez and Mahlin 1986). Testicular ultrasound is also useful in the search of nonpalpable testicular tumors, serial examination of high risk testicles, and surgical planning in the setting of testis surgery (Nachtsheim et al. 1983). Testicular tumors may occasionally present with pain or a history of trauma, and approximately 10–15% are detected incidentally during ultrasonography of the acute scrotum (Wittenberg et al. 2006; Dogra et al. 2003).

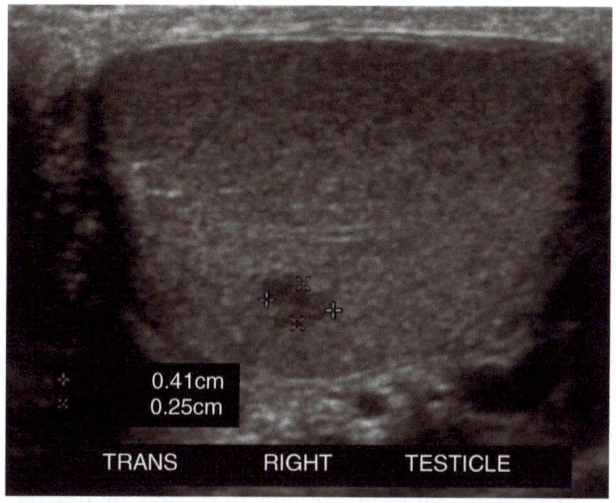


**Fig. 4.1** Sonogram of a 4 mm nonpalpable testicular lesion which turned out to be seminoma

Ultrasonography is performed using high-frequency sound waves emitted from a portable transducer and aimed at the intended tissues - in this case the testes. The sonographic images may be produced in any anatomic plane by adjusting the orientation of the transducer. As the acoustic waves pass through the testis, they are reflected, refracted, and absorbed by the infrastructure of the scrotum and testis prior to returning to the receiver probe where they are processed and ultimately displayed in several ways including gray-scale, duplex Doppler, and color Doppler diagnostic images (Dogra et al. 2003). Solid structures within the testis that reflect more acoustic waves than normal are termed hyperechoic and appear brighter on the monitor. Structures that reflect less acoustic waves are hypoechoic. Water and cysts are anechoic since they do not reflect any acoustic waves.


M. De Santis (✉)
Center for Oncology and Hematology, Ludwig Boltzmann Institute for Applied Cancer Research, Vienna, Austria



M.P. Laguna et al. (eds.), *Cancer of the Testis*,
DOI: 10.1007/978-1-84800-370-5_4, © Springer-Verlag London Limited 2010

Ultrasound frequencies are measured in one million cycles per second and referred to as megahertz (MHz). As the frequency of a transducer is increased, the wavelength of the emitted waves decreases and the resolution of the imaging improves. "High" frequency probes (typically ≥5 MHz) yield the greatest spatial resolution in tissue, but have limited depth of tissue penetration due to the shorter sound waves. Low frequency probes (<3.5 MHz) emit longer sound waves to allow deeper tissue penetration such as required for the adult abdomen, but the result is lower resolution. Since the testis and scrotum are superficial, high frequency transducers in the range of 7.5–12 MHz are used, and at these frequencies, they provide extremely detailed resolution of the returning echoes from the intratesticular contents.

Doppler ultrasound is a variant that records the movement of the acoustic echoes and allows for detection and characterization of intratesticular blood flow. While Doppler is primarily used in the diagnosis of testicular torsion, Doppler settings can occasionally provide additional information that can supplement the gray-scale findings of an intratesticular mass, particularly in the differentiation between tumors and hematomas (Varsamidis et al. 2001; Atkinson et al. 1992). In some instances, Doppler has successfully been used to distinguish between inflammatory and malignant lesions (Horstman et al. 1992). While experiments have examined the use of contrast agents for vascular ultrasonography, there is no role for contrast ultrasonography in the setting of testicular ultrasound.

In performing a testicular ultrasound, the testis should be examined in the transverse and longitudinal planes. The asymptomatic testis should be examined first to adjust the gain and Duplex settings for maximal visualization prior to examining the affected side. The size and echogenicity of the affected side should be compared to the normal testis, and any palpable lesions should be examined with a finger placed under the nodule and the transducer placed directly on the nodule (Howlett et al. 2000).

Compared to alternative imaging modalities, ultrasound has the advantages of being portable, noninvasive, and inexpensive (Schwerk et al. 1987; Benson et al. 1989; Rifkin et al. 1985). US limitations are rare, but on occasion, the ultrasound examination may be limited by the patient's body habitus or other physical conditions that preclude firm transducer contact with the scrotum (Howlett et al. 2000). While the sensitivity of ultrasound is near perfect in the detection of pathology, intratesticular mimics of malignancy such as abscesses, orchitis, and hematomas may occasionally confound the examiner. It is therefore important to correlate US findings with clinical history. Even if an infectious process is highly likely, it is important to follow up the testis with an additional ultrasound to exclude a tumor and document resolution of the abnormal process. Rarely, additional modalities such as MRI, CT, or nuclear imaging may aid in the uncertain diagnosis, but most commonly the radiographic diagnosis is made with repeat ultrasound. Equivocal testicular masses have to be explored surgically (inguinal exploration) (Albers et al. 2006).

#### 4.2.1.1 Normal and Abnormal US Findings

The normal adult testis is approximately 3–5 cm long, 2–3 cm thick, and ovoid in shape (Akin et al. 2004). A prepubertal testicle is much smaller at 1–2 cm length. On sonogram, the testis has a homogeneous medium echo level and is easily differentiated from the epididymis anatomically. Gray-scale imaging of normal testicular parenchyma demonstrates a "speckled" texture representing the seminiferous tubules, which fill the testis, and are separated into lobes by hyperechoic fibrous septa and covered by a hyperechoic testicular capsule called the tunica albuginea (Fig. 4.2). Simple cysts are a common finding in the testicular parenchyma and appear anechoic (black) and thin-walled and have distal acoustic shadowing. No further follow-up is required once a diagnosis of simple cyst is made. Outside the testicular parenchyma lies the isoechoic epididymis, which sits posterior and lateral to the testicle and connects the testicle to the vas deferens.

Testicular tumors as a rule are located within the testicular parenchyma, but large lesions may extend into the epididymis and up the spermatic cord. Lesions that are located solely outside of the testis are not testicular cancer by definition, but can on occasion represent rare malignancies, such as paratesticular sarcomas. On gray-scale imaging, testicular tumors are of variable sizes and shapes, but they are characteristically hypoechoic compared to normal parenchyma. On Doppler imaging, these lesions can be hyper - or hypovascular. As a general rule, the Doppler vascularity

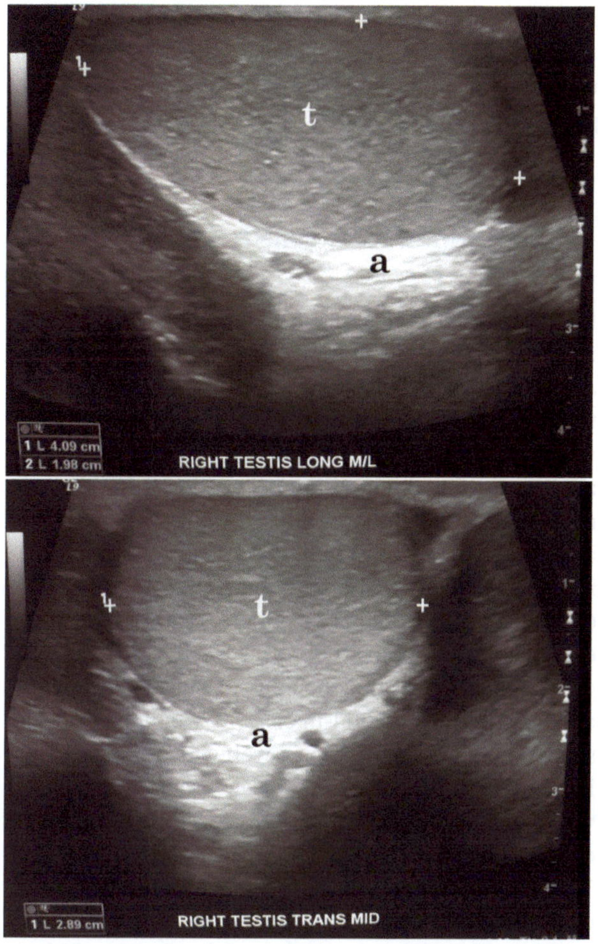


**Fig. 4.2** Normal testicular ultrasound in longitudinal and transverse sections. Normal testis (t) has a speckled echotecture and is surrounded by a dense tunica albuginea (a) capsule

within a testicular tumor depends more on the tumor size than any other criteria. Studies show that lesions <1.5 cm have decreased vascularity, while lesions >1.5 cm typically demonstrate increased blood flow, regardless of histology (Varsamidis et al. 2001; Horstman et al. 1992). It is very difficult to predict tumor histology based strictly on sonographic criteria (Nachtsheim et al. 1983; Kim et al. 2007); however, certain "textbook" sonographic patterns are described.

*Seminomas* are classically well defined tumors with sharply demarcated sonographic borders. They tend to be round to oval in shape on US, and they are hypoechoic and homogeneous compared to the surrounding normal testicular parenchyma (Nachtsheim et al. 1983) (Fig. 4.3). Seminomas classically do not have cystic areas or foci of calcification on US

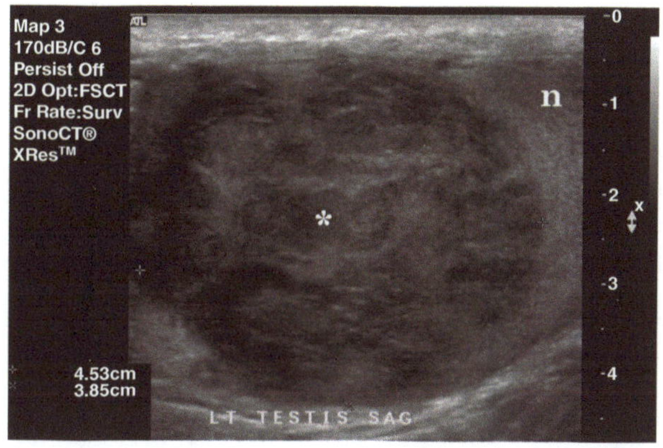


**Fig. 4.3** Sonogram of a pure seminoma (*asterisk*) which is hypoechoic clearly demarcated from the normal (n) parenchyma

(Fig. 4.3). *Embryonal, chorioncarcinoma, and yolk-sac tumors* all have similar appearances to each other and cannot be distinguished from one another. Typically they are all hypoechoic, but as a group they tend to be more heterogeneous and poorly demarcated compared to seminomas. Sonographically, the nonseminomatous germ cell tumors frequently show cystic areas of necrosis (30%), focal hyperechoicity, and acoustic shadowing due to hemorrhage (Nachtsheim et al. 1983) (Fig. 4.4). Embryonal carcinomas are more likely to distort the testis and have tunica vaginalis invasion (Grantham et al. 1985). *Teratomas* sonographically appear as a well defined mass. Internally, they may have an inhomogeneous echo texture containing cystic areas, calcification, and shadowing representative of the mixture of cysts, cartilage, and fibrous components of the teratoma (Grantham et al. 1985; Benson 1988). *Stromal tumors* are highly variable in appearance. Smaller Sertoli and Leydig tumors tend to be hypoechoic, while some larger tumors may have a complex architecture composed of necrosis and hemorrhage (Mazlin et al. 2004). Leydig cell tumors may have circumferential blood flow on Doppler US (Mazlin et al. 2004).

*Lymphomas* appear hypoechoic and homogeneous and frequently bilateral (Nachtsheim et al. 1983). They may present as a well defined mass or as a completely infiltrating tumor that replaces the entire parenchyma. Doppler ultrasound typically demonstrates increased vascularity to the mass regardless of tumor size (Mazzu et al. 1995). Cysts and areas of necrosis as well as hemorrhage are rare in lymphoma. *Leukemia* has a

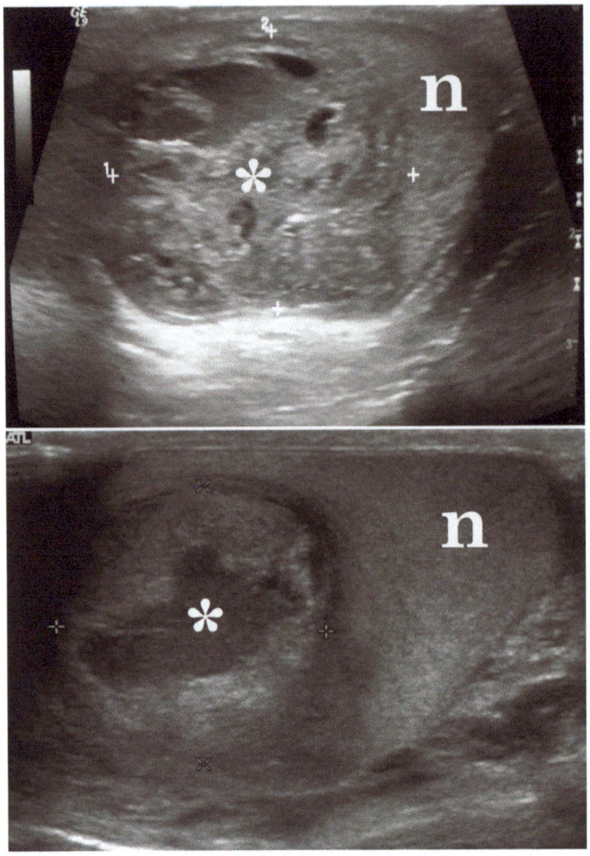


**Fig. 4.4** Sonograms of different nonseminomatous germ cell tumors (*asterisk*) displacing normal (n) testicular parenchyma. The tumors are hypoechoic and demonstrate necrosis, hemorrhage, and cystic spaces. The *top image* contained mixed choriocarcinoma, teratoma, and seminoma on pathology. The *bottom image* was predominantly embryonal

similar sonographic appearance to lymphoma and is often bilateral. In patients with lymphoma and leukemia, ultrasound can serve as an important marker in assessing the efficacy of chemotherapy, or in the detection of early recurrence (Fuse et al. 1990).

Rarely, patients present with advanced disease without a recognizable primary tumor in the testis on physical exam. Some of these may *be extragonadal germ cell tumors (EGCTs)*, whereas others may represent a nonpalpable or a burned-out primary testicular tumor (Scholz et al. 2002). Testicular ultrasound is a crucial diagnostic component in the work-up of EGCT, and all patients with a presumed diagnosis of EGCT require a formal testicular ultrasound to rule out a nonpalpable primary lesion or a burned-out testicular tumor. Evidence of a burned-out primary tumor typically appears as a small echogenic focus within the testis that demonstrates acoustic shadowing within normal parenchyma but lacks a tissue or vascular component (Glazer et al. 1982; Shawker et al. 1983).

## 4.2.2 Magnetic Resonance Imaging

MRI can be useful as a problem solving tool if the ultrasonographic images are of suboptimal quality or if a discrepancy between the clinical and sonographic findings arises (Kubik-Huch et al. 1999). MRI can identify various lesions in the testis and can occasionally aid in the differentiation between a solid testis mass and an inflammatory or fibrotic lesion. MRI is also the recommended imaging modality for identifying and evaluating intrabdominal undescended testis (Kim et al. 2007). Otherwise there is no major difference between the sensitivity of US and MRI.

Malignant as well as benign solid testicular tumors are characterized by mid-intense T1-weighted (fat sensitive) signals, which compare well with normal testicular tissue, and T2-weighted (water sensitive) signals, which are lower than that of normal testis tissue (Hricak et al. 1995). The tunica albuginea is best defined on T2-weighted images as a low-intensity line (Noone et al. 1997). Gadolinium enhancement has not proven to add any information for characterizing lesions (Hricak et al. 1995; Cramer et al. 1991), but it helps to differentiate the epididymis from the testis on T2-weighted images.

As with ultrasound, primary tumor grading and staging is possible with MRI with only moderate accuracy. On MRI, pure seminomas are characterized by a homogeneous hypo-intense T2-weighted signal without a capsule, whereas NSGCTs produce a heterogeneous T2-weighted hypo-intense signal with a capsule (Fig. 4.5). A variety of exceptions to these rules, however, do not permit reliable differentiation of benign from malignant tumors or seminoma from NSGCTs with sufficient certainty. For instance, necrosis may cause heterogenic areas within seminomas and mimic NSGCT (Hricak et al. 1995; Cramer et al. 1991; Johnson et al. 1990; Oyen et al. 1993) and inflammatory reactions can mimic tumor infiltration of the spermatic cord. Tumor infiltration into the tunica albuginea, which generates a consistently low signal, is difficult to differentiate on MRI (Baker et al. 1987). As a result,

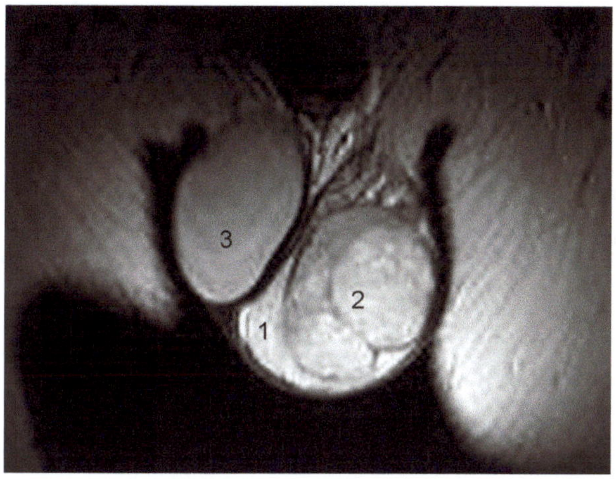


**Fig. 4.5** T2-weighted testicular MRI. *1*: Normal testicular tissue. *2*: Inhomogeneous, mainly hyperintense tumor, histologically classical seminoma. *3*: Hypo-intense testicular prosthesis

the staging accuracy of testicular primaries with MRI is between 63 and 87% (Johnson et al. 1990; Thurnher et al. 1988). In the case of an extragonadal primary tumor and suspected cryptorchidism or testicular agenesis, MRI is superior to palpation and ultrasonography, especially if the ectopic location is the abdominal cavity rather than the inguinal canal.

## 4.3 Radiographic Staging

### 4.3.1 Staging Techniques

Thorough imaging of chest, abdomen, and pelvis are required to complete the work-up and staging of a newly diagnosed testicular tumor. Together with tumor marker levels, radiographic staging provides the basis for tumor staging according to the UICC- and IGCCCG-classifications (Pollock et al. 2004; International Germ Cell Cancer Collaborative 1997) (Tables 4.1 and 4.2).

CT is the imaging modality of choice for evaluation of the chest, abdomen, and pelvis (Dalal et al. 2006). In some centers, CT of the chest is replaced by plain-films of the chest in the setting of negative abdominal scans (see below). MRI has not shown any superiority compared to CT with regard to radiographic staging (Ellis et al. 1984). However, MRI has the advantage that it does not deliver ionizing radiation and that it can be used whenever CT is contraindicated. US is not a useful staging modality.

### 4.3.2 Abdominal and Pelvic Imaging

*Abdominal CT* is the procedure of choice for evaluation of the abdominal viscera and staging of the retroperitoneal lymph nodes. In addition, CT also provides anatomic and functional information about the kidneys and surrounding soft tissues and crucial information about tumor soft tissue and vascular invasion relevant for surgical planning. CT imaging for testis cancer patients should be performed with oral and intravenous contrast as a standard procedure, provided renal and thyroid functions permit its use. Problems and pitfalls when intravenous contrast is omitted are listed below. They are mainly caused by the misinterpretation of vessels due to anatomic variants within the expected tumor landing zones (Royal and Callen 1979; Moul et al. 1992; Dixon et al. 1986; Brener et al. 1974; Pick and Anson 1940; Dubowitz 1997; Bass et al. 2000; Meanock et al. 1988).

Possible anatomic variants include:

1. Variable prevalences of a circumaortic and retroaortic left renal vein
2. Supernumerary left renal vein
3. Doubled vena cava
4. Normal asymmetry of common iliac veins (left common iliac vein larger with an at least twofold difference)
5. Insufficiently opacified bowel loops
6. Anatomic variant of the testicular veins.

The distribution of retroperitoneal lymph node metastases in testicular carcinoma patients follows the lymphatic drainage of the testis. Left sided testicular primaries are expected to metastasize first to the left renal hilar nodes, the pre- and paraaortic (upper part) and left common iliac regions, whereas pre-, para-, and interaortocaval as well as right common iliac node groups are considered to be the primary lymphatic spread of right sided testicular tumors (Ray et al. 1974; Donohue et al. 1982; Mason et al. 1991; Bradey et al. 1987; Bosl and Motzer 1997) (Fig. 4.6a, b).

Modern CT scanners can identify lymph node deposits along paraaortic landing zones, including all

**Table 4.1** TNM-classification of germ cell tumors (Stephenson et al. 2005)

| | |
|---|---|
| Primary tumor (T) | |
| pTX | Primary tumor cannot be assessed |
| pT0 | No evidence of primary tumor |
| pTis | Intratubular germ cell neoplasia (carcinoma in situ) |
| pT1 | Tumor limited to the testis and epididymis without vascular/lymphatic invasion; tumor may invade into the tunica albuginea but not the tunica vaginalis |
| pT2 | Tumor limited to the testis and epididymis with vascular/lymphatic invasion, or tumor extending through the tunica albuginea with involvement of the tunica vaginalis |
| pT3 | Tumor invades the spermatic cord with or without vascular/lymphatic invasion |
| pT4 | Tumor invades the scrotum with or without vascular/lymphatic invasion |
| Regional lymph nodes (R) | |
| *Clinical* | |
| NX | Regional lymph nodes cannot be assessed |
| N0 | No regional lymph node metastasis |
| N1 | Metastasis with a lymph node mass 2 cm or less in greatest dimension; or multiple lymph nodes, none more than 2 cm in greatest dimension |
| N2 | Metastasis with a lymph node mass more than 2 cm but not more than 5 cm in greatest dimension; or multiple lymph nodes, any one mass greater than 2 cm but not more than 5 cm in greatest dimension |
| N3 | Metastasis with a lymph node mass more than 5 cm in greatest dimension |
| *Pathologic (pN)* | |
| pNX | Regional lymph nodes cannot be assessed |
| pN0 | No regional lymph node metastasis |
| pN1 | Metastasis with a lymph node mass 2 cm or less in greatest dimension and less than or equal to five nodes positive, none more than 2 cm in greatest dimension |
| pN2 | Metastasis with a lymph node mass more than 2 cm but not more than 5 cm in greatest dimension; or more than five nodes positive, none more than 5 cm; or evidence of extranodal extension of tumor |
| pN3 | Metastasis with a lymph node mass more than 5 cm in greatest dimension |
| Distant metastasis (M) | |
| MX | Distant metastasis cannot be assessed |
| M0 | No distant metastasis |
| M1 | Distant metastasis |
| M1a | Nonregional nodal or pulmonary metastasis |
| M1b | Distant metastasis other than to nonregional lymph nodes and lungs |
| Serum tumor markers (S) | |
| SX | Marker studies not available or not performed |
| S0 | Marker study levels within normal limits |
| S1 | LDH <1,5 × UNL and hCG (mIU/mL) <5,000 and AFP (ng/mL) <1,000 |
| S2 | LDH 1,5–10 × UNL or hCG (mIU/mL) 5,000–50,000 or AFP (ng/mL) 1,000–10,000 |
| S3 | LDH >10 × UNL or hCG (mIU/mL) >50,000 or AFP (ng/mL) >10,000 |

**Table 4.2** Prognostic classification according to the IGCCCG 1997 (Moul et al. 1992)

| Groups | Nonseminoma | Seminoma |
|---|---|---|
| *Good prognosis* | *56% of cases* | *90% of cases* |
| Five-year progression-free survival | 89% | 82% |
| Five-year survival | 92% | 86% |
| With all of | Testis/retroperitoneal primary<br>No nonpulmonary visceral metastases<br>AFP <1,000 ng/mL and<br>hCG <5,000 mIU/L (1,000 ng/mL) and<br>LDH <1,5× upper limit of normal | Any primary site<br>No nonpulmonary visceral metastases<br>Normal AFP<br>Any hCG<br>Any LDH |
| *Intermediate prognosis* | *28% of cases* | *10% of cases* |
| Five-year progression-free survival | 75% | 68% |
| Five-year survival | 80% | 73% |
| With all of | Testis/retroperitoneal primary<br>No nonpulmonary visceral metastases<br>AFP ≥1,000 and ≤10,000 ng/mL or<br>hCG ≥5,000 and ≤50,000 mIU/L or<br>LDH >= 1,5 and ≤10× upper limit of normal | Any primary site<br>Nonpulmonary visceral metastases<br>Normal AFP<br>Any hCG<br>Any LDH |
| *Poor prognosis* | *16% of cases* | *No patients classified as poor prognosis* |
| Five-year progression-free survival | 41% | |
| Five-year survival | 48% | |
| With any of | Mediastinal primary<br>Nonpulmonary visceral metastases<br>AFP > 10,000 ng/mL or hCG > 50,000 mIU/L or LDH > 10× upper limit of normal | |

the way up to the crus of the diaphragm, and it can identify individual lymph nodes in these crucial locations. The size of normal retroperitoneal lymph nodes in healthy people varies substantially (6–20 mm) due to methodological differences and variations in size at different anatomic locations (Leibovitch et al. 1995; Lien et al. 1986). The combined measurement of long and short diameters of the largest lymph nodes in different retroperitoneal regions did not add to accuracy (Forsberg et al. 1986). Thresholds for physiologic minimum (short axis) diameters in different anatomic locations are shown in Table 4.3. Usually, the short diameter on axial sections is used, although no consensus has been defined so far for standard measurements of retroperitoneal lymph nodes. In clinical studies different measurements have been used and their pro and cons have extensively been discussed (World Health Organization 1979; Therasse et al. 2000; Jaffe 2006). CT diagnosis is not only based on size. In the literature several criteria have been discussed controversially. The following were among them: the shape and the potential absence of a fatty center, inhomogeneities, strong enhancement after contrast administration reflecting hypervascularization, which may be due to tumor or inflammation (Lien et al. 1987). The strongest correlation of CT-enlarged retroperitoneal nodes with malignancy, however, is their location within the primary landing zone (Leibovitch et al. 1995).

The staging accuracy of CT scans at presentation of stage I and II GCT is about 70% (Lien et al. 1986; Fernandez et al. 1994; Donohue et al. 1995; Stephenson et al. 2005). Of all clinical stage II patients 20–30% turn out to be stage I pathologically, whereas 30% of clinical stage I patients are understaged by CT (Donohue et al. 1995; Gatti and Stephenson 1998).

Paraaortic lymph nodes of >10 mm are suspect of metastatic involvement in any case of GCT. A cut-off value as low as 4 mm (short axis) has been suggested for paraaortic nodes anterior to the midportion of the

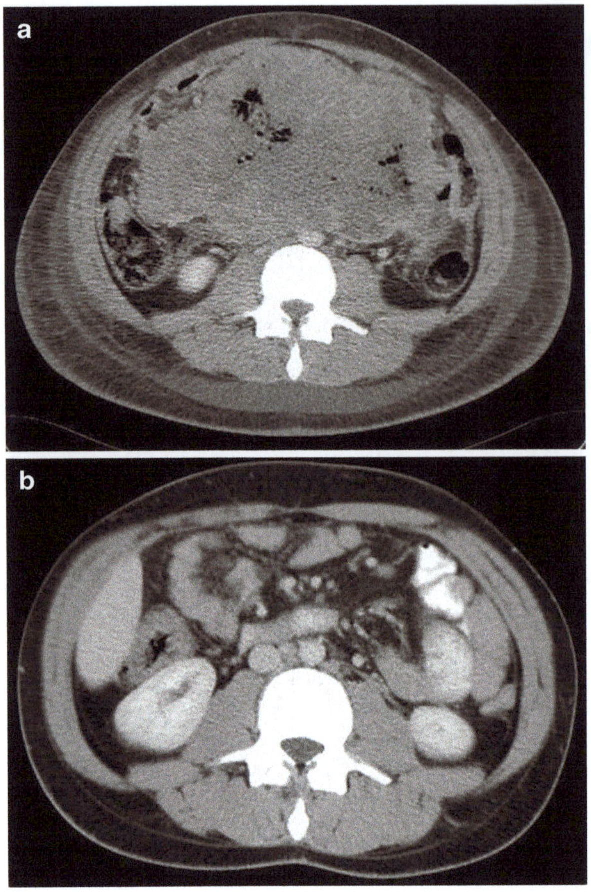

**Fig. 4.6** Abdominal CTs with i.v. and oral contrast. (**a**) Bulky retroperitoneal disease at presentation (intermediate prognosis). High image noise due to intensive care unit conditions and distinctive anasarca of patient. (**b**) Same patient after four courses of cisplatin-containing chemotherapy. Partial remission, tumor-marker negative, histologically necrosis and mature teratoma at residual tumor resection

aorta in patients with NSGCT (Forsberg et al. 1986; Hilton et al. 1997; Dorfman et al. 1991) (Table 4.4). Other authors suggested a repeat CT scan after 6–8 weeks following the detection of 8–10 mm retroperitoneal lymph nodes in the ipsilateral landing zone (Leibovitch et al. 1995; Stephenson and Sheinfeld 2005). In such cases the additional radiation burden should be weighed against the diagnostic and therapeutic benefit.

In summary, any number of nodes within the expected primary/ ipsilateral landing zone, irrespective of their size, should raise serious suspicion of occult metastases (Leibovitch et al. 1995; Lien et al. 1986; Fernandez et al. 1994; Hilton et al. 1997; Donohue et al. 1993; Stomper et al. 1987; Moul 1995).

The prevalence of *pelvic nodes* in testicular cancer patients is low (only 8%) and the additional radiation burden of a pelvic CT scan is high with an increase of the effective dose equivalent (EDE) by 2.6 mSv (74%). In a retrospective analysis bulky abdominal disease was found to be the strongest single risk factor. Therefore, CT of the pelvis should be included only in the primary staging procedures. Further pelvic CT scans for restaging and follow-up are recommended only for patients at high risk of pelvic disease (Ray et al. 1974; Mason et al. 1991; White et al. 1997; MacVicar 1993). Previous inguinal or scrotal surgery is a known risk factor for the uncommon spread to the inguinal and pelvic nodes (White et al. 1997; Busch et al. 1965). Retroperitoneal hematoma following bleeding from an inappropriately ligated vessel at orchidectomy is a possible source of false-positive pelvic CT findings (Page et al. 1990; Kullmann and Lien 1987; Tran et al. 1989).

**Table 4.3** After Prokop 2003, page 623 (Wood et al. 1996)

| Location | Threshold diameter (mm) |
|---|---|
| Retrocrural nodes | 6 |
| Gastrohepatic nodes | 8 |
| Pancreaticoduodenal nodes | 10 |
| Mesenteric nodes | 10 |
| High preaortic and celiac nodes | 10 |
| Paraaortocaval nodes | 11 |

**Table 4.4** Abdominal CT for GCT staging according to size cut-off and relation to the abdominal aorta: after Hilton et al. (1997); (Choi et al. 2000)

| Node size: cut-off (mm) | Specificity (%) | Sensitivity (%) |
|---|---|---|
| >10 | 37 | 100 |
| >8 | 47 | 100 |
| >6 | 67 | 83 |
| >4 | 93 | 58 |

### 4.3.3 Chest and Mediastinal Imaging

Posteroanterior and lateral chest radiographs should be performed in all patients with a new diagnosis of testicular cancer. These films provide initial evaluation of the lung parenchyma and mediastinal structures for metastatic disease. CXR is generally sufficient for staging of the chest in the setting of low suspicion of pulmonary disease (See and Hoxie 1993), although many advocate the use of CT Chest in place of CXR. Opponents of routine chest CT scan argue that screening all patients with testicular cancer with chest CTs will increase false-positive chest CT results and lead to unnecessary reevaluations with CT scanning associated with an increase in the radiation dose delivered or the risks of invasive procedures (Lien et al. 1986; Naidich et al. 1998).

In a study comparing staging with CXR vs. CT Chest in 120 patients with testicular cancer, tomography detected only one case (0.8%) of lung involvement that was not detected on conventional chest plain films (Jochelson et al. 1984). Another study compared chest computerized tomography to chest X-ray on the basis of abnormal CT scan findings in 92 patients with testis cancer. The authors found that in patients with negative abdominal CT, the chest CT failed to increase diagnostic sensitivity above chest radiography alone. Importantly, however, in patients with positive abdominal masses, chest CT identified abnormalities missed on routine, standard chest radiography alone. As a result, these authors concluded that CXR is the preferred initial staging study in patients with negative abdominal imaging, while CT chest is mandatory in patients with pathology detected on abdominal imaging (See and Hoxie 1993).

Many authorities including the European Association of Urology recommend a chest CT be obtained routinely in all patients with NSGCT histology (Albers et al. 2006; Schmoll et al. 2004) (Fig. 4.7), as it is estimated that 17–25.7% of NSGCT patients harbor intrathoracic disease (See and Hoxie 1993; Lien et al. 1988; White et al. 1999; Williams et al. 1987), and 10% have isolated intrathoracic involvement (Cagini et al. 1998). In the setting of negative tumor markers, a clear retroperitoneum, and suspected lung metastases, all pulmonary nodules, regardless of their size, are suspect and require biopsy. Only calcified foci are a safe exception to this rule (Fig. 4.8a, b).

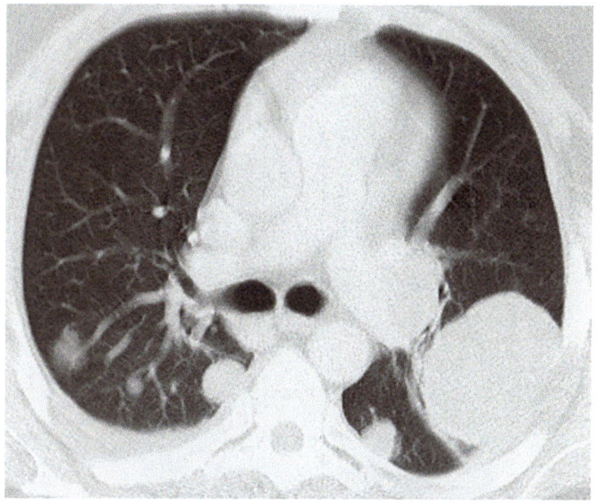

**Fig. 4.7** Chest CT with i.v. and oral contrast; lung window. NSGCT with poor prognosis; multiple intrapulmonary lesions

The most common sites of supradiaphragmatic nodal involvement are the paraesophageal, subcarinal, and posterior mediastinal areas (Meyer and Conces 2002; Wood et al. 1996). The association with pulmonary metastases is seen in 12–25% of patients (White et al. 1999; Cagini et al. 1998), whereas isolated mediastinal involvement is relatively uncommon in NSGCT (9%). It is, however, more frequently seen in pure SGCT (Williams et al. 1987).

A normal-sized lymph node in all thoracic regions has been reported to be 10 mm with one exception: subcarinal lymph nodes with a 12 mm short axis have been rated as the upper limit of normal (Naidich et al. 1998). Measurement of intrathoracic lymph nodes is usually based on the short-axis diameter, as it is the use in the retroperitoneum. Chest CT for diagnosing metastases of GCT has excellent sensitivity but relatively poor specificity with an overall accuracy that does not exceed 70%. The advantages and draw backs of plain chest X-rays vs. chest CTs for staging have been extensively discussed in the literature (Moul 1995; MacVicar 1993; See and Hoxie 1993; Lien et al. 1988; White et al. 1999).

Pure seminomas (SGCT) are the most common malignant GCT of the mediastinum. They may contain small low density areas due to hemorrhage or necrosis within usually large homogeneous masses (Marchevsky and Kaneko 1992; Nichols 1991; Lee et al. 1989) (Fig. 4.9a, b). Hemorrhage and necrosis are common

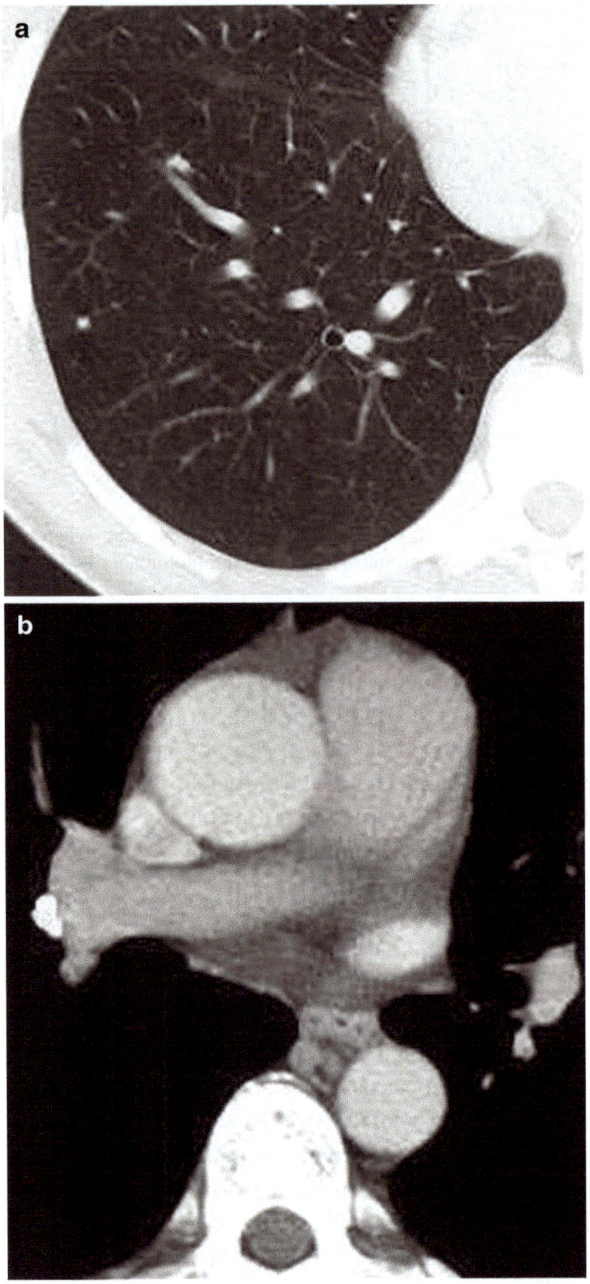

Fig. 4.8 Chest CT with i.v. and oral contrast. Patient with stage Ib NSGCT. (**a**) Small pulmonary lesions at follow-up. (**b**) Same patient. Calcified hilus lymph node, supporting the hypothesis of nonrecent tuberculosis rather than pulmonary metastases

and sometimes responsible for up to 50% of the tumor volume in NSGCT (Rosado-de-Christenson et al. 1992; Levitt et al. 1984).

In the setting of an EGCT, CT imaging of the chest on rare occasions may uncover a primary lesion, typically within the mediastinum. Primary mediastinal germ cell tumors are defined by the absence of a gonadal and retroperitoneal tumor manifestation (Williams et al. 1987; Nichols 1991). CT of the chest is the diagnostic tool of choice for diagnosis. MRI has no specific role for routine staging of the mediastinum. Primary mediastinal GCT mostly emerge in the anterior mediastinum within or adjacent to the thymic gland.They are rarely located in the posterior mediastinum. Mature teratomas can also be found in the mediastinum as primary tumors (Marchevsky and Kaneko 1992; Nichols 1991; Brown and Aughenbaugh 1991). These are typically well defined masses with cystoid components of low density and fatty tissue in about half of the cases (Naidich et al. 1998; Brown and Aughenbaugh 1991; Suzuki et al. 1983). Calcifications are typical features, followed by fat/fluid levels (Brown and Aughenbaugh 1991; Fulcher et al. 1990; Seltzer et al. 1984). Soft tissue is usually not the major component of a mediastinal mature teratoma

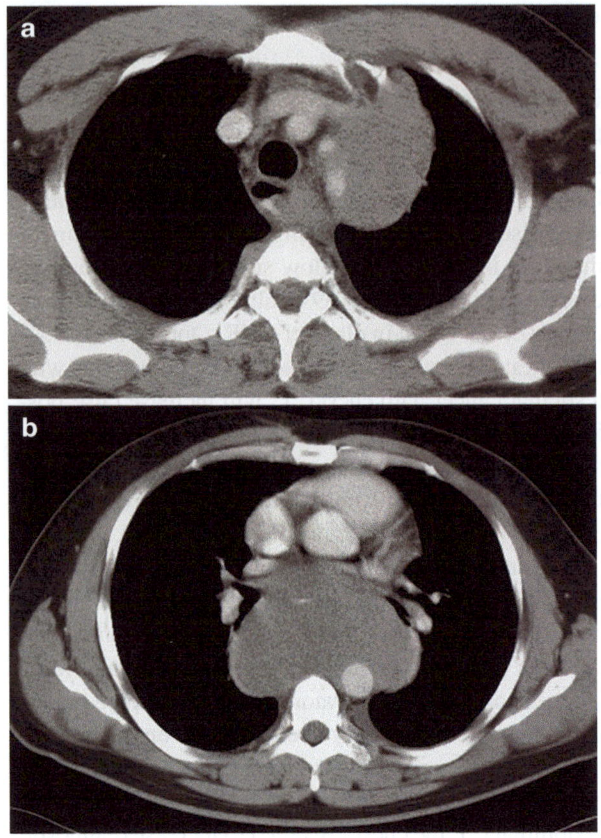

Fig. 4.9 Chest CT with i.v. and oral contrast. Primary mediastinal seminoma. (**a**) Mass in the anterior mediastinum. (**b**) Posterior mediastinal mass

(Rosado-de-Christenson et al. 1992). The presence of all three components, fat, fluid, and calcifications within a single mediastinal lesion allows a high degree of histologic certainty that teratoma is present. The growth pattern of malignant teratomas can be very aggressive with infiltration of the chest wall and metastatic spread (Lee et al. 1989; Rosado-de-Christenson et al. 1992; Levitt et al. 1984).

*Chest CT pitfalls*: including normal structures and variants and different coincidental conditions:

1. Thymic hyperplasia (for thymic rebound phenomenon)
2. Normal pericardial recesses mistaken for nodal metastases (both structures may be low density) (White et al. 1999)
3. Large transverse sinus of the superior pericardium simulating a paratracheal lymph node (Choi et al. 2000)
4. Posterior pericardial recess and oblique sinus of the pericardium simulating a low-density subcarinal or paraesophageal node (Budoff et al. 2000)
5. The cisterna chyli (Gollub and Castellino 1996)
6. Coincidental presence of *sarcoidosis:*

Typical findings on chest CT (better still on high-resolution CT) images that are sources of potential errors in GCT imaging, but *suspicious of sarcoidosis,* are (Webb et al. 2000)

- Small, well defined nodules in relation to the pleural surfaces, interlobular septa, centrilobular structures
- Large nodules (>1 cm) or consolidation
- Lymph node enlargement, usually symmetrical.

## 4.3.4 Brain Imaging

CNS imaging is not recommended in all GCT patients, but only in those with neurologic signs and symptoms (Bosl and Motzer 1997) as well as in asymptomatic patients with "intermediate" or "poor" prognosis according to the IGCCCG classification (International Germ Cell Cancer Collaborative Group) (International Germ Cell Cancer Collaborative 1997). Patients with histologic evidence of chorionic carcinoma in addition to poor prognostic features carry increased risk of cerebral metastases (Hartmann et al. 1999; Kollmannsberger et al. 2000).

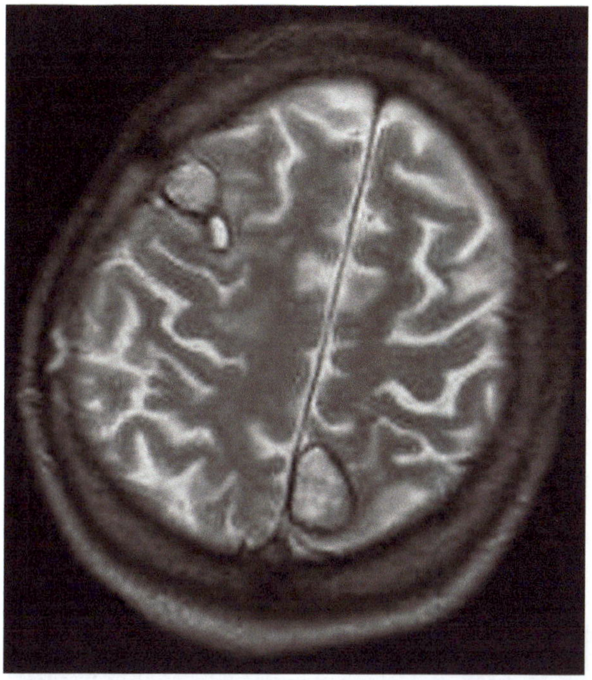

**Fig. 4.10** T2-weighted MRI of the brain. Three brain metastasis, surrounded by hemosiderin deposits due to hemorrhage

CNS metastases occur in only 1% of all GCT patients and in 10% of those with advanced disease. MRI of the CNS is the diagnostic method of choice. Advantages of MRI (Fig. 4.10) for CNS imaging compared to CT (Fig. 4.11) are the higher sensitivity (Davis et al. 1991) and, therefore, the chance to detect additional small lesions as well as the radioprotection of the ocular lens. The detection of brain metastases at initial staging in GCT patient has an important role compared to other tumor entities because the long-term survival rate of these patients with adequate treatment is up to 30–40% (Bokemeyer et al. 1997; Fossa et al. 1999).

## 4.3.5 Skeletal Imaging

There is no role for routine skeletal surveys in patients with testicular cancer. In the event of advanced disease and symptomatic bone pain, a bone scan or skeletal series may aid in the diagnosis of bone metastases, however these lesions are very rare (Dalal et al. 2006).

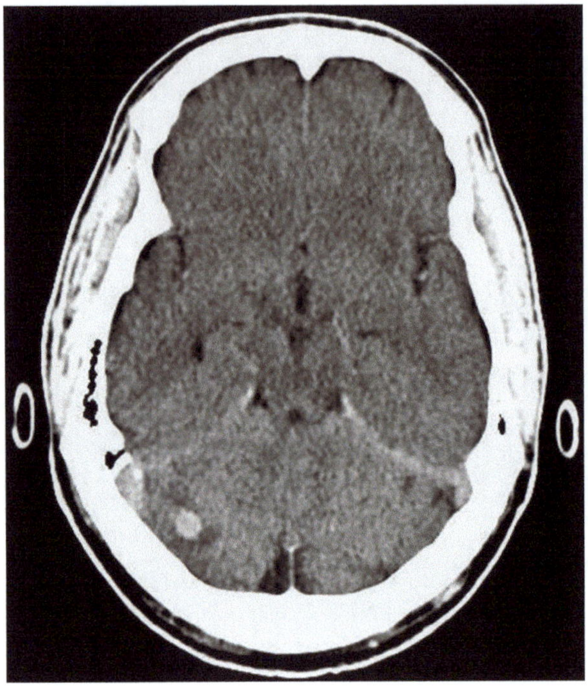

**Fig. 4.11** Brain CT. Contrast-enhancing metastasis and perifocal edema

### *4.3.6 Visceral Organ Imaging*

CT scanning of the abdomen is the standard diagnostic tool for abdominal visceral staging as mentioned above. CT of the abdomen is useful for the detection of hydronephrosis, bowel obstruction, vascular invasion, and visceral organ metastases including the liver. *Liver metastases* in NSGCT are known to carry poor prognosis (International Germ Cell Cancer Collaborative 1997). They occur in about 6%. Patients with poor prognostic features (Table 4.2) or advanced bulky disease should be carefully examined to make sure that liver involvement is not missed. According to the European Guidelines (Schmoll et al. 2004) MRI provides the best imaging of the liver and may be useful in the characterization of unclear lesions in the liver, especially in the case of uncertainties or in order to clarify specific questions. Whenever the liver lesion is the only poor prognostic feature and would therefore prompt a different classification and treatment strategy, the diagnosis should be established by a biopsy, provided the lesion is accessible. Standard MRI protocols for the liver include the administration of gadolinium chelate. Metastases from GCT may vary in their MRI appearance even within one and the same patient due to different histologic components. According to Semelka et al., the main advantage of MRI imaging of the liver is that it collects many different types of data (Semelka and Helmberger 2001). Therefore, it is the imaging technique with the strongest likelihood of detecting liver metastases of different sizes and histologic components. In comparisons of current MRI with current CT techniques, MRI has been rated as being more accurate than CT for detecting liver metastases (Semelka et al. 1996; Vassiliades et al. 1991). Gray-scale and Doppler ultrasound of the liver has poor sensitivity and specificity for detecting liver metastases. Some investigators have experimented with contrast enhanced ultrasound techniques using microbubbles and are reporting results comparable to CT (Albrecht et al. 2004), however, further studies are required and this is not a recommended staging modality at this time.

## 4.4 Role of Positron Emission Tomography (PET) in Germ Cell Tumors (GCT)

$^{18}$F-FDG PET relies on the uptake and metabolism of glucose which distinguishes metabolically active from inactive cells. Thus there is potential to differentiate viable cancer from nonviable tissue (necrosis or fibrosis) making it a useful tool in the staging and monitoring of tumor response to therapy (Bomanji et al. 2001). Most data involving PET and germ cell tumors is in the field of monitoring response to therapy particularly in seminoma (Kollmannsberger et al. 2002) whilst tumor markers and CT are well-established methods in the same setting. CT offers information on size and anatomy of residual masses but provides limited functional information. CT may aid decision-making following chemotherapy when combined with tumor markers and initial histology (Steyerberg et al. 2000); however, CT is a poor predictor of viability of residual masses (Kollmannsberger et al. 2002). The ability to identify and predict tumor activity is the main advantage provided by $^{18}$F-FDG PET.

European Association of Urology guidelines on testicular cancer recommend (PET) in metastatic seminoma after chemotherapy (Albers et al. 2006) citing it as a valid tool with which to detect vital residual tumor based on numerous studies (De Santis et al. 2004; Johns Putra et al. 2004; Becherer et al. 2005). The picture is not so clear in NSGCT with regard to PET. Although the efficacy of chemotherapy in NSGCT can be measured by documenting the reduction of markers (Wilson et al. 1995), such markers are unlikely to replace imaging because of the relatively high number of tumors with negative markers. The relapsed tumor can also differ biologically, with marker-negative relapses occurring even in cases where the tumor was initially positive (Stephens et al. 1996). In approximately 50% of patients who have residual masses following chemotherapy for NSGCT, the masses will have only necrotic or fibrous tissue.(Steyerberg et al. 1995; Stenning et al. 1998) A diagnostic tool that is more accurate at predicting the composition of postchemotherapy masses would spare selected patients potentially unnecessary surgery that carries high morbidity(Beck et al. 2002). Unfortunately PET has not proven to be definitive and offer unambiguous information over CT because of the inconsistent uptake of teratoma and confusion with fibrosis (Rutherford et al. 2006), giving a high positive predictive value but low negative predictive value (Johns Putra et al. 2004).

### 4.4.1 Tracers in GCT

In oncology, 2-$^{18}$fluoro-2-deoxy-D-glucose (FDG) is currently the most widely used tracer because it selectively accumulates in cancer cells. On account of regionally increased blood flow and elevated activity of glucose transporters (GluT1) and intracellular hexokinase, cancer cells are avid glucose seekers. $^{18}$F-substitution at the C2 of the glucose structure turns $^{18}$FDG-6-phosphate into a polar molecule, which cannot be further metabolized and, as cancer cells contain little glucose-6-phosphatase, is trapped in them. These mechanisms contribute to distinguishing active tumor from nonneoplastic cells by its increased tracer uptake (Bomanji et al. 2001; Lienhard et al. 1992; Nabi and Zubeldia 2002).

#### 4.4.1.1 Physiologic FDG Uptake

FDG also actively accumulates in normal tissues of the brain, the myocardium, the liver, the smooth muscles, and the bone marrow and is eliminated along renal and urinary pathways. Three-dimensional imaging and iterative reconstruction help to differentiate these superimposed structures from neoplastic tissue (Vesselle and Miraldi 1998).

PET–CT is now the gold standard providing simultaneously obtained CT and PET images which may then delineate the exact anatomic location of the lesion with a resolution of 5 mm.

### 4.4.2 False-Positive FDG PET Results

High FDG uptake is not totally tumor-specific. It is well known that inflammatory and granulomatous tissue such as sarcoidosis show extensive tracer uptake caused by elevated macrophage activity (Cremerius et al. 1998; Nuutinen et al. 1997; Strauss 1996). This is also true for inflammatory reactions up to several months after irradiation (Engenhart et al. 1992; Haberkorn et al. 1991). Active $^{18}$F-FDG uptake by phagocytes within abscesses or by granulation tissue surrounding abscesses causes false-positive results, whereas chemically sterile abscesses do not accumulate FDG (Kubota et al. 1992). Macrophage accumulation due to resorption of necrotic post-treatment tumor tissue will cause false-positive FDG PET studies. Most importantly, there may be a metabolic flare within the first days after chemotherapy. Therefore, PET should not be performed too early in germ cell residual tumors after chemotherapy, i.e., within 2–4 weeks postchemotherapy (Nuutinen et al. 1997; Cohade and Wahl 2002; Hain et al. 2000).

### 4.4.3 False-Negative FDG PET Results

The timing of PET studies is of utmost importance in GCT. FDG uptake by neoplastic tissue may be reduced within 2 weeks of exposure to cytostatics (Cremerius et al. 1998). This phenomenon is tumor- and treatment specific. The size of the lesions to be evaluated is important as well. Due to the limited resolution we do not expect FDG PET to be positive in low-volume disease, e.g., lesions <5 mm. But PET may detect extremely active lesions between 5 and 10 mm in size (Wilson et al. 1995; Albers et al. 1999; Cremerius et al. 1999; Hofer et al. 2001; Muller-Mattheis et al. 1998; Spermon et al. 2002; Tsatalpas et al. 2002; de Wit et al. 2005).

## 4.4.4 PET for Diagnosis of Testicular Tumors

At present FDG PET has no role in addition to ultrasound in the primary diagnosis of testicular tumor (Kitajima et al. 2007). Interestingly, PET was used to diagnose an NSGCT in a patient with elevated tumor markers despite a left orchidectomy and negative imaging (testicular ultrasound and CT). Significant pathological FDG uptake in the right testis was found and histology confirmed a teratoma and embryonal carcinoma (Wolf et al. 2003).

## 4.4.5 PET for Noninvasive Tumor Staging

Consistent prospective data have established the clinical role of FDG PET in oncology particularly for staging nonsmall-cell lung cancer, colorectal cancer, and melanoma, for evaluating single pulmonary lesions, for detecting liver metastases, and for staging cancers with unknown primaries (Bomanji et al. 2001; Nabi and Zubeldia 2002; Eary 1999; Hustinx et al. 1998; Lowe et al. 1998; Moog et al. 1998; Regelink et al. 2002). In Non-Hodgkin's lymphoma and Hodgkin's disease PET has become crucial for staging, treatment evaluation, early detection of relapse, and most recently for distinguishing aggressive and indolent disease (Spaepen et al. 2002; Jerusalem et al. 1999, 2003; Kostakoglu et al. 2002; Schoder et al. 2005; Juweid et al. 2005).

## 4.4.6 FDG PET in Germ Cell Tumors (GCT)

Germ cell tumors as well as their secondaries are generally characterized by high FDG uptake. This very fact led to extensive investigations to elucidate the clinical role of FDG PET in GCT.

For clear metastatic disease on conventional CT with or without elevated tumor markers, there is no clinical need for additional staging tools. As for clinical stage I or equivocal clinical stage II disease, additional information would be helpful to decide the appropriate treatment strategies.

## 4.4.7 PET for Staging at Presentation

### 4.4.7.1 Nonseminomatous and Seminomatous Germ Cell Tumors (NSGCT and SGCT)

The role of FDG PET in initial staging in unselected NSGCT and SGCT patients was the subject of investigation in several trials (Wilson et al. 1995; Cremerius et al. 1998, 1999; Hain et al. 2000; Albers et al. 1999; Hofer et al. 2001; Muller-Mattheis et al. 1998; Spermon et al. 2002; Tsatalpas et al. 2002), two of which (Hain et al. 2000; Tsatalpas et al. 2002) reported a higher sensitivity for PET vs. CT. The specificities of the two methods were comparable. No clinical consequences were drawn. Recently, a German group investigated the sensitivity, specificity, and accuracy of FDG PET in stage I/II NSGCT patients scheduled for primary retroperitoneal lymph node dissection (RPLND). There was no difference between CT and FDG PET in terms of false-negative results, especially in small lesions (de Wit et al. 2005).

In most of the studies PET failed to detect small (<1 or <0.5 cm) retroperitoneal lymph nodes (Wilson et al. 1995; Albers et al. 1999; Cremerius et al. 1999; Hofer et al. 2001; Muller-Mattheis et al. 1998; Spermon et al. 2002; Tsatalpas et al. 2002; de Wit et al. 2005) and mature teratomas (Albers et al. 1999; Spermon et al. 2002). One of the positive PET scans in one trial was attributable to sarcoidosis (Cremerius et al. 1998). None of the trials unequivocally established a benefit of PET vs. conventional staging with tumor markers and CT at presentation.

In summary, there is no benefit in the use of FDG PET for staging at presentation.

### 4.4.7.2 The Role of FDG PET in Clinical Stage I Nonseminomatous Germ Cell Tumors (NSGCT)

After orchidectomy, about 30% of clinical stage I NSGCT patients staged with conventional CT scans will relapse within the first 2 years after the diagnosis. In high risk stage I NSGCT patients (with vascular invasion, pT2) the relapse rate is known to be up to 50%. No matter if surveillance, risk adapted treatment, or staging lymphadenectomy is the physician`s strategy of choice, improved staging tools would be of utmost importance in this clinical setting.

Three of four trials examining FDG PET for staging clinical stage I NSGCT patients with no more than a total of 27 patients, correlated PET data with histopathology data obtained from subsequent RPLND (Albers et al. 1999; Muller-Mattheis et al. 1998; Spermon et al. 2002). In all 3 trials PET failed to improve clinical staging. Of 22 negative PET scans, 7 proved to be false-negative (NPV 68%): in 6 patients the histologically positive lymph nodes were smaller than 0.5 cm and in the remaining patient PET failed to detect a mature teratoma. PET (sensitivity 42%) correctly identified no more than 5 out of 12 metastasizing patients (Albers et al. 1999; Muller-Mattheis et al. 1998; Spermon et al. 2002). In the fourth study by Lassen et al. (Lassen et al. 2003), PET data of 46 patients were compared to clinical follow-up data collected during surveillance. In this prospective trial, by contrast, 7 out of 10 relapses were correctly predicted (sensitivity 70%) and no more than 3 out of 39 negative PET scans proved to be false-negative (NPV 92%). This prompted the authors to conclude that FDG PET had improved clinical staging in their patients. A CT review later on classified two patients to be stage II, who finally had to be removed from the analysis. After that, the sensitivity of FDG PET in this study fell to 50% (Lassen et al. 2003). Based on the initial results of this trial (Lassen et al. 2000), the Medical Research Council initiated a prospective large-scale trial to investigate the role of FDG PET in high-risk clinical stage I NSGCT. PET-positive patients enrolled in this trial were subjected to adjuvant chemotherapy, while those with negative PET scans were put on surveillance. The study was closed early in 2005, after 33 out of 88 PET negative patients had relapsed, with a 1 year relapse free rate of 63.3% instead of the expected 2 year relapse free rate of >90% (Huddart et al. 2007).

*Summary*: FDG PET has no role in staging or early detection of micrometastases in clinical stage I NSGCT.

#### 4.4.7.3 Clinical Stage I Seminoma

Clinical stage I seminoma patients overall run a relapse risk of 18% (Warde et al. 2002) without further adjuvant treatment. Patients are usually offered adjuvant chemotherapy or standard radiation therapy or rarely may be placed on a surveillance protocol. Adjuvant chemotherapy with carboplatin now has mounting evidence of its efficacy with longer term data being published.. Any kind of adjuvant treatment in clinical stage I seminoma causes an overtreatment rate of about 80%.

So far, no scientific evidence is available for a positive role of PET in this clinical setting. Albers et al. (1999and Müller-Matheis et al. 1998) described 31 clinical stage I seminoma patients, all of them with negative PET scans. But as all of them had undergone adjuvant radiotherapy, there is no way of telling whether the PET data was correct or not.

The role of PET in an adjuvant setting should be analyzed in patients on surveillance.

*Summary:* FDG PET has no advantage over CT in staging clinical stage I SGCT.

#### 4.4.7.4 Clinical Stage II Disease/NSGCT

In clinical stage II, particularly in stage IIa disease, pathologic staging with RPLND shows that in up to 25% of cases patients are overstaged by CT (Donohue et al. 1995). FDG PET data for this clinical situation are contradictory: in a study by Albers et al. (1999) CT staging was false-positive in 4 out of 9 clinical stage II NSGCT patients, while PET correctly staged all 9 patients. Of the 7 patients with clinical stage II disease contributed by Spermon et al. (2002), all were correctly staged by CT, while PET failed to detect metastatic embryonic carcinoma in a retroperitoneal lymph node 1.2 cm in size and metastatic mature teratoma in another.

*Summary:* There is no evidence-based support for the use of FDG PET in stage II NSCGT.

## References

Akin EA, Khati N, Hill MC (2004) Ultrasound of the scrotum. Ultrasound Quarterly 20(4):181–200

Albers P, Bender H, Yilmaz H, Schoeneich G, Biersack HJ, Mueller SC (1999) Positron emission tomography in the clinical staging of patients with Stage I and II testicular germ cell tumors. Urology 53(4):808–811

Albers P, Albrecht W, Algaba F et al (2005) Guidelines on testicular cancer. Eur Urol 48(6):885–894

Albrecht T, Hohmann J, Oldenburg A, Skrok J, Wolf KJ (2004) Detection and characterization of liver metastases. Eur Radiol 14(supp 8):25–33

Atkinson GO, Patrick LE, Ball TI, Stephenson CA, Broecker BH, Woodwatd JR (1992) The normal and abnormal scrotum in

children: evaluation with color Doppler sonography. AJR Am J Roentgenol 158(3):613–617
Baker LL, Hajek PC, Burkhard TK et al (1987) MR imaging of the scrotum: pathologic conditions. Radiology 163(1): 93–98
Bass JE, Redwine MD, Kramer LA, Huynh PT, Harris JH Jr (2000) Spectrum of congenital anomalies of the inferior vena cava: cross-sectional imaging findings. Radiographics 20(3):639–652
Becherer A, De Santis M, Karanikas G et al (2005) FDG PET is superior to CT in the prediction of viable tumour in post-chemotherapy seminoma residuals. Eur J Radiol 54(2): 284–288
Beck SD, Foster RS, Bihrle R et al (2002) Teratoma in the orchiectomy specimen and volume of metastasis are predictors of retroperitoneal teratoma in post-chemotherapy nonseminomatous testis cancer. J Urol 168(4 pt 1):1402–1404
Benson CB (1988) The role of ultrasound in the diagnosis and staging of testicular cancer. Semin Urol 6:189–202
Benson CB, Doubilet PM, Richie JP (1989) Sonography of the male genital tract. AJR Am J Roentgenol 153(4):705–713
Bokemeyer C, Nowak P, Haupt A et al (1997) Treatment of brain metastases in patients with testicular cancer. J Clin Oncol 15(4):1449–1454
Bomanji J, Costa D, Ell P (2001) Clinical role of positron emission tomography in oncology. Lancet Oncol 2(3):157–164
Bosl GJ, Motzer RJ (1997) Testicular germ-cell cancer. N Engl J Med 337(4):242–253
Bradey N, Johnson RJ, Read G (1987) Abdominal computed tomography in teratoma of the testis: its accuracy in stage I disease and an assessment of the distribution of retroperitoneal lymph-node metastases in other stages of the disease. Br J Radiol 60(713):487–491
Brener BJ, Darling RC, Frederick PL, Linton RR (1974) Major venous anomalies complicating abdominal aortic surgery. Arch Surg 108(2):159–165
Brown LR, Aughenbaugh GL (1991) Masses of the anterior mediastinum: CT and MR imaging. AJR Am J Roentgenol 157(6):1171–1180
Budoff MJ, Lu B, Mao S et al (2000) Evaluation of fluid collection in the pericardial sinuses and recesses: noncontrast-enhanced electron beam tomography. Invest Radiol 35(6): 359–365
Busch FM, Sayegh ES, Chenault OW Jr (1965) Some uses of lymphangiography in the management of testicular tumors. J Urol 93:490–495
Cagini L, Nicholson AG, Horwich A, Goldstraw P, Pastorino U (1998) Thoracic metastasectomy for germ cell tumours: long term survival and prognostic factors. Ann Oncol 9(11): 1185–1191
Carroll BA, Gross DM (1983) High-frequency scrotal sonography. AJR Am J Roentgenol 140(3):511–515
Choi YW, McAdams HP, Jeon SC, Seo HS, Hahm CK (2000) The "High-Riding" superior pericardial recess: CT findings. AJR Am J Roentgenol 175(4):1025–1028
Cohade C, Wahl RL (2002) PET scanning and measuring the impact of treatment. Cancer J 8(2):119–134
Cramer BM, Schlegel EA, Thueroff JW (1991) MR imaging in the differential diagnosis of scrotal and testicular disease. Radiographics 11(1):9–21
Cremerius U, Effert PJ, Adam G et al (1998) FDG PET for detection and therapy control of metastatic germ cell tumor. J Nucl Med 39(5):815–822
Cremerius U, Wildberger JE, Borchers H et al (1999) Does positron emission tomography using 18-fluoro-2-deoxyglucose improve clinical staging of testicular cancer? – Results of a study in 50 patients. Urology 54(5):900–904
Dalal PU, Sohaib S, Huddart R (2006) Imaging of testicular germ cell tumors. Cancer Imaging 6:124–134
Davis PC, Hudgins PA, Peterman SB, Hoffman JC Jr (1991) Diagnosis of cerebral metastases: double-dose delayed CT vs contrast-enhanced MR imaging. AJNR 12(2): 293–300
De Santis M, Becherer A, Bokemeyer C et al (2004) 2-18fluoro-deoxy-D-glucose positron emission tomography is a reliable predictor for viable tumor in postchemotherapy seminoma: an update of the prospective multicentric SEMPET trial. J Clin Oncol 22(6):1034–1039
de Wit M, Brenner W, Hartmann M et al (2008) [18F]-FDG-PET in clinical stage I/II non-seminomatous germ cell tumours: results of the German multicentre trial. Ann Oncol19(9): 1619–23
Dixon AK, Ellis M, Sikora K (1986) Computed tomography of testicular tumours: distribution of abdominal lymphadenopathy. Clin Radiol 37(6):519–523
Dogra VS, Gottlieb RH, Oka M et al (2003) Sonography of the scrotum. Radiology 227:18–36
Donohue JP, Zachary JM, Maynard BR (1982) Distribution of nodal metastases in nonseminomatous testis cancer. J Urol 128(2):315–320
Donohue JP, Thornhill JA, Foster RS, Rowland RG, Bihrle R (1993) Primary retroperitoneal lymph node dissection in clinical stage A non-seminomatous germ cell testis cancer. Review of the Indiana University experience 1965-1989. Br J Urol 71(3):326–335
Donohue JP, Thornhill JA, Foster RS, Bihrle R, Rowland RG, Einhorn LH (1995) The role of retroperitoneal lymphadenectomy in clinical stage B testis cancer: the Indiana University experience (1965 to 1989). J Urol 153(1):85–89
Dorfman RE, Alpern MB, Gross BH, Sandler MA (1991) Upper abdominal lymph nodes: criteria for normal size determined with CT. Radiology 180(2):319–322
Dubowitz DJ (1997) Problem in diagnostic imaging. Clin Anat 10(4):279–282
Eary JF (1999) Nuclear medicine in cancer diagnosis. Lancet 354(9181):853–857
Ellis JH, Bies JR, Kopecky KK, Klatte EC, Rowland RG, Donohue JP (1984) Comparison of NMR and CT imaging in the evaluation of metastatic retroperitoneal lymphadenopathy from testicular carcinoma. J Comput Assist Tomogr 8(4):709–719
Engenhart R, Kimmig BN, Strauss LG et al (1992) Therapy monitoring of presacral recurrences after high-dose irradiation: value of PET, CT, CEA and pain score. Strahlenther Onkol 168(4):203–212
Fernandez EB, Moul JW, Foley JP, Colon E, McLeod DG (1994) Retroperitoneal imaging with third and fourth generation computed axial tomography in clinical stage I nonseminomatous germ cell tumors. Urology 44(4):548–552
Forsberg L, Dale L, Hoiem L et al (1986) Computed tomography in early stages of testicular carcinoma. Size of normal

retroperitoneal lymph nodes and lymph nodes in patients with metastases in stage II A. A SWENOTECA study: Swedish-Norwegian Testicular Cancer Project. Acta Radiol Diagn (Stockh) 27(5):569–574

Fossa SD, Bokemeyer C, Gerl A et al (1999) Treatment outcome of patients with brain metastases from malignant germ cell tumors. Cancer 85(4):988–997

Fulcher AS, Proto AV, Jolles H (1990) Cystic teratoma of the mediastinum: demonstration of fat/fluid level. AJR Am J Roentgenol 154(2):259–260

Fuse H, Shimazaki J, Katayama T (1990) Ultrasonography of testicular tumors. Eur Urol 17(4):273–275

Gatti JM, Stephenson RA (1998) Staging of testis cancer. Combining serum markers, histologic parameters, and radiographic imaging. Urol Clin North Am 25(3):397–403

Glazer HS, Lee JK, Melson GL (1982) Sonographic detection of occult testicular neoplasms. AJR Am J Roentgenol 138: 673–675

Gollub MJ, Castellino RA (1996) The cisterna chyli: a potential mimic of retrocrural lymphadenopathy on CT scans. Radiology 199(2):477–480

Grantham JG, Charboneau J, James EM (1985) Testicular neoplasms: 29 tumors studied by high-resolution ultrasound. Radiology 157:775–780

Guthrie JA, Fowler R (1992) Ultrasound diagnosis of testlar tumors presenting as epididymal disease. Clin Radiol 46:397–400

Haberkorn U, Strauss LG, Dimitrakopoulou A et al (1991) PET studies of fluorodeoxyglucose metabolism in patients with recurrent colorectal tumors receiving radiotherapy. J Nucl Med 32(8):1485–1490

Hain SF, O'Doherty MJ, Timothy AR, Leslie MD, Harper PG, Huddart RA (2000) Fluorodeoxyglucose positron emission tomography in the evaluation of germ cell tumours at relapse. Br J Cancer 83(7):863–869

Hartmann JT, Kanz L, Bokemeyer C (1999) Diagnosis and treatment of patients with testicular germ cell cancer. Drugs 58(2):257–281

Hilton S, Herr HW, Teitcher JB, Begg CB, Castellino RA (1997) CT detection of retroperitoneal lymph node metastases in patients with clinical stage I testicular nonseminomatous germ cell cancer: assessment of size and distribution criteria. AJR Am J Roentgenol 169(2):521–525

Hofer C, Kubler H, Hartung R, Breul J, Avril N (2001) Diagnosis and monitoring of urological tumors using positron emission tomography. Eur Urol 40(5):481–487

Horstman WG, Melson GL, Middleton WD, Andriole GL (1992) Testiculat tumors: findings with color Doppler US. Radiology 185(3):733–737

Horstman WG, Haluszka MM, Burkhard TK (1994) Management of testicular masses incidentally discovered by ultrasound. J Urol 151:1263–1265

Howlett DC, Marchbank ND, Sallomi DF (2000) Ultrasound of the testis. Clin Radiol 55:595–601

Hricak H, Hamm B, Bohyun K (1995) Imaging of the scrotum. Raven, New York

Huddart RA, O'Doherty MJ, Padhani A et al (2007) 18fluorodeoxyglucose positron emission tomography in the prediction of relapse in patients with high-risk, clinical stage I nonseminomatous germ cell tumors: preliminary report of MRC Trial TE22–the NCRI Testis Tumour Clinical Study Group. J Clin Oncol 25(21):3090–3095

Hustinx R, Paulus P, Jacquet N, Jerusalem G, Bury T, Rigo P (1998) Clinical evaluation of whole-body 18F-fluorodeoxyglucose positron emission tomography in the detection of liver metastases. Ann Oncol 9(4):397–401

International Germ Cell Cancer Collaborative Group (1997) International Germ Cell Consensus Classification: a prognostic factor-based staging system for metastatic germ cell cancers. J Clin Oncol 15(2):594–603

Jaffe CC (2006) Measures of response: RECIST, WHO, and new alternatives. J Clin Oncol 24(20):3245–3251

Jerusalem G, Beguin Y, Fassotte MF et al (1999) Whole-body positron emission tomography using 18F-fluorodeoxyglucose for posttreatment evaluation in Hodgkin's disease and non-Hodgkin's lymphoma has higher diagnostic and prognostic value than classical computed tomography scan imaging. Blood 94(2):429–433

Jerusalem G, Beguin Y, Fassotte MF et al (2003) Early detection of relapse by whole-body positron emission tomography in the follow-up of patients with Hodgkin's disease. Ann Oncol 14(1):123–130

Jochelson MS, Garnick MB, Balikian JP, Richie JP (1984) The efficacy of routine whole lung tomography in germ cell tumors. Cancer 54(6):1007–1009

Johns Putra L, Lawrentschuk N, Ballok Z et al (2004) 18F-fluorodeoxyglucose positron emission tomography in evaluation of germ cell tumor after chemotherapy. Urology 64(6):1202–1207

Johnson JO, Mattrey RF, Phillipson J (1990) Differentiation of seminomatous from nonseminomatous testicular tumors with MR imaging. AJR Am J Roentgenol 154(3):539–543

Juweid ME, Wiseman GA, Vose JM et al (2005) Response assessment of aggressive non-Hodgkin's lymphoma by integrated International Workshop Criteria and fluorine-18-fluorodeoxyglucose positron emission tomography. J Clin Oncol 23(21):4652–4661

Kim W, Rosen MA, Langer JE, Baner MP, Siegelman ES, Ramchandani P (2007) US MR imaging correlation in pathologic conditions of the scrotum. Radiographics 27(5): 1239–1253

Kitajima K, Nakamoto Y, Senda M, Onishi Y, Okizuka H, Sugimura K (2007) Normal uptake of (18)F-FDG in the testis: an assessment by PET/CT. Ann Nucl Med 21(7): 405–410

Kollmannsberger C, Nichols C, Meisner C, Mayer F, Kanz L, Bokemeyer C (2000) Identification of prognostic subgroups among patients with metastatic 'IGCCCG poor-prognosis' germ-cell cancer: an explorative analysis using cart modeling. Ann Oncol 11(9):1115–1120

Kollmannsberger C, Oechsle K, Dohmen B et al (2002) Prospective comparison of [$^{18}$F]fluorodeoxyglucose positron emission tomography with conventional assessment by computed tomography scans and serum tumor markers for the evaluation of residual masses in patients with nonseminomatous germ cell carcinoma. Cancer 94(9):2353–2362

Kostakoglu L, Coleman M, Leonard JP, Kuji I, Zoe H, Goldsmith SJ (2002) PET predicts prognosis after 1 cycle of chemotherapy in aggressive lymphoma and Hodgkin's disease. J Nucl Med 43(8):1018–1027

Kubik-Huch RA, Hailemariam S, Hamm B (1999) CT and MRI of the male genital tract: radiologic-pathologic correlation. Eur Radiol 9(1):16–28

Kubota R, Yamada S, Kubota K, Ishiwata K, Tamahashi N, Ido T (1992) Intratumoral distribution of fluorine-18-fluorodeoxyglucose in vivo: high accumulation in macrophages and granulation tissues studied by microautoradiography. J Nucl Med 33(11):1972–1980

Kullmann G, Lien HH (1987) Intraabdominal hematoma following orchiectomy: a potential pitfall in using CT for staging of testicular cancer. Radiology 163(1):129–130

Lassen U, Daugaard G, Rorth M, Eigtved A, Hojgaard L (2000) Positron emission tomography with 18F-fluoro-deoxyglucose in clinical stage I non-seminomatous germ cell tumors. ASCO Annual Meeting abstract no 1337

Lassen U, Daugaard G, Eigtved A, Hojgaard L, Damgaard K, Rorth M (2003) Whole-body FDG-PET in patients with stage I non-seminomatous germ cell tumours. Eur J Nucl Med Mol Imaging 30(3):396–402

Lee KS, Im JG, Han CH, Han MC, Kim CW, Kim WS (1989) Malignant primary germ cell tumors of the mediastinum: CT features. AJR Am J Roentgenol 153(5):947–951

Leibovitch L, Foster RS, Kopecky KK, Donohue JP (1995) Improved accuracy of computerized tomography based clinical staging in low stage nonseminomatous germ cell cancer using size criteria of retroperitoneal lymph nodes. J Urol 154(5):1759–1763

Levitt RG, Husband JE, Glazer HS (1984) CT of primary germ-cell tumors of the mediastinum. AJR Am J Roentgenol 142(1):73–78

Lien HH, Stenwig AE, Ous S, Fossa SD (1986) Influence of different criteria for abnormal lymph node size on reliability of computed tomography in patients with non-seminomatous testicular tumor. Acta Radiol Diagn (Stockh) 27(2): 199–203

Lien HH, Lindskold L, Stenwig AE, Ous S, Fossa SD (1987) Shape of retroperitoneal lymph nodes at computed tomography does not correlate to metastatic disease in early stage non-seminomatous testicular tumors. Acta Radiol 28(3): 271–273

Lien HH, Lindskold L, Fossa SD, Aass N (1988) Computed tomography and conventional radiography in intrathoracic metastases from non-seminomatous testicular tumor. Acta Radiol 29(5):547–549

Lienhard GE, Slot JW, James DE, Mueckler MM (1992) How cells absorb glucose. Sci Am 266(1):86–91

Lowe VJ, Fletcher JW, Gobar L et al (1998) Prospective investigation of positron emission tomography in lung nodules. J Clin Oncol 16(3):1075–1084

MacVicar D (1993) Staging of testicular germ cell tumours. Clin Radiol 47(3):149–158

Marchevsky A, Kaneko M (1992) Surgical pathology of the mediastinum. Raven, New York

Mason MD, Featherstone T, Olliff J, Horwich A (1991) Inguinal and iliac lymph node involvement in germ cell tumours of the testis: implications for radiological investigation and for therapy. Clin Oncol 3(3):147–150

Mazlin ZV, Belenky A, Kunichezky M, Sandbank J, Strauss S (2004) Leydig cell tumors of the testis: gray scale and color Doppler sonographic appearance. J Ultrasound Med 23(7): 959–964

Mazzu D, Jeffrey RB, Ralls PW (1995) Lymphoma and leukemia involving the testicles: findings on gray-scale and color Doppler soography. AJR Am J Roentgenol 164(3):645–647

Meanock CI, Ward CS, Williams MP (1988) A potential pitfall of pelvic computed tomography. Br J Radiol 61(727):584–585

Meyer CA, Conces DJ (2002) Imaging of intrathoracic metastases of nonseminomatous germ cell tumors. Chest Surg Clin N Am 12(4):717–738

Moog F, Bangerter M, Kotzerke J, Guhlmann A, Frickhofen N, Reske SN (1998) 18-F-fluorodeoxyglucose-positron emission tomography as a new approach to detect lymphomatous bone marrow. J Clin Oncol 16(2):603–609

Moul JW (1995) Proper staging techniques in testicular cancer patients. Tech Urol 1(3):126–132

Moul JW, Maggio MI, Hardy MR, Hartman DS (1992) Retroaortic left renal vein in testicular cancer patient: potential staging and treatment pitfall. J Urol 147(2):454–456

Muller-Mattheis V, Reinhardt M, Gerharz CD et al (1998) Positron emission tomography with [18 F]-2-fluoro-2-deoxy-D-glucose (18FDG-PET) in diagnosis of retroperitoneal lymph node metastases of testicular tumors. Urologe A 37(6):609–620

Nabi HA, Zubeldia JM (2002) Clinical applications of (18)F-FDG in oncology. J Nucl Med Technol 30(1):3–9; quiz 10–11

Nachtsheim DA, Scheible F, Gosink B (1983) Ultrasonography of testis tumors. J Urol 129(5):978–981

Naidich D, Webb W, Müller N, Krinsky G, Zerhouni E (1998) Computed tomography and magnetic resonance of the thorax, 3rd edn. Lippincott Williams & Wilkins, Philadelphia

Nichols CR (1991) Mediastinal germ cell tumors. Clinical features and biologic correlates. Chest 99(2):472–479

Noone T, Huch-Böni R, Semelka RC (1997) MRI of the abdomen and pelvis. Wiley-Liss, New York

Nuutinen JM, Leskinen S, Elomaa I et al (1997) Detection of residual tumours in postchemotherapy testicular cancer by FDG-PET. Eur J Cancer 33(8):1234–1241

Oyen R, Verellen S, Drochmans A et al (1993) Value of MRI in the diagnosis and staging of testicular tumors. J Belge Radiol 76(2):84–89

Page JE, Prendergast CM, King DM (1990) Retroperitoneal haematoma following orchidectomy: implications for staging computed tomography. Br J Radiol 63(750):490–492

Pick J, Anson BJ (1940) The renal vascular pedicle: an anatomical study of 430 body halves. J Urol 44:411–434

Pollock RE, Doroshow JH, Khayat D (2004) UICC manual of clinical oncology, 8th edn. Wiley, Hoboken

Prokop M, Galanski M. Spiral and Multislice Computed tomography of the Body, Thieme, 2003

Ray B, Hajdu SI, Whitmore WF Jr (1974) Proceedings: distribution of retroperitoneal lymph node metastases in testicular germinal tumors. Cancer 33(2):340–348

Regelink G, Brouwer J, de Bree R et al (2002) Detection of unknown primary tumours and distant metastases in patients with cervical metastases: value of FDG-PET versus conventional modalities. Eur J Nucl Med Mol Imaging 29(8):1024–1030

Rifkin MD, Kurtz AB, Pasto ME, Goldberg BB (1985) Diagnostic capabilities of high-resolution scrotal ultrasonography: prospective evaluation. J Ultrasound Med 4(1):13–19

Rosado-de-Christenson ML, Templeton PA, Moran CA (1992) From the archives of the AFIP. Mediastinal germ cell tumors: radiologic and pathologic correlation. Radiographics 12(5):1013–1030

Royal SA, Callen PW (1979) CT evaluation of anomalies of the inferior vena cava and left renal vein. AJR Am J Roentgenol 132(5):759–763

Rutherford EE, Ferguson JL, Geldart TR, Mead GM, Smart JM, Tung KT (2006) Late relapse of metastatic non-seminomatous testicular germ cell tumours. Clin Radiol 61(11):907–915

Sanchez S, Mahlin M (1986) Simultaneous bilateral testicular tumors, one side clinically occult: detection by ultrasound. J Urol 135:591–592

Schmoll HJ, Souchon R, Krege S et al (2004) European consensus on diagnosis and treatment of germ cell cancer: a report of the European Germ Cell Cancer Consensus Group (EGCCCG). Ann Oncol 15(9):1377–1399

Schoder H, Noy A, Gonen M et al (2005) Intensity of 18fluorodeoxyglucose uptake in positron emission tomography distinguishes between indolent and aggressive non-Hodgkin's lymphoma. J Clin Oncol 23(21):4643–4651

Scholz M, Zehender M, Thalmann GN, Borner M, Thoni H, Studer UE (2002) Extragonadal retroperitoneal germ cell tumor: evidence of origin in the testis. Ann Oncol 13(1):121–124

Schwerk WB, Schwerk WN, Rodeck G (1987) Testicular tumors: prospective analysis of real-time US patterns and abdominal staging. Radiology 164(2):369–374

See WA, Hoxie L (1993) Chest staging in testis cancer patients: imaging modality selection based upon risk assessment as determined by abdominal computerized tomography scan results. J Urol 150(3):874–878

Seltzer SE, Herman PG, Sagel SS (1984) Differential diagnosis of mediastinal fluid levels visualized on computed tomography. J Comput Assist Tomogr 8(2):244–246

Semelka RC, Helmberger TK (2001) Contrast agents for MR imaging of the liver. Radiology 218(1):27–38

Semelka RC, Schlund JF, Molina PL et al (1996) Malignant liver lesions: comparison of spiral CT arterial portography and MR imaging for diagnostic accuracy, cost, and effect on patient management. J Magn Reson Imaging 6(1):39–43

Shawker TH, Javadpour N, O'Leary T et al (1983) Ultrasound detection of "burned-out" primary testicular tumor in clinically normal testis. J Ultrasound Med 2:477–479

Spaepen K, Stroobants S, Dupont P et al (2002) Early restaging positronemissiontomographywith(18)F-fluorodeoxyglucose predicts outcome in patients with aggressive non-Hodgkin's lymphoma. Ann Oncol 13(9):1356–1363

Spermon JR, De Geus-Oei LF, Kiemeney LA, Witjes JA, Oyen WJ (2002) The role of (18)fluoro-2-deoxyglucose positron emission tomography in initial staging and re-staging after chemotherapy for testicular germ cell tumours. BJU Int 89(6):549–556

Stenning S, Parkinson M, Fisher C et al (1998) Postchemotherapy residual masses in germ cell tumor patients. Cancer 83(7):1409–1419

Stephens A, Gonin R, GD H, Einhorn L (1996) Positron emission tomography evaluation of residual radiographic abnormalities in postchemotherapy germ cell tumor patients. J Clin Oncol 14(5):1637–1641

Stephenson AJ, Sheinfeld J (2005) Management of patients with low-stage nonseminomatous germ cell testicular cancer. Curr Treat Options Oncol 6(5):367–377

Stephenson AJ, Bosl GJ, Motzer RJ et al (2005) Retroperitoneal lymph node dissection for nonseminomatous germ cell testicular cancer: impact of patient selection factors on outcome. J Clin Oncol 23(12):2781–2788

Steyerberg E, Keizer H, Fossa S et al (1995) Prediction of residual retroperitoneal mass histology after chemotherapy for metastatic nonseminomatous germ cell tumor: multivariate analysis of individual patient data from Six Study Groups. J Clin Oncol 13(5):1177–1187

Steyerberg E, Keizer H, Sleijfer D et al (2000) Retroperitoneal metastases in testicular cancer: role of CT measurements in decision making for resection after chemotherapy. Radiology 215(2):437–444

Stomper PC, Fung CY, Socinski MA, Jochelson MS, Garnick MB, Richie JP (1987) Detection of retroperitoneal metastases in early-stage nonseminomatous testicular cancer: analysis of different CT criteria. AJR Am J Roentgenol 149(6):1187–1190

Strauss LG (1996) Fluorine-18 deoxyglucose and false-positive results: a major problem in the diagnostics of oncological patients. Eur J Nucl Med 23(10):1409–1415

Suzuki M, Takashima T, Itoh H, Choutoh S, Kawamura I, Watanabe Y (1983) Computed tomography of mediastinal teratomas. J Comput Assist Tomogr 7(1):74–76

Therasse P, Arbuck SG, Eisenhauer EA et al (2000) New guidelines to evaluate the response to treatment in solid tumors. European Organization for Research and Treatment of Cancer, National Cancer Institute of the United States, National Cancer Institute of Canada. J Natl Cancer Inst 92(3):205–216

Thurnher S, Hricak H, Carroll PR, Pobiel RS, Filly RA (1988) Imaging the testis: comparison between MR imaging and US. Radiology 167(3):631–636

Tran T, Grech P, Crofton ME (1989) Computed tomographic staging of testicular tumours: an unexpected source of error. Br J Radiol 62(742):942–944

Tsatalpas P, Beuthien-Baumann B, Kropp J et al (2002) Diagnostic value of 18F-FDG positron emission tomography for detection and treatment control of malignant germ cell tumors. Urol Int 68(3):157–163

Varsamidis K, Varsamidou E, Marvropoulos G (2001) Doppler ultrasonography in testicular tumors presenting with acutescrotal pain. Acta Radiol 42(2):230–233

Vassiliades VG, Foley WD, Alarcon J et al (1991) Hepatic metastases: CT versus MR imaging at 1.5T. Gastrointest Radiol 16(2):159–163

Vesselle HJ, Miraldi FD (1998) FDG PET of the retroperitoneum: normal anatomy, variants, pathologic conditions, and strategies to avoid diagnostic pitfalls. Radiographics 18(4):805–823; discussion 23–24

Warde P, Specht L, Horwich A et al (2002) Prognostic factors for relapse in stage I seminoma managed by surveillance: a pooled analysis. J Clin Oncol 20(22):4448–4452

Webb W, Müller N, Naidich D (2000) High-resolution CT of the lung, 3rd edn. Lippincott Williams & Wilkins, Philadelphia

White PM, Howard GC, Best JJ, Wright AR (1997) The role of computed tomographic examination of the pelvis in the management of testicular germ cell tumours. Clin Radiol 52(2):124–129

White PM, Adamson DJ, Howard GC, Wright AR (1999) Imaging of the thorax in the management of germ cell testicular tumours. Clin Radiol 54(4):207–211

Williams MP, Husband JE, Heron CW (1987) Intrathoracic manifestations of metastatic testicular seminoma: a comparison of chest radiographic and CT findings. AJR Am J Roentgenol 149(3):473–475

Wilson C, Young H, Ott R et al (1995) Imaging metastatic testicular germ cell tumours with F18-FDG positron emission tomography: prospects for detection and management. Eur Nucl Med 22(6):508–513

Wittenberg AF, Tobias T, Rzeszotarski M, Minotti AJ (2006) Sonography of the acute scrotum: the four T's of testicular imaging. Curr Probl Dign Radiol 35(1):12–21

Wolf G, Aigner RM, Schwarz T, Krippl P, Samonigg H (2003) Diagnosis of a contralateral second testicular carcinoma by F18-FDG PET. Onkologie 26(2):155–157

Wood A, Robson N, Tung K, Mead G (1996) Patterns of supra-diaphragmatic metastases in testicular germ cell tumours. Clin Radiol 51(4):273–276

World Health Organization (1979) Handbook for reporting results of cancer treatment. WHO Offset Publication No 48. WHO, Geneva

# Staging and Prognostic Systems

# 5

Graham M. Mead, W. Bedford Waters, and Wesley M. White

## 5.1 Introduction

Testis cancer is a relatively uncommon tumor that is wholly curable in the vast majority of cases. Of the estimated 8,250 new cases of testicular cancer that would have been diagnosed in 2006, close to 90% of these patients would have achieved long-term survival (American Cancer 2006; Landis et al. 1998). And while the multimodal treatment of testis tumors represents the quintessential approach to cancer management, one must not overlook how important the development, implementation, and refinement of staging have been in this triumph. Indeed, the utilization and modification of staging systems since the early 1950s set the groundwork for much of the critical treatment discoveries that were to follow (Boden and Gibb 1951). In the modern era of testis cancer treatment, clinical staging is predicated on an orderly and thorough history and physical examination, radiographic evaluation of the chest and retroperitoneum, laboratory determination of biochemical tumor marker assays, and the pathologic evaluation of the testis and, in some cases, the retroperitoneal lymph nodes. An ordered and systematic approach to the staging of testis cancer leads to informed and appropriate treatment decisions and yields important prognostic information that often shapes those decisions. This pragmatic and logical approach to staging is the focus of this chapter.

G.M. Mead (✉)
Department of Medical Oncology, Southampton General Hospital, Southampton, UK

## 5.2 Clinical and Surgical Staging

The staging of any cancer begins with the search for malignant disease. In the case of testis cancer, the history and physical examination marks the beginning of this search. A thorough examination will define for the physician and the patient the nature of any testicular anomaly. The index of suspicion for malignancy will be based on this initial assessment and, as a result, the necessity of additional imaging and serum laboratory tests. Once the patient has been thoroughly evaluated clinically, diagnostic and therapeutic surgical exploration and extirpation may follow. These staging strategies foster optimal treatment decisions that affect cure rates of more than 90% in most patients. This section of the chapter details optimal, evidence-based guidelines for clinical and surgical staging and how staging of an exacting nature ultimately proffers significant predictive value.

### *5.2.1 History and Physical Examination*

Testis tumors most commonly present as a painless testicular mass in one gonad, dense testicular firmness, and/or diffuse scrotal swelling. Some 10–30% of patients will report scrotal pain or "heaviness" as their presenting complaint. Acute testicular pain is rarely the chief complaint and tends to occur in the setting of intratesticular hemorrhage and/or epididymitis (Richie 1993; Preti and Logothetis 1993). Seventy-five percent of testis tumors are discovered by the patient or his partner on self-examination. Another fifteen percent are discovered by physician examination, and the remaining patients present with symptoms of diffuse disease (Kennedy et al. 1987).

M.P. Laguna et al. (eds.), *Cancer of the Testis*,
DOI: 10.1007/978-1-84800-370-5_5, © Springer-Verlag London Limited 2010

While nearly 50% of patients present with metastatic disease, symptoms, as previously stated, are present in only 10% of cases (Bosl et al. 1981). Patients may exhibit constitutional symptoms such as weight loss and fatigue or symptoms referable to the locoregional spread of disease, notably supraclavicular lymphadenopathy, dyspnea or coughing (pulmonary metastases), abdominal pain or fullness (bulky retroperitoneal lymphadenopathy or disease), nervous system dysfunction (central or peripheral nervous system involvement), and lower extremity swelling (venous obstruction or thrombosis). Gynecomastia is present in approximately 5% of patients owing to elevated or imbalanced levels of β-human chorionic globulin, androgens, prolactin, and/or estrogens (Richie 1993; Bosl et al. 1981). This rate may approach 40% among those with Sertoli and Leydig cell tumors (Caldamone et al. 1979). Infertility is a rare but well-documented presentation (Raman et al. 2005).

The duration of symptoms varies greatly. Most patients present in a delayed fashion owing to patient denial or ignorance or, unfortunately, physician's error. Indeed, studies have consistently reported a delay in diagnosis of nearly 2–3 months from the onset of symptoms. This delay produces an advanced stage of disease and, among those with a delay of more than 6 months, a doubled mortality rate (Bosl et al. 1981; Nizkas et al. 1990). There is an apparent need for patient and provider education that tenders earlier diagnosis and treatment of disease.

Physical examination begins with a thorough evaluation of the diseased gonad and the remaining scrotal contents. While seated, the examiner should palpate the testicle between the thumb and first two fingers of the examining hand. The normal contralateral testis should be examined first as this will provide the examiner with a baseline testis size, contour, and consistency to which the diseased testis may be compared. The normal testis should be uniform in its consistency, movable, and easily separated from the epididymis. Any areas of firmness, nodularity, or inhomogeneity should be noted and considered malignant until proven otherwise. Involvement of the spermatic cord, epididymis, and/or scrotal skin must be noted, as approximately 10–15% of patients will present with invasion of these two former structures (Kennedy et al. 1987). An ipsilateral varicocele may imply retroperitoneal venous congestion. A reactive hydrocele is sometimes present, making a thorough exam of the testicle difficult. Any suspicious findings and/or those with difficult examinations should be sent for scrotal ultrasonography.

The remainder of the physical exam should focus on the presence of systemic disease. The abdomen should be palpated for bulky adenopathy and visceral disease. The supraclavicular lymph nodes should be examined. Any evidence of gynecomastia should be noted. The chest should be auscultated for the presence of intrathoracic disease.

### 5.2.2 Differential Diagnosis

The finding of an abnormal testicular mass and/or an enlarged and firm testis should be considered cancer until proven otherwise. However, the differential diagnosis of testicular firmness, irregularity, and/or discomfort is myriad. Epididymitis, epididymo-orchitis, testicular torsion, and benign paratesticular lesions may all present with features suggestive of malignancy. The presence of a hernia or hydrocele often confuses the clinical picture by preventing a thorough testicular exam, but they rarely present with frank testicular findings reminiscent of cancer. When it is difficult to differentiate malignant from benign pathology, or when any concern exists regarding the nature or extent of a testicular anomaly, imaging is mandatory.

### 5.2.3 Testicular Imaging

Any testicular mass requires prompt and apposite imaging. In the modern era, several modalities exist for precise and accurate imaging, among them ultrasonography and magnetic resonance imaging (MRI). These techniques, when in experienced hands, offer a degree of confidence regarding the nature of any testicular lesion. But despite their ability to identify and in some cases accurately characterize testicular lesions, these techniques offer little help in the staging of testis tumors.

Sonographic evaluation of the scrotum is widely recognized as the standard of care for the evaluation of testicular masses. Ultrasonography in this setting is accurate, readily available, noninvasive, of relatively low-cost, and avoids ionizing radiation. The introduction of high-frequency transducers (5–10 MHz) has made the identification of even extremely small intratesticular lesions (1–2 mm) possible and, as a result, made ultrasound the single best test when assessing for testicular pathology. Ultrasound is exquisitely sensitive in delineating intratesticular vs. extratesticular anomalies, a critical differentiation when assessing masses of a potentially paratesticular nature (Benson 1988). The addition of Doppler Color ultrasonography has further improved reliability by imbuing the technique with dynamic function that is often necessary in differentiating among the myriad causes of acute scrotal pain (Hortsman 1997).

Findings on ultrasound characteristic of testis tumors include intratesticular masses that are usually hypervascular on Doppler examination. A region of normal testicular parenchyma is usually identifiable, even in cases of extremely large tumors that one would expect to replace the entirety of the testicle. Tumors are of varying consistencies based in part on the histologic type of the tumor (Richie et al. 1982a; Schwerk et al. 1987; Marth et al. 1990). While studies have proven the reliability of ultrasound in distinguishing between seminoma and nonseminomatous germ cell tumors (NSGCT), these patterns are not pathognomonic and should rightly be interpreted with sage clinical judgment and in the context of the patient's entire clinical picture (Marth et al. 1990).

The sonographic appearance of seminoma is characterized by a well- circumscribed mass that is uniform in appearance and is generally less echogenic than the surrounding gonadal parenchyma (Fig. 5.1) (Richie et al. 1982a). Calcifications and cystic changes are unusual findings (Schwerk et al. 1987). Conversely, NSGCTs are generally poorly circumscribed lesions that are of a nonuniform consistency. These lesions may be hypoechoic, isoechoic, hyperechoic, or some combination thereof owing to intratumoral calcifications, cysts, necrosis, and hemorrhage (Fig. 5.2). The architecture of the testicle may be badly distorted (Benson 1988; Richie et al. 1982a; Schwerk et al. 1987; Marth et al. 1990). Some academic distinction between the various histologic subtypes of NSGCT may be made, but these have been unreliable in controlled studies. Embryonal carcinomas exhibit the prototypical appearance of NSGCT, namely an inhomogeneous mass intermixed with calcifications and cysts. Choriocarcinoma typically appears sonographically as a small primary intratesticular lesion that is largely hypoechoic with admixed areas of calcification and hemorrhage. Conversely, teratoma exhibits a predominantly cystic pattern with areas of hypoechogenecity (Gash Book).

Ultrasound generally lacks reliability in accurately staging testicular tumors. Studies by Marth et al. found that ultrasound accurately staged testis tumors in only 10% of cases (1990). The homogeneous nature of seminomas may afford some improved sensitivity in staging, but not to an unacceptable threshold. The inability of

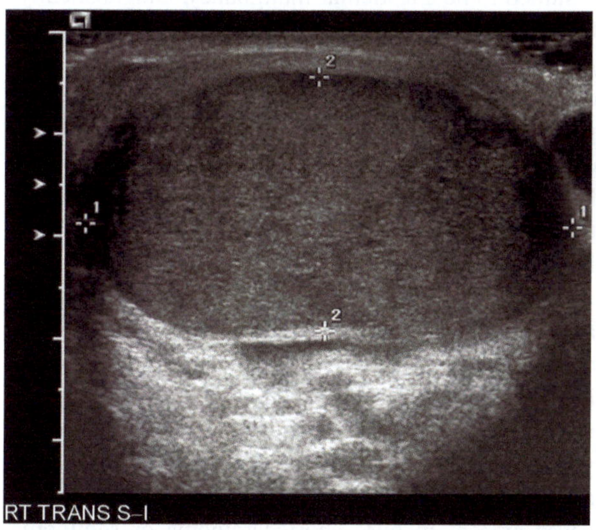


Fig. 5.1 Sonographic appearance of seminoma

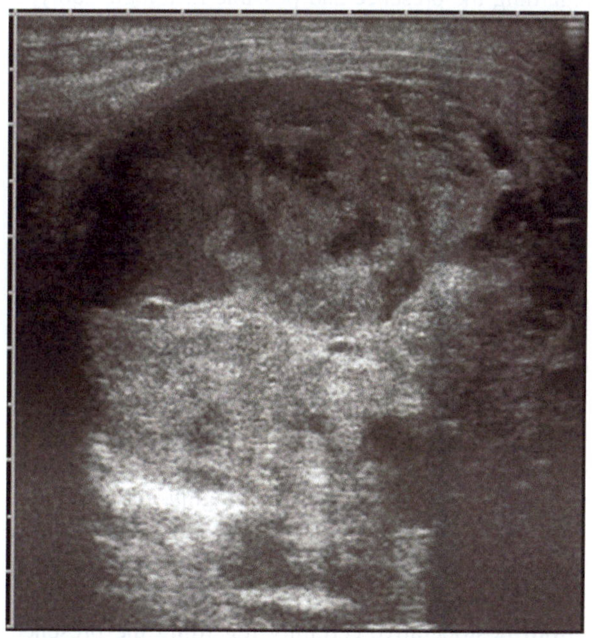

Fig. 5.2 Sonographic appearance of nonseminomatous germ cell tumor

ultrasound to reliably stage testis tumors is born of its failure to accurately define the tunica albuginea and mediastinum testis (Thurnher et al. 1988). Given these limitations and the need for histologic confirmation, surgical exploration is a necessity.

The use of MRI for the evaluation and staging of testis cancer has remained largely academic. While its expense and lack of superiority over ultrasound have rendered it investigative, excellent intrascrotal images can still be obtained (Oyen et al. 1993). Normal testicular parenchyma appears homogenous on both T1-weighted and T2-weighted imaging. Testicular tumors are generally difficult to identify on T1-weighted imaging, but reliably exhibit loss of signal intensity on standard T2 imaging and enhance on T2 imaging with the use of gadolinium (Hricak et al. 1995). Like ultrasound, distinguishing seminoma from NSGCT has been studied and noted to be poor. While seminomas typically appear homogeneous on MRI and NSGCTs are usually inhomogeneous, no study has found these features to be significantly predictive of tumor histology (Thurnher et al. 1988; Oyen et al. 1993). Similarly, while the tunica albuginea is easily distinguished on MRI, the ability to accurately stage the primary tumor is unreliable. Thurnher et al. assigned the correct stage based on MRI in only 63% of cases (1988). Again, while MRI may provide adequate diagnostic information regarding the presence and possible histologic subtype of a testis tumor, little staging information is provided.

### 5.2.4 Tumor Markers

The presence of a concerning testicular mass on physical exam and/or the finding of an intratesticular lesion on ultrasound, mandates both surgical exploration of the testis and the preoperative measurement of biochemical serum tumor markers. Tumor markers have become an integral part of testis cancer staging, so much so that the AJCC Testicular Cancer Staging System was most recently revised to include serum tumor markers as a part of its staging classification. Not only do these markers provide helpful clues regarding the presence of malignancy and the possible histologic nature of that malignancy, but they also afford postoperative certainty regarding the presence and/or persistence of metastatic disease, and offer additional benefit in diagnosing the 5–7% of germ cell tumors that present as extragonadal primaries (Bokemeyer et al. 2003; Klein 1993).

Three tumor markers are of diagnostic and prognostic importance in testicular cancer; beta human chorionic gonadotropin (hCG), alpha-fetoprotein (AFP), and lactate dehydrogenase (LDH). Each of these oncologic markers proffers valuable information in the setting of germinal tumors. All are of adequate sensitivity to detect both primary tumors and subclinical recurrence, but are not of adequate specificity to afford population screening (Bower and Rustin 2000). Each is readily measured, most commonly via radioimmunoassay (Bagshawe and Searle 1977). The half-lives of each of the respective markers are short enough to aid in the detection of residual tumor burden and/or reflect the adequacy of treatment. In the setting of a concomitant testicular mass, the presence of elevated tumor markers is virtually diagnostic of malignancy. All of these features are of significant benefit when managing patients with an unknown testicular mass or those with established testis cancer.

Elevated levels of serum beta-hCG may be seen in a host of malignant processes, among them liver, pancreas, gastric, breast, bladder, and kidney cancers. However, concentrations greater than 10,000 mIU/mL are indicative of germ cell tumors, some primary cancers of the stomach, pregnancy, or gestational trophoblastic disease (Richie and Steele 2002). While lower levels of hCG by itself lacks sufficient sensitivity to definitively diagnose testis cancer without histologic confirmation, its elevation in a young male must be assumed to be a testicular malignancy. Diagnostically, hCG is elevated in approximately 50% of patients with germ cell tumors. Specifically, all patients with choriocarcinoma exhibit elevation of hCG, close to 80% of patients with embryonal carcinoma have elevated levels, and about 10% of patients with seminoma have hCG elevation. The origin of beta-hCG elevation in these settings is the syncytiotrophoblastic cells. Its half life is 24–36 h (Klein 1993).

Like beta-hCG, AFP elevation postnatally is noted in a host of malignant processes. Levels above 10,000 kU/L are found almost exclusively in germ cell tumors and liver cancer (Bower and Rustin 2000). In general, elevated levels are found in pure embryonal carcinoma, yolk sac tumors (endodermal sinus tumors), teratoma, and combined NSGCTs (e.g., teratocarcinoma). AFP is never present in pure choriocarcinoma or seminoma (Klein 1993). However, some cases of advanced metastatic seminoma may exhibit histologic evidence of nonseminomatous dedifferentiation that is therefore capable of elaborating AFP (Javadpour 1980). The origin of AFP elevation in these settings is trophoblastic cells. Its half life is 5–7 days (Richie and Steele 2002).

LDH is elevated in numerous illnesses, among them testis cancer. As it lacks a strong tendency for any single histologic subtype, its diagnostic value is somewhat limited. By itself, LDH is the sole biochemical abnormality in only 10% of cases, and little histologic information can be gleaned from this elevation (Richie and Steele 2002). Despite these limitations, repeated multivariate analyses have found LDH to be of prognostic value, especially as it pertains to tumor burden. A study by Boyle and Samuels found a linear relationship between measured LDH values of greater than 2,000 U/L and significant tumor burden. Further, a rising LDH was found to be indicative of disease relapse. It is these, prognostic and surveillance roles for which LDH is utilized (Boyle and Samuels 1977; Mencel et al. 1994).

Several additional tumor markers of arguable value include placental alkaline phosphatase (PLAP) and gamma-glutamyl-transpeptidase (GGTP). While both markers have relatively poor sensitivity, small studies have demonstrated that their combined use may be of some diagnostic value (Javadpour 1983). However, their use is both uncommon and generally unnecessary with the concomitant assessment of hCG and AFP.

The clinical use of serum tumor markers is, as stated before, of both diagnostic and prognostic importance. Practically, serum values of LDH, AFP, and beta-hCG should be determined preoperatively and postoperatively. Preoperative values can offer clues as to the presence and histologic nature of the suspected testicular tumor as stipulated above, and in the setting of planned postoperative surveillance, provides a requisite baseline (Richie and Steele 2002). Regarding the presence of disease, hCG and AFP are elevated in 85–90% of testis cancers, regardless of their clinical stage (Barzell and Whitmore 1979). Therefore, an additional 10–15% of patients with testis cancer (especially NSGCTs) will present with normal serum levels of these markers. In addition, patients with early stage (stage I) testis cancers are more likely to present with less profound elevations as marker sensitivity is proportional to tumor burden (Bosl et al. 1981).

Postoperatively, serum values should be evaluated and should decline based on the aforementioned half-lives of AFP and hCG. Persistent elevation is indicative of metastatic disease, often beyond the retroperitoneum. A slow rate of marker decline may be of prognostic significance as it reflects tumor volume and viability (Lange and Raghavan 1983). This is of even greater importance postchemotherapy in which case, persistent marker elevation is indicative of an incomplete response. Delayed tumor recurrence often presents initially with tumor marker elevation and therefore effects earlier treatment. Undetectable postoperative levels may imply localized control, but retroperitoneal radiographic and, in some cases, surgical staging is still essential as between 10 and 20% of patients treated with platinum-based combination chemotherapy and subsequent retroperitoneal lymph node dissection exhibit normalized serum tumor markers despite pathologic evidence of viable tumor (Richie and Steele 2002). As always, tumor markers must be interpreted in the context of the patient's entire clinical picture so as to avoid misinterpretations (i.e., false-positives) that could result in unnecessary adjuvant treatment.

### 5.2.5 Orchiectomy and Testicular Pathology

The first step in the surgical staging of testis cancer comes at the time of radical inguinal orchiectomy. Orchiectomy provides not only a definitive diagnosis but also provides local control of the primary tumor. While the details of this procedure are beyond the scope of this chapter (see Chap. 6), its role in staging is extremely important.

An appropriately processed testis specimen should comment specifically on the histologic type of the tumor and should be broadly divided into seminoma or nonseminoma (Richie and Steele 2002). In the case of NSGCT, the presence and percentage of the varying histologic subtypes must be mentioned as these components are of profound prognostic importance (Bower and Rustin 2000). In addition to the type of tumor, comment should be made regarding the extent of the tumor, specifically its T stage and the presence or absence of lymphatic and vascular invasion. The 1997 AJCC Testicular Cancer Staging System is found in Tables 5.1–5.3 and defines explicitly the nature and extent of T stages for testis cancer. Schematic representations are included in Figs. 5.3–5.5. A representative surgical specimen is labeled as Fig. 5.6.

**Table 5.1** Corresponding T (tumor) and N (node) stages TNM staging system 2002 from AJCC

| | |
|---|---|
| Primary tumor (T) | |
| pT0 | No evidence of primary tumor |
| pTis | Intratubular germ cell neoplasia (carcinoma in situ) |
| pT1 | Tumor limited to the testis and epididymis without vascular/lymphatic invasion; tumor may invade into the tunica albuginea but not the tunica vaginalis |
| pT2 | Tumor limited to the testis and epididymis with vascular/lymphatic invasion, or tumor extending through the tunica albuginea with involvement of the tunica vaginalis |
| pT3 | Tumor invades the spermatic cord with or without vascular/lymphatic invasion |
| pT4 | Tumor invades the scrotum with or without vascular/lymphatic invasion |
| Regional lymph nodes (N) | |
| *Clinical* | |
| NX | Regional lymph nodes cannot be assessed |
| N0 | No regional lymph node metastasis |
| N1 | Metastasis with a lymph node mass 2 cm or less in greatest dimension; or multiple lymph nodes, none more than 2 cm in greatest dimension |
| N2 | Metastasis with a lymph node mass more than 2 cm but not more than 5 cm in greatest dimension; or multiple lymph nodes, any one mass greater than 2 cm but not more than 5 cm in greatest dimension |
| N3 | Metastasis with a lymph node mass more than 5 cm in greatest dimension |
| *Pathologic* | |
| pNX | Regional lymph nodes cannot be assessed |
| pN0 | No regional lymph node metastasis |
| pN1 | Metastasis with a lymph node mass 2 cm or less in greatest dimension and less than or equal to five nodes positive, none more than 2 cm in greatest dimension |
| pN2 | Metastasis with a lymph node mass more than 2 cm but not more than 5 cm in greatest dimension; or more than five nodes positive, none more than 5 cm; or evidence of extranodal extension of tumor |
| pN3 | Metastasis with a lymph node mass more than 5 cm in greatest dimension |

**Table 5.2** Corresponding M (metastases) and S (serum tumor markers) of the TNM staging system 2002 from AJCC

| | |
|---|---|
| Distant metastasis (M) | |
| MX | Distant metastasis cannot be assessed |
| M0 | No distant metastasis |
| M1 | Distant metastasis |
| M1a | Nonregional nodal or pulmonary metastasis |
| M1b | Distant metastasis other than to nonregional lymph nodes and lungs |
| Serum tumor markers (S) | |
| SX | Marker studies not available or not performed |
| S0 | Marker study levels within normal limits |
| S1 | LDH < 1.5× **AND**<br>hCG (mIu/mL) <5,000 **AND**<br>AFP (ng/mL) <1,000 |
| S2 | LDH 1.5–10× **OR**<br>hCG (mIu/mL) 5,000–50,000 **OR**<br>AFP (ng/mL) 1,000–10,000 |
| S3 | LDH > 10× **OR**<br>hCG (mIu/mL) >50,000 **OR**<br>AFP (ng/mL) >10,000 |

Significant research has focused on elements of the testis specimen that are predictive of either retroperitoneal spread, risk of tumor relapse, or treatment response. For patients with pure seminoma, the overall risk of metastatic disease is less than 30%, of which less than 5% will have distant disease. Conversely, patients with NSGCTs tend to present equally with localized disease, retroperitoneal metastases, and distant disease (International Germ Cell Cancer Collaborative Group 1997). As seminoma typically exhibits a low metastatic potential, an indolent natural history, and very rare cases of metastatic disease, little focus has been placed on the predictive value of the primary stage of seminoma. Conversely, given the risk of metastasis with NSGCTs and the variability of histologic subtypes among these tumors, directed research was conducted to predict the likelihood of retroperitoneal metastasis based on features of the orchiectomy specimen. Studies by Fung, Moul, and Rodriguez, among others, demonstrated that the presence of vascular invasion, primary stage pT2 or greater, and an embryonal composition of greater than 30% are all proven adverse prognostic features in patients with nonseminomatous tumors (Fung et al. 1988; Rodriguez et al. 1986; Klepp et al. 1990; Wishnow et al. 1989; McLeod et al. 1991; Moul et al. 1993,

**Table 5.3** Equivalence between the original Staging Grouping of Boden and Gibb and the TNM of the AJCC

| Stage grouping | | | | |
|---|---|---|---|---|
| Stage 0 | pTis | N0 | M0 | S0 |
| Stage I | pT1–4 | N0 | M0 | SX |
| Stage IA | pT1 | N0 | M0 | S0 |
| Stage IB | pT2 | N0 | M0 | S0 |
| | pT3 | N0 | M0 | S0 |
| | pT4 | N0 | M0 | S0 |
| Stage IS | Any pT/Tx | N0 | M0 | S1–3 |
| Stage II | Any pT/Tx | N1-3 | M0 | SX |
| Stage IIA | Any pT/Tx | N1 | M0 | S0 |
| | Any pT/Tx | N1 | M0 | S1 |
| Stage IIB | Any pT/Tx | N2 | M0 | S0 |
| | Any pT/Tx | N2 | M0 | S1 |
| Stage IIC | Any pT/Tx | N3 | M0 | S0 |
| | Any pT/Tx | N3 | M0 | S1 |
| Stage III | Any pT/Tx | Any N | M1 | SX |
| Stage IIIA | Any pT/Tx | Any N | M1a | S0 |
| | Any pT/Tx | Any N | M1a | S1 |
| Stage IIIB | Any pT/Tx | N1–3 | M0 | S2 |
| | Any pT/Tx | Any N | M1a | S2 |
| Stage IIIC | Any pT/Tx | N1-3 | M0 | S3 |
| | Any pT/Tx | Any N | M1a | S3 |
| | Any pT/Tx | Any N | M1b | Any S |

1994). On the contrary, the presence of a high percentage of teratoma and yolk sac elements has been noted to portend a more favorable outcome (Klepp et al. 1990). Current research focuses on the predictive value of molecular and genetic features of testis tumors (Bosl et al. 1989; de Graaff et al. 1993; Rodriguez et al. 1992; Austenfield et al. 1992). While these techniques are promising, they have not been proven to be reliable and of true benefit, and have thus been reserved primarily for academic investigation (Bower and Rustin 2000).

### 5.2.6 Retroperitoneal Staging

Surgical removal of the testicle confirms the presence and primary stage of malignancy and offers local control of disease. As with any staging protocol, determination of the extent of disease follows. In the case of testicular cancer, this search for metastatic disease begins in the retroperitoneum. The predilection of testis cancer to spread through lymphatic channels and for metastatic testis cancer to land primarily in the retroperitoneum makes evaluation of this area mandatory. The initial studies by Donohue et al. deftly described the "landing zones" for tumors of both the left and right sides (Fig. 5.7) (1982). Their study demonstrated that right-sided tumors preferentially metastasize to the interaortocaval lymph nodes followed by the precaval and paraaortic lymph nodes. Left-sided tumors, however, preferentially metastasize to the paraaortic and preaortic lymph nodes followed by the interaortocaval lymph nodes with advanced disease. Moreover, it was noted that right-sided tumors are more likely to

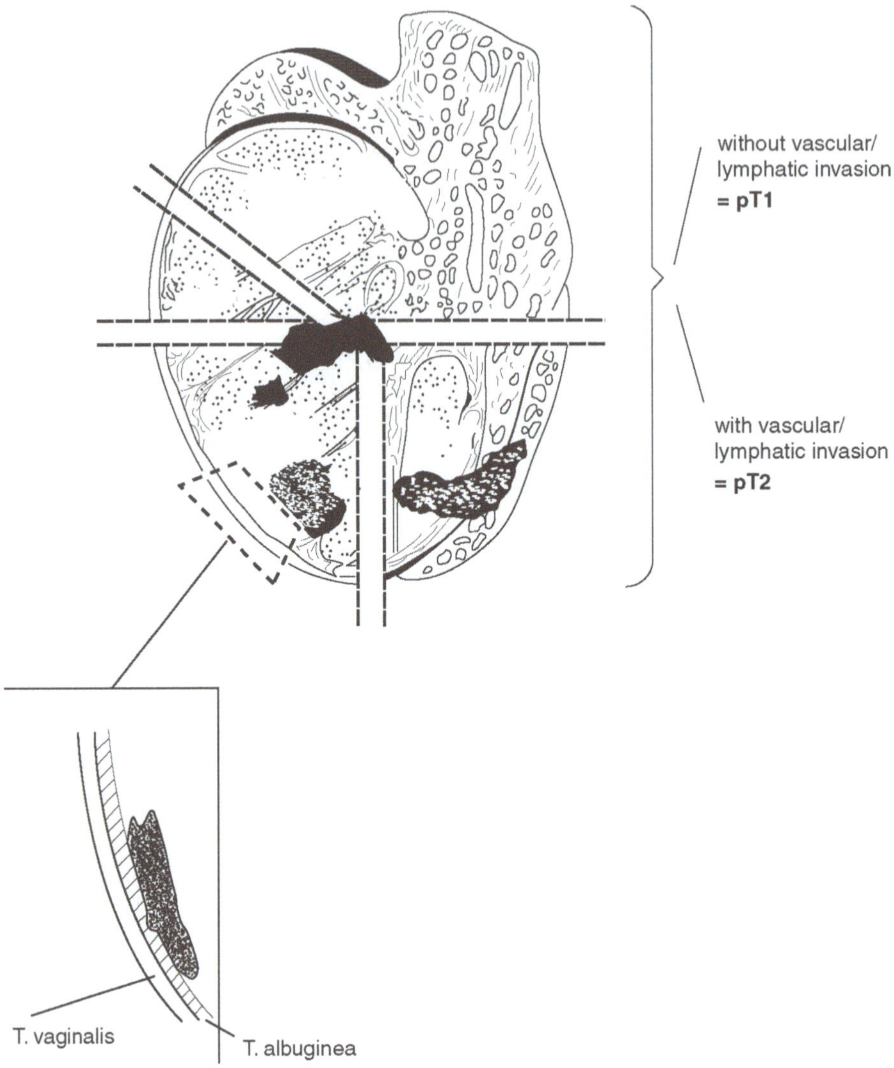


**Fig. 5.3** Schematic representation of T1/T2 primary testis tumor. (Used with the permission of the American Joint Committee on Cancer (AJCC), Chicago, Illinois. The original source for this material is the AJCC Cancer Staging Manual, 6th edn (2002) published by Springer New York, www.springeronline.com)

metastasize to the left side than left-sided tumors are to the right. This general pattern of spread is typical of nearly all germ cell tumors. However, there are notable exceptions to this pattern of lymphatic drainage, among them the vascular propagation of choriocarcinoma (Bower and Rustin 2000).

Computed tomography (CT) is the most commonly employed radiographic tool in staging evaluation of the retroperitoneum. In general, CT offers good sensitivity and accuracy in the identification and description of retroperitoneal pathology, principally soft tissue and visceral disease and lymph nodes greater than 2 cm (Richie and Steele 2002). With the introduction of spiral CT and advanced multidetector systems, CT will likely remain the imaging modality of choice. However, CT is not without its limitations. The false-negative rate at the traditional cut-off of 1 cm approaches 50% owing largely to its inability to detect occult micrometastatic disease (McLeod et al. 1991; Richie et al. 1982b; Hilton et al. 1997). This is of profound importance in the setting of NSGCTs in which occult disease is found in as many as 30% of men. This issue was explicitly evaluated by Sameulssom, Richie and others by comparing CT abnormalities with rendered pathology from retroperitoneal lymph node dissection. Again, the accuracy of CT in predicting retroperitoneal disease was between 50 and 90%, again reflecting the inherent limitation of CT in reliably identifying micrometastatic disease (Richie et al. 1982b; Sameulssom et al. 1986).

Yet another important determinant of CT's utility and adequacy is the assignment of a nodal size that is considered abnormal. This arbitrary threshold profoundly

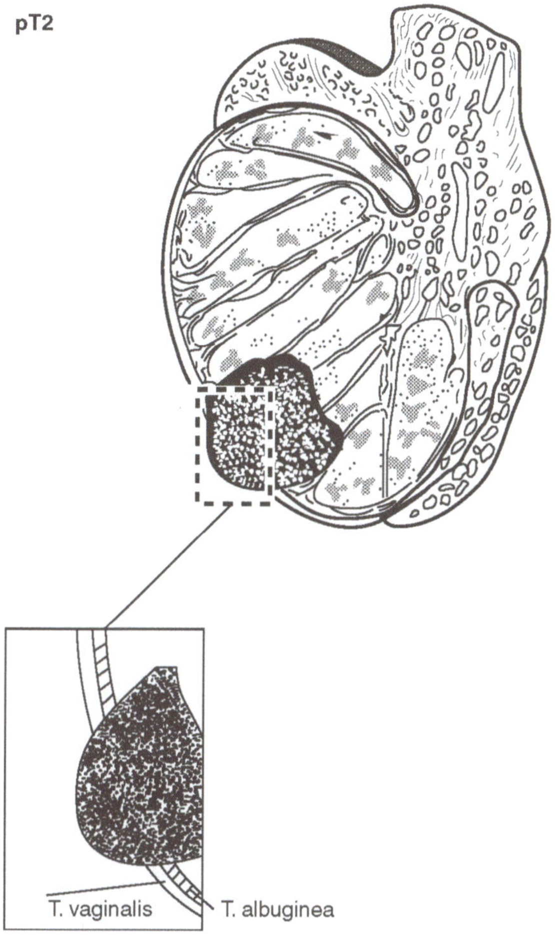


Fig. 5.4 Schematic representation of T2 primary testis tumor

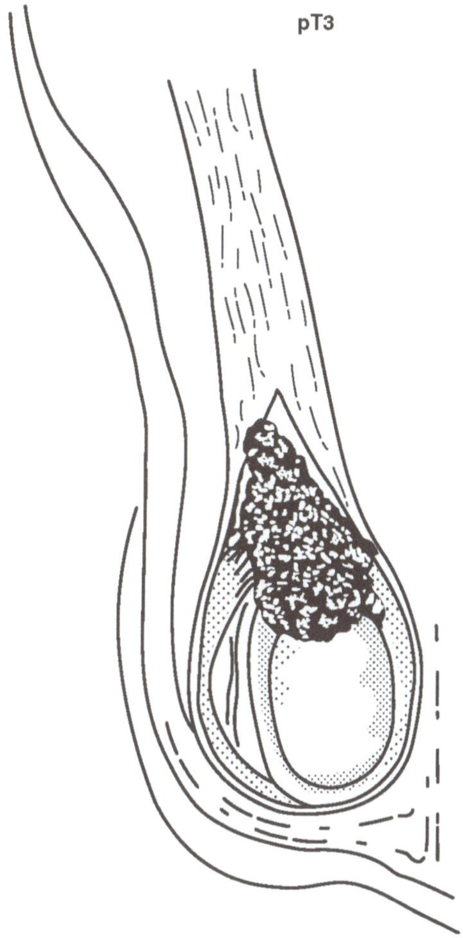


Fig. 5.5 Schematic representation of T3 primary testis tumor

impacts the specificity of CT in detecting retroperitoneal disease. The plurality of institutions considers lymph nodes larger than 10 mm to be abnormal. However, if this threshold is set at 5 mm, the false-negative rate drops significantly but often at the expense of unnecessary therapy (Socinki and Stomper 1988). Conversely, if the threshold is set at 15 mm, the false-negative rate is significantly higher, perhaps delaying the treatment of potentially curable, early-stage metastatic disease (Bower and Rustin 2000; Socinki and Stomper 1988). While studies from Indiana University have found the highest accuracy at a cut-point of 8 mm, the conventional cut-off remains 1 cm (Leibovitch et al. 1995). This point is controversial.

Lymphangiography was utilized for many years in the assessment of retroperitoneal disease. While its use

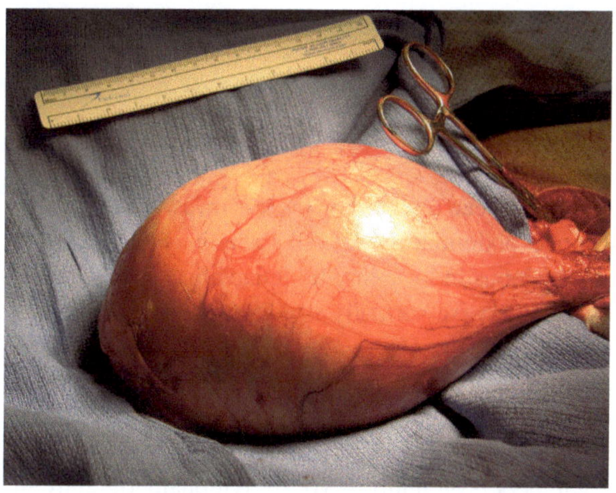

Fig. 5.6 Intraoperative photograph of testis tumor during radical inguinal orchiectomy

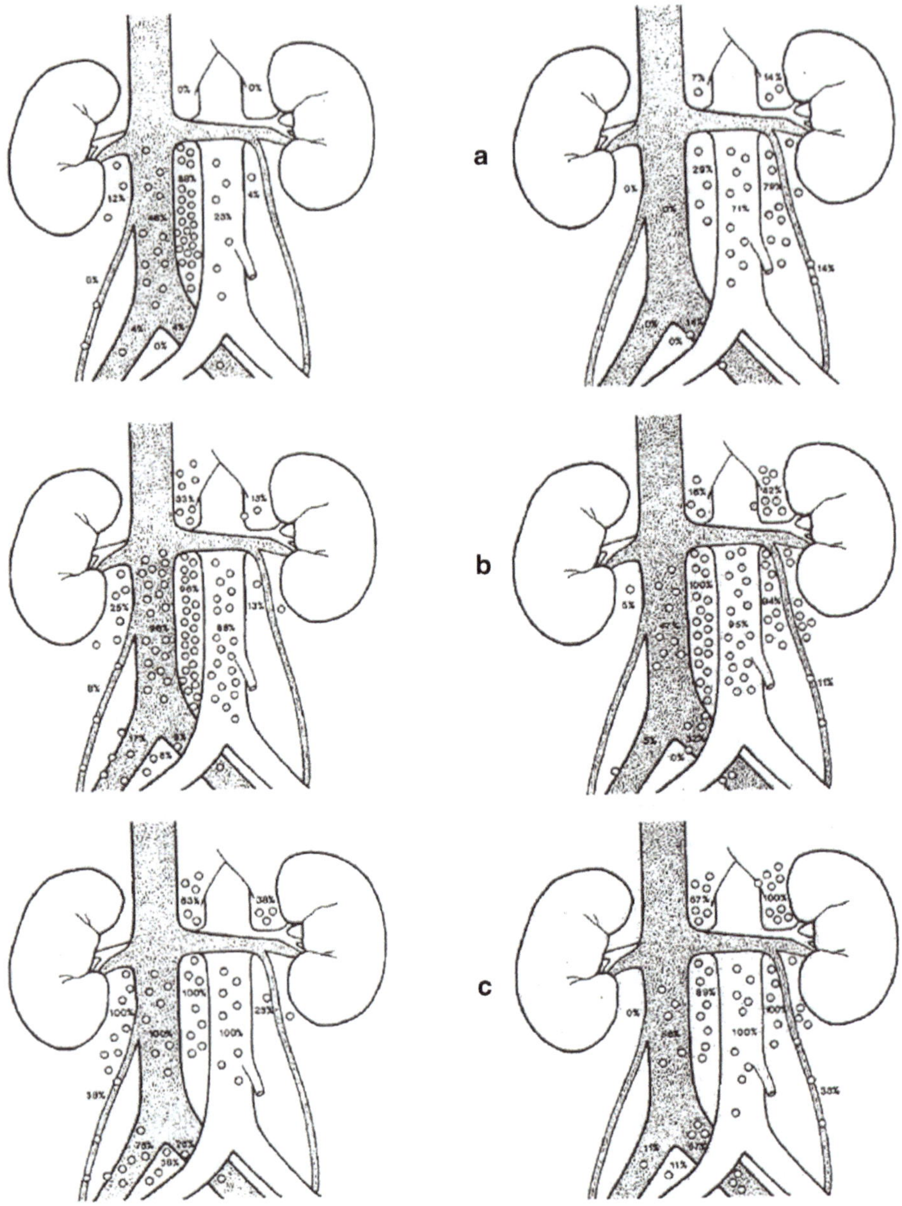


**Fig. 5.7** Schematic representation of metastatic landing zones. (**a**) Stage B1 (*right* and *left*). (**b**) Stage B2 (*right* and *left*). (**c**) Stage B3 (*right* and *left*). (Reprinted with permission from Donohue et al. (1982)

has largely been replaced by the less invasive yet equally accurate abdominopelvic CT scan, it is nevertheless advantageous in its ability to define abnormal architecture in otherwise normally sized lymph nodes (Thomas et al. 1981; Chagnon et al. 1989). However, the risks associated with the procedure, primarily lymphadenitis, wound infection, and pain have essentially prohibited its use (Bower and Rustin 2000). Despite these risks, some researchers profoundly advocate lymphangiography in the evaluation of patients with seminoma preparing for retroperitoneal radiotherapy (Marks et al. 1991).

MRI has been evaluated in limited studies and has been found to offer little advantage over CT in staging of the retroperitoneum. Its accuracy and false-negative rate parallel that of CT, but with prolonged imaging time and at considerable expense (Ellis et al. 1984; Hogeboom et al. 1993).

Positron emission tomography (PET) offers considerable promise but is not yet a viable staging technique. Thus far, its merit in the staging of the retroperitoneum has been proven in only one small study. While this study was limited by some incongruities, it nevertheless found the sensitivity and specificity of PET in detecting retroperitoneal disease to be superior to CT (Cremerius et al. 1999). This data has as yet not been replicated. It appears that the more valuable utility of PET remains the differentiation between teratoma, viable tumor, and necrosis in the setting of a radiographically-detected postchemotherapy mass (Becherer et al. 2005). PET's utility as a functional study has additionally been evaluated in the setting of rising tumor markers after chemotherapy in which no definitive mass can be defined on traditional imaging. Again, its use in this setting is experimental (Hoh et al. 1998). One interesting avenue of possible future investigation may include the combined use of PET-CT as a formal staging modality. While studies of PET have shown no advantage over CT given its inability to detect micrometastatic disease, improved technology and evolving radiotracers may make combined PET-CT a viable technique in the future.

The gold standard for staging of retroperitoneal disease remains retroperitoneal lymph node dissection. All current knowledge of the patterns of disease spread as well as the true incidence of occult retroperitoneal micrometastatic disease was a result of RPLND (Rowland et al. 1982; Donohue et al. 1993). Studies comparing the true incidence of occult disease discovered during RPLND against that predicted radiographically have consistently found an approximate error rate of 20% with imaging (McLeod et al. 1991; Richie et al. 1982b). RPLND thus reveals those patients with micrometastatic disease who are destined to fail surveillance. Not only does RPLND provide optimal diagnostic information but also yields considerable therapeutic benefit as very few patients treated with RPLND experience disease recurrence (Fig. 5.8) (Bower and Rustin 2000). Moreover, the less than 10% of patients that recur after RPLND are almost universally salvaged with chemotherapy.

However valuable RPLND appears as a staging and treatment modality, controversy exists regarding its necessity. Regardless of the limitations of diagnostic imaging in accurately predicting retroperitoneal disease, some have argued that surveillance of stage I NSGCTs should be favored over RPLND (Peckham et al. 1982). This argument is born of the considerable morbidity imbued by RPLND compared to the relatively low risk of micrometastatic disease and the impressive efficacy of chemotherapy in the treatment of surveillance failures. This argument has led to improvements in surgical technique including, but not limited to, nerve-sparing and/or modified operative templates (Jewett and Torbey 1988; Donohue et al. 1990).

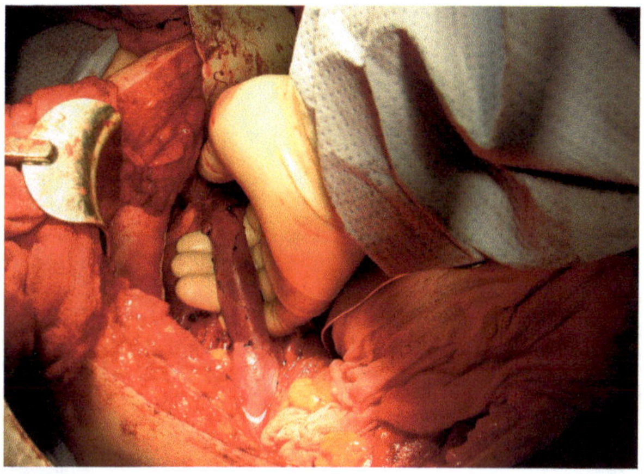

**Fig. 5.8** Intraoperative photograph demonstrating complete retroperitoneal lymph node dissection utilizing a modified right-sided template

The morbidity of open RPLND has led some to advocate laparoscopic RPLND as a less invasive but equally effective diagnostic and therapeutic tool. While the laparoscopic technique certainly reduces the morbidity associated with RPLND and has been proven to decrease postoperative pain and hospital stay, its therapeutic role has been questioned (Klotz 1994). In its current form, laparoscopic RPLND can tender valuable diagnostic information, especially in those with poor prognostic features who decline traditional RPLND (Bhayani et al. 2004). Unfortunately, many pundits criticize the ability of laparoscopic RPLND to duplicate the oncologic efficacy of its open counterpart (Bower and Rustin 2000; Foster 2006). This critical short-coming, coupled with prolonged operative times and the risk of major vessel injury, have thus far limited its widespread acceptance. It appears that while the advent of robotics and the continued maturation of laparoscopic surgeons may eventually allow laparoscopic RPLND to have a prominent role in the staging and treatment of testis cancer in the future, its current role remains controversial and experimental (Davol et al. 2006).

### 5.2.7 Chest Staging

The spread of metastatic disease traditionally follows lymphatic channels to the aforementioned landing zones of the retroperitoneum (Donohue et al. 1982). In cases of advanced disease, the metastases are very

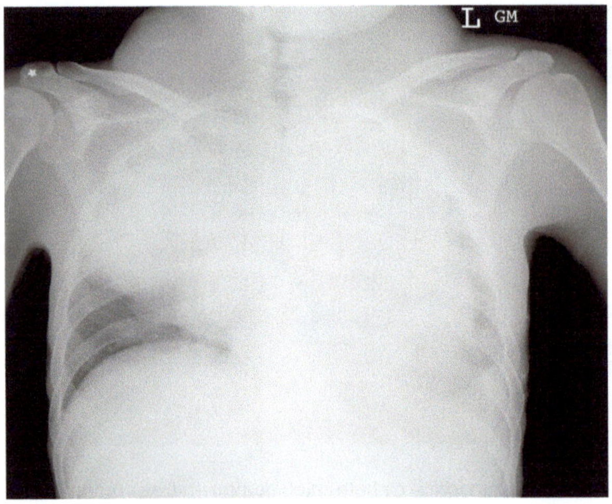


**Fig. 5.9** Chest radiograph demonstrating diffuse metastatic disease

commonly found in the chest. For this reason, staging of the chest is the next requisite step.

Imaging is the most appropriate means of staging the chest owing to its noninvasiveness and overall sensitivity. The only controversial aspect of this issue is the means by which the chest is imaged. Traditionally, chest radiograph and chest tomography were employed with nearly identical sensitivity. As the former is by far the less involved imaging technique, tomography has largely been abandoned (Jochelson et al. 1984). CT of the chest offers improved sensitivity over its counterparts, but is both more expensive and invasive. Determination of the optimal imaging modality was born of a study conducted by See and Hoxie. They determined that the likelihood of chest disease was only 4% in those with negative abdominal CT scans while those with positive abdominal CT scans exhibited chest disease in nearly 40% (Fig. 5.9). As the former group of patients is best served by a test with high specificity, chest radiograph is the most appropriate imaging technique. Conversely, those in the latter group are best served by a test of high sensitivity which in this setting is CT of the chest (See and Hoxie 1993; Steinfeld and Macher 1990).

## 5.3 Staging Systems and Prognostic Models

Staging systems for malignancy exist for essentially two reasons; first, to offer universality of nomenclature, and second, to provide prognostic information based on the presence and extent of disease. In 1951, Boden and Gibb crafted what is widely recognized as the first clinical staging system for testis cancer (Boden and Gibb 1951). In this original system, stage I testis cancer was confined to the testis alone, stage II disease was confined to the retroperitoneum, and stage III disease was beyond the retroperitoneal lymph nodes. And while myriad refinements and subcategories have been created in recent years, current testis cancer staging systems continue to reflect Boden and Gibb's original system.

The staging of seminoma and nonseminomatous germ cell tumors is radically different, as was reflected in the methods by which staging information is collected. NSGCTs are staged both with clinical and surgical modalities while seminomas are staged entirely on a clinical basis. Much of the justification for the differences in the staging of these two types of disease is due to the natural history of the subtypes and the relative success in treatment of each subtype. As varying institutions employed different treatment regimens, especially for metastatic disease, myriad independent staging systems also evolved. In an attempt to consolidate these numerous systems, the American Joint Committee on Cancer (AJCC) created a consensus classification system that was applicable to both seminoma and nonseminomatous tumors. Not only did this initial effort in 1997 help to standardize the nomenclature of testis cancer stages, but it also provided uniformity for research studies. Most notably, the 1997 AJCC staging system introduced a serum tumor marker category for the first time. The ultimate benefit of this "T, N, M, S" system, therefore, was the ability to predict prognosis stage by stage. This is of the utmost importance among those with metastatic disease.

### 5.3.1 Staging systems: Metastatic disease

Prognostic factors for metastatic germ cell cancer are quite unlike those for other solid tumors, particularly in the case of nonseminoma. For example, it became apparent early after the development of effective, cisplatin containing, chemotherapy that the degree of elevation of the serum markers AFP and HCG were more important prognostically than disease bulk or conventional stage. Thus it soon became clear that stage IV disease diagnosed on the basis of lung metastases may have no prognostic significance if markers are low.

Similarly bulky retroperitoneal disease with low serum markers may have an excellent prognosis when modest chemotherapy is combined with surgery for what often proves to predominantly comprise mature teratoma.

During the 1980s multiple prognostic factor classifications were designed by single institutions, national and international groups with a resulting spate of publications (Medical Research Council Working Party on testicular tumours 1985; Mead and Stenning 1992; Bosl et al. 1983; Stoter et al. 1987; Birch et al. 1986). Whilst each of these classifications were demonstrated to be effective on retrospective series, they were rarely tested prospectively. Trials using these classifications around the world could not be compared, with conflicting claims made about the efficacy of different therapies. Indeed a number of publications began to appear comparing classifications and advocating one classification over another (Bajorin et al. 1988).

During this period of time, it was clearly documented that prognosis was rapidly improving as a result of the widespread acceptance that BEP or related regimens were standard therapy and also as a result of increasing experience worldwide in the medical and surgical management of these cases.

## 5.4 The International Germ Cell Collaborative Group

In 1991, the International Germ Cell Cancer Collaborative Group (IGCCCG) was formed. This was led by the United Kingdom Medical Research Council and including clinicians from multiple large institutions and collaborative groups' worldwide (International Germ Cell Cancer Collaborative Group 1997). Early on it was agreed to pool data on patients with metastatic germ cell cancer from the entire platinum treatment era. Furthermore it was agreed that the group would not seek to find the "best fit" amongst the eight or ten classifications in use at that time, but rather would make a fresh start with the new large volumes of data available. In total the data base comprised 5,202 patients with nonseminoma, with a median follow up time of surviving patients of 5 years, and with 75% survival at this time. In addition 660 patients with seminoma were included in the data base, with comparable follow up and 81% five-year survival.

The nonseminoma group was sufficiently large to allow a random 70/30% split of the data, with the larger group used as a "test" set for prognostic classifications, and the smaller group a "validation" set. The data base on seminoma was insufficiently large to allow this data manipulation. The underlying theme of this collaboration was that any classification derived should be user friendly for both clinicians and patients, should include both seminoma and teratoma as the chemotherapy treatment options, which were regarded as comparable, and should also be pertinent to the clinical trial questions considered important at that time.

The study was strengthened by the additional availability of recently acquired separately analyzed data from MRC/EORTC trials in both good and poor prognosis disease and a co-operative group American study in patients with poor prognosis disease.

To fulfill the criteria described above it was considered preferable, where possible; to use objective data (e.g., tumor markers, presence/absence of involvement of a tumor site) rather than more subjective information, e.g., mass size or pathological classification.

Eventually the classification in Table 5.4 was devised and agreed (International Germ Cell Cancer Collaborative Group 1997). Remarkably within 1 year this was adopted worldwide, both for routine clinical use, but also by clinical trial groups, and has dominated clinical practice since.

Any compromise classification of this type can be seen to have areas of weakness, particularly after years of use. The IGCCC classification analyses included patients treated with metastatic disease using carboplatin as a single agent (in seminoma) or in combination in nonseminoma. It is now widely accepted that there may be a survival disadvantage to the use of this drug in these settings (Bokemeyer et al. 2000; Horwich et al. 1997). LDH was confirmed in this study as being an important prognostic factor. There were problems with measurement of this enzyme as assay conditions vary considerably worldwide. It was considered best to measure the degree of elevation of LDH when compared with the upper limit of normal range in any lab. LDH levels were divided into <1.5× upper limit of normal, 1.5–10× upper limit of normal and >10× upper limit of normal. This latter group was small comprising of only 1% of patients with nonseminoma. However, almost half of these cases (5% of the poor risk group) were characterized as high risk on the basis of LDH alone and indeed had poor long term

**Table 5.4** Prognostic based staging system for metastatic Germ Cell Cancer of the IGCCCG (International Germ Cell Cancer Collaborative Group)

| Nonseminoma | Seminoma |
|---|---|
| **Good prognosis** | |
| Testis/retroperitoneal primary<br>Good markers – all of<br>AFP <1,000 ng/mL,HCG<5,000 IU/L<br>LDH < 1.5× upper limit of normal<br>58% of nonseminomas<br>5 year PFS 89%<br>5 year survival 92% | Any primary site<br>No nonpulmonary visceral metastases<br>Normal AFP, any HCG any LDH<br>90% of seminomas<br>5 year PFS 82%<br>5 year survival 86% |
| **Intermediate prognosis** | |
| Testis/retroperitoneal primary<br>No nonpulmonary visceral metastases<br>Intermediate markers – any of<br>AFP ≥1,000 and ≤10,000 ng/mL<br>HCG >5,000 IU/L and <50,000 IU/L<br>LDH ≥1.5× N and ≤10× N<br>28% of nonseminomas<br>5 year PFS 75%<br>5 year survival 80% | Any primary site<br>Nonpulmonary visceral metastases<br>Normal AFP, any HCG, any LDH<br>10% of seminomas<br>5 year PFS 67%<br>5 year survival 72% |
| **Poor prognosis** | |
| Mediastinal primary<br>Nonpulmonary visceral metastases<br>Poor markers – any of<br>AFP >10,000 ng/mL or HCG>50,000 IU/L<br>LDH >10× upper limit of normal<br>16% of nonseminomas<br>5 year PFS 41%<br>5 year survival 48% | No patients classified as poor prognosis |

PFS: pression free survival
AFP: alfa feto protein
HCG : human chorionic gonadotrophin
LDH: lactate dehydrogenase.

survival (3 year progression free survival 42%). A further perceived weakness of the classification was the relatively small numbers of patients with metastatic seminoma – this however reflecting the lower incidence of metastatic disease in patients with this primary histology.

The IGCCCG classification passed its first tests well. Complete IGCCCG data was available on 202 of the patients entered into the previously mentioned co-operative ECOG / SWOG / CALGB trial. These patients were included on the basis of advanced disease according to the Indiana classification and were randomized between BEP and VIP chemotherapy (Hinton et al. 2003). Remarkably, within this group and using the then new IGCCC classification, 14% of patients were considered good prognosis, with a 2-year progression free survival (PFS) of more than 80%. Over 30% were considered intermediate risk, with a 2-year progression free survival of 74% and just over half were classified as poor prognosis with a 2-year progression free survival of 50%.

In a second study from the MRC / EORTC, reported in 1998 (Kaye et al. 1998), patients were reclassified in a similar fashion. Two hundred and fifty two patients were entered into this study on the basis of poor prognosis disease using an MRC classification in use at that time (Mead and Stenning 1992). Comparable data to the US study was obtained, as 39% of patients proved to have good / intermediate prognosis disease with a 1 year PFS rate of 71%, the remaining poor prognosis patients having a PFS of 49%.

To some extent, the IGCCC classification has driven trial development. In particular, the EORTC conducted a study in 812 patients with good prognosis disease which compared 3 vs. 4 courses of BEP chemotherapy (de Wit et al. 2001). The treatment results in this study population were excellent with a 90% PFS at 2 years and overall survival of 97%. The group demonstrated convincingly that three cycles of BEP should now be standard therapy, and also confirmed that this therapy was equally effective given over 3 or 5 days.

The EORTC/MRC are currently conducting separate randomized trials in patients with intermediate and poor prognosis disease. In the former group 4 cycles of BEP are being compared with four cycles of BEP + paclitaxel. In the latter group the EORTC are conducting a trial comparing four cycles of standard dose BEP against four cycles of VIP – the last three cycles given at high dose with stem cell support. Finally, in the 2006 ASCO meeting a co-operative group trial by the Memorial Sloan – Kettering Cancer Center, ECOG, SWOG and CALGB was reported (Fossa et al. 1997). This study randomized 219 patients with intermediate or poor prognosis germ cell cancer using the IGCCC classification. Patients were randomized to receive either four cycles of BEP or two cycles of BEP followed by two cycles of high dose chemotherapy.

Complete remission rates at 1 year were reported respectively as 52% and 48% ($P=0.53$) approximating those anticipated from the classification.

### 5.4.1 New Prognostic Models: Seminoma

Seminoma is less common than nonseminoma and relatively small numbers in the IGCCC study precluded as comprehensive review as was possible for nonseminoma. This cancer differs in a number of ways from nonseminoma and is far less commonly metastatic. This disease comparatively rarely involves the viscera and is exquisitely chemo-sensitive. Tumor marker elevations are generally modest and confined to HCG and LDH. Finally, a proportion of patients will have been previously irradiated for stage I or early stage II disease but will only receive chemotherapy at relapse. Patients with seminoma are a median 10 years older than patients with nonseminoma.

A number of attempts have been made since the IGCCC classification to re-look at seminoma, with attempts to exploit these possible prognostic factors in a new classification.

Fossa et al. (1997) studied 286 patients with advanced seminoma and in many cases had much more detailed data than was available to the IGCCC; 50 of these patients had been treated with prior radiotherapy. The median age of the patients was 40 years. All patients were treated with platin containing chemotherapy; in 58 cases this was carboplatin given as a single agent. LDH levels were not available in all patients. The 3 year survival rate was 85%. Prognostic models derived from this patient population were tested on a separate data set of 166 patients entered into MRC / EORC trials current at that time. On multivariable analysis the most important adverse feature was, as in the IGCCC classification, the presence of nonpulmonary visceral metastases. LDH provided initial prognostic discrimination when handled as a binary variable (<2× upper limit of normal vs. ≥ × normal range). Prior radiotherapy was shown to be associated with a poorer prognosis. Further analysis suggested that this related to the use of extended field irradiation in the earliest treatment era analyzed, with presumed resulting bone marrow damage and impaired chemotherapy delivery. Since such widefield irradiation has now been abandoned it was decided to omit these patients from the analyses.

Two possible classifications were devised by Fossa et al. The favored classification is shown below.

| | |
|---|---|
| Group I | Stage II any LDH or stage III LDH <2× normal or |
| | stage IV PVM with LDH <2× normal |
| Group II | Stage III LDH ≥2× normal or |
| | Stage IV PVM with LDH ≥2× normal or<br>Stage IV NPVM with any LDH |
| | PVM = pulmonary visceral metastases only |
| | NVPM = nonpulmonary visceral metastases |

The results of the analyses of the test and validation data used in this classification are shown in Table 5.5.

In a further attempt to improve prognostic discrimination in patients with seminoma, Bokemeyer et al. (2000) presented a poster at the ASCO meeting in 2000 in which accumulated data from 566 patients with seminoma entered into prospective trials by the MRC and were analyzed in France and Germany. Thirty-five percent of these patients had been treated with single agent carboplatin and the remainder with cisplatin containing combinations. Remarkably 28% of the patients had an extra-gonadal primary site.

At a median follow up of 4 years 86% of the patients were alive and disease free. Univariate analysis revealed the following negative factors for progression free and overall survival ($P<0.05$): age >50 years,

**Table 5.5** Survival in the classification proposed by Fossa et al, 1997) for advanced Seminoma

| Group | No. | % | 3 Year PFS |
|---|---|---|---|
| *Test set* | 198 | | |
| Group I | 160 | 84 | 94 |
| Group II | 38 | 16 | 56 |
| *Validation set* | 118 | | |
| Group I | 104 | 88 | 87 |
| Group II | 14 | 12 | 64 |

previous irradiation, presence of visceral metastases (only overall survival), presence of pulmonary metastases and two or more metastatic sites. Carboplatin was shown to be less effective than cisplatin in terms of progression free survival but not overall survival. The data was also examined using the IGCCC criteria in which the division into good / intermediate prognosis was 92% vs. 8% of patients.

The data presented from Fossa et al. (1997) Bokemeyer et al. (2000) provided interesting new insights into the prognostic factors determining treatment outcome. To date these have not been widely adopted. What is quite clear is that outlook for this condition is excellent – and probably still improving.

### 5.4.2 Nonseminoma: Reviews of the Functionality of the IGCCC

The IGCCC classification was, as described, deliberately developed as a user friendly and relatively noncomplex formulation of prognosis. A number of potential weaknesses were later identified in the classification. For example the absence of weighting of the poor prognostic features (where the presence of any one feature, e.g., mediastinal primary or liver metastases put the patient into this group) and similarly the potential loss of discrimination between patients having one or more than one adverse feature.

A number of studies have explored this aspect of the IGCCC to see if it could be refined, or made more flexible. van Dijk et al. (2004a) applied prognostic weighting to the different components of the IGCCC patient population using complex statistical modeling. Interestingly they found that AFP, as used in the IGCCC cut-offs was a less useful discriminator of prognosis than HCG or LDH, and similarly found that the presence of nonpulmonary visceral metastases (NPVM) was the least important amongst the poor prognosis prognostic factors. This group derived a number of possible alternative models to the IGCCC using these weightings, particularly in the poor prognosis group, but failed to demonstrate a clear discriminatory improvement. Their predominant proposal was a division of the poor prognostic groups into potentially three groups.

Kollmannsberger et al. (2000) also chose to examine the IGCCC poor prognosis population in more detail. They used the classification – and – regression tree modeling (CART) on a group of 332 patients entered into poor prognosis studies in Germany and the USA between 1984 and 1997, and examined the subgroup found retrospectively to be poor prognosis using IGCCC criteria. This study was regarded as exploratory. The two most important adverse prognostic features for progression free survival were the presence of a mediastinal primary, followed by the presence of NPVM. However when survival was examined (and in contrast to the van Dijk study) NPVM became the most important function. Kollmannsberger et al. then proceeded to divide the poor prognosis population into three groups with 2 years survival varying between 49% in the worse group and 84% in the best group – this latter having a gonadal / retroperitoneal primary site without visceral metastases. The classification derived was then tested by van Dijk in a separate publication (van Dijk et al. 2004b) using the IGCCC patient data set. They also re-examined this data using CART methodology. They noted that the outlook in the German / American study was markedly better than the IGCCC outcome, probably relating to the fact that this was a more recent patient population. van Dijk found that neither regression tree functioned at all well in further dividing this patient population.

Whilst these latter studies are of great intrinsic interest the author would wish to note that this is a rare patient population - comprising in the IGCCC grouping only 14% of patients – and almost certainly diminishing. Recent trials have had considerable difficulty accruing patients with poor prognosis disease even when the overall group is used as a randomization factor. Therefore, further division of poor prognosis patients in this fashion is almost not worthwhile other than in the interest of the individual patient or clinician.

Extra-cranial, extra-gonadal, germ cell cancers comprise only a tiny proportion (perhaps 2–5%) of metastatic germ cell cancer. Retroperitoneal extragonadal cancers (which may in perhaps half of cases derive from an occult testicular primary) were found in the IGCCC to have no detriment in outlook compared with their gonadal counterpart. By contrast mediastinal nonseminoma is recognized worldwide as having a poor outlook – in marked contrast to mediastinal seminoma which can be regarded as having a good prognosis in the absence of NPVM.

In a remarkable study Hartmann et al. (2002) accumulated multicenter data on 635 patients with extragonadal germ cell cancer, comprising 104 patients with seminoma and 524 with nonseminoma (7 were not specified). Fifty-four percent of the patients were found to have a mediastinal primary. Data was obtained from 11 centers worldwide by a standard questionnaire and analyzed using a standard Cox model and CART.

All patients with extra-gonadal seminoma proved to have an excellent (89% 5 year) survival. The non-seminomatous population fared less well and were divided into three populations. Scoring was applied as follows: score 1 each for the presence of liver or lung metastase or the presence of an elevated HCG, score 2 for CNS metastases or a mediastinal primary. The patients population was divided into score 0 (seminoma) / 1, 2/3, or >3 risk factors with the resulting 5 year survival respectively of 94%, 90%, 80% and 49%. This study, like the previous studies in poor prognosis disease, can however be criticized as examining a rare patient group, with little practical relevance to clinical trials. Again this may be useful data with regard to individual patients and their prognosis.

In summary it can be stated that the IGCCC, for all its perceived faults, has functioned well and been a driver for clinical trials. Subsequent studies described above have proved invaluable in interrogating this and other data sets but have not substantially moved things forward in clinical practice.

## 5.5 Conclusions

The evolution in our understanding and management of germ cell cancers in the last 30 years has been one of the outstanding achievements in modern oncology practice. The vast majority of patients are now cured, and their appropriate management is now highly accurately guided by the prognostic models described for early and advanced disease. The diminishing number of randomized trials currently underway in this disease is a testimony to the effectiveness of these modern therapies.

New biological markers of prognosis are under development, but as always in clinical medicine these must be robustly tested and proven to be accurate, affordable, and widely applicable.

## References


American Cancer Society (2006) Cancer facts and figures 2006. American Cancer Society, Atlanta

Austenfield M, Bilhartz D, Nativ O et al (1992) Flow cytometric DNA ploidy pattern for predicting metastasis of clinical stage I nonseminomatous germ cell testicular tumors. Proc Natl Acad Sci USA 41:379–383

Bagshawe K, Searle F (1977) Tumour markers. In: Marks C, Hale C (eds) Essays in medical biochemistry, vol 3. Biochemical Society, London, pp 25–74

Bajorin D, Katz A, Chan E et al (1988) Comparison of criteria for assigning germ cell tumor patients to "good risk" and "poor risk" studies. J Clin Oncol 6:786–792

Barzell W, Whitmore W Jr (1979) Clinical significance of biological markers: Memorial Hospital experience. Semin Oncol 6:48–52

Becherer A, DeSantis M, Karanikas G et al (2005) FDG PET is superior to CT in the prediction of viable tumour in post-chemotherapy seminoma residuals. Eur J Radiol 54:284–288

Benson C (1988) The role of ultrasound in diagnosis and staging of testicular cancer. Semin Urol 6:189–202

Bhayani S, Allaf M, Kavoussi L (2004) Laparoscopic RPLND for clinical stage I nonseminomatous germ cell testicular cancer: current status. Urol Oncol 22:145–148

Birch R, Williams S, Cone A et al (1986) Prognostic factors for favorable outcome in disseminated germ cell tumors. J Clin Oncol 4:400–407

Boden G, Gibb R (1951) Radiotherapy and testicular neoplasms. Lancet 2:1195–1197

Bokemeyer C, Kollmannsberger C, Flechon A et al (2000) Prognostic factors in patients with advanced metastatic seminoma (SEM) treated with either single agent carboplatin (CP) or cisplatin based (DDP) combination chemotherapy (CTX): a meta-analysis of prospective European trials. Proc ASCO 2000; 19 Abstr 740

Bokemeyer C, Hartmann J, Fossa S et al (2003) Extragonodal germ cell tumors: relation to testicular neoplasia and management options. APMIS 111:49–63

Bosl G, Vogelzang N, Goldman A et al (1981) Impact of delay in diagnosis on clinical stage of testicular cancer. Lancet 2: 970–973

Bosl GJ, Geller NL, Cirrincione C et al (1983) Multivariate analysis of prognostic variables in patients with metastatic testicular cancer. Cancer Res 43:3403–3407

Bosl G, Dmitrovsky E, Reuter V et al (1989) Isochromosome of chromosome 12: clinically useful marker for male germ cell tumors. J Natl Cancer Inst 81:874–878

Bower M, Rustin G (2000) Serum tumor markers and their role in monitoring germ cell cancers of the testis. In: Vogelzang N, Scardino P, Shipley W, Coffey D (eds) Comprehensive textbook of genitourinary oncology, 2nd edn. Lippincott Williams and Wilkins, Philadelphia, pp 927–938

Boyle L, Samuels M (1977) Serum LDH activity and isoenzyme patterns in nonseminomatous germinal (NSG) testis tumors. Proc Am Soc Lin Oncol 18:278

Caldamone A, Altebarmakian V, Frank I et al (1979) Leydig cell tumor of testis. Urology 14:39–43

Chagnon S, Cochand-Priollet B, Gzall M et al (1989) Pelvic cancers: staging of 139 cases with lymphangiography and fine-needle aspiration biopsy. Radiology 173:103–106

Cremerius U, Wildberger J, Borchers H et al (1999) Does positron emission tomography using 18-fluoro-2-deoxyglucose improve clinical staging of testicular cancer? Results of a study of 50 patients. Urology 54:900–904

Davol P, Sumfest J, Rukstalis D (2006) Robotic-assisted laparoscopic retroperitoneal lymph node dissection. Urology 67:199

de Graaff W, van Echten-Arends J, Oosterhuis J et al (1993) Cytogenetic abnormalities and clinical stage in testicular nonseminomatous germ cell tumors. Cancer Genet Cytogenet 70:12–16

de Wit R, Roberts T, Wilkinson M et al (2001) Equivalence of three or four cycles of bleomycin, etoposide and cisplatin chemotherapy and of a 3- or 5- day schedule in good prognosis germ cell cancer: a randomized study of the European Organization for Research and Treatment of Cancer Genitourinary Tract Cancer Cooperative Group and the Medical Research Council. J Clin Oncol 19:1629–1640

Donohue J, Zachary J, Maynard B (1982) Distribution of nodal metastases in nonseminomatous testis cancer. J Urol 128: 315–320

Donohue J, Foster R, Rowland R et al (1990) Nerve sparing retropertioneal lymphadenectomy with preservation of ejaculation. J Urol 144:287–291

Donohue J, Thornhill J, Foster R (1993) Retroperitoneal lymphadenopathy for clinical stage A testis cancer (1965-1989): modifications of technique and impact on ejaculation. J Urol 149:237–243

Ellis J, Bies J, Kopecky K et al (1984) Comparison of NMR and CT imaging in the evaluation of metastatic retroperitoneal lymphadenopathy from testicular carcinoma. J Comput Assist Tomogr 8(4):709–719

Fossa SD, Oliver RTD, Stenning SP et al (1997) Prognostic factors for patients with advanced seminoma treated with platinum based chemotherapy. Eur J Cancer 33:1380–1387

Foster R (2006) Point and counterpoint: treating stage I testis cancer – should laparoscopic RPLND replace open RPLND as the standard of care? Cont Urol :29-38.

Fung C, Kalish L, Brodsky G et al (1988) Stage I nonseminomatous germ cell testicular tumor: prediction of metastatic potential by primary histopathology. J Clin Oncol 6:1467–1473

Hartmann JT, Nichols CR, Droz JP et al (2002) Prognostic variables for response and outcome in patients with extragonadal germ cell tumors. Ann Oncol 13:1017–1028

Hilton S, Herr H, Teitcher J et al (1997) CT detection of retroperitoneal lymph node metastasis in patients with clinical stage I testicular nonseminomatous germ cell cancer: assessment of size and distribution criteria. AJR 149:1187–1190

Hinton S, Catalano PJ, Einhorn LH et al (2003) Cisplatin, etoposide and either bleomycin or ifosfamide in the treatment of disseminated germ cell tumors. Final analysis of an Intergroup trial. Cancer 97:1869–1875

Hogeboom W, Koekstra H, Mooyaart E et al (1993) Magnetic resonance imaging of retroperitoneal lymph node metastases of nonseminomatous germ cell tumors of the testis. J Surg Oncol 19:429–437

Hoh C, Seltzer M, Franklin J et al (1998) Positron emission tomography in urological oncology. J Urol 159:347–356

Hortsman W (1997) Scrotal imaging. Urol Clin North Am 24: 653–668

Horwich A, Sleijfer DT, Fossa SD et al (1997) Randomised trial of bleomycin, etoposide and cisplatin compared with bleomycin, etoposide and carboplatin in good prognosis metastatic nonseminomatous germ cell cancer: a Multiinstitutional Medical Research Council/European Organization for Research and Treatment of Cancer Trial. J Clin Oncol 15:1844–1952

Hricak H, Hamm B, Kim B (1995) Imaging of the scrotum: textbook and atlas. Raven press, New York, pp 49–93

International Germ Cell Cancer Collaborative Group (1997) International Germ Cell Consensus Classification: a prognostic factor-based staging system for metastatic germ cell cancers. J Clin Oncol 15:594–603

Javadpour N (1980) Significance of elevated serum alphafetaproteins (AFP) in seminoma. Cancer 45:2166–2168

Javadpour N (1983) Multiple biochemical tumour markers in testicular cancer. Cancer 52:887–889

Jewett M, Torbey C (1988) Nerve sparing techniques in retroperitoneal lymphadenectomy in patients with low stage testicular cancer. Semin Urol 6:233–237

Jochelson M, Garnick M, Balikian J, Richie J (1984) The efficacy of routine whole lung tomography in germ cell tumors. Cancer 54:1007–1009

Kaye SB, Mead GM, Fossa S et al (1998) Intensive induction-sequential chemotherapy with BOP/VIP-B compared with treatment with BEP/EP for poor prognosis metastatic nonseminomatous germ cell tumor: a randomized Medical Research Council/European Organization for Research and Treatment of Cancer study. J Clin Oncol 16:692–701

Kennedy B, Schmidt J, Winchester D et al (1987) National survey of patterns of care for testis cancer. Cancer 60:1921–1930

Klein E (1993) Tumor markers in testis cancer. Urol Clin North Am 20:67–73

Klepp O, Olsson A, Henrikson H et al (1990) Prognostic factors in clinical stage I nonseminomatous germ cell tumors of the testis: multivariate analysis of a protective multicenter study. J Clin Oncol 8:509–518

Klotz L (1994) Laparoscopic retroperitoneal lymphadenectomy for high-risk stage I nonseminomatous germ cell tumor: a report of four cases. Urology 43:752–756

Kollmannsberger C, Nichols C, Meisner C et al (2000) Identification of prognostic subgroiups among patients with metastatic IGCCCG poor prognosis germ cell cancer: an explorative analysis using cart modelling. Ann Oncol 11:1115–1120

Landis S, Murray T, Bolden S et al (1998) Cancer statistics, 1998. CA Cancer J Clin 48:6–29

Lange P, Raghavan D (1983) Clinical application of tumor markers in testicular cancer. In: Donohue J (ed) Testis tumor. Williams and Wilkins, Baltimore, pp 111–130

Leibovitch I, Foster R, Kopecky K et al (1995) Improved accuracy of computerized tomography based clinical staging in low stage nonseminomatous germ cell cancer using size criteria of retroperitoneal lymph nodes. J Urol 154: 1759–1763

Marks L, Shipley W, Walker T et al (1991) Role of lymphangiograpy in staging testicular seminoma. Urology 38: 264–266

Marth D, Scheidegger J, Studer U (1990) Ultrasonography of testicular tumors. Urol Int 45:237–240

McLeod D, Weiss R, Stablein D et al (1991) Staging relationships and outcome in early stage testicular cancer: a report from the Testicular Cancer Intergroup Study. J Urol 145: 1178–1183

Mead GM, Stenning SP, Parkinson MC et al (1992) The second Medical Research Council Study of prognostic factors in nonseminomatous germ cell tumors. J Clin Oncol 10: 85–94

Medical Research Council Working Party on testicular tumours (1985) Prognostic factors in advanced non-seminomatous germ cell testicular tumours: results of a multi-centre study. Lancet 1:8–11

Mencel P, Motzer R, Mazumdar M et al (1994) Advanced seminoma; treatment results, survival, and prognostic factors in 142 patients. J Clin Oncol 12:120–126

Moul J, Foely J, Hitchcock C et al (1993) Flow cytometric and quantitative histological parameters to predict occult disease in clinical stage I nonseminomatous testicular germ cell tumors. J Urol 150:879–883

Moul J, McCarthy W, Fernandez C et al (1994) Percentage of embryonal carcinoma and vascular invasion predicts pathological stage in clinical stage I nonseminomatous testicular cancer. Cancer Res 54:362–364

Nizkas D, Champion A, Fox M (1990) Germ cell tumors of testis: prognostic factors and results. Eur Urol 18:242–247

Oyen R, Verellen S, Drochmans A et al (1993) Value of MRI in the diagnosis and staging of testicular tumors. J Belge Radiol 76:84–89

Peckham M, Barrett A, Husband J et al (1982) Orchidectomy alone in testicular stage I non-seminomatous germ-cell tumours. Lancet 2:678–680

Preti H, Logothetis C (1993) Testicular carcinoma. In: Pazdur R (ed) Medical oncology. PRR, Huntington, NY, pp 295–312

Raman J, Nobert C, Goldstein M (2005) Increased incidence of testicular cancer in men presenting with infertility and abnormal semen analysis. J Urol 174:1819–1822

Richie J (1993) Advances in the diagnosis and treatment of testicular cancer. Clin Invest 11:670–675

Richie J, Steele G (2002) Neoplasms of the testis. In: Walsh P, Retik A, Vaughan E, Wein A (eds) Campbell's urology, 8th edn. Saunders, Philadelphia, pp 2876–2919

Richie J, Birnholz J, Garnick M (1982a) Ultrasonography as a diagnostic adjunct for the evaluation of masses in the scrotum. Surg Gynecol Obstet 154:695–698

Richie J, Garnick M, Finberg H (1982b) Computerized tomography: how accurate for abdominal staging of testis tumors? J Urol 127:715–717

Rodriguez P, Hafez G, Messing E (1986) Nonseminomatous germ cell tumor of the testicle: does extensive staging of the primary tumor predict the likelihood of metastatic disease? J Urol 136:604–608

Rodriguez E, Mathew S, Mukherjee A et al (1992) Cytogenetic analysis of 124 prospectively ascertained male germ cell tumors. Cancer Res 52:2285–2291

Rowland R, Weisman D, Williams S et al (1982) Accuracy of preoperative staging in stage A and B nonseminomatous germ cell testis tumors. J Urol 127:718–720

Sameulssom L, Fosberg L, Olsson A (1986) Accuracy of radiological staging procedures in nonseminomatous testis cancer compared with findings from surgical exploration and histopathological studies of extirpated tissue. Br J Radiol 59: 131–134

Schwerk W, Schwerk W, Rodeck G (1987) Testicular tumors: prospective analysis of real-time US patterns and abdominal staging. Radiology 164:369–374

See W, Hoxie L (1993) Chest staging in testis cancer patients: imaging modality selection based upon risk assessment as determined by abdominal computerized tomography scan results. J Urol 150:874–878

Socinki M, Stomper P (1988) Radiologic evaluating of nonseminomatous germ cell tumor of the testis. Semin Urol 6: 203–215

Steinfeld A, Macher M (1990) Radiologic staging of chest in testicular seminoma. Urology 36:428–436

Stoter G, Sylvester R, Sleijfer DT et al (1987) Multivariate analysis of prognostic factors in patients with disseminated nonseminomatous testicular cancer. Results from a European Organization for Research on Treatment of Cancer multiinstitutional Phase III study. Cancer Res 47:2714–2718

Thomas J, Bernardino M, Bracken R (1981) Staging of testicular carcinoma: comparison of CT and lymphangiography. Am J Roentgenol 137:991–996

Thurnher S, Hricak H, Carroll P et al (1988) Imaging the testis: comparison between MR staging and US. Radiology 167: 633–636

van Dijk MR, Steyerberg EW, Stenning SP, Dusseldorp E, Habbema JDF (2004) Survival of patients with nonseminomatous germ cell cancer: a review of the IGCC classification by Cox regression and recursive partitioning. Br J Cancer 90:1176–1183

van Dijk MR, Steyerberger EW, Stenning SP, Habbema JDF (2004b) Identifying subgroups among poor prognosis patients with nonseminomatous germ cell cancer by tree modelling: a validation study. Ann Oncol 15:1400–1405

Wishnow K, Johnson D, Swanson D et al (1989) Identifying patients with low-risk clinical stage I nonseminomatous testicular tumors who should be treated by surveillance. Urology 34:339–343

# 6 CIS and Bilateral Cancer: Clinical Presentation and Diagnostics

Paul J. Turek, Ewa Rajpert-De Meyts, Gedske Daugaard, and Niels E. Skakkebaek

## 6.1 Introduction

Although a rare disease, the incidence of testis cancer is increasing in many countries, exhibiting an average annual rate of rise of 2–5% (Bray et al. 2006). Moreover, patients with testis cancer have a significantly higher risk of developing a second germ cell tumor in the remaining testis, as a preinvasive neoplasm can be found in the contralateral testis at the time of primary orchiectomy in approximately 5% of cases. Combined with a very high cure rate, these observations make the topic of secondary testis cancer a timely issue for study. In addition, knowledge of secondary germ cell cancers may improve our understanding of etiologic factors and mechanisms of tumor development. This chapter focuses on the prevalence, diagnosis, treatment, and etiology of bilateral testis cancer.

## 6.2 Prevalence

The prevalence of bilateral testicular germ cell tumor (TGCT) varies between 1 and 5% of testis cancer cases (Hentrich et al. 2005). Secondary germ cell tumors can occur either as synchronous lesions, occurring simultaneous (i.e., within 2 months) to the original tumor, or metachronously, in which a second tumor is detected after the diagnosis of the original tumor. In a review of the world literature published in 2005, bilateral cancers were detected in 2.5% of patients ($n=28{,}689$) with germ cell tumors (Hentrich et al. 2005). Among the 700 bilateral cancers reviewed, 16% were synchronous and 84% were metachronous. Therefore, synchronous tumors constituted 0.4% of all germ cell tumor cases and metachronous tumors comprised 2.1% of cancer cases. The median time to develop a contralateral tumor in metachronous cases from one report of 1,180 germ cell tumor cases is 71 months after the original tumor is diagnosed (Hentrich et al. 2005).

Additionally, although not presenting as overt cancer, the contralateral testis may harbor a precancerous condition termed carcinoma in situ of the testis (CIS), also known as intratubular germ cell neoplasia (ITGCN) or testicular intraepithelial neoplasia (TIN). CIS was first proposed as a precursor for TGCT in 1972 (Skakkebaek 1972) and, a few years later, it was observed to occur in the contralateral testes of 5% of Danish patients with unilateral TGCT in the same group (Berthelsen et al. 1979, 1982; Von der Maase et al. 1986a). The prevalence of contralateral CIS has been subsequently investigated in numerous studies. The largest recent study from Germany confirms that approximately 5% of patients with unilateral testis cancer are affected (Dieckmann et al. 2007). There is no reliable prevalence data from the US, where contralateral biopsies are rarely performed.

## 6.3 Risk Factors

As detailed elsewhere in this chapter, the best-established risk factor for the development of subsequent testis cancer is the finding of CIS/TIN in the contralateral testis. In roughly 50% of cases, CIS of the contralateral testis will develop into overt testis cancer within 5 years (Von der Maase et al. 1986a; Dieckmann and Loy 1996). This has led to controversy concerning

P.J. Turek (✉)
The Turek Clinic, 55 Francisco st, suite 300,
San Francisco, CA 94133, USA
e-mail: Dr Paul Turek@gmail.com

M.P. Laguna et al. (eds.), *Cancer of the Testis*,
DOI: 10.1007/978-1-84800-370-5_6, © Springer-Verlag London Limited 2010

whether the contralateral testis should undergo biopsy at the time of treatment of the original tumor. In general, other risk factors for the development of testis cancer are prior cryptorchidism, infertility, testis microlithiasis or atrophy (<12 mL), and genetic predisposition. These are also considered risk factors for the development of second germ cell tumors based on the fact that each condition leads to increased risk of CIS in contralateral testis (Harland et al. 1998). However, with the exception of CIS, the exact weight of these risk factors in the development of second germ cell tumors has not been well elucidated. In addition, despite the presence of these risk factors, the majority of patients with testicular cancer do not harbor CIS in the remaining testis and the reason for cancer development in these cases is less clear. Lastly, it is also apparent that cytotoxic treatment of the first tumor does not protect against the development of subsequent germ cell tumors (Wanderas et al. 1997a; Fossa and Aass 1989). In summary, based more on biological than clinical evidence, the risk factors for the development of a second testis cancer are similar to those outlined for first tumors.

Similar to other cancers, the country of origin of patients may also be a risk factor for the development of a second germ cell tumor. Depending on the country of origin, European men have a 12- to 38-fold increase risk of developing a second testis cancer compared to men from the general population (Fossa et al. 2005). This risk is up to 17-fold higher than the relative risk of developing a subsequent nongerm cell cancer (Wanderas et al. 1997b). In U.S. men, the cumulative risk of developing a metachronous contralateral testis cancer is 12.4-fold higher relative to the general population, with a crude prevalence rate of 1.9% at 15 years of age (see Table 6.1) (Fossa et al. 2005). This prevalence rate is lower than those reported for most European studies with comparable information (except for Sweden). Given that the differences between European and U.S. men in second germ cell tumor risk are based on population studies, explanations for the differences in findings include:

1. European studies often include patients with extragonadal germ cell tumors that have a particularly high incidence of metachronicity (Hartmann et al. 2001).
2. Some studies may include patients with synchronous testis tumors in the analysis.
3. Most studies include patients who were treated before cisplatin based chemotherapy was introduced in 1970s.
4. There may be real as yet unexplained variations in testis cancer rates between countries.

There is also risk data that address the time to secondary germ cell tumors, the age of the patient, and the type of primary tumor. The cumulative risk of secondary germ cell tumors reaches a plateau 15–20 years after original diagnosis (Wanderas et al. 1997a). This pattern is distinct from that of the cumulative risk of nongerm cell cancers developing, which continues to increase with time. In addition, according to Norwegian data, an age of <30 years at first cancer diagnosis places the patient at higher risk of subsequent germ cell tumors: 7.8% (CI 3.1–10.4%) risk in men <30 years old, compared to 2.1% (CI 1.2–3.0%) in men >30 years (Wanderas et al. 1997a). Although confirmed in a U.S. based study (Fossa et al. 2005), it is important to note that age analyses are biased by the age distribution of cancer cases from different studies. Finally, the risk of a second germ cell tumor is higher for those with a nonseminomatous germ cell tumor

**Table 6.1** Crude estimates of bilateral testis cancer prevalence by country

| Country | Number patients | Synchronous (%) | Metachronous (%) | Cumulative risk | References |
|---|---|---|---|---|---|
| US | 29,515 | 0.6 | 1.0 | 15 year: 1.9% | Fossa et al. (2005) |
| Netherlands | 1,909 | 0.2 | 1.0 | 15 year: 2.4% | van Leeuwen et al. (1993) |
| Hungary | 2,386 | 0.8 | 2.2 | N/A | Geczi et al. (2003) |
| France | 2,383 | 0.6 | 1.3 | N/A | Theodore et al. (2004) |
| Denmark | 2,850 | 0.2 | 2.4 | 20 year: 5.2% | Osterlind et al. (1991) |
| Norway | 2,201 | 0.4 | 2.7 | 15 year: 3.9% | Wanderas et al. (1997b) |
| Sweden | 4,650 | N/A | 0.9 | N/A | Dong et al. (2001) |

*Source*: Data from Fossa et al. (2005), with permission

(NSGCT) as a first tumor: men with NSGCT had a 5% (CI 3.1–6.9%) risk of secondary tumors at 15 years, compared to men with seminomas (3.4% at 15 years, CI 2.1–4.6%) (Wanderas et al. 1997a). Despite this difference in risk based on first tumor type, the relative risk of having seminoma and NSGCT in secondary cancers appears equal (Wanderas et al. 1997a).

## 6.4 Diagnosis

In general, the diagnostic approach for second germ cell tumors is the same as for primary cancers. One large difference is the role of the diagnostic testis biopsy in predicting the evolution of second germ cell tumors in the contralateral testis. Arguments supporting the use of prophylactic, contralateral testis biopsy at the time of the original diagnosis have been recently summarized by von der Maase (2005) from Denmark and include:

1. The real goal of testis biopsy and a CIS diagnosis is not to improve overall survival but to avoid another radical orchiectomy (in favor of irradiation or partial orchiectomy).
2. The cancer follow-up for biopsied patients is the same as that associated with the primary cancer and no more intense. This is because the chance of invasive cancer associated with a negative biopsy is <0.5% (von der Masse et al. 1987).
3. The knowledge of CIS on biopsy is useful as it can be "cured" by radiation therapy and reduces patient stress. In addition, sperm can be banked before such treatment and preserve fertility options.
4. The quality of life cost of sterility after prophylactic radiation to the CIS testis is less than that associated with bilateral anorchia, mainly because hormonal function can be preserved with radiation.

Arguments against the role of routine testis biopsy at the time of the original cancer diagnosis have been summarized by Hentrich et al. (2005) from Germany and include:

1. The prognosis for bilateral metachronous testis cancer disease is excellent and insignificantly different from primary tumors (see Table 6.2) (Fossa et al. 2005).
2. Follow-up examinations are mandatory for testis cancer patients regardless of CIS status.
3. The knowledge of CIS may be stressful to patients and greatly affects patient quality of life.
4. Fertility may be maintained in the absence of radiation treatment for CIS. Infertility is a sure consequence of this treatment for CIS.

An additional variable is the fact that the contralateral biopsies may not show CIS (false-negative biopsy) due to the focal nature of CIS in some cases (Dieckmann et al. 2007; Kliesch et al. 2003; Pamenter et al. 2003). To increase the sensitivity of CIS detection, the performance of multiple biopsies has been suggested (Dieckmann et al. 2007), but the value of this approach has been questioned (Pamenter et al. 2003). Since the relative risk of secondary germ cell cancers varies with the specific study population, including the country of origin, the type of primary tumor, the age of the patient and other risk factors, a reasonable solution to this controversy is to recommend that high risk patients (especially those not likely to receive chemotherapy) undergo a contralateral testis biopsy at the time of the primary tumor diagnosis. However, low risk patients could be encouraged to perform regular testicular self examination and possibly undergo testis ultrasound at regular intervals to find subsequent tumors at an early stage amendable to testis sparing surgery (Fossa et al. 2005). One solution for this diagnostic dilemma could involve a sensitive, reliable, and noninvasive assay to detect CIS or tumor cells in the ejaculate of affected patients. We have reported the feasibility of identifying protein markers specific to CIS in ejaculated cells (e.g., AP-2 gamma or OCT-3/4); however, we currently find assay sensitivity to be unacceptably low for routine clinical practice (Hoei-Hansen et al. 2007).

**Table 6.2** 10-Year survival with unilateral, synchronous, and metachronous testis cancer ($n = 29{,}515$ cases)

| Extent of disease | Unilateral cancer | Synchronous cancer | Metachronous cancer |
|---|---|---|---|
| Local | 95% (CI 94.5–95.4) | Overall | Overall |
| Regional | 90% (CI 88.8–91) | 85% (CI 78–90) | 93% (CI 88–96) |
| Metastatic | 65% (CI 63–67.1) | | |

*Source*: Data from Fossa et al. (2005)

## 6.5 Treatment of Secondary Testis Cancer

In principle, the treatment of secondary testis cancers does not differ from treatment of primary tumors. However, in light of the specific therapy given to the primary tumor, special consideration should be given to treatment of subsequent tumors. If radiation therapy was given at standard doses for treatment of the primary tumor, then it may not be indicated for treatment of a secondary tumor. Similarly, if retroperitoneal lymph node dissection (RPLND) was given for the primary tumor, then altered lymphatic drainage may result. In this case, radiation therapy might not be indicated for the second tumor. Recognize also that RPLND may be a more difficult surgical procedure in a previously irradiated field. Finally, as discussed elsewhere in this volume, organ sparing surgery is successful in selected cases of small T1 cancers with no infiltration of the rete testis or vasculature and in the setting of normal preoperative testosterone and luteinizing hormone levels. In fact, a review of 29,515 cases of testis cancer cases in the U.S. suggested that 36% of men with metachronous cancers will have second tumors <20 mm in size that may qualify for testis sparing surgery (Fossa et al. 2005). Importantly, this fraction of cases is likely to increase with improved surveillance, particularly in high risk patients, in the future.

## 6.6 Treatment of Contralateral CIS

Three treatment options exist for contralateral CIS: radical orchiectomy, radiotherapy, and surveillance. Orchiectomy and radiotherapy offer definitive treatment for CIS and also eliminate the potential for future fertility. Since the interval between the diagnosis of CIS and the development of an overt testicular tumor can be lengthy, surveillance strategies can be offered to patients who seek to father children shortly after orchiectomy. If surveillance is chosen, evaluation of the CIS bearing testicle at regular intervals by ultrasound for the development of overt tumor is mandatory.

It is clear that CIS can be eradicated by fractionated radiotherapy. Biopsies after irradiation revealed complete eradication of CIS cells and germ cells with reasonable preservation of both Sertoli cells and Leydig cells (von der Maase et al. 1986b). In addition, several studies have examined the relationship between radiotherapy dose and testosterone balance trying to optimize cancer cure rates and quality of life. The largest published study to examine this issue included 48 patients with unilateral testicular germ cell cancer and contralateral CIS (Petersen et al. 2002). The CIS-bearing testis was treated with daily irradiation doses of 2 Gy, 5 days a week, to a cumulative dose of 20 Gy (21 patients), 18 Gy (3 patients), 16 Gy (10 patients), and 14 Gy (14 patients). All patients treated at dose levels from 16 to 20 Gy achieved histologically verified complete CIS remission and exhibited no evidence of recurrence after at least 5 years of follow-up. One of 14 patients treated with 14 Gy relapsed with CIS 20 months after irradiation. Leydig cell function was examined before and regularly after radiotherapy in 44 of 48 patients. Testosterone levels were lower after radiotherapy than before treatment and showing a linear decrease for 5 years after treatment (decreasing at 3.6% per year). This trend in testosterone levels was independent of the radiotherapy dose given. As expected, luteinizing hormone and follicle-stimulating hormone levels increased after radiotherapy. The need for androgen substitution therapy was similar at all radiation dose levels studied.

In smaller series, relapse of CIS or the development of invasive cancers has been described with 16, 18, and 20 Gy radiotherapy in patients with at least 2 years of follow-up (Dieckmann et al. 2002; Classen and Dieckmann 2002). Two explanations for this phenomenon are that (1) a small fraction of radio-resistant CIS cells is able to overcome irradiation injury and progress to germ cell cancer with time, or (2) alternatively, technical issues such as inaccurate targeting during treatment or treatment of a radio-resistant germ cell tumor leads to radiotherapeutic failure.

Chemotherapy has also been used to treat men with contralateral CIS, mainly in the setting of advanced disease. Chemotherapy leads to the disappearance of CIS cells, but probably only temporarily, as the cumulative risk of CIS relapse 5 and 10 years after chemotherapy in these patients is estimated to be 21 and 42%, respectively (Christensen et al. 1998). This data suggests that the combination of chemotherapy and surveillance does not reduce CIS recurrence. Since it has not been documented that fertility is preserved after chemotherapy in this population of patients, adjuvant chemotherapy cannot be recommended for the treatment of CIS. Given our current understanding of the biology of CIS, the optimal treatment is local radiotherapy to the CIS-bearing testis.

## 6.7 Prognosis

The overall prognosis for men who develop secondary germ cell tumors is excellent, largely because the second primary tumors are in most cases caught at an early stage. The most recent and comprehensive data on overall survival in men who developed bilateral testis cancers is based on a U.S. registry ($n = 29,515$ cases) and is outlined in Table 6.2. Conclusions derived from this work include the fact that the development of metachronous testis cancers do not increase the overall mortality risk beyond that associated with unilateral cancers. In addition, there appears to be no decrease in overall survival with metachronous cancers when compared to unilateral cancers (Fossa et al. 2005). Lastly, cisplatin-based chemotherapy does not completely eliminate metachronous tumor risk. Thus, the "treatability" of bilateral testis cancer, whether synchronous or metachronous, is high and very encouraging in general.

## 6.8 Etiology

The study of bilateral testis cancer allows for interesting speculation regarding etiologic factors in cancer development. The fact that seminomas and NSGCTs occur with equal prevalence among secondary tumors (Wanderas et al. 1997a) suggests that they may share a common developmental pathway (Skakkebaek and Berthelsen 1981). However, the finding that NSGCT patients have a younger median age at diagnosis of second tumors than do seminoma patients suggests that the carcinogenic process associated with NSGCT development is faster or more intense than that associated with seminomas (Møller 1993). In addition, the theory that NSGCT's have a faster growth rate than do seminomas and that this may guide the order of clinical presentation is supported by the fact that primary seminomas are commonly followed by secondary NSGCTs, but seminomas seldom occur after an initial diagnosis of NCGCT (Wanderas et al. 1997a). Lastly, the lack of real differences in the relative risk of secondary tumors according to type of treatment suggests that the type of cytotoxic treatment is not an important carcinogenic factor in cancer development. In summary, the early onset and significant second tumor associations in testis cancer cases suggest a prenatal or early postnatal predisposition to the disease, as discussed elsewhere in this volume (Skakkebaek et al. 1987).

Indeed, our basic science research in the molecular genetics of testis cancer supports a prenatal disposition to develop germ cell tumors (Andrews, 1998). Indeed, the presence of embryonic genes, the so-called "onco-fetal antigens," was described within germ cell tumors a decade ago [reviewed in Looijenga et al. 2003a]. Recently, the pluripotency-related transcription factor, OCT-3/4, and other embryonic stem cell genes have also been detected in germ cell tumors (Looijenga et al. 2003a; Sperger et al. 2003; Clark et al. 2004). In addition, we have now demonstrated that several novel human embryonic stem cell genes, *NANOG* and two of its neighboring genes, *STELLAR* and *GDF3* (Growth and Differentiation Factor 3), map to 12p (the chromosomal region that is abnormal and overexpressed in the vast majority of germ cell tumors) and are 4- to 12-fold overexpressed in seminomas relative to normal testis tissue (Clark et al. 2004). These embryonic genes are located exclusively in germ cells in the ovary and testis and are critical for the regulation and maintenance of pluripotency in human embryonic stem cells. Similar to TGCT's, we have also shown that a marked overexpression of embryonic genes is observed in CIS (Almstrup et al. 2004), reflecting the primordial germ cell/gonocyte-like phenotype of the CIS cell (Rajpert-De Meyts et al. 2003). The expression of embryonic genes has since been confirmed in other studies of germ cell tumors (Ezeh et al. 2005; Skotheim et al. 2005; Korkola et al. 2006). Based on these findings, we hypothesize that the inappropriately prolonged expression of pluripotency genes in adult germ cells, genes that are normally down-regulated during the transition from fetal gonocytes to infantile spermatogonia, is a novel pathway for the development of human germ cell tumors (Clark et al. 2004; Rajpert-De Meyts 2006).

In a parallel work that supports a prenatal timeframe for early development of testis cancer, we sought to further characterize the specific seminoma cell type using a library of both embryonic and spermatogenesis genes. We and others have observed that seminomas are phenotypically and genotypically more closely related to early perimigratory germ line stem cells such as primordial germ cells, than to later, differentiated spermatogenic cells found in the adult testis (Ezeh et al. 2005; Korkola et al. 2006; Almstrup et al. 2005). Indeed, similar to what is surmised from clinical studies of bilateral testis cancer, this research suggests that tumors arise early on during development, as seminomas appear to be derived from cells similar to those of the inner cell mass, cells arising during germ cell specification of the first trimester human embryo. Additionally, the relatively frequent detection of *c-KIT* mutations in these tumors lends further evidence that testis tumors arise at the primordial germ cell stage, before germ cell migration to the gonads (Looijenga et al. 2003b). KIT is a tyrosine kinase receptor for stem cell factor, which is essential for survival of early germ cells. If "gain-of-function" mutations were to occur in the c-*KIT* gene, first detected in seminomas by Tian et al. (1999), this would encourage proliferation of primordial germ cells. *KIT* mutations are now known to occur in subsets of familial and sporadic testicular tumors, primarily in seminomas, and much less frequently in nonseminomas (Looijenga et al. 2003b; Madani et al. 2003; Kemmer et al. 2004; Rapley et al. 2004; McIntyre et al. 2005). Thus molecular genetic findings agree with clinical, population-based research regarding the origin of testis tumors in humans.

The familial predisposition of bilateral TGCTs could also provide information regarding the genetic aspects of these cancers. In one study from the U.K., the relative risk of testicular malignancy in family members of patients with bilateral TGCT was investigated (Harland et al. 2007). Preliminary results suggest that there is a slight excess of TGCT in brothers of patients with bilateral tumors; however, the difference did not achieve significance. Confounding issues that complicate this analysis include exposure to environmental factors, as brothers may share not only genes, but also environmental risk (Hemminki and Li 2004; Ottesen et al. 2004). Although further studies may support a familial nature of bilateral testis cancers, we believe that most bilateral cancers are similar to unilateral tumors regarding their origin and pathogenesis. Although a mutational defect could underlie some tumors, the likely genetic mechanism operating in most TGCTs (both unilateral and bilateral) is the differential response of polymorphic genes or their products to the environment (Rajpert-De Meyts 2006; Skakkebaek et al. 1998). These mechanisms are undoubtedly multi-factorial, and will be difficult to dissect and define, but are likely the primary drivers of the events of early testis development.

## References


Almstrup K, Hoei-Hansen CE, Wirkner U et al (2004) Embryonic stem cell-like features of testicular carcinoma in situ revealed by genome-wide gene expression profiling. Cancer Res 64: 4736–4743

Almstrup K, Hoei-Hansen CE, Nielsen JE et al (2005) Differences in genome-wide gene expression profiles of testicular carcinoma in situ and invasive germ cell tumours. Br J Cancer 92: 1934–1941

Andrews PW (1998) Teratocarcinomas and human embryology: pluripotent human EC cell lines. APMIS 106:158–168

Berthelsen JG, Skakkebaek NE, Mogensen P et al (1979) Incidence of carcinoma in situ of germ cells in contralateral testis of men with testicular tumours. Br Med J 2:363–364

Berthelsen JG, Skakkebæk NE, von der Maase H et al (1982) Screening for carcinoma in situ of the contralateral testis in patients with germinal testicular cancer. Br Med J 285: 1683–1686

Bray F, Ferlay J, Devesa SS et al (2006) Interpreting the international trends in testicular seminoma and nonseminoma incidence. Nat Clin Pract Urol 3:532–543

Christensen TB, Daugaard G, Geertsen PF et al (1998) Effect of chemotherapy on carcinoma in situ of the testis. Ann Oncol 9:657–660

Clark AT, Rodriguez RT, Bodnar MS et al (2004) Human STELLAR, NANOG and GDF3 genes are expressed in pluripotent cells and map to chromosome 12p13, a hotspot for teratocarcinoma. Stem Cells 22:169–179

Classen J, Dieckmann KP (2002) Radiotherapy of carcinoma-in-situ of the testis. J Clin Oncol 20:3559–3560

Dieckmann K-P, Loy V (1996) Prevalence of contralateral testicular intraepithelial germ cell neoplasia in patients with testicular germ cell neoplasms. J Clin Oncol 14:3126–3132

Dieckmann KP, Lauke H, Michl U, Winter E, Loy V (2002) Testicular germ cell cancer despite previous local radiotherapy to the testis. Eur Urol 41:643–649; discussion 649–650

Dieckmann KP, Kulejewski M, Pichlmeier U et al (2007) Diagnosis of contralateral testicular intraepithelial neoplasia (TIN) in patients with testicular germ cell cancer: systematic two-site biopsies are more sensitive than a single random biopsy. Eur Urol 51:175–183

Dong C, Lonnstedt I, Hemminki K (2001) Familial testicular cancer and second primary cancers in testicular cancer patients by histological type. Eur J Cancer 37:1878–1885

Ezeh UI, Turek PJ, Reijo Pera RA et al (2005) Seminoma and breast cancer have expression profiles similar to pluripotent stem cells. Cancer 104:2255–2265

Fossa SD, Aass N (1989) Cisplatin-based chemotherapy does not eliminate the risk of a second testicular cancer. Br J Urol 63:531–534

Fossa SD, Chen J, Schonfeld SJ et al (2005) Risk of contralateral testicular cancer: a population-based study of 29515 U.S. men. J Natl Cancer Inst 97:1056–1066

Geczi L, Gomez F, Bak M et al (2003) The incidence, prognosis, clinical and histological characteristics, treatment, and outcome of patients with bilateral germ cell testicular cancer in Hungary. J Cancer Res Clin Oncol 129:309–315

Harland SJ, Cook PA, Fossa SD et al (1998) Intratubular germ cell neoplasia of the contralateral testis in testicular cancer: defining a high risk group. J Urol 160:1353–1357

Harland SJ, Rapley EA, Nicholson PW (2007) Do all patients with bilateral testis cancer have a hereditary predisposition? Int J Androl 30(4):251–255; discussion 255

Hartmann JT, Fossa SD, Nichols CR et al (2001) Incidence of metachronous testicular cancer in patients with extragonadal germ cell tumors. J Natl Cancer Inst 93:1733–1738

Hemminki K, Li X (2004) Familial risk in testicular cancer as a clue to a heritable and environmental aetiology. Br J Cancer 90:1765–1770

Hentrich M, Weber N, Bergsdorf T et al (2005) Management and outcome of bilateral testicular germ cell tumors: twenty five year experience in Munich. Acta Oncol 44:529–536

Hoei-Hansen CE, Carlsen E, Jørgensen N et al (2007) Towards a non-invasive method for early detection of testicular neoplasia in semen samples by identification of fetal germ cell-specific markers. Hum Reprod 22:167–173

Kemmer K, Corless CL, Fletcher JA et al (2004) KIT mutations are common in testicular seminomas. Am J Pathol 164:305–313

Kliesch S, Thomaidis T, Schutte B et al (2003) Update on the diagnostic safety for detection of testicular intraepithelial neoplasia (TIN). APMIS 111:70–74; discussion 75

Korkola JE, Houldsworth J, Chadalavada RS et al (2006) Down-regulation of stem cell genes, including those in a 200-kb gene cluster at 12p13.31, is associated with in vivo differentiation of human male germ cell tumors. Cancer Res 66: 820–827

Looijenga LH, Stoop H, de Leeuw HP et al (2003a) *POU5F1* (OCT3/4) identifies cells with pluripotent potential in human germ cell tumors. Cancer Res 63:2244–2250

Looijenga LHJ, De Leeuw PJC, Van Oorschot M et al (2003b) Stem cell factor receptor (c-KIT) codon 816 mutations predict development of bilateral testicular germ cell tumors. Cancer Res 63:7674–7678

Madani A, Kemmer K, Sweeney C et al (2003) Expression of KIT and epidermal growth factor receptor in chemotherapy refractory non-seminomatous germ-cell tumors. Ann Oncol 14:873–880

McIntyre A, Summersgill B, Grygalewicz B et al (2005) Amplification and overexpression of the KIT gene is associated with progression in the seminoma subtype of testicular germ cell tumors of adolescents and adults. Cancer Res 65: 8085–8089

Møller H (1993) Clues to the aetiology of testicular germ cell tumours from descriptive epidemiology. Eur Urol 23:8–15

Osterlind A, Berthelsen JG, Abildgaard N et al (1991) Risk of bilateral testicular germ cell cancer in Denmark: 1960-1984. J Natl Cancer Inst 83:1391–1395

Ottesen AM, Rajpert-De Meyts E, Holm M et al (2004) Cytogenetic and molecular analysis of a family with three brothers afflicted with germ cell cancer. Clin Genet 65: 32–39

Pamenter B, De Bono JS, Brown IL et al (2003) Bilateral testicular cancer: a preventable problem? Experience from a large cancer centre. BJU Int 92:43–46

Petersen PM, Giwercman A, Daugaard G et al (2002) Effect of graded testicular doses of radiotherapy in patients treated for carcinoma in situ. J Clin Oncol 20:1537–1543

Rajpert-De Meyts E (2006) Developmental model for the pathogenesis of testicular carcinoma in situ: environmental and genetic aspects. Hum Reprod Update 12:303–323

Rajpert-De Meyts E, Bartkova J, Samson M, Hoei-Hansen CE, Frydelund-Larsen L, Bartek J, Skakkebaek NE (2003) The emerging phenotype of the testicular carcinoma in situ germ cell. APMIS 111:267–279

Rapley EA, Hockley S, Warren W et al (2004) Somatic mutations of KIT in familial testicular germ cell tumours. Br J Cancer 90:2397–2401

Skakkebaek NE (1972) Possible carcinoma-in-situ of the testis. Lancet 2:516–517

Skakkebaek NE, Berthelsen JG (1981) Carcinoma-in-situ of the testis and invasive growth of different types of germ cell tumours. A revised germ cell theory. Int J Androl 4(Suppl 4):26–34

Skakkebaek NE, Berthelsen JG, Giwercman A et al (1987) Carcinoma-in-situ of the testis: possible origin from gonocytes and precursor of all types of germ cell tumours except spermatocytoma. Int J Androl 10:19–28

Skakkebaek NE, Rajpert-De Meyts E, Jørgensen N et al (1998) Germ cell cancer and disorders of spermatogenesis: an environmental connection? APMIS 106:3–12

Skotheim RI, Lind GE, Monni O et al (2005) Differentiation of human embryonal carcinomas in vitro and in vivo reveals expression profiles relevant to normal development. Cancer Res 65:5588–5598

Sperger JM, Chen X, Draper JS et al (2003) Gene expression patterns in human embryonic stem cells and human pluripotent germ cell tumors. Proc Natl Acad Sci U S A 100: 13350–13355

Theodore Ch, Terrier-Lacombe MJ, Laplanche A et al (2004) Bilateral germ-cell tumours: 22-year experience at the ****Institut Gustave Roussy. Br J Cancer 90:55–59

Tian Q, Frierson HF Jr, Krystal GW et al (1999) Activating c-kit gene mutations in human germ cell tumors. Am J Pathol 154:1643–1647

van Leeuwen FE, Stiggelbout AM, van den Belt-Dusebout AW et al (1993) Second cancer risk following testicular cancer: a follow-up study of 1,909 patients. J Clin Oncol 11: 415–424

von der Maase H (2005) Is a contralateral testicular biopsy in patients with unilateral germ cell testis cancer indicated as a routine procedure? Acta Oncol 44:523–525

Von der Maase H, Rorth M, Walbom-Jorgensen S et al (1986a) Carcinoma in situ of contralateral testis in patients with testicular germ cell cancer: study of 27 cases in 500 cases. Br Med J 293:1398–1401

von der Maase H, Giwercman A, Skakkebaek NE (1986b) Radiation treatment of carcinoma in situ of testis. Lancet 1:624–625

von der Masse H, Giwercman A, Muller J et al (1987) Management of carcinoma in-situ of testis. Int J Androl 10:209–220

Wanderas EH, Fossa SD, Tretli S (1997a) Risk of a second germ cell cancer after treatment of a primary germ cell cancer in 2201 Norwegian male patients. Eur J Cancer 33: 244–252

Wanderas EH, Fossa SD, Tretli S (1997b) Risk of subsequent non-germ cell cancer after treatment of germ cell cancer in 2006 Norwegian male patients. Eur J Cancer 33:253–262

# Part III

# Primary Surgery

# Radical Orchiectomy and Testis Sparing Procedures for the Management of Germ Cell Tumors

7

Brett S. Carver, Axel Heidenreich, and Pramod Sogani

## 7.1 Introduction

Testicular cancer represents the most common malignancy in males 15–35 years old. The American Cancer Society estimates that in the United States, approximately 7,920 new cases of testicular cancer would have been diagnosed and 380 men would have died of this disease in 2007 (American Cancer Society 2007). Although there is considerable geographic variation in the incidence of testicular cancer, with Scandinavia and Switzerland having the highest rates, there has been a world-wide increase in the incidence of testicular cancer over recent years (Huyghe et al. 2003; McKiernan et al. 1999). Germ cell tumors (GCT) of the testis occur predominantly in Caucasian males and are rarely seen in African-Americans (Daniels et al. 1981).

Testicular cancer has become one of the most curable solid tumors and serves as a paradigm for the multidisciplinary approach for the management of malignancy. The dramatic improvement in survival resulting from the combination of improved diagnostic techniques, effective chemotherapeutic agents, and appropriate modifications of surgical techniques has led to a decrease in patient mortality from more than 50% before 1970 to less than 5% in 2006. Through successful implementation of clinical trials, treatment protocols for men with all stages of testicular cancer have been evaluated to maximize therapeutic efficacy while minimizing morbidity.

GCT comprise approximately 95% of all intratesticular masses with the remaining 5% representing benign tumors of the testis, such as Leydig cell tumors, Sertoli cell tumors, and epidermoid cysts. GCT of the testis can be divided into two major subgroups based on histology: seminoma and nonseminoma. Seminoma accounts for approximately 50% of all GCT and most frequently appears in the fourth decade of life. The remainder of GCT comprises nonseminomatous histology (embryonal cell carcinoma, yolk sac tumor, choriocarcinoma, and teratoma) and frequently presents in the third decade of life. Most nonseminomatous tumors are mixed, composed of two or more cell types, of which seminoma may be a component; however, the definition of a pure seminoma excludes the presence of any nonseminomatous elements or an elevated serum alpha-fetoprotein.

Radical inguinal orchiectomy is the initial standard surgical procedure for almost all testicular neoplasms and serves both a diagnostic and therapeutic role for the management of testicular malignancies. In this chapter, we discuss the initial diagnosis and staging of testicular GCT, the role of radical orchiectomy for the management of GCT of the testis, the surgical procedure in detail, and the potential role of testis sparing procedures for select patients.

## 7.2 Clinical Presentation and Diagnosis

The most common symptom at the time of diagnosis is painless swelling or enlargement of the testis. Acute testicular pain is reported to occur in approximately 10% of patients with testicular cancer and often represents infarction or hemorrhage within the tumor (Richie 1993). At initial presentation, symptoms manifesting secondary to metastatic disease occur in approximately 20% of patients and include, a mass in the left neck, pulmonary complaints such as hemoptysis or dyspnea,

B.S. Carver (✉)
Department of Surgery, Division of Urology, Memorial Sloan-Kettering Cancer Center, New York, NY, USA

M.P. Laguna et al. (eds.), *Cancer of the Testis*,
DOI: 10.1007/978-1-84800-370-5_7, © Springer-Verlag London Limited 2010

abdominal mass, or back pain that can often be disabling (Bosl et al. 1981). In approximately 5% of patients, gynecomastia or tenderness of the breast is reported. A delay in diagnosis has been reported in the literature ranging from 2.5 to 4.4 months and is associated with a more advanced clinical stage at the time of diagnosis (Nikzas et al. 1990). Reasons for delay in diagnosis are multifactorial but may include both a physician and patient component. Previous reports have shown that approximately 18–33% of patients with testicular cancer were initially treated for epididymitis by their physician (Moul et al. 1990; Moul and Moellman 1992). Patients have also been initially misdiagnosed, undergoing unnecessary mastectomy or exploratory laparotomy which ultimately delays and increases the burden of therapy (Bosl et al. 1981; Stephenson et al. 2004).

Testicular ultrasonography is the initial imaging modality of choice with a greater than 95% sensitivity and specificity in identifying intratesticular lesions (Benson 1988). The serum tumor markers (STM) alpha-fetoprotein (AFP), human chorionic gonadotropin (HCG), and lactate dehydrogenase (LDH) have a clear role in both the diagnosis and clinical management of testicular GCT. Elevation of one or both markers occurs in 80% of metastatic GCT of the testis.

## 7.3 Clinical Staging

Staging evaluation must include a thorough history and physical exam, with particular attention to possible sites of metastases and the contralateral testis. STM should be obtained prior to and following radical orchiectomy. The STM are necessary for diagnosis, staging, and risk classification. While a normal post-orchiectomy STM does not preclude the finding of metastatic disease, an elevation of either AFP or HCG does signify the presence of metastasis.

AFP is a glycoprotein produced in the liver, gastrointestinal tract, and fetal yolk sac, and its secretion in GCT is restricted to nonseminomatous histology. Therefore, any patients with histologic pure seminomas and an elevated serum AFP are classified and managed like those with nonseminomatous germ cell tumors (NSGCT). AFP is elevated in approximately 60% of patients with metastatic NSGCT and 20% of patients with clinical stage I NSGCT. HCG is a glycoprotein produced by the synctiotrophoblasts and is elevated in approximately 15% of pure seminomas, and in 40% of advanced nonseminomas. The serum half-life of AFP and HCG is approximately 5 days and 24 h respectively. LDH comprises multiple isoenzymes, but in clinical practice the total LDH value is utilized for decision making. Increases in serum LDH correlate with tumor burden, growth rate, and cellular proliferation. Elevation of LDH is present in approximately 60% of patients with advanced NSGCT, and 80% of patients with metastatic seminoma.

The initial staging evaluation should include a CT scan of the chest, abdomen, and pelvis. This staging evaluation is preferably performed prior to the treatment of the primary tumor, as significant retroperitoneal hematomas - a known complication of radical orchiectomy - may be misinterpreted as metastatic disease on staging CT scan and result in unnecessary treatment (Bochner et al. 1995). CT is the most effective radiographic technique for identifying metastatic disease both above and below the diaphragm. The abdominal CT scan is normal in approximately 70% of patients with seminoma and 30% of patients with NSGCT. Lymph nodes in the primary landing zone measuring 10–20 mm are positive for GCT approximately 70% of the time, and nodes measuring 5–10 mm are involved approximately 50% of the time (Leibovitch et al. 1995a; Hilton et al. 1997).

MRI, like CT scan, is capable of identifying lymphadenopathy with similar sensitivity and specificity. MRI may provide additional information preoperatively regarding the vascular anatomy and patency of the great vessels in patients with bulky retroperitoneal disease; however, overall, it contributes little to the management of most patients with GCT.

In 1997, the American Joint Committee on Cancer revised the TNM staging system for testicular cancer, and for the first time STM were incorporated into the staging criteria (see Chap. 5) (Fleming 1998). Broadly, stage I refers to disease confined to the testis, stage II metastases restricted to the retroperitoneum, and stage III metastases to nonretroperitoneal sites.

The International Germ Cell Cancer Collaborative Group (IGCCCG) evaluated independent prognostic factors for predicting progression-free survival in men with GCT and stratified these patients into three risk classifications: good, intermediate, and poor risk disease (see Chap. 5) (IGCCCG 1997). This risk classification has been utilized for clinical decision making in patients with advanced GCT, and for the design of clinical trials.

## 7.4 Radical Orchiectomy

A radical orchiectomy with high ligation of the spermatic vessels at the level of the internal ring is the first procedure for the management of patients with testicular neoplasms. This procedure provides histologic diagnosis and pathologic tumor characterization (pT, see Chap. 5) (Fleming 1998). A properly performed radical orchiectomy is associated with minimal morbidity and provides excellent local control of the primary tumor in the vast majority of patients. Once the decision to proceed with radical orchiectomy is made based on clinical history, physical examination, and radiologic evaluation, risks and benefits of the surgery should be discussed with the patient.

## 7.5 Operative Procedure

The procedure may be performed using general, spinal, or local anesthesia on an outpatient basis. After induction of anesthesia and administration of peri-operative antibiotics, the patient is positioned in supine on the operating table and prepped and draped in a sterile fashion, such that the ipsilateral inguinal region and scrotum are exposed in the surgical field. A 5–7 cm oblique skin incision is made in the inguinal region approximately 2 cm superior to the pubic tubercle. This incision may be extended onto the upper scrotum to facilitate resection of larger testicular tumors. Camper's and Scarpa's fascia are incised to the level of the external oblique fascia, which is then incised in the direction of its fibers to the level of the internal ring. The ilioinguinal nerve is then identified, dissected free from the spermatic cord, and preserved. The spermatic cord is isolated and occluded with either a non-crushing clamp or a 0.5 in. penrose tourniquet at the level of the internal ring. The testis and its surrounding tunics are delivered into a carefully draped off field as the gubernacular attachments are divided. Radical orchiectomy is completed by mobilizing the spermatic cord 1 cm into the internal inguinal ring and individually ligating the vas deferens and spermatic vessels between separate clamps. The cord vessels are secured with silk ligatures to facilitate identifying the cord stump if a retroperitoneal lymph node dissection is performed in the future. The wound and scrotum are thoroughly irrigated and meticulous hemostasis is obtained. A testicular prosthesis may be placed at this time. The external oblique fascia and Scarpa's fascia are closed individually using absorbable suture. The skin edges may be reapproximated using staples or a subcuticular suture. Sterile compressive fluff dressings and scrotal support minimize postoperative edema.

## 7.6 Surgical Complications

Every effort should be made to minimize potential surgical complications related to the radical orchiectomy as approximately 33–70% of patients with testicular GCT present with metastatic disease requiring additional therapy, which may be unnecessarily delayed in the presence of a postoperative complication. The most common complication following a radical orchiectomy is postoperative bleeding, which may occasionally result in a scrotal or retroperitoneal hematoma (Bochner et al. 1995). This complication has the potential to delay future therapy, and may be misinterpreted as metastatic disease during clinical staging. Wound infection and paresthesia of the scrotum are less common postoperative complications.

## 7.7 Scrotal Violation

Prior inguinal or scrotal surgery may alter the normal lymphatic drainage of the testis. Suboptimal approaches to the management including scrotal orchiectomy, transscrotal biopsy, or fine needle aspiration are reported in approximately 4–17% of patients with testicular GCT (Capelouto et al. 1995; Leibovitch et al. 1995b). A meta-analysis of patients with a history of scrotal violation at initial therapy demonstrated the local recurrence rate was 2.9% compared to 0.4% for patients undergoing an inguinal radical orchiectomy (Capelouto et al. 1995). However, no difference was observed with regard to systemic relapse or survival rates. Therefore, current recommendations for the management of scrotal violation are: (1) In patients with low-stage seminoma, the radiation portals should be extended to include the ipsilateral inguinal region and scrotum. (2) In patients with low-stage NSGCT, the scrotal scar should be widely excised with the spermatic cord at the time of RPLND. (3) Patients receiving induction chemotherapy for metastatic disease should have the cord stump excised at the time of PC-RPLND; however, given the relative absence of local relapse after systemic chemotherapy, an extensive inguinal dissection or hemiscrotectomy should not be performed. (4) While patients with a history of scrotal violation are not appropriate candidates for surveillance, those on surveillance protocols should be monitored closely with additional CT imaging of the pelvis and thorough physical examination of the ipsilateral groin and scrotum.

## 7.8 Delayed Radical Orchiectomy

A small subset of patients with advanced metastatic GCT may undergo systemic chemotherapy prior to radical orchiectomy based on diagnosis from extragonadal biopsies and STM evaluation. Rarely, postoperative complications have resulted in delays in initiating systemic chemotherapy following radical orchiectomy. Following completion of chemotherapy, a delayed orchiectomy should be performed as approximately 25% of patient will harbor viable GCT and 30% will harbor teratomatous elements in the primary testis (Simmonds et al. 1995).

## 7.9 Testis Sparing Surgery

While radical orchiectomy remains the therapeutic "gold standard" for the management of testicular masses, testis sparing surgery has become an important option for select patients with testicular disease. Patients with bilateral GCT, patients with benign lesions, and prepubertal children with testis lesions are potential candidates for organ-sparing procedures. In case of benign testicular lesions such as epidermoid cysts, Leydig cell tumors, etc. organ sparing surgery can be performed without increased risk of local or systemic recurrence (Heidenreich et al. 1990, 2001). In patients with bilateral GCT of the testis, radical orchiectomy was considered to represent the treatment option of choice. Only in cases of a second metachronously or synchronously occurring testicular cancer, a testicular tumor developing in a solitary testis or a benign testis tumor, might an organ-sparing approach be considered, to maintain endogenous testosterone synthesis, to preserve fertility, and to improve quality of life in these long-term survivors. Since the original reports of small patient cohorts by Heidenreich et al. and Weißbach, numerous case reports, small series, and the large experience by the German Testicular Cancer Study Group (GTCSG) have been published (Heidenreich et al. 1995, 1997, 2001; Weißbach 1995; Kazem and Danella 1999; Steiner et al. 2003; Sheynkin et al. 2004). According to a recent analysis of 115 patients undergoing tumor enucleation, it became evident that the majority of men developed metachronous second cancer in the remaining testicle 6–125 months after primary orchiectomy. Only 21% and 8% of the patients underwent organ sparing surgery for a synchronous bilateral tumor or a tumor developing in a solitary testis, respectively. Based on the experience of the GTCSG and the recommendations of the European Germ Cell Cancer Consensus Group, organ sparing surgery should be considered early in the management of patients with bilateral testicular cancer or testicular tumors developing in a solitary testis (Schmoll et al. 2004).

In general, organ sparing surgery with preservation of enough testicular parenchyma for endogenous testosterone production may be considered if $\geq$50% parenchyma will remain after surgery. Preoperative endocrinological work-up including measurement of testosterone and luteinizing hormone (LH) – serum levels is mandatory, since normal androgen levels in the presence of elevated LH-levels indicate compensated Leydig cell insufficiency which might decompensate after tumor enucleation. In any patient considered for an organ sparing approach several preoperative Guidelines identified by the German Testicular Cancer Intergroup based on results from more than 115 patients with a testicular germ-cell tumor and a mean follow-up of 85 months are outlined in Box 7.1. However, it must be emphasized that tumor enucleation for testicular germ-cell tumors should be the exception for the few patients presenting with bilateral testicular cancer.

**Box 7.1 Guidelines for Organ Preserving Surgery of Bilateral Testicular GCT**

Organ confined tumor ≤50% of the testicular volume
Intraoperative biopsies of the tumor bed negative for cancer
Normal serum levels of testosterone and LH preoperatively
High compliance by both patients and physicians
Close follow-up with regular oncological and endocrinological screening
Management at a tertiary referral center for testis cancer

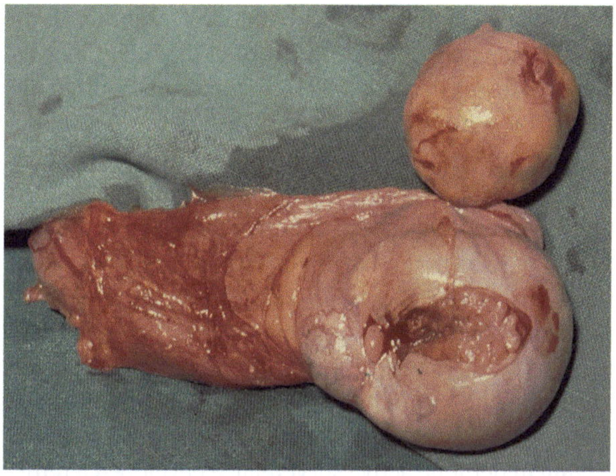

**Fig. 7.1** Organ preserving surgery in a testicle with solitary lesion; the pseudocapsule of the tumor can be easily identified

## 7.10 Surgical Procedure

The testicle is explored via an inguinal approach; after appropriate draping of the surgical field, the tumor bearing testis is delivered and the tunica vaginalis is opened longitudinally without clamping the spermatic cord. Usually, the tunica albuginea is incised above the palpable tumor; if the tumor cannot be palpated due to central location or a small diameter, intraoperative ultrasonography with a 7.5 MHz or a 10 MHz ultrasound probe is mandatory. In most cases, the tumor demonstrates a pseudocapsule without infiltrative growth and the adjacent testicular parenchyma can be easily swept away with a small sponge stick. This procedure can be easily performed in the presence of solitary tumor but also if multiple small tumors are present (Fig. 7.1). Tumor infiltrating blood vessels should be coagulated with the use of a bipolar forceps in order to spare as much vascularization of the remaining parenchyma as possible. Once the tumor has been completely excised, it is sent for frozen section examination. In addition, 2–4 biopsies of the tumor bed are taken and analyzed by frozen section examination to guarantee negative surgical margins. If surgical margins are positive, additional parenchyma has to be excised. Since it is well known that every GCT is accompanied by testicular intraepithelial neoplasia (TIN) in the adjacent testicular parenchyma, it is not necessary to take a biopsy from the peripheral testicular tissue. The tumor bed is coagulated with bipolar forceps before the tunica albuginea and the tunica vaginalis are closed by running sutures and the testis is delivered intrascrotally. Postoperatively, analgesics and antiphlogistics should be delivered for a couple of days. Postoperative follow-up should consist of regular ultrasonographic examinations by the treating physician and routine self-palpation by the patient. The first scrotal ultrasound should be obtained as early as 4 weeks postoperatively to identify intraparenchymatous changes due to edema and scars; afterward ultrasonography is sufficient at 3 month intervals.

## 7.11 Treatment Outcome

Recently, the long-term results after a median follow-up of 85 (4–185) months of 115 patients treated by some centers of the GTCSG have been evaluated (Heidenreich et al. 2006). Histology of the resected tumors revealed classical seminoma in 57%, whereas an embryonal carcinoma, mature teratoma, and mixed GCT were identified in 20, 15, and 9%, respectively. The median diameter of the enucleated tumors was 15.9 (4–40) mm which was significantly smaller than the primary tumor with a median diameter of 29.5 (15–82) mm. The majority of patients presented with a pT1 (89%) tumor and clinical stage I (85%).

Since all GCT are accompanied by TIN, postoperative adjuvant radiation therapy with 18 Gy is recommended which was performed in 87 (75.6%) patients within 4 weeks after surgery. In the remaining 28 patients, local radiation therapy was either postponed due to the wish to father a child in the presence of only slightly impaired spermatogenesis in 10 (8.7%) men or due to patient's denial in 18 (15.6%) patients. During the follow-up period of 85 months, 7 men fathered a child.

Local recurrences developed in seven (6.3%) patients and were successfully treated by secondary radical orchiectomy. Of these, six recurrences developed in the group of 28 men not having undergone adjuvant radiation therapy and one recurrence developed after local radiation of a mature teratoma with positive surgical margins. Still, 21/28 (75%) of men not having undergone adjuvant local irradiation are without a local recurrence. Four (3.1%) patients with clinical stage I NSGCT having undergone active surveillance developed a retroperitoneal relapse after a mean interval of 17 (6–32) months and were successfully managed by systemic chemotherapy. One patient (0.9%) died due to local and systemic relapse and very poor compliance.

The testosterone serum levels were within the normal range in 92 (81%) patients and only 19 men needed androgen substitution due their hypogonadal status. It appears that a cancer diameter ≥20 mm is significantly associated with the risk of developing hypergonadotropic hypogonadism.

## References


American Cancer Society (2007) Cancer facts and figures 2007. American Cancer Society, Atlanta

Benson CB (1988) The role of ultrasound in the diagnosis and staging of testicular cancer. Semin Urol 6:189–202

Bochner BH, Lerner SP, Kawachi M, Williams RD, Scardino PT, Skinner DG (1995) Postradical orchiectomy hemorrhage: should an alteration in staging strategy for testicular cancer be considered? Urology 46:408–411

Bosl G, Goldman A, Lange P, Vogelzang N, Fraley E, Levitt S (1981) Impact of delay in diagnosis on clinical stage of testicular cancer. Lancet 2:970–973

Capelouto C, Clark P, Ransil B, Loughlin K (1995) A review of scrotal violation in testicular cancer: is adjuvant local therapy necessary? J Urol 153:1397–1401

Daniels J, Stutzman R, McLeod D (1981) A comparison of testicular tumors in black and white patients. J Urol 125:341–342

Fleming I (ed) (1998) AJCC cancer staging handbook. Lippincott-Raven, Philadelphia

Heidenreich A, Engelmann UH, von Vietsch H et al (1990) Organ preserving surgery in testicular epidermoid cysts. J Urol 153:1147–1150

Heidenreich A, Bonfig R, Derschum W, von Vietsch H, Wilbert DM (1995) A conservative approach to bilateral testicular germ cell tumors. J Urol 153:1147–1150

Heidenreich A, Moul JW, Srivastava S, Engelmann UH (1997) Synchronous bilateral testicular tumor: nonseminomatous germ cell tumors and contralateral benign tumors. Scand J Urol Nephrol 31:389–392

Heidenreich A, Weißbach L, Höltl W, Albers P, Kliesch S, Köhrmann KU et al (2001) Organ sparing surgery for malignant germ cell tumor of the testis. J Urol 166:2161–2165

Heidenreich A, Albers P, Krege S (2006) Management of bilateral testicular germ cell tumors – experience of the German Testicular Cancer Study Group. Eur Urol Suppl 5:97; abstract no. 299

Hilton S, Herr H, Teitcher J, Begg C, Castellino R (1997) CT detection of retroperitoneal lymph node metastases in patients with clinical stage I testicular nonseminomatous germ cell cancer: assessment of size and distribution criteria. Am J Roentgenol 169:521–525

Huyghe E, Matsuda T, Thonneau P (2003) Increasing incidence of testicular cancer worldwide: a review. J Urol 170:5–11

IGCCCG (1997) International germ cell consensus classification: a prognostic factor-based staging system for metastatic germ cell cancers. J Clin Oncol 15:594–603

Kazem I, Danella JF (1999) Organ preservation for the treatment of contralateral testicular seminoma. Radiother Oncol 53: 45–47

Leibovitch I, Foster R, Kopecky K, Donohue J (1995a) Improved accuracy of computerized tomography based clinical staging in low stage nonseminomatous germ cell cancer using size criteria of retroperitoneal lymph nodes. J Urol 154:1759–1763

Leibovitch I, Baniel J, Foster RS, Donohue JP (1995b) The clinical implications of procedural deviations during orchiectomy for nonseminomatous germ cell cancer. J Urol 154:935–939

McKiernan J, Goluboff E, Liberson G, Golden R, Fisch H (1999) Rising risk of testicular cancer by birth cohort in the United States from 1973 to 1995. J Urol 162:361–363

Moul J, Moellman J (1992) Unnecessary mastectomy for gynecomastia in a testicular cancer patient. Mil Med 157: 433–434

Moul J, Paulson D, Dodge R, Walther P (1990) Delay in diagnosis and survival in testicular cancer: impact of effective therapy and changes during 18 years. J Urol 143:520–523

Nikzas D, Champion AE, Fox M (1990) Germ cell tumours of the testis: prognostic factors and results. Eur Urol 18:242–247

Richie JP (1993) Advances in the diagnosis and treatment of testicular cancer. Cancer Invest 11:670–675

Schmoll HJ, Souchon R, Krege S et al (2004) European consensus on diagnosis and treatment of germ cell cancer: a report of the European Germ Cell Cancer Consensus Group (EGCCCG). Ann Oncol 15:1377–1399

Sheynkin YR, Sukkarieh T, Lipke M, Cohen HL, Schulsinger DA (2004) Management of nonpalpable testicular tumors. Urology 63:1163–1167

Simmonds PD, Mead GM, Lee AH et al (1995) Orchiectomy after chemotherapy in patients with metastatic testicular cancer. Is it indicated? Cancer 75:1018–1024

Steiner H, Höltl L, Maneschg C, Berger AP, Rogatsch H, Bartsch G, Hobisch A (2003) Frozen section analysis guided organ sparing approach in testicular tumors: technique, feasibility and long-term results. Urology 62:508–513

Stephenson AJ, Russo P, Kaplinsky R, Sheinfeld J (2004) Impact of unnecessary exploratory laparotomy on the treatment of patients with metastatic germ cell tumor. J Urol 171: 1474–1477

Weißbach L (1995) Organ preserving surgery of malignant germ cell tumors. J Urol 153:90–93

# Diagnostic and Therapeutic Laparoscopic Retroperitoneal Lymph Node Dissection in Low Stages Nonseminomatous GCC: The American View

8

Brian A. VanderBrink, Ernesto Reggio, Lee Richstone, and Louis R. Kavoussi

## 8.1 Introduction

Minimally invasive techniques have revolutionized current surgical practice across all subspecialties. Specifically in urology, laparoscopic approaches to adrenal and renal pathology have evolved into not only acceptable alternatives but indeed the preferred surgical technique at select centers. The decreased morbidity and convalescence time following laparoscopic procedures compared to traditional open technique has provided the stimulus to apply a laparoscopic approach for the treatment of an increasing spectrum of urologic conditions.

Laparoscopic retroperitoneal lymph node dissection (RPLND) was initially described by Rukstalis and Chodak in 1992 (Janetschek et al. 1994). It was performed only for staging purposes, with no dissection of nodes posterior to the lumbar vessels. Subsequent reports followed demonstrating its safety and feasibility (Stone et al. 1993; Rukstalis and Chodak 1992). Initially, laparoscopic RPLND was employed for staging purposes with the goal of reducing the incidence of relapse in patients being considered for surveillance protocols. However, at select centers, laparoscopic RPLND has evolved into an identical replication of the open technique. Thus, laparoscopic RPLND can be performed with therapeutic intent, offering control of the retroperitoneum with all the inherent benefits of a laparoscopic approach (Allaf et al. 2005). This chapter will describe our current operative technique when performing laparoscopic RPLND.

L.R. Kavoussi (✉)
Urology Department, Arthur Smith Institute for Urology, New Hyde Park, NY, USA

## 8.2 Indications and Contraindications

The goal of performing laparoscopic RPLND in patients with stage I nonseminomatous germ cell tumor (NSGCT) is to accurately stage the approximately 25–30% of men who harbor retroperitoneal metastases and provide therapeutic control of the retroperitoneum. Our current indications for laparoscopic RPLND are outlined in Box 8.1. Relative contraindications to laparoscopic RPLND are no different from that of other laparoscopic procedures. Postchemotherapy laparoscopic RPLND is technically more challenging than primary RPLND and should be performed by those with significant experience in laparoscopic procedures as rates of open conversion are higher (Permpongkosol et al. 2007; Gerber et al. 1994).

Contraindications to laparoscopic RPLND include patients with elevated serum tumor markers as a significant percentage harbor distant metastases and should receive systemic chemotherapy. Patients with prior abdominal surgery, even prior open RPLND, have successfully undergone laparoscopic RPLND and should not be considered excluded from laparoscopic approach depending upon surgeon experience (Lima et al. 2005).

### Box 8.1 Indications for Laparoscopic RPLND

- Clinical stage I nonseminomatous testis tumor
- Select clinical stage II nonseminomatous testis tumor
- Residual retroperitoneal mass following chemotherapy in presence of normal serum tumor markers
- Clinical stage I paratesticular rhabdomyosarcoma
- Clinical stage I Leydig cell tumor

M.P. Laguna et al. (eds.), *Cancer of the Testis*,
DOI: 10.1007/978-1-84800-370-5_8, © Springer-Verlag London Limited 2010

## 8.3 Patient Preparation

All patients should undergo mechanical bowel preparation to decompress the bowel. Type and cross of blood products should be performed as the risk of intraoperative hemorrhage, particularly in postchemotherapy RPLND, is significant (Permpongkosol et al. 2007). Autologous blood donation should be considered for similar rationale. Patients who have received bleomycin are at risk of pulmonary complications and preoperative pulmonary function tests can assist in both identification of such patients and in postoperative management. Utilizing modified retroperitoneal template dissection can preserve antegrade ejaculation; however, preoperative sperm banking should be discussed (Donohue et al. 1990).

## 8.4 Patient Positioning and Port Placement

Sequential pneumatic compression devices are used throughout the procedure. Following induction of anesthesia the patient should be secured in the supine position with both arms tucked to the side. Prophylactic broad-spectrum intravenous antibiotics are administered. Nasogastric tube and Foley catheter are inserted and secured. The patient's abdomen is prepped and draped in a sterile fashion from the nipples to mid thigh.

Standard laparoscopic instruments are used throughout the procedure, including a 10-mm 30° laparoscope, Veress needle, atraumatic grasping forceps, scissors, clip appliers, and irrigation/suction device. Specific equipment is as follows:

- Laparoscopic paddle retractor
- Radiolucent polypropylene clips (Hem-o-Lock, Weck Closure Systems, Triangle Park, NC)
- Needle driver loaded with 4-0 Prolene suture
- Oxidized cellulose (Surgicel, Ethicon, Piscataway, NJ)
- Bipolar coagulation

The operating room set-up for a left LRPLND is shown in Fig. 8.1.

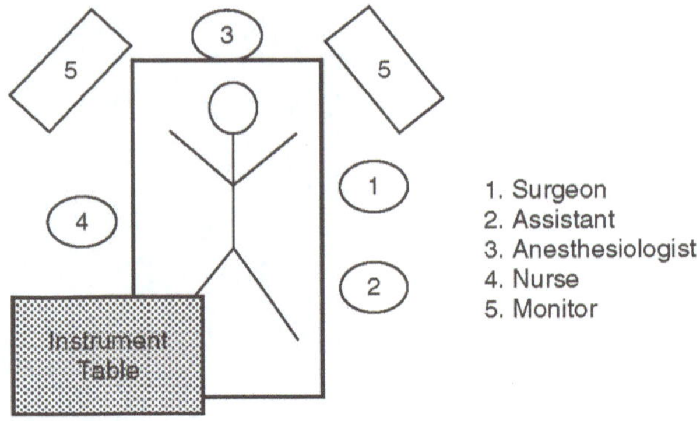


Fig. 8.1 Operating room setup for laparoscopic RPLND

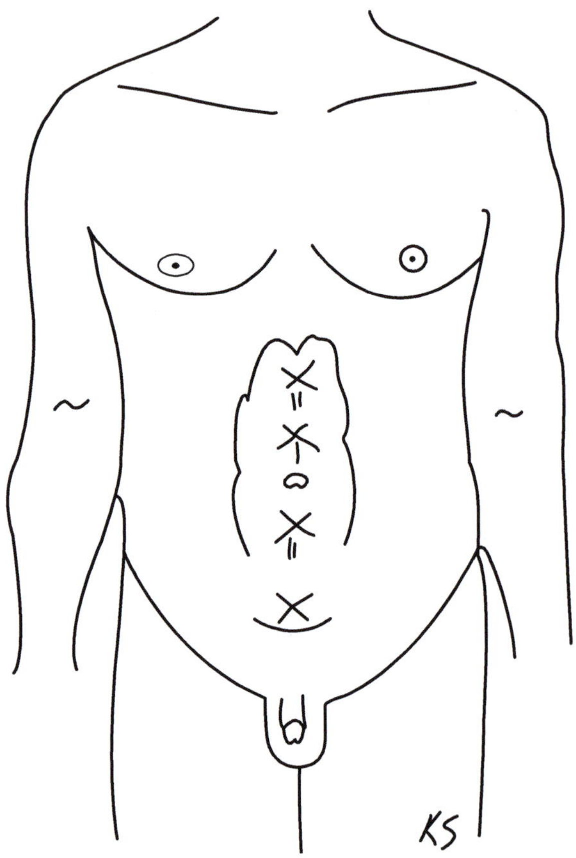


Fig. 8.2 Diagram demonstrating port site placement for laparoscopic RPLND

Pneumoperitoneum is established using a Veress needle placed via the umbilicus. Four equally spaced 12-mm laparoscopic ports are placed in the midline beginning 2–4 cm below the xiphoid process (Fig. 8.2). The large port size allows for the introduction of larger instruments from varying angles throughout the procedure. An additional 5-mm port may be placed in the mid-axillary line midway between the iliac crest and ribs for additional retraction, if needed. The bed is rotated to allow the bowel segments to fall away from the operative field.

## 8.5 Surgical Templates

When performing a right-sided template LRPLND, the limits of dissection include the right ureter laterally, the renal vessels superiorly, the aorta (including the preaortic nodes), and the common iliac artery inferiorly. Extension of this template to include the paraaortic nodes as well as the performance of a nerve-sparing bilateral dissection can routinely be performed. The limits of a left-sided template LRPLND include the ureter laterally, the vena cava (including precaval nodes), the common iliac artery, and the renal vessels (Donohue et al. 1993) (Fig. 8.3). Similarly, extension to a full bilateral LRPLND may be performed. Our typical approach is to perform a template dissection as described above; if metastatic disease is suspected intraoperatively, a bilateral modified template dissection is performed, in accordance with accepted oncologic principles. In both templates, the inferior mesenteric artery is spared.

The removal of tissue behind the aorta and vena cava is controversial with some authors arguing that this tissue is rarely a landing site for metastatic disease (Steiner et al. 2004). However, we believe that the removal of this tissue is an exact replication of the open RPLND and may reduce the risk of retroperitoneal recurrence thus providing a better oncological outcome for these patients. Therefore, complete removal of all retrocaval and retroaortic LN tissue is performed in all cases.

## 8.6 Right-Sided Dissection

Wide access to the retroperitoneum is necessary for LRPLND. A 10-mm 30° laparoscope is inserted through the umbilical port. The lower-most port is used to retract the bowel medially in order to expose the great vessels. This maneuver is usually done by the assistant, using the laparoscopic paddle retractor. Initially, the primary

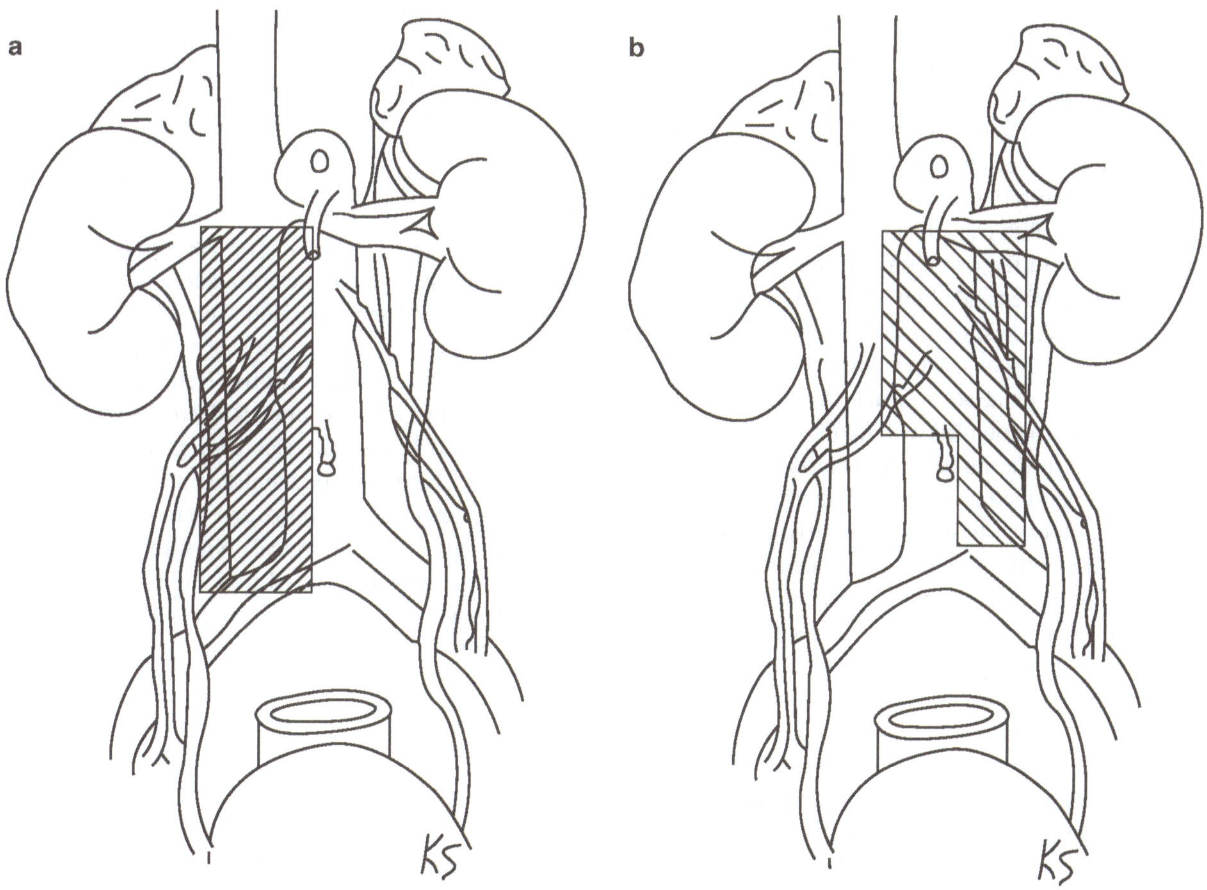


**Fig. 8.3** Surgical dissection templates for (**a**) right- and (**b**) left-sided laparoscopic RPLND

surgeon uses the three most cephalad ports to begin the dissection.

Dissection begins by incising the line of Told from the iliac vessels to the hepatic flexure and the colon is mobilized away from the abdominal wall. Care must be taken to avoid injury of the mesenteric vessels. On the right side, the surgeon defines the duodenum and an extensive Kocher's maneuver is carried out. This reflects the head of pancreas medially and allows adequate exposure not only of the anterior surfaces of the inferior vena cava and right renal vein, but also medially to visualize the contralateral renal hilum.

After colon mobilization, the ipsilateral internal inguinal ring is identified; the spermatic cord remnant is dissected and completely excised. The gonadal vein and surrounding lymphatics are then dissected in a cephalad direction to its insertion into the inferior vena cava. At this point it is doubly clipped and divided, thus excising the entire gonadal vein and associated lymphatics. Special care must be taken during right-sided dissections to avoid avulsion of the gonadal vein off of the inferior vena cava. The spermatic artery is clipped and transected where it crosses over the vena cava. The ureter is then identified as it crosses the iliac vessels.

All of the lymphatic tissue between the ureter and the great vessels is excised, using the "split/roll" technique. The tissues overlying precaval/preaortic are split laterally from cranial to caudal, superiorly to the renal vein, and inferiorly to the common iliac vessels. The lateral nodal tissue is lifted and blunt dissection is carried down to the lumbar vessels, which are clipped and transected. The underlying psoas fascia is preserved. At this point, the lower pole renal arteries may be encountered and should not be confounded with lumbar vessels.

Cephalad to the inferior mesenteric artery, the dissection is continued along the left margin to the aorta. The interaortocaval tissue is cautiously dissected, taking care to identify all vascular branches off the great vessels. The anterior spinous ligament represents the posterior boundary of the interaortocaval dissection and should be clearly visualized. The right renal artery and left renal vein must always be identified. As with open RPLND, it is essential to rule-out the presence of a retroaortic left renal vein on preoperative imaging, as failure to do so may result in continued cephalad dissection along the aorta and potential injury to the superior mesenteric artery. Small blood and lymphatic vessels are clipped. The entire package is gently dissected off the surface of the great vessels using the irrigation/suction device. Special care must be taken when dissecting posteriorly to the inferior vena cava as the efferent sympathetic nerves fibers may be injured.

We perform the retrocaval and retroaortic dissections as exact replications of open RPLND. The inferior vena cava is lifted with atraumatic instruments such as a laparoscopic DeBakey forceps, and all lymphatic tissue is teased off the retrocaval space. Posterior lumbar vessels are clipped and transected. The caudal point of dissection is the point where the ureter crosses the iliac vessels. At this point the entire nodal package is clipped distally and can be removed.

## 8.7 Left-Sided Dissection

On the left side, the peritoneum is incised along the line of Told from the iliac vessels to the splenic flexure. The splenocolic and phrenicocolic ligaments are divided. The colon is then mobilized medially until the anterior surface of the aorta and vena cava are exposed. The spermatic vein is identified and dissected proximally with associated lymphatic tissue toward to the left renal vein, where it is doubly clipped and divided. The left renal artery is then identified, paying close attention to the lumbar vein draining into the left renal vein, which can be injured. The spermatic artery is clipped at its origin from the aorta and transected. The ureter is identified and separated. The nodal package is dissected free in a similar way as to the right side, according to the template limits. Retroaortic dissection is performed as in the open RPLND. Care must be taken with the lumbar arteries during this step. The sympathetic chain must be identified and spared.

The specimen is entrapped and removed using an Endocatch device (US Surgical, Norwalk, CT). Intra-abdominal pressure is lowered to 5 mmHg in order to evaluate possible bleeding. A drain is not routinely placed. Port sides are endoscopically closed under direct vision.

## 8.8 Complications and Prevention

Potential complications during LRPLND include injury to surrounding visceral structures including bowel, pancreas, liver, spleen, and the kidneys.

However, the most common major complication during LRPLND is hemorrhage. Careful dissection of the great vessels and their branches, along with the advent of new equipment, allows for the prevention of most hemorrhagic events. Furthermore, the magnification provided by the laparoscope facilitates the tissue dissection, preventing injuries. Anatomical landmarks, potential risks of injury, and the maneuvers to prevent and treat some complications are described as follows:

- Lumbar vessels can be injured mainly during retrocaval and retroaortic dissection. The vessels encountered must be carefully ligated and divided. An important point is to leave a long vessel stump, in case a clip dislodges, making bleeding control easier. Hemorrhage from lumbar vessels that retract into the iliopsoas can usually be managed with pressure or a figure-of-eight stitch placed deep into the muscle.
- Accessory lower pole renal arteries may be found and should not be confounded with lumbar vessels. The right renal artery and left renal vein should also not be confused with lumbar vessels at the interaortocaval dissection.
- Lacerations of the inferior vena cava and aorta do not demand open conversion. As in open surgery, acute bleeding, mainly from venous bleeding, can be stopped by direct pressure applied with a surgical sponge. Most venous bleeding can be stopped with the help of fibrin glue. Clips, bipolar cautery, or intracorporeal suturing, using 3-0 monofilament nonabsorbable sutures, may be used to control arterial bleeding.
- On the right side, dissection of the duodenum and the head of the pancreas must be gentle, using sharp movements and avoiding thermal energy.
- Meticulous ligation of lymphatic channels with laparoscopic clip applier throughout the procedure can minimize the risk of postoperative lymphocele formation. Use of ultrasound shears is not recommended as the sealing of large lymphatic channels is improbable.
- Retrograde ejaculation has been reported at a rate similar to that seen with open RPLND, using the template introduced by Donohue and colleagues. Efferent sympathetic nerve fibers, passing posteriorly to the inferior vena cava, should be identified and carefully dissected. On the left side, the dissection is limited to a level 5 cm inferior to the renal vessels to spare the lumbar splanchnic nerves.

## 8.9 Postoperative Care

The nasogastric tube is removed in the operating room and the urethral catheter is removed as soon as the patient is alert, oriented, and ambulatory. Postoperative pain can be managed with oral analgesics. Diet is restarted immediately with clear fluids and advanced as tolerated. We advise our patients to consume a low-fat, medium chain fatty acid diet to minimize the risk of chylous ascites in the initial weeks after surgery as others have described (Steiner et al. 2004). Most patients are ready to be discharged home on postoperative day 2 and can resume normal activity between 10 and 20 days.

## 8.10 Results

Similar to other laparoscopic urologic procedures, reports of intra- and perioperative outcomes of laparoscopic RPLND have demonstrated a reduction in morbidity, shorter length of stay and convalescence time, and improved cosmesis when compared to open series. However, an important distinction exists between European and U.S. centers with respect to the primary role of laparoscopic RPLND in the treatment of NSGCT. European opinion is to apply laparoscopic RPLND chiefly as a diagnostic staging procedure, whereas centers of laparoscopic expertise in America believe that the operation serves a therapeutic as well as staging purpose.

The technical challenges of performing laparoscopic RPLND have led some investigators to pursue the value of lymph node dissection behind the aorta or vena cava as this represents the most difficult portion of the operation. Höltl et al. (2002) have reported that in 29 patients with clinical Stage I disease who underwent laparoscopic RPLND with removal of tissue anterior and posterior to great vessels, no lymph node dorsal to great vessels contained viable germ cell tumor. On the basis of these findings, the authors have omitted retroaortic/retrocaval dissection within the same template for patients with clinical Stage I disease. Of 49 patients with this approach followed for mean 28 months no retroperitoneal recurrences have been identified leading the authors to conclude that the reduction of the diagnostic lymph node dissection to the lymphatic tissue ventral to the lumbar vessels does not result in an increased incidence of local recurrence (Höltl et al. 2002).

The results of Höltl et al. provide evidence to exclude retroaortic and retrocaval dissection without compromising oncologic efficacy; however, our philosophy has been that laparoscopy is merely an alternative technique to perform surgery that traditionally has been performed with open technique. We believe that replication of all aspects of RPLND utilizing laparoscopic techniques allows for the true duplication of open RPLND and outcomes. Consequently, laparoscopic RPLND can be considered in this way as a therapeutic procedure, limiting relapses inside the template, analogous to the open counterpart.

The therapeutic efficacy of laparoscopic RPLND has been difficult to ascertain at the current time. It has been reported that up to 65% of patients with low volume retroperitoneal disease treated by open RPLND are cured of disease with surgery alone (Donohue et al. 1995). Many patients with pathologic Stage IIa disease in laparoscopic RPLND series have undergone chemotherapy making it difficult to truly assess the therapeutic benefit of the surgery. However, in a multi-institutional study of laparoscopic RPLND outcomes, Nielsen et al. (2007) identified ten patients with pathologic stage II disease who had clinical stage I disease preoperatively and declined postoperative chemotherapy. In this cohort with a mean follow-up of 37 months, not one retroperitoneal recurrence was discovered while two distant recurrences occurred; one in the chest and the other with elevated tumor markers and negative imaging.

While the study by Nielsen et al. is a retrospective study and has its inherent flaws, it does provide the initial evidence of the adequacy and therapeutic efficacy of the retroperitoneal dissection during laparoscopic RPLND. Recurrence in the retroperitoneum would be expected during this 3 year surveillance period if laparoscopic RPLND resulted in an inadequate dissection. Larger numbers of patients found to have pathologic stage IIa disease will need to be placed on a surveillance protocol instead of receiving immediate chemotherapy to determine if equivalent advantage exists as in open RPLND. A randomized trial between open and laparoscopic RPLND, though the best way to demonstrate oncologic equivalence, is unlikely to be performed given the relatively low incidence of testicular cancer and reluctance of some tertiary centers to incorporate advanced laparoscopic techniques.

Post operatively, patients treated with laparoscopic RPLND have benefited from shorter hospitalization

**Table 8.1** Summary of results from contemporary laparoscopic RPLND series

| Author | No. patients | Success rate (%) | Mean blood loss (mL) | Mean hospital stay (days) | Recurrence (%) | | Complication rate (%) | |
|---|---|---|---|---|---|---|---|---|
| | | | | | RP | Distant | Minor | Major |
| Rassweiler et al. (2000) | 34 | 88 | – | – | 0 | 5.9 | 8.8 | 5.9 |
| Bhayani et al. (2003) | 29 | 93 | 389 | 2.6 | 0 | 10 | 6.8 | 6.8 |
| Steiner et al. (2004) | 185 | | | | | | | |
| | Stage I 113 | 94 | 159 | 4.1 | 0.8[a] | 3.5 | 13.3 | 5.3 |
| | StageII 72 | 100 | 78 | 3.7 | 1.6[b] | 0 | | 0 |
| Neyer et al. (2007)[c] | 136 | 95 | 50 | 4.1 | 0 | 5.9 | 19.8 | 5.1 |
| Nielsen et al. (2007)[d] | 120 | NR | NR | NR | 0 | 7.5 | NR | NR |

*RP* retroperitoneum, *NR* not reported

[a]Recurrent disease found on contralateral side outside surgical template

[b]Recurrent disease found on ipsilateral side outside surgical template

[c]Includes patients from Steiner et al.

[d]Includes patients from Bhayani et al.

and convalescence as well as the obvious improved cosmesis in select series. However, in tertiary care centers of excellence for open RPLND, the difference between length of stay and time to resume diet for open and laparoscopic RPLND patients may not be as disparate. Beck et al. (2007) from Indiana University reported on 75 patients undergoing primary open RPLND from 2003 to 2005 and mean time to begin clear liquids and hospitalization was 1 and 2.8 days, respectively.

Another important postoperative variable that is gaining attention in the surgical outcomes literature is patient quality of life (QoL). Poulakis et al. (2006) reported the only study comparing QoL after laparoscopic and open RPLND. In this study, median hospital stay for the 21 patients undergoing laparoscopic RPLND was 2 days versus 7 for the 29 patients undergoing open RPLND. A higher incidence of early and late postoperative complications was also observed in the open group. As measured by SF-36™ and the European Organisation for the Research and Treatment of Cancer QLQ-C30, quality of life was significantly better for laparoscopy than for open RPLND, although the study population in the two groups was small.

A summary of outcomes from recent reports in the literature of laparoscopic RPLND is presented in Table 8.1.

## 8.11 Conclusions

Laparoscopic RPLND offers excellent diagnostic and therapeutic performance, with local control of the retroperitoneum in line with the established benchmarks of open RPLND. We feel that in offering treatment options to patients with Stage I NSGCT, laparoscopic RPLND should be offered as an option without reservation on the basis of current literature.

## References

Allaf ME, Bhayani SB, Link RE, Schaeffer EM, Varkarakis JM, Shadpour P, Lima G, Kavoussi LR (2005) Laparoscopic retroperitoneal lymph node dissection: duplication of open technique. Urology 65:575–577

Beck SD, Peterson MD, Bihrle R, Donohue JP, Foster RS (2007) Short-term morbidity of primary retroperitoneal lymph node dissection in a contemporary group of patients. J Urol 178:504–506

Bhayani SB, Ong A, Oh WK, Kantoff PW, Kavoussi LR (2003) Laparoscopic retroperitoneal lymph node dissection for clinical stage I nonseminomatous germ cell testicular cancer: a long-term update. Urology 62:324–327

Donohue JP, Foster RS, Rowland RG, Bihrle R, Jones J, Geier G (1990) Nerve-sparing retroperitoneal lymphadenectomy with preservation of ejaculation. J Urol 144:287–291

Donohue JP, Thornhill JA, Foster RS, Rowland RG, Birhle R (1993) Retroperitoneal lymphadenectomy for clinical stage A testis cancer (1965 to 1989): modifications of technique and impact on ejaculation. J Urol 149:237–243

Donohue JP, Thornhill JA, Foster RS, Bihrle R, Rowland RG, Einhorn LH (1995) The role of retroperitoneal lymphadenectomy in clinical stage B testis cancer: the Indiana University experience (1965-1989). J Urol 153:85–89

Gerber GS, Bissada NK, Hulbert JC, Kavoussi LR, Moore RG, Kantoff PW, Rukstalis DB (1994) Laparoscopic retroperitoneal lymphadenectomy: multi-institutional analysis. J Urol 152:1188–1191

Höltl L, Peschel R, Knapp R, Janetaschek G, Steiner H, Rogatsch H, Hittmair A, Rogatsch H, Bartsch G, Hobisch A (2002) Primary lymphatic metastatic spread in testicular cancer occurs ventral to the lumbar vessels. Urology 59:114–118

Janetschek G, Reissigl A, Peschel R, Hobisch A, Bartsch G (1994) Laparoscopic retroperitoneal lymph node excision in clinical stage I non-seminomatous testicular cancer. Urologe A 33:24–30

Lima GC, Kohanim S, Rais-Bahrami S, Kavoussi LR (2005) Laparoscopic retroperitoneal lymph node dissection after prior open retroperitoneal lymphadenectomy and chemotherapy. Urology 66:1319

Neyer M, Peschel R, Akkad T, Springer-Stöhr B, Berger A, Bartsch G, Steiner H (2007) Long-term results of laparoscopic retroperitoneal lymph-node dissection for clinical stage I nonseminomatous germ-cell testicular cancer. J Endourol 21:180–183

Nielsen ME, Lima G, Schaeffer EM, Porter J, Cadeddu JA, Tuerk I, Kavoussi LR (2007) Oncologic efficacy of laparoscopic RPLND in treatment of clinical stage I nonseminomatous germ cell testicular cancer. Urology 70:1168–1172

Permpongkosol S, Lima GC, Warlick CA, Allaf ME, Varkarakis IM, Bagga HS, Kohanim S, Kavoussi LR (2007) Postchemotherapy laparoscopic retroperitoneal lymph node dissection: evaluation of complications. Urology 69:361–365

Poulakis V, Skriapas K, de Vries R, Dillenburg W, Ferakis N, Witzsch U, Becht E (2006) Quality of life after laparoscopic and open retroperitoneal lymph node dissection in clinical Stage I nonseminomatous germ cell tumor: a comparison study. Urology 68:154–160

Rassweiler JJ, Frede T, Lenz E, Seemann O, Alken P (2000) Long-term experience with laparoscopic retroperitoneal lymph node dissection in the management of low-stage testis cancer. Eur Urol 37:251–260

Rukstalis DB, Chodak GW (1992) Laparoscopic retroperitoneal lymph node dissection in a patient with stage 1 testicular carcinoma. J Urol 148:1907–1909

Steiner H, Peschel R, Janetschek G, Höltl L, Berger AP, Bartsch G, Hobisch A (2004) Long-term results of laparoscopic retroperitoneal lymph node dissection: a single-center 10-year experience. Urology 63:550–555

Stone NN, Schlussel RN, Waterhouse RL, Unger P (1993) Laparoscopic retroperitoneal lymph node dissection in stage A nonseminomatous testis cancer. Urology 42:610–614

# 9 Diagnostic and Therapeutic Laparoscopic Retroperitoneal Lymph Node Dissection in Low-Stage Nonseminomatous GCC: The European View

Günter Janetschek and Reinhold P. Zimmermann

## 9.1 Introduction

Efficacious treatment of nonseminomatous germ cell tumor (NSGCT) consists of two treatment modalities – retroperitoneal lymph node dissection and chemotherapy – of which the timing and combination is of utmost importance. However, the concepts differ to some extent between Europe and the US, and only the European standpoint is discussed in this chapter.

The role of RPLND in clinical stage I has been demonstrated in many publications and is well established. In Europe, RPLND is considered as a diagnostic procedure only, and adjuvant chemotherapy following RPLND in clinical stage I/pathologic stage II is strongly recommended by the 2007 EAU guidelines. In the US, the concept for clinical stage I/pathologic stage II differs substantially, and RPLND is seen as a definitive therapeutic measure despite the high relapse rates ranging from 8 to 55% (2–6, Table 9.1). It has to be realized that diagnostic and therapeutic RPLND substantially differ in regard to the template, which is not only important oncologically but also has implications for the risk of loss of antegrade ejaculation. Therefore, clear description of the template of RPLND is of utmost importance. With the unilateral diagnostic template (Weissbach and Boedefeld 1987), antegrade ejaculation is preserved so that no additional nerve sparing is required, whereas it is at risk with larger therapeutic templates. This is true for both open surgery and laparoscopy.

It was always our goal to duplicate open RPLND without any compromise because of the laparoscopic technique. Therefore, we performed exactly the same dissection within the same template as previously with open surgery. As a consequence, all the tissue behind the aorta and vena cava was removed in our first 30 laparoscopic cases (Janetschek et al. 1999). However, in an analysis of our patients, we could demonstrate that the primary landing site of lymph node metastases is always ventral to the lumbar vessels; dorsal metastases are always due to further spread from the primary metastasis (Holtl et al. 2002). Since the goal of diagnostic RPLND is removal of the primary landing site only, we stopped to transect all lumbar vessels to remove all tissue behind the aorta and vena cava, which is still required for therapeutic RPLND.

There are different concepts to treat clinical stage II. The combination of both surgery and chemotherapy is highly efficacious, but carries substantial morbidity. In our concept, we could maintain efficacy while reducing morbidity by replacing open surgery with laparoscopy and by reducing the dose of chemotherapy, the effect of which was controlled by surgery anyway. In a consecutive series of stage IIb tumors (2–5 cm prior to chemotherapy), excellent results could be achieved with minimal morbidity (Janetschek et al. 1999). In stage IIc, this concept is applied to selected patients only (Albqami and Janetschek 2005).

## 9.2 Indications

### 9.2.1 Clinical Stage I

In the new guidelines of the EAU (Albers et al.), RPLND is considered second-line therapy for both low and high NSGCT. First-line therapy is either

G. Janetschek (✉)
Department of Urology, Paracelsus Medical University, Salzburg, Austria
e-mail: g.janetschek@salk.at

M.P. Laguna et al. (eds.), *Cancer of the Testis*,
DOI: 10.1007/978-1-84800-370-5_9, 

**Table 9.1** Relapse rates after RPLND for clinical stage I/pathologic stage II

| | IIa | IIb | IIa+b |
|---|---|---|---|
| Javadpour 1984 | – | – | 24% ($n=50$) |
| Williams et al. 1987 | – | – | 49% ($n=98$) |
| Richie and Kantoff 1991 | 8% ($n=39$) | – | – |
| Pizzocaro et al. 1994 | 29% ($n=51$) | 34% ($n=71$) | – |
| Donohue et al. 1995 | 26% ($n=27$) | 55% ($n=20$) | – |

wait-and-see (low risk) or primary chemotherapy (high risk). There are, however, still several arguments in favor of RPLND. A relapse may be difficult to detect in a marker-negative patient. Therefore, wait-and-see is not a valid option in this situation. The same is true in a patient with poor compliance. Primary chemotherapy carries the risk of late recurrence with NSGCT containing chemoresistant tumor (Ronnen et al. 2005). In summary, the indications for laparoscopic RPLND are the same as for open surgery. Previous surgery or obesity was never considered a contraindication and neither resulted in conversion in our series.

### 9.2.2 Stage II After Chemotherapy

#### 9.2.2.1 Stage IIa

This stage is treated similar as clinical stage I with primary chemotherapy, and additional RPLND is usually not indicated.

#### 9.2.2.2 Stage IIb

Tumor size in this stage is 2–5 cm prior to chemotherapy. Therapy is started with two cycles of PEB. Further chemotherapy, which is usually given to increase safety but has no more therapeutic impact once there is no more vital tumor, is replaced by laparoscopic RPLND. The benefit of this approach is twofold. The patient is spared unnecessary chemotherapy, and in a substantial proportion of patient chemoresistant mature teratoma will be removed as well. Thereby, the effect of chemotherapy is well documented. Normalization of markers is a prerequisite to perform surgery. In our experience, morbidity of laparoscopic RPLND is clearly less than morbidity of further chemotherapy. It has to be realized in this context that morbidity of chemotherapy increases exponentially after each cycle.

#### 9.2.2.3 Stage IIc

Laparoscopic surgery is only indicated in selected smaller tumors where a unilateral surgical template is considered sufficient. The template has to include all visible tumors prior to chemotherapy. Three cycles PEB are administered initially. We not only remove a residual tumor but also always dissect the complete unilateral template.

## 9.3 Surgical Technique

The technique of laparoscopic RPLND has been described in detail by Dr.Brian A. VanderBrink in this chapter. To avoid redundancy, only those aspects are discussed where our technique differs.

### 9.3.1 Patient Positioning

The patient is placed with the ipsilateral side elevated 45° off the operating table. The operating table is then slightly flexed at the level of the umbilicus. By rotating the table, the patient can be placed into a supine or lateral decubitus position. If necessary, the Trendelenburg or anti-Trendelenburg position is used.

### 9.3.2 Trocar Position

The first trocar is placed at the umbilicus for the laparoscope; two secondary trocars are placed at the lateral edge of the rectus muscle 8 cm above and below the umbilicus for the surgeons' instruments. A fourth trocar is placed laterally at the anterior axillary line in the best point for retraction decided by the surgeon (Fig. 9.1); Trocar of 5 and 11-mm size are used.

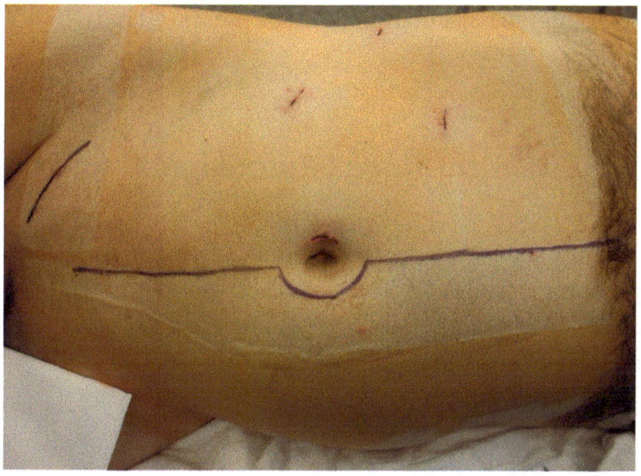

**Fig. 9.1** Position of trocars (scars: *right side*). For comparison, the incision lines of right orchiectomy and alternative open RPLND are marked with ink

### 9.3.3 Surgical Templates

For diagnostic RPLND, the specimen to be removed has to include all primary retroperitoneal lymph node metastases. We strictly adhere to the templates described by Weissbach for clinical stage I (Weissbach and Boedefeld 1987). The right and left template will hold at least 97 and 95%, respectively, of all primary landing sites. Interestingly, Donohue, who initially described larger templates, also later changed to a smaller left template sparing interaortocaval dissection (Donohue et al. 1993). Since the primary landing site is never dorsal to the lumbar vessels, the tissue behind the vena cava and aorta does not need to be removed (Holtl et al. 2002). Therefore, transection of the lumbar vessels is not required.

*Right template:* It includes the tissues ventral to the vena Cava, the right paracaval, the interaortocaval and the preaortic tissue between the renal left vein and the inferior mesenteric artery. The cranial border is delineated by the renal vessels, and the caudal border by the crossing of the ureter with the iliac artery. The spermatic vessels are removed in their entire length (Fig. 9.2a).

*Left template:* It does not include the interaortocaval tissue but all tissue lateral to the aorta as well as the tissue ventral to the aorta between the renal vessels and the origin of the inferior mesenteric artery. The upper boarder are the renal vessels, the lower boarder is the crossing of the ureter with the common iliac artery (Fig. 9.2b).

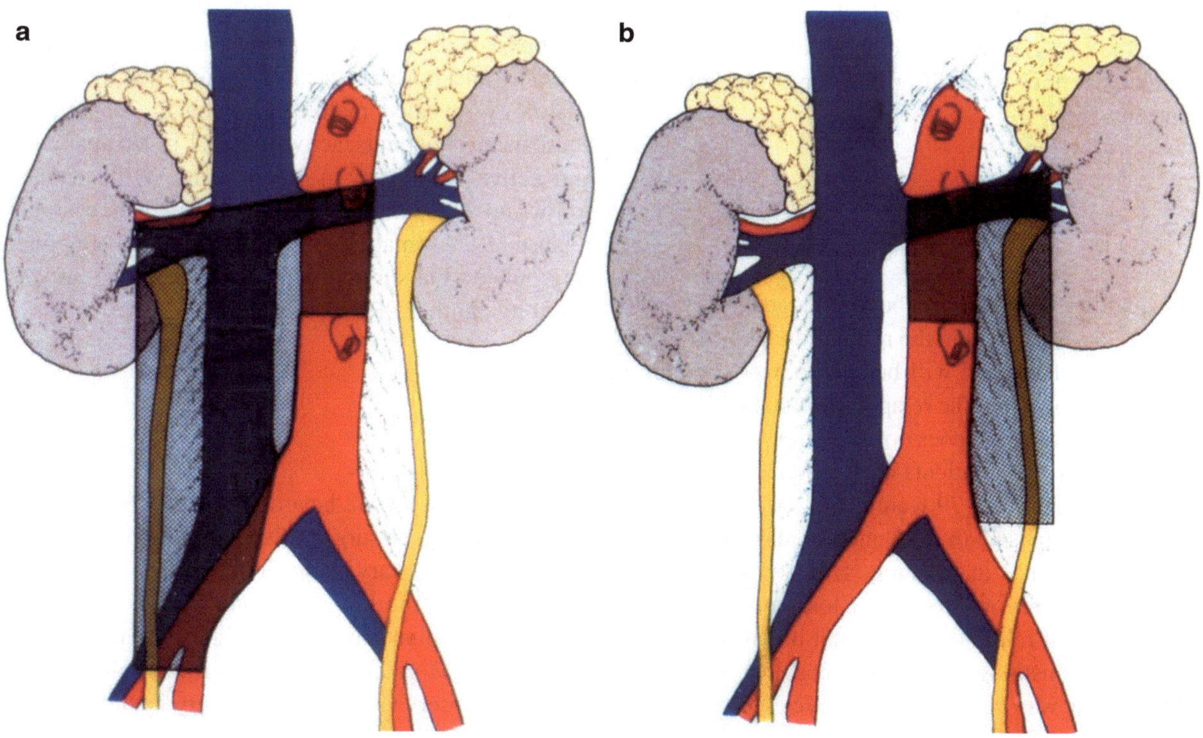

**Fig. 9.2** Templates of diagnostic unilateral RPLND (**a**) *right side* (**b**) *left side*

## 9.4 Stage II After Chemotherapy

Unilateral RPLND for stage II after chemotherapy is performed within the same templates as used for clinical stage I disease. Previous chemotherapy renders identification of the tissue layers more difficult. This problem, however, does not depend so much on the number of chemotherapeutic cycles, but more on the initial tumor size and tumor type. Mature teratoma is usually well delineated whereas tumor-free residuals after embryonal carcinoma may be tightly adherent to the surrounding structures. This is particularly true for the vena Cava. Small venous branches draining the tumor have to be meticulously dissected before they are clipped and transected. A small bipolar dissector as well as a small surgical sponge held by a grasper proved most useful for this purpose. Small vessels to the vena Cava can also be coagulated and cut without previous clipping when there is a long stump.

## 9.5 Results

Data on surgical efficiency and morbidity are presented by Dr. Brian A. VanderBrink in the previous chapter. Therefore, only data on oncologic efficacy are presented since they may differ because of the different concepts.

### 9.5.1 Clinical Stage I/Pathologic Stage I

The quality of RPLND can be best judged by analysis of the relapse rate within the retroperitoneum, because any tumor left behind will become obvious within a short period of time. The relapse rate outside the retroperitoneum, however, does not rely on surgery. Among 115 clinical stage I patients operated between August 1992 and April 2006, 79 were pathologic stage I. The mean follow-up is 63 (6–113) months. There were five relapses (5.8%), 3 in the lung, 1 marker only, and 1 (1.15%) in the retroperitoneum. Closer analysis of this retroperitoneal relapse revealed that it was not due to insufficient histology, but false-negative histology. This patient was cured with two cycles of PEB and laparoscopic RPLND on the contralateral side.

Antegrade ejaculation could be preserved in 104/105 patients (99%).

### 9.5.2 Clinical Stage I/Pathologic Stage II

Twenty six out of one-hundred and five patients were pathologic stage II. They all received two cycles of adjuvant chemotherapy (PEB). There was not a single relapse after a mean follow-up of 47 (4–97) months.

### 9.5.3 Pathologic Stage II After Chemotherapy

Between February 1995 and April 2006, laparoscopic RPLND was performed in 47 consecutive stage IIb patients and 18 selected stage IIc patients. There was not a single conversion among the 65 patients which is in contrast to the 2.7% conversion rate in clinical stage I. A single major complication occurred – a delayed bleeding which was managed laparoscopically. In seven patients, a chylous ascites occurred which was always managed conservatively (low-fat diet, middle-chain triglycerides). We now start diet postoperatively in every patient over a period of 3 weeks and have not seen this complication since. Histology revealed mature teratoma in 24 patients, necrosis in 39 patients, active NSGCT in 1/64 patients, and active seminoma in 1/1 patients. With a mean follow-up of 38 (3–73) months, there was a single relapse (1.5%) (mature teratoma at the inner inguinal ring outside the surgical template). That patient was cured by another PRLND.

## 9.6 Discussion

Surgical efficiency of laparoscopic RPLND at least equals that of open surgery. Direct comparison of data with a contemporary, large, open series shows that operative time and blood loss and operative time are equal, but hospital stay is clearly shorter (Heidenreich et al. 2003). More importantly, the rate of major complications observed with open surgery is significantly higher (5.4%), including severe complications such as nephrectomy due to a lesion of the renal artery, bowel necrosis requiring colostomy following a lesion of the superior mesenteric artery, and an ileus followed by relaparotomy. The rate of minor complications was 14.2% in the open group.

The major long-term morbidity consists in loss of antegrade ejaculation. Dissection within the unilateral diagnostic templates results in injury of the ipsilateral sympathetic chain only, whereas the contralateral side remains intact. It is known since a long time that preservation of one sympathetic chain is sufficient to maintain normal antegrade ejaculation (Whitelaw and Smithwick 1951). Therefore, nerve-sparing as described by Donohue is not required (Donohue et al. 1993).

The quality of diagnostic RPLND is best judged by the rate of retroperitoneal relapse in pathologic stage I. This rate was 1.15% in our series compared to 1.8% after open RPLND (Heidenreich et al. 2003). The value of laparoscopic RPLND after chemotherapy is well documented by the low relapse rate, complication rate, and relapse rate.

We performed a quality of life study including 112 patients after either laparoscopic or open RPLND. Half of the patients in each group also received adjuvant chemotherapy. All the patients answered a questionnaire containing 39 questions, and the interview was not performed by the surgeon but a psychiatrist. It could be shown that open surgery impairs quality of life much more than laparoscopy. Surprisingly, not only laparoscopy was favored over chemotherapy but open surgery as well.

## References


Albers P, Albrecht W, Algaba F, Bokemeyer C, Cohn-Cedermark G, Horvich A et al (2009) EAU Working group on Testis Cancer. EAU guidelines on testicular cancer. In EAU-guidelines edition pp 1–46

Donohue JP, Thornhill JA, Foster RS et al (1995) The role of retroperitoneal lymphadenectomy in clinical stage B testis cancer: The Indiana University experience (1965 to 1989). J Urol 153:85–89

Holtl L, Peschel R, Knapp R, Janetschek G (2002) Primary lymphatic metastatic spread in testicular cancer occurs ventral to the lumbar vessels. Urol 59:114–118

Janetschek G, Hobisch A, Höltl L et al (1996) Retroperitoneal lymphadenectomy for clinical stage I nonseminomatous testicular tumor: Laparoscopy versus open surgery and impact of Iearning curve. J Urol 156:89–93

Javadpour N (1984) Predictors of recurrence in stage II nonseminomatous testicular cancer after lymphadenectomy: Implications for adjuvant chemotherapy. J Urol 135:629

Pizzocaro G, Nicolai N, Salvioni R (1994) Evolution and controversies in the management of low- stage nonseminomatous germ-cell tumors of the testis. World J. Urol 12: 113–119

Richie JP, Kantoff PW (1991) Is adjuvant chemotherapy necessary for patients with stage I testicular cancer? J Clin Oncol 9:1393–1396

Weissbach L, Boedefeld EA (1987) Testicular Tumor Study Group: Localization of solitary and multiple metastases in stage II nonseminomatous testis tumor as basis for a modified staging lymph node dissection in stage I. J Urol 138: 77–82

Williams SD, Stablein DM, Einhorn LH, Muggia FM, Weiss RB, Donohue JP et al (1987) Immediate adjuvant chemotherapy versus observation with treatment at relapse in pathological stage II testicular cancer. N Engl J Med 317:1433–1438

# Part IVA

## Treatment of Stage I

# Treatment of Nonseminoma: Stage I

# 10

Michael A.S. Jewett, Jerome P. Richie, and Peter Albers

## 10.1 Introduction

Testicular cancer, afflicting 1 in 30,000 men per year, represents the most common malignancy in men between the ages of 20 and 34. The management of nonseminomatous germ cell tumors has undergone significant and dramatic changes in the past 30 years. The combination of improved staging modalities, surgical approaches, and chemotherapy has been largely responsible for enhanced survival with appropriate reductions in morbidity.

Appropriate management begins with establishing the primary tumor histopathology as well as the clinical stage of disease. Radical inguinal orchiectomy establishes the diagnosis as well as controls the primary tumor, regardless of local tumor growth or histologic pattern. Careful histologic examination, including step-sectioning of the testicle, will establish the histologic diagnosis. The most common tumor of the testicle is seminoma, followed by embryonal carcinoma, teratoma, and choriocarcinoma. Combinations of different tumor types occur in up to 40% of patients.

According to regional cancer registries in Europe, about 90% of patients present with low-stage disease (TNM stages I–IIB). Most (61–78%) have clinical stage I disease confined to the testis with normalized markers after orchidectomy (Powles et al. 2005; Sonneveld et al. 1999). Patients with clinical stage I testis cancer are expected to be cured in nearly 100% of cases. The changes in treatment options after orchidectomy have been documented by the implementation of interdisciplinary guidelines-based treatment recommendations (Schmoll et al. 2004, 2009 Wood et al. 2010 ). This chapter focuses on (1) the modern treatment of the primary tumor including organ-sparing surgery, Wood L, (2) research on prognostic factors to predict those patients who will relapse with clinical stage I, and (3) the current treatment recommendations in nonseminoma after the publication of several large randomized trials.

## 10.2 Staging

Clinical staging should be performed at the earliest convenience (if possible, before orchidectomy). It includes serum tumor markers (alpha fetoprotein, human chorionic gonadotropin, and lactate dehydrogenase), computed tomography staging of the chest and abdomen, and ultrasound of the contralateral testis if not already done. After orchidectomy, markers should normalize, although, the AFP normalization may take some weeks (half-time 5–7 days). With normalized markers and no metastases found on the CT scans, patients are classified as clinical stage I.

Details on clinical staging are covered in Chap. 5 and imaging in diagnosis and staging is covered in Chap. 14. In spite of the advancing technology, with faster generation of CT scans, tumor markers, positron emission tomography (PET) scans, etc., there are severe limitations to the ability of clinical staging to predict retroperitoneal involvement. Although extensive pulmonary disease or nonpulmonary visceral metastases are readily identified, identification of minimal retroperitoneal nodal disease remains suboptimal. A significant false-negative rate exists because of the patients with microscopic or limited macroscopic nodal involvement. The false-positive rate is very low.

M.A.S. Jewett (✉)
Departments of Surgery and Surgical Oncology, Princess Margaret Hospital, University Health Network, University of Toronto, Toronto, ON, Canada

M.P. Laguna et al. (eds.), *Cancer of the Testis*,
DOI: 10.1007/978-1-84800-370-5_10, © Springer-Verlag London Limited 2010

The clinical staging error cannot yet be overcome by modern generation imaging techniques. Radiologists have generally utilized size criteria to describe abnormal lymph nodes in the retroperitoneum. Most radiologists utilize a 1-cm size cutoff. In a retrospective blinded study, radiologists utilized different CT size criteria ranging from 4 to 10 mm (Hilton et al. 1997). However, at a 4-mm size criteria, the sensitivity increased to 93% but the specificity dropped to 58% (Hilton et al. 1997). The combination of histopathologic/immunohistochemical evaluation with expert review of the CT may diminish the false-negative staging error, but this approach is preserved for specialized centers (Leibovitch et al. 1998). PET improves the specificity of imaging and this is more important for clinical stage II disease (Albers et al. 1999; Hain et al. 2000; Lassen et al. 2003). If the CT is normal on expert review, a PET scan probably will not improve sensitivity.

The main issue in the adjuvant treatment of patients with clinical stage I NSGCT is to minimize overall morbidity of treatment without reducing the survival chances for those 28% of patients who have occult metastatic disease (Table 10.1). Based on the historical literature, active surveillance of all patients, i.e., without risk stratification, will result in delayed treatment of recurrence in up to 30% of patients, usually with multiple courses of chemotherapy and resection of residual masses. The other options, retroperitoneal lymph node dissection (RPLND) and primary chemotherapy without risk stratification, will overtreat at least 70% of patients. Identification of prognostic or risk factors for occult metastatic disease is a priority in the management of stage I NSGCT.

**Table 10.1** Surveillance management of patients with clinical stage I nonseminoma (trials >100 patients)

| References | Number of patients | Recurrences (%) |
|---|---|---|
| Freedman et al. (1987) | 259 | 70 (29) |
| Swanson et al. | 100 | 31 (31) |
| Sturgeon et al. (1992) | 105 | 37 (35) |
| Read et al. (1992) | 373 | 100 (27) |
| Fossa et al. | 102 | 22 (22) |
| Gels et al. (1995) | 154 | 42 (27) |
| Sogani et al. (1998) | 105 | 27 (26) |
| Sharir et al. (1999) | 170 | 48 (28) |
| Oliver et al. | 234 | 71 (30) |
| Colls et al. (1999) | 115 | 34 (30) |
| Francis et al. (2000) | 183 | 52 (28) |
| Atsu et al. (2003) | 132 | 32 (24) |
| Total | 2,032 | 566 (28) |

## 10.3 Prognostic Factors in NSGCT I

The UK Medical Research Council (MRC) performed the first major study to identify the risk factors for relapse (Freedman et al. 1987). The multivariate analysis revealed four prognostic factors for recurrence: vascular and lymphatic invasion in the primary tumor, the presence of embryonal carcinoma, and the absence of yolk sac tumor. A prospective MRC trial based on these prognostic variables found the presence of at least three of these four factors to be predictive for relapse in 48% of patients (Read et al. 1992). Vascular invasion was the most significant factor. This was confirmed in several retrospective analyses and prospective trials that used vascular invasion to identify the high-risk group that subsequently was treated with adjuvant chemotherapy (Albers et al. 2006; Cullen et al. 1996a; Klepp et al. 1997; Pont et al. 1996; Ondrus et al. 1998; Böhlen et al. 2001; Maroto et al. 2005). The relapse rate for patients without vascular invasion who were managed by observation ranged between 14 and 22%. In most prospective clinical series, the high-risk population was treated, so the predictive value of vascular invasion could not be evaluated. The German Testicular Study Group performed a randomized trial with risk-factor analysis using all available predictors (Albers et al. 2003). One goal of this trial was to define risk factors that more accurately predict high risk for recurrence. One hundred and sixty-five patients who underwent RPLND (pathological stage I, follow-up >12 months) or surveillance and a mean follow-up of 3 years have been prospectively evaluated by reference pathology. After multivariate analysis, three adverse prognostic parameters had been identified: (1) vascular invasion, (2) proliferation rate by MIB-1 immunostaining (>70% positively stained tumor cells), and (3) percentage embryonal carcinoma (>50%) as a component of the primary tumor. A combination of all the three factors predicted 64% of patients with occult metastatic disease. Patients without vascular invasion and a low MIB score (<70%) had only a 13% chance of retroperitoneal metastatic disease. In addition, risk factors of recurrence have been systematically reviewed in a meta-analysis (Vergouwe et al. 2003). Based on these new prognostic factor combinations, risk-adapted treatment strategies have been introduced to select patients for adjuvant treatment with a much higher risk of relapse (Amato et al. 2004; Chevreau et al. 2004). Studies from the MD Anderson Cancer Center and from Toulouse combined at least vascular invasion with embryonal carcinoma to define a high-risk group of patients.

Table 10.2 includes a summary of the variables that have been identified as statistically significant predictors of relapse in NSGCT surveillance subjects. In studies that performed both univariate and multivariate analyses, only those features that were significant on multivariate analysis are listed. Vascular invasion of the primary tumor was the most consistent prognostic feature identified (Read et al. 1992; Klepp et al. 1997; Alexandre et al. 2001; Colls et al. 1999; Daugaard et al. 2003; Fossa et al. 1994; Gels et al. 1995; Hao et al. 1998; Hoskin et al. 1986; Ondrus and Hornak 1994; Peckham and Brada 1987; Sogani et al. 1998; Sturgeon et al. 1992; Thompson et al. 1988; Wishnow et al. 1989). However, pathological interpretation varies between venous invasion, lymphatic invasion or lymphovascular invasion (Pont et al. 1990). Predominantly embryonal carcinoma histology and T stage were also frequently associated with rate of relapse (Hao et al. 1998; Hoskin et al. 1986; Peckham and Brada 1987; Sogani et al. 1998; Wishnow et al. 1989; Atsu et al. 2003; Dunphy et al. 1988; Nicolai and Pizzocaro 1995; Raghavan et al. 1988). Absence of yolk sac tumor in the primary specimen, occasionally represented by surrogate low alpha-fetoprotein levels was another unfavorable prognostic feature (Read et al. 1992; Sturgeon et al. 1992; Wishnow et al. 1989). Other histopathologic adverse prognostic features identified include undifferentiated histology, spermatic cord involvement, and the presence of mature teratoma (Alexandre et al. 2001). Nicolai and Pizzocaro identified trans-scrotal violation as an independent predictor of relapse although others have suggested that this may alter the pattern of spread without increasing the risk of recurrence (Read et al. 1992; Nicolai and Pizzocaro 1995; Ernst et al. 2005).

In summary, risk factors have been identified that define a low-risk and a high-risk group of patients with a risk for relapse of 13 and 64%, respectively. These factors have led to a risk-adapted approach of treatment in Europe favoring surveillance for patients with low risk and chemotherapy for patients with high risk of recurrence. In America, the high-risk patients frequently undergo RPLND.

## 10.4 Treatment of the Primary Tumor and Organ-Sparing Surgery

Standard treatment of a testicular cancer with a normal contralateral testis is orchidectomy via an inguinal approach. This allows for an exact histopathological diagnosis and, in true stage I patients, orchidectomy is the only necessary treatment for the patient.

According to the current European guidelines, the patient should be informed about the possibility of a contralateral biopsy and this should be recommended for patients with risk factors for a testicular intraepithelial neoplasia testicular intraepithelial neoplasia (TIN) such as cryptorchidism, and history of maldescendent testis (Schmoll et al. 2004; Albers et al. 2005; Harland et al. 1998). The incidence of TIN in the contralateral testis is about 5% (Dieckmann and Loy 1996). Internationally, however, there is still a debate of whether an immediate biopsy at the time of orchidectomy is necessary regarding the excellent 10-year survival figures of patients with metachronous contralateral tumors (Hoei-Hansen et al. 2005; Fossa et al. 2005).

### 10.4.1 *Small Intratesticular Lesions*

Intratesticular lesions present a special clinical problem. The exact diagnosis is rarely made by imaging techniques alone and histological verification is necessary. However, in benign lesions, orchidectomy is overtreatment and, at least in solitary testes, low-volume malignant lesions may be managed by organ-sparing surgery (Albers et al. 2005).

Nongerm cell tumors (e.g., Leydig cell tumors, Sertoli cell tumors, granulosa cell tumors) represent less than 5% of all intratesticular lesions. However,

**Table 10.2** Summary of surveillance outcomes for clinical stage I NSGCT

| References | *n* | Median FU | # Relapse (%) | # Late relapse (%) | # Marker only relapse (%) | # Palpable relapse (%) | Prognostic features identified | Deaths (%) |
|---|---|---|---|---|---|---|---|---|
| Hoskin et al. (1986) | 126 | 42 months | 36 (0.29) | NR | NR | NR | LI, emb | 1 (0.01) |
| Peckham and Brada (1987) | 132 | 43 months | 35 (0.27) | 2 (0.02) | 8 (0.06) | 0 (0.00) | LI, emb | 1 (0.01) |
| Dunphy et al. (1988) | 93 | 34 months | 28 (0.30) | 0 (0.00) | 8 (0.09) | 0 (0.00) | VLI, emb | 0 (0.00) |
| Raghavan et al. (1988) | 46 | 40 months | 13 (0.28) | 2 (0.04) | 1 (0.02) | NR | Tstage | 2 (0.04) |
| Thompson et al. (1988) | 36 | 36 months | 12 (0.33) | 2 (0.06) | 1 (0.03) | 1 (0.03) | LI | 1 (0.03) |
| Wishnow et al. (1989) | 82 | NR | 24 (0.29) | NR | NR | NR | Emb, VI, low AFP | NR |
| Liedke et al. (1990) | 107 | 38 months | 37 (0.35) | NR | NR | NR | Tstage | NR |
| Rorth et al. (1991) | 77 | 64 months | 23 (0.30) | 4 (0.05) | 2 (0.03) | 0 (0.00) | None | 0 (0.00) |
| Read et al. (1992) | 373 | 60 months | 100 (0.27) | 8 (0.02) | 13 (0.04) | 3 (0.01) | Venous Invasion, undiff, NYS | 5 (0.01) |
| Sturgeon et al. (1992) | 105 | 60 months | 37 (0.35) | NR | 6 (0.06) | 3 (0.03) | VI | 1 (0.01) |
| Ondrus and Hornak (1994) | 80 | >60 months | 29 (0.36) | 5 (0.06) | NR | NR | VI | 4 (0.05) |
| Freiha (1994) | 28 | >24 months | 4 (0.14) | 0 (0.00) | 0 (0.00) | 0 (0.00) | – | 0 (0.00) |
| Fossa et al. (1994) | 102 | 47 months | 22 (0.22) | 0 (0.00) | 4 (0.04) | 1 (0.01) | VLI | 1 (0.01) |
| Nicolai and Pizzocaro (1995) | 85 | 132 months | 25 (0.29) | 3 (0.04) | 1 (0.01) | 2 (0.02) | Emb, Tstage, scrot viol | 3 (0.04) |
| Tekgul et al. (1995) | 58 | 39 months | 17 (0.29) | 0 (0.00) | 8 (0.14) | 0 (0.00) | None | 0 (0.00) |
| Gels et al. (1995) | 154 | 84 months | 42 (0.27) | 0 (0.00) | 8 (0.05) | 2 (0.01) | VI | 2 (0.01) |
| Boyer et al. (1997) | 77 | 58 months | 27 (0.35) | 2 (0.03) | 3 (0.04) | 3 (0.04) | – | 2 (0.03) |
| Klepp et al. (1997) | 106 | 40 months | 20 (0.19) | 2 (0.02) | 3 (0.03) | NR | VI, low AFP | 0 (0.00) |
| Ondrus et al. (1998) | 49 | 37 months | 7 (0.14) | 0 (0.00) | NR | NR | – | 0 (0.00) |
| Hao et al. (1998) | 76 | 46 months | 28 (0.37) | 2 (0.03) | 6 (0.08) | 2 (0.03) | Emb, VI | 3 (0.04) |
| Sogani et al. (1998) | 105 | 136 months | 27 (0.26) | 0 (0.00) | 2 (0.02) | 0 (0.00) | VI, emb | 3 (0.03) |
| Jones (1999) | 31 | 47 months | 15 (0.48) | 0 (0.00) | 2 (0.06) | 1 (0.03) | – | 0 (0.00) |
| Sharir et al. (1999) | 170 | 76 months | 48 (0.28) | 0 (0.00) | 4 (0.02) | 2 (0.01) | – | 1 (0.01) |

| | | | | | | | | |
|---|---|---|---|---|---|---|---|---|
| Colls et al. (1999) | 248 | 53 months | 70 (0.28) | 1 (0.00) | 17 (0.07) | 3 (0.01) | VLI | 4 (0.02) |
| Francis et al. (2000) | 183 | 70 months | 52 (0.28) | 2 (0.01) | 14 (0.08) | 2 (0.01) | – | 2 (0.01) |
| Alexandre et al. (2001) | 88 | 52 months | 24 (0.27) | 0 (0.00) | 7 (0.08) | 0 (0.00) | VI, mature teratoma | 1 (0.01) |
| Roeleveld (2001) | 90 | 97 months | 23 (0.26) | 3 (0.03) | 1 (0.01) | 2 (0.02) | VI | 1 (0.01) |
| Kakehi et al. (2002) | 39 | 46 months | 11 (0.28) | 3 (0.08) | 4 (0.10) | 0 (0.00) | – | 2 (0.05) |
| Daugaard et al. (2003) | 301 | 60 months | 86 (0.29) | 9 (0.03) | NR | NR | VLI | 0 (0.00) |
| Atsu et al. (2003) | 132 | 38 months | 32 (0.24) | 0 (0.00) | 10 (0.08) | 0 (0.00) | Emb | 1 (0.01) |
| Oliver et al. (2004) | 234 | 84 months | 71 (0.30) | 5 (0.02) | NR | NR | – | 6 (0.03) |
| Total | 3,613 | | 1,025 (0.28) | 55 (0.02) | 133 (0.05) | 20 (0.01) | | 47 (0.01) |

*LI* lymphatic invasion; *LVI* lymphovascular invasion; *Emb* embryonal carcinoma; *Tstage* primary tumor stage; *Undiff* undifferentiated; *NYS* nonyolk sac; *Scrot viol* scrotal violation biopsy or surgery instead of standard inguinal lymphadenectomy suspicion of a nongerm cell tumor might be derived from specific ultrasound features and, in rare cases, special endocrine profiles (like luteinizing hormone depression) (Fig. 10.1). Most of the nongerm cell tumors are sharp round lesions on ultrasound and have a hypoechogenic feature. They are to be differentiated from other peripheral lesions like Tunica albuginea cysts and epidermoid cysts. Biopsy is not recommended for these lesions and open surgery should be performed (Albers et al. 2005). The typical ultrasound feature should direct the surgical strategy to an organ-sparing approach. In some cases, frozen section analysis is able to safely diagnose the nongerm cell lesions (Elert et al. 2002). However, there is no need to strictly use frozen section analysis for diagnosis. After an organ-sparing complete resection of the tumor, paraffin histology is safer and, in the unusual case of a malignant tumor on the final histology, secondary surgery (e.g., orchidectomy) can be performed without any harm for the patient apart from the second surgical intervention. After a nongerm cell testicular tumor has been confirmed in final histology, there is no need to locally treat the remaining testicle. However, there is an ongoing debate on whether staging (and in some cases therapeutic) RPLND should be recommended. About 10% of patients will present with metastatic disease and usually they cannot be cured by surgery, chemotherapy or radiotherapy. With the complete resection of low-volume disease, however, this small cohort of patients usually is cured. Ninety percent of patients, however, do not need this adjuvant surgery. The reported number of patients is yet too small to present prognostic features of metastatic disease one can rely on. Old age, high mitotic activity of the primary tumor, high volume of the primary tumor and vascular invasion are bad prognostic parameters that have been reported. At least these patients should be recommended to undergo RPLND.

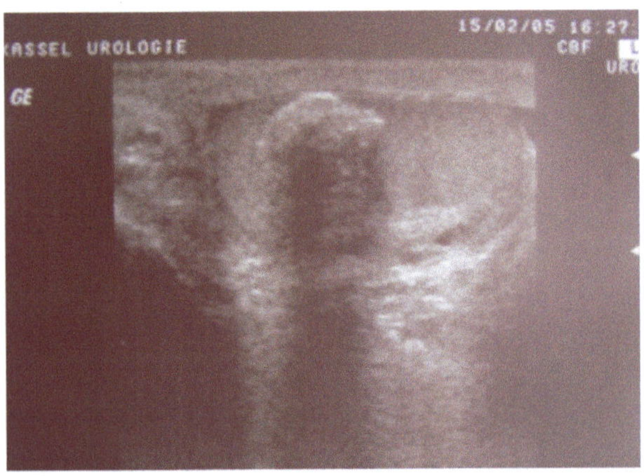


**Fig. 10.1** Testicular ultrasound image of a benign intratesticular lesion

### 10.4.2 Malignant Lesions

Current European guidelines recommend the organ-sparing approach for malignant tumors in solitary testis with certain precautions. The original technique of organ-sparing surgery was published by Weissbach (1995). Using these technical recommendations, the German Testicular Cancer Study Group (GTCSG) published their experience with the technique in more than 70 patients in 2001 (Weissbach 1995; Heidenreich et al. 2001). This experience was updated for the EAU meeting 2006 with 101 patients (Heidenreich et al. 2006). The bottom line of this experience is that organ-sparing surgery in malignant lesions can be recommended in the following situation:

- Solitary testis
- Volume of the lesion < 2 cm (respectively ~30% of the testicular volume) (Fig. 10.1)
- Adjuvant radiotherapy of the remaining testicular parenchyma with 20 Gy
- Normal preoperative serum testosterone values
- Patient and urologist fully informed about risks and benefits as well as the follow-up strategy of the organ-sparing approach
- Surgical experience with the approach

In more than 83% of patients, testosterone production was preserved and local recurrences are rare (4%). Local recurrences are due to the remnant testicular intraepithelial neoplastic (TIN) cells (when no adjuvant radiotherapy was given) or due to teratoma left behind in the remaining parenchyma. Some patients were able to father a child by postponing radiotherapy.

### 10.4.3 TIN in the Remaining Testis

In malignant lesions, the remaining testicular parenchyma always harbors the precursor lesion TIN. These precursor cells of a malignant germ cell tumor need to be treated. In solitary testes, this is usually performed by radiotherapy. However, the time of treatment needs to be discussed. First, the normal testosterone level needs to be confirmed postoperatively (at several occasions, at least 3 months or longer after organ-sparing surgery). Second, the patient has to be aware that radiotherapy will lead to irreversible infertility (Classen et al. 2003). Thus, the patient needs to be informed that treatment may be delayed until all fertility issues have been clarified. Third, even with the reduced dose of 18–20 Gy of testicular radiation, about 30% of patients will develop Leydig cell insufficiency that demands testosterone substitution (Fig. 10.2) (Petersen et al. 2002).

### 10.4.4 Historical Perspectives

Careful anatomic studies at the turn of the century identified lymphatic drainage of the testis with primary drainage for right-sided tumors located in the interaortocaval region and left paraaortic region for left-sided tumors just below the left renal hilum. Crossover does exist more so from the right side to the left side of the aorta. These anatomical studies have provided the basis for regional control after local control by radical orchiectomy. In 90% of the cases, the first presentation of metastatic spread is in the retroperitoneal lymph nodes.

In America, RPLND was established as primary therapy for patients with nonseminomatous germ cell tumors by Lewis (1948). Sentinel work by Kimbrough and Cook fostered the approach of inguinal orchiectomy and RPLND as preferred treatment for patients with clinically localized testis cancer (Kimbrough and Cook 1953). This practice continues in many centers. In Europe, radiation therapy was utilized as the primary therapy for the retroperitoneum. This has given way to the use of initial active surveillance or chemotherapy use a risk adapted approach.

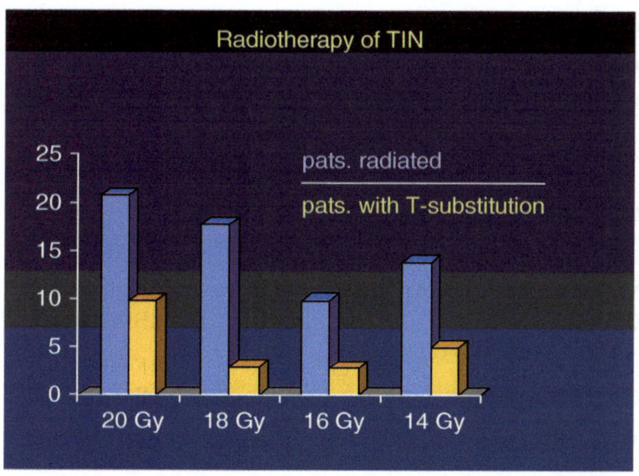


**Fig. 10.2** Long-term follow-up after radiotherapy for testicular intra-epithelial neoplasia (TIN) demonstrating that, of patients receiving scrotal irradiation of 18–20 Gy, a significant % require testosterone substitution (T-substitution) (Petersen 2002)

## 10.5 Treatment Options for NSGCT I

### 10.5.1 Active Surveillance

Active surveillance implies delayed therapy for relapse after orchiectomy. Based on a literature search, relapse occurs in 28% of patients and cause-specific survival is 98% (Groll et al. 2007).

Surveillance involves varying regimens of serial clinical examinations, serologic studies and imaging studies after orchiectomy. Proponents of surveillance emphasize that potentially toxic treatments are avoided in the majority of patients with this approach. Orchidectomy alone followed by a surveillance regimen was first reported by Peckham in 1982 as a management option for stage I NSGCT (Peckham et al. 1982). A combination of concurrent factors served as the impetus for this management strategy. Improved accuracy of clinical staging with CT and tumor markers, a better understanding of prognostic features, and confidence that chemotherapy could offer a reliable salvage therapy for patients who progressed to metastatic disease provided patients and physicians with motivation to adopt surveillance and, at least initially, defer potentially avoidable treatment. In the late 1980s, surveillance strategies were also implemented for stage I seminoma.

When Peckham et al. first abandoned adjuvant radiotherapy in favor of surveillance for NSGCT in 1979, it was estimated that 60–80% of patients would be cured by orchidectomy alone and this prediction has been supported. Early studies reported relapse rates from 27 to 36% and these numbers improved slightly over time as prognostic features were identified and risk-adapted therapy was introduced (Read et al. 1992; Hoskin et al. 1986; Ondrus and Hornak 1994; Peckham and Brada 1987; Sturgeon et al. 1992; Thompson et al. 1988;

Wishnow et al. 1989; Dunphy et al. 1988; Raghavan et al. 1988; Liedke et al. 1990; Rorth et al. 1991). Oliver et al. reported a 36% relapse rate for unselected surveillance patients in the era prior to adjuvant chemotherapy and 27% in those selected based on risk from 1986 onward (Oliver et al. 2004). Studies with the largest cohorts and longest follow-up durations reported relapse rates in a narrower range of 26–30% and a pooled analysis documents 1,025 relapses in 3,613 NSGCT or 28% of surveillance patients (Table 10.1) (Read et al. 1992; Colls et al. 1999; Daugaard et al. 2003; Gels et al. 1995; Sogani et al. 1998; Nicolai and Pizzocaro 1995; Groll et al. 2007; Oliver et al. 2004; Francis et al. 2000; Sharir et al. 1999; Tekgul et al. 1995).

Most relapses are detected simultaneously by more than one modality with abdominal/pelvic CT scan, the predominant sole indicator of disease. One followup regime used by one of the authors in Toronto is shown in Table 10.3 (Sharir et al. 1999). No relapses have been detected with chest X-ray alone in this series. However, Daugaard et al. reported that 4 of 86 relapses in their large series were detected by chest X-ray alone (Daugaard et al. 2003). In the Toronto series, chest radiography was the initial indicator of disease recurrence in 8.3% of patients. Positive serum tumor markers and clinical examination were the sole indicators of progression in 8.3 and 4.2% of relapsing patients, respectively, in the Toronto series (Sharir et al. 1999). In the pooled review, roughly 5% of all NSGCT surveillance patients (and 18% of all relapsing patients) relapse with elevated serum markers as the only sign of disease. This protocol is currently under revision to reduce the number of CT scans.

The proportion of cases reported that demonstrated recurrence only by physical examination of palpable disease is 1% of all patients and 3% of all relapsing patients (Groll et al. 2007). Palpable recurrent disease, albeit rare, typically manifests as supraclavicular or inguinal adenopathy. Inguinal metastases do not represent normal anatomic patterns of lymphatic spread, and often occur after trans-scrotal violation or other surgical disruption of pelvic lymphatics. In a study by Boyer et al., all the three of the documented palpable relapses were detected by patients, all of whom had prior scrotal violation, between scheduled surveillance appointments (Boyer et al. 1997). Several studies document the development of contralateral testis tumors in 1–2% of surveillance patients, but these should be considered separate primary malignancies and not recurrences (Read et al. 1992; Alexandre et al. 2001; Colls et al. 1999; Oliver et al. 2004; Fossa et al. 2005). It should be noted that the site of initial recurrence of NSGCT, the modality detecting recurrence, and the documented time to recurrence may be influenced by the frequency of surveillance investigations.

The majority of NSGCT progression is detected within the first year on surveillance. Late relapse for NSGCT is typically defined as the detection of disease after being free of disease for 2 years following orchidectomy and appears to be uncommon. A pooled analysis identified 55 cases, which was 2% of all surveillance patients from studies that reported late relapse and 6% of all relapses (Groll et al. 2007). The highest late relapse rate was 8% reported by Kakehi in a relatively small series (3 of 39 subjects) (Kakehi et al. 2002). There were only seven reported recurrences after 5 years on surveillance (Colls et al. 1999; Daugaard et al. 2003; Nicolai and Pizzocaro 1995; Rorth et al. 1991). One large study by Daugaard et al. reported four very late relapses ranging from 74 to 171 months post-orchidectomy one of which was seminomatous (Daugaard

**Table 10.3** Surveillance protocol used at Princess Margaret Hospital, Toronto

| | Month 2 | Month 4 | Month 6 | Month 8 | Month 10 | Month 12 |
|---|---|---|---|---|---|---|
| Year 1 | MARKERS CXR | MARKERS CXR CT ABD + pelvis | MARKERS CXR | MARKERS CXR CT ABD + pelvis | MARKERS CXR | MARKERS CXR CT ABD + pelvis |
| Year 2 | MARKERS CXR | MARKERS CXR CT ABD + pelvis | MARKERS CXR | MARKERS CXR CT ABD + pelvis | MARKERS CXR | MARKERS CXR CT ABD + pelvis |
| Year 3 | | MARKERS CXR | | MARKERS CXR | | MARKERS CXR |
| Year 4 | | | MARKERS CXR | | | MARKERS CXR |
| Year 5 | | | | | | MARKERS CXR |

*MARKERS* AFP, hCG, LDH; *CXR* chest X-ray

et al. 2003). In a recent series, 3 of 305 patients relapsed at 28 months, 10 and 12 years with the later two presenting with symptoms (Duran et al. 2007). Despite these rare occurrences, most clinicians seem comfortable with discharging patients from surveillance after five progression-free years.

Patients with clinical stage I NSGCT have an excellent prognosis irrespective of management strategy. The main rationale for surveillance is that salvage therapy is highly successful. Cause-specific survival for clinical stage I NSGCT managed by surveillance is more than 95% in all studies. The overall pooled cause-specific survival is 98.6% (47 deaths of 3,424 patients in papers that reported mortality outcomes) (Groll et al. 2007). While these results reflect effectiveness, surveillance efficacy may, in fact, be underestimated as several authors noted that patients who died of disease were often those who dropped out of surveillance or refused salvage treatment.

In a recent report from Toronto, 305 patients were placed on an active surveillance protocol between 1981 and 2004 (Duran et al. 2007). Importantly, they were not stratified by risk and only received treatment on the event of a relapse. This experience demonstrates the overall natural history of stage I disease without modification by selective treatment. Recurrence rates, time to relapse, risk factors predictive for recurrence, disease specificity and overall survival were determined. For the analysis by time period, patients were divided in to two groups based on diagnosis date. (Initial = 1981–1992 [$n=141$] and recent = 1993–2004 [$n=164$].) With a median follow-up of 6.3 years, 77/305 patients (25%) relapsed; 46/141 patients (32.6%) in the initial group and 31/164 (18.9%) in the recent. This is the lowest overall relapse rate reported for nonrisk-adapted surveillance and may reflect stage migration due to modern imaging. All but 3 (4%) relapses occurred within 2 years after orchiectomy with a median time to relapse of 7 months. A multivariate analysis established lymphovascular invasion ($P<0.01$) and pure embryonal carcinoma ($P=0.03$) as independent predictors of recurrence. Overall, 104/305 (34.1%) patients were designated as "high-risk" based on the presence of one/both of these factors. In the initial group, 60/141 (42.6%) patients were high-risk and 32/60 (53%) relapsed vs. 14/81 (17.3%) low-risk ($P=0.047$). In the recent group, 44/164 (26.8%) patients were high-risk and 17/44 (38.6%) recurred, vs. 14/120 (11.7%) low-risk ($P<0.001$). There were 2 (0.7%) deaths due to testis cancer. The estimated 5-year disease-specific survival was 98.9% in the initial group and 100% in the recent one. The authors concluded that surveillance is an effective strategy for the management of all stage I NSGCT and a risk-adapted policy would result in more than 50% of the patients being unnecessarily treated.

At the present time, risk-adapted surveillance is widely practiced especially for low-risk patients. High-risk patients are generally not managed by surveillance but this may gain popularity if the above Toronto experience is validated by others. The total burden of therapy and the Kollmansberger experience in terms of cycles of chemotherapy, RPLNDs and imaging may well support nonrisk-adapted surveillance for all new stage I patients (Duran et al. 2007).

Intuitively, compliance with a surveillance regimen would seem vital to its success; however, little research has been done to address the issue of compliance and its impact on clinical outcomes of testis cancer surveillance patients. The earliest study that addressed compliance with NSGCT surveillance was a cross-sectional chart review/questionnaire study by Young et al. (1991). Although the sample size was small ($n=25$), chart review demonstrated that surveillance patients were significantly less compliant with follow-up compared to those treated with chemotherapy. None of the surveillance patients were 100% compliant and over half were less than 80% compliant (i.e., attended less than 80% of scheduled investigations or follow-up visits). To attempt to explain compliance patterns, a questionnaire was subsequently administered to both surveillance and chemotherapy stage I NSGCT patients addressing perceptions of illness severity, susceptibility to relapse and the benefits and difficulties of follow-up. Surveillance patients generally found it difficult to attend follow-up visits and considered their disease less dangerous than chemotherapy patients. Fossa et al. note that administrative problems at their institution such as excessive staff workload and breakdown of CT scanners likely account for the fact that 27 of 80 (34%) recurrence-free NSGCT surveillance patients had fewer than the four recommended CT scans during the first year (Fossa et al. 1994). Despite this, a policy of immediately tracing and contacting patients who miss surveillance visits has led to the authors' impression that noncompliance has not been a major problem, especially during the first year.

Hao et al. conducted a chart-review assessing NSGCT patient compliance with surveillance, potential predictors of compliance and the impact of compliance on clinical outcomes such as relapse and mortality (Hao et al. 1998). Based on perceived clinical relevance, the authors defined noncompliance a priori as missing two or more consecutive clinic visits, tumor marker measurements or chest X-rays, or missing one or more CT scans at any time during the first 2 years of surveillance. Overall, compliance in this cohort was deemed poor. Compliance with clinical evaluations was 62% in year one and 36% in year two, and compliance with CT scanning was 25 and 12% in years one and two, respectively. The authors attribute the disturbing CT noncompliance rate to the need for preparation the night before and the fact that a separate trip to the hospital was required. The most common reason was unspecified scheduling conflicts, but other explanations in decreasing frequency include discretionary changes by physician, work or school, travel or moving, transportation difficulties, dissatisfaction with surveillance, wedding, and fear of attendance. The only statistically significant predictor of noncompliance by univariate analysis was diagnosis before 1990. There was no statistically significant difference in relapse rates between compliant and noncompliant patients and the small number of deaths in this cohort did not permit a meaningful analysis of the impact of compliance on mortality. Ernst et al. recently published a retrospective report on NSGCT surveillance compliance at seven Canadian treatment centers using the very rigid definition of compliance previously defined by Hao et al. (Ernst et al. 2005). The compliance rate for clinical visits ranged from 68 to 94% (median 79%) and the compliance for CT scanning ranged from 32 to 100% (median 64%). The same center reported the highest rate of clinical and CT appointment compliance and this center's protocol had the lowest frequency of follow-up and investigations. The overall disease-free survival across all the centers in this study was 100% and compliance rates were not significantly correlated with rates of relapse.

Studies addressing compliance are inherently limited by selection bias, both at the level of treatment decision making and study recruitment. Anticipated compliance based on personality, psychological profile and geographical proximity to treatment center is often a criterion for bringing patients into a surveillance program (Sogani et al. 1998). Furthermore, patients that consent to studies that measure compliance by self-report or questionnaire are probably more compliant with follow-up. It is important to recognize that these phenomena would result in an overestimation of compliance if any differential effect is observed.

### 10.5.2 Primary Retroperitoneal Lymphadenectomy

In the United States, surgical removal of retroperitoneal lymph nodes has been the mainstay of treatment for clinical low-stage testicular cancer. Chemotherapy has been reserved as an adjunct. RPLND is an important staging as well as a therapeutic procedure for patients with nonseminomatous germ cell tumors. With a meticulous RPLND, cure rate for patients with stage I or low-stage II testis cancer is exceedingly high. Even before adjunctive radiation therapy or chemotherapy, Staubitz demonstrated a 5-year survival of 75% for clinical stage I and stage II patients with RPLND alone (Staubitz 1970). Therefore, removal of retroperitoneal lymph nodes can be therapeutic as well as diagnostic.

RPLND can be therapeutic because retroperitoneal lymph node involvement is usually the first and often the only evidence of spread outside the testis. Testicular cancer is one of the few malignancies in which removal of involved regional lymph nodes can result in a high cure rate. Cure rate for patients with pathologically confined stage I disease approaches 93–95% with surgery alone. Patients who relapse generally do so with pulmonary metastasis or marker elevation.

RPLND via a transabdominal approach is generally a 2–3 h operation with limited morbidity. The mortality rate is less than 1%. Morbidity is usually related to pulmonary problems, ileus, lymphocele, or pancreatic inflammation.

The classic RPLND involved extensive dissection of retroperitoneal lymph nodes. Although the cure rate was high, patients experienced loss of ejaculatory function and fertility. With better elucidation about the distribution of nodal metastases, as well as the neuroanatomy of the retroperitoneal sympathetic chain, modifications in surgical technique have allowed preservation of ejaculatory function. Ejaculation is mediated by postganglionic sympathetic fibers emerging from the sympathetic chain at L-2 to L-5. These postganglionic fibers cross posterior to the vena cava but anterior to the aorta crossing over the aortic bifurcation. Based upon the patterns of nodal spread reported by Donohue et al. in pathologic stage II patients, template methods to avoid damage to the contralateral postganglionic sympathetic nerves for ejaculation below the level of the inferior mesenteric artery have been advocated and successfully utilized (Donohue et al. 1982). Jewett and Donohue have described nerve-sparing techniques resulting in the preservation of ejaculation in virtually 100% of patients (Jewett et al. 1988; Donohue et al. 1990).

Even for patients with high-risk disease (high percentage of embryonal carcinoma with or without lymphovascular invasion), RPLND alone results in long-term cure rates of 70–75% without the need for adjunctive chemotherapy.

Primary retroperitoneal lymphadenectomy for stage I NSGCT is the gold standard nodal staging technique and a therapeutic procedure. Approximately, one-quarter of patients are upstaged from surgical pathology. RPLND has evolved in efforts to minimize the morbidity of the procedure without compromising completeness of cancer resection and therapeutic benefit. Currently, most consider a "nerve-sparing" technique to be mandatory to curtail the risk of damaging sympathetic nerves responsible for seminal emission and ejaculatory function, a problematic surgical complication historically. With the practice of nerve-sparing RPLND, long-term reported antegrade ejaculation rates range from 95 to 100% in the face of minimal retroperitoneal disease recurrence and essentially zero mortality (Albers et al. 2003; Jewett et al. 1988; de Bruin et al. 1993; Donohue and Foster 1998; Jewett 1990). Other potential complications from RPLND include general surgical complications such as wound infection, ileus and pulmonary embolism, and procedure-specific complications such as lymphocele, chylous ascites, and hydronephrosis (Albers et al. 2003). In a recent series of 75 patients having undergone primary RPLND at Indiana University, the morbidity of surgery was assessed with a mean blood loss of about 200 cc, no short-term complications and a mean hospital stay of 2.8 days as a reference for competing surgical procedures such as laparoscopic RPLND (Beck 2007).

### 10.5.3 Adjuvant Chemotherapy

To date, the best prognostic model for patients with clinical stage I NSGCT indicates an approximate 64% of relapse. It is generally accepted to treat these patients as high-risk for metastatic disease. Importantly, 36% of this cohort will not harbor disease. In the United States, therefore, these patients are offered RPLND to better determine pathological stage. In most European countries, these patients are recommended to get adjuvant chemotherapy.

Thus, adjuvant chemotherapy with two cycles of bleomycin, etoposide and cisplatin (BEP) is usually reserved for stage I NSGCT with "high-risk" features such as vascular invasion, or if conditions against surveillance exist. With chemotherapy, 95–97% of patients remain free of relapse and the overall cure rate approaches 100%. There are, however, concerns of chemo-resistance in patients who relapse after receiving adjuvant chemotherapy rendering them difficult to cure.

The Austrian group was one of the first who started adjuvant treatment of high-risk patients (based on vascular invasion) with two cycles of cisplatin, etoposide, and bleomycin (PEB) in a controlled, prospective trial in 1985. In 1996, they reported on 42 patients with two relapses and one patient who had died of disease (Pont et al. 1996). In the same year, the MRC published their experience with 114 patients at high risk, 93 had been followed for more than 2 years (Cullen et al. 1996a). Two of 114 patients had a relapse (1.8%) and one patient had died of disease. Klepp et al. (1997), Ondrus et al. (1998), Hendry et al. (2000), and Böhlen et al. (2001) confirmed these data with 32, 18, 60, and 59 high-risk patients, respectively. However, some of them used three cycles of PEB for the adjuvant treatment of the high-risk group. Remarkably, in most of these series single deaths have occurred in patients with clinical stage I disease. The MD Anderson experience was finally published in 2004 with 99 patients at high risk (vascular invasion or >80% embryonal carcinoma or AFP >80 ng/dL) (Amato et al. 2004). These patients got two cycles of carboplatin, etoposide, and bleomycin on an outpatient basis and none of them experienced relapse. Comparable results have recently been published by Chevreau et al. who treated a total of 40 patients with either vascular invasion or the presence of embryonal carcinoma in the primary tumor (Chevreau et al. 2004). After two cycles of cisplatin, vinblastin, and bleomycin or PEB, no relapse was seen after an extended follow-up of nearly 10 years. In summary, adjuvant chemotherapy with two cycles of PEB in the group of patients with vascular invasion provides a long-term progression-free survival of at least 97% (Cullen et al. 1996a) The German and Swedish experience with one cycle of BEP is excellent as well with reduced morbidity (Albers et al. 2006 and Jewett et al.).

#### 10.5.3.1 Toxicity of Adjuvant Chemotherapy

Since more than 50% of patients with vascular invasion as the only risk factor for high-risk are still overtreated by this risk-adapted approach, long-term toxicity assessment is crucial. There is a considerably high rate of unfavorable changes in blood pressure and body mass index which consecutively results in a twofold increased risk of cardiovascular disease in patients after chemotherapy for testis cancer (Huddart et al. 2003; Sagstuen et al. 2005). Unfortunately, only a few studies of two cycles of adjuvant chemotherapy evaluated long-term toxicities. Reports on the rate of nephrotoxicity, neurotoxicity, vascular toxicity, and high serum triglyceride levels do not differentiate between different dosages of chemotherapy (Boyer and Raghavan 1992; Bokemeyer et al. 1996; Meinardi et al. 2000; Nuver et al. 2005). Thus, valid conclusions on the impact of long-term toxicity of adjuvant chemotherapy cannot be drawn.

Secondary leukemia is a typical risk of high-dose etoposide treatment (Kollmannsberger et al. 1998). The development of other secondary cancers after long-term survival after testis cancer treatment has intensively been studied and suggests an increased probability of various secondary malignancies with radiotherapy and chemotherapy (Travis et al. 1997, 2005; Bokemeyer and Schmoll 1993). Especially, patients with both treatments have a relative risk of 2.9 to develop solid malignancies like mesothelioma, cancers of the esophagus, lung, colon, bladder, and pancreas with no difference between seminoma and nonseminoma patients. The cumulative risk for a 35-year-old patient treated with radiotherapy and chemotherapy to develop a solid tumor 40 years later is 36% compared to controls (23%). Again, no long-term data are available for the group of patients with only two cycles of PEB. Fertility was assessed in the studies of Cullen et al. (1996a), Pont et al. (1990), and Böhlen et al. (2001). However, semen analysis was only available in a minority of patients before and after treatment. Only 24 of 114 patients in the study of Cullen et al., 18 of 42 patients in the study of Pont et al., and 27 of 59 patients in the study of Böhlen et al. had post-chemotherapy semen analysis. Hence, the conclusion of these series that adjuvant chemotherapy has no effect on long-term fertility is based on only a few cases. In a recent report from Norway, Brydoy et al. report on 1,814 men followed up for paternity with different kinds of testicular cancer treatment. Patients with surveillance achieved a paternity rate of up to 92%. Even in patients who had undergone high-dose chemotherapy treatment, paternity was achieved in 48% (Rorth et al. 1991). As long as no long-term data on fertility after adjuvant BEP chemotherapy are available, cryoconservation before chemotherapy is recommended (Magelssen et al. 2005).

In summary, long-term studies in patients with advanced disease have indicated that there is some long-term toxicity of chemotherapy. Extrapolation of these data suggests no significant long-term toxicities of two cycles of PEB. But there is lack of long-term data in the group of patients with adjuvant treatment. This demands a long-term follow-up of these patients.

In order to reduce toxicity, Oliver et al. started to reduce adjuvant treatment to one single cycle of PEB chemotherapy (Oliver et al. 1992). This approach was published by Corti Ortiz et al. with 18 patients and a median follow-up of 47 months and Schefer et al. with 42 patients and a median follow-up of more than 24 months for 31 of them (Corti Ortíz et al. 1997; Schefer et al. 2000). The Swiss group experienced one relapse and the patient unfortunately died because of salvage treatment.

The German Testicular Study Group randomized 382 nonrisk-adapted patients to either RPLND or one course of adjuvant PEB chemotherapy (Albers et al. 2006). Adjuvant PEB could significantly reduce the recurrence rate to 1.1% as opposed to 7.5% using RPLND and adjuvant chemotherapy in cases of pathological stage II. Adjuvant chemotherapy with only one course of BEP, therefore, is active and more efficacious in the reduction of recurrence rates than surgery and represents a less toxic adjuvant treatment as compared to two cycles of BEP.

Future studies should concentrate on the reduction of treatment for the high-risk group and a better staging, e.g., by molecular parameters in order to avoid toxicity for those who do not need treatment.

## 10.6 Practice Pattern and Management Preferences

When several management options with comparable outcomes are available for a given disease, management preferences and physician practice patterns will likely be influenced by a variety of interrelated factors. There have been few reports that address these issues. Cullen et al. investigated preferences among NSGCT patients, oncologists and controls (Cullen et al. 1996b). Aware of equivalent mortality outcomes, management preferences of stage I NSGCT between surveillance, adjuvant chemotherapy and deference of decision making to a physician at various hypothetical recurrence risk thresholds were assessed. Trends of management preference by recurrence risk level, the upper limit of recurrence risk for which surveillance was chosen ("surveillance limit"), the lower limit of recurrence risk for which chemotherapy was chosen ("chemotherapy limit"), and the range of risk level between which deference to a physician is preferred ("uncertainty range") were reported comparatively between groups. There was wide variability of management preference and corresponding risk thresholds both within and across groups. Patients, who had remained disease-free on surveillance, reported both the highest median surveillance limit (40% recurrence risk) and the highest chemotherapy limit (70% recurrence risk), demonstrating a preference for surveillance even with high hypothetical risk of relapse. Interestingly, the median surveillance limit was the lowest (10% recurrence risk) for patients who had progressed on a surveillance regimen. Stiggelbout et al. designed a decision analysis to assess the relapse rate at which adjuvant chemotherapy would be preferred by both patients and clinicians (Stiggelbout et al. 1996). Probabilities of various outcomes and utilities of potential disease states were incorporated into the decision tree and the maximum quality-adjusted life expectancy (QALE) determined the preferred management. Surveillance was preferred over chemotherapy by patients in the baseline quality-adjusted analysis although QALEs for surveillance and chemotherapy were not drastically different. Preference shifted from surveillance to chemotherapy at a relapse rate of 51%. Some discordance was demonstrated between patient and clinician utilities and preferences. Clinicians also preferred surveillance to chemotherapy and had a higher threshold for chemotherapy, shifting preference at a relapse rate of 74%. The findings in these studies shed light on the subjective influence of prognostic statistics on patient treatment preferences and indicate that for stage I NSGCT optimal management may be highly individualized (Fig. 10.3).

### 10.6.1 Impact on Sex and Fertility

There has been abundant research on the morbidity of adjuvant treatment for testicular cancer with respect to sexual function and fertility. The effect of chemotherapy on fertility remains poorly understood. Relatively few studies, however, have addressed the impact of orchidectomy alone and surveillance on sex and fertility. Blackmore conducted a cross-sectional questionnaire study comparing three groups with respect to body image, sexual drive and sexual satisfaction (Blackmore 1988). No statistically significant differences were noted between testis cancer patients

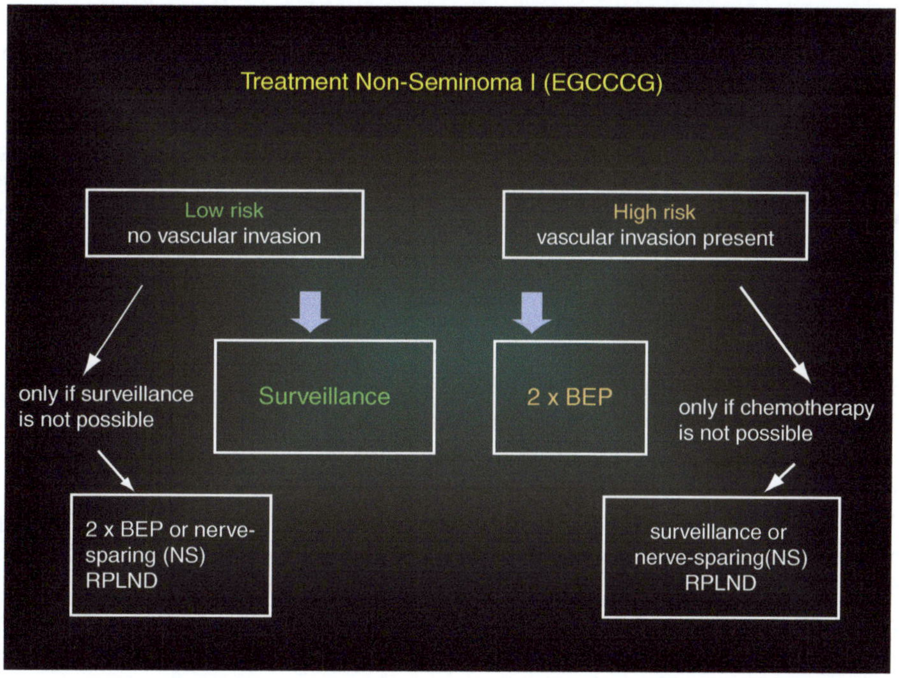


**Fig. 10.3** Algorithm of treatment of clinical stage I nonseminoma as recommended by the first European Germ Cell Cancer Consensus Group (Schmoll et al. 2004)

following unilateral orchidectomy and surveillance individuals who had previous orchidectomy for other reasons and controls. This study was the first identified to address this topic; however, it suffered from selection and response bias in addition to a relatively small sample size. Another cross-sectional study used self-administered questionnaires to compare sexuality and fertility between testicular cancer survivors grouped by treatment modality (combination RPLND and chemotherapy, chemotherapy alone, radiotherapy and surveillance) (Arai et al. 1997). The only statistically significant differences related to ejaculatory function and semen volume which were predictably lower in the RPLND group. Interestingly, sexual drive, erectile function, and sexual satisfaction were no better in the surveillance group compared to those who underwent more toxic therapies. Roughly, 20% of surveillance patients reported some loss of sexual drive and one-third felt that erectile potential and orgasm intensity was reduced even several years after orchidectomy. Although not statistically significant, there was a trend towards a greater sense of decreased attractiveness and more desire for testicular prosthesis in the surveillance group. Jonker-Pool et al. conducted a cross-sectional questionnaire study evaluating sexual function of testicular cancer survivors by treatment modality and found that those on surveillance reported less decrease in sexual function and activity compared to other treatments (Jonker-Pool et al. 1997). Almost one-quarter of surveillance patients, however, did report some degree of sexual dysfunction which appears to be higher than the general age-matched population, although a direct comparison was not made. It is concluded that clinicians should not discount the fact that patients on active surveillance may experience significant sexual side effects from orchidectomy alone, which may in part be mediated by psychological factors.

Jonker-Pool et al. also recently assessed informational and supportive needs regarding sexuality, comparing testicular cancer patients to malignant lymphoma patients (Jonker-Pool et al. 2004). An existing questionnaire was adapted to assess patients' evaluation of both retrospective sexual information and support in addition to current informational and supportive needs. Although reported sexual dysfunction was similar in both groups, testicular cancer survivors were less satisfied with information and support concerning sexuality compared to survivors of lymphoma. Over half of testicular cancer patients surveyed felt in retrospect that both information and support regarding sexual issues offered at the time of treatment was insufficient and roughly two-thirds of these individuals report a current need for information concerning sexuality several years later. Testicular cancer patients managed on surveillance reported similar dissatisfaction with information and support received compared to those undergoing treatment, except for the fact that radiotherapy patients recalled support during treatment as more sufficient and that patients who received both chemotherapy and RPLND expressed a higher current need for support. The authors discuss the merits of inviting testicular cancer patients to discuss their concerns regarding sexuality regardless of stage of disease or management strategy and that further research is warranted to learn how to offer information and support to patients not only in sufficient amounts but "in the right way."

While chemotherapy and retroperitoneal surgery may have direct physiologic effects that impact sexual function and potentially fertility, the impact of losing a testicle and psychological issues associated with long-term surveillance should be appreciated as potential problems for the testicular cancer surveillance population. A large comparative study looking at paternity rates in testicular cancer survivors stratified by treatment type found the highest conception rates in the surveillance group (81%) and the lowest in the high-dose chemotherapy group (38%) with low-dose chemotherapy and post-radiotherapy rates in-between (62 and 65%, respectively). Conception rates post-RPLND approached surveillance rates (77%) and are likely underestimated as the data included cases prior to the adoption of nerve-sparing techniques (Jonker-Pool et al. 2004). It should also be recognized that there is an increased incidence of testicular cancer in men presenting with infertility and abnormal semen analysis (Raman et al. 2005) and that the pretreatment semen quality (concentration, motility, and morphology) is impaired in a significant proportion of testicular cancer patients (Bussen et al. 2004).

### 10.6.2 Quality of Life and Psychosocial Issues

It can be argued that in simple terms quality of life and mental well-being are the most important outcomes in any illness. That being said, they are outcomes that are less straightforward to reliably measure than outcomes such as relapse, fertility and mortality. Testicular cancer typically affects young men who are at a stage in their lives when relationships, family, education and work are of peak importance or uncertainty. The impact of testicular cancer and its management on quality of life and psychosocial welfare at various stages of illness is important to understand, and several investigators have contributed to knowledge on this topic.

Moynihan used mixed quantitative and qualitative methods to determine the prevalence of psychosocial morbidity in testis cancer patients and their relatives several years after diagnosis, and to compare psychological outcomes by treatment regimen (Moynihan 1987). A relatively high prevalence of psychological morbidity, especially anxiety, was demonstrated among testicular cancer patients compared to population findings from community studies. Health worries, fear of relapse, and employment and financial difficulties were factors relating to psychological morbidity. Treatment modality was not significant in predicting psychological problems by univariate analysis. The majority of survivors reported that they continued to be unreasonably prone to attribute any new symptom to cancer recurrence despite recognizing their good prognosis. This phenomenon was equally experienced by patients in all the treatment groups. Other "worry areas" identified were fear of death, testicular loss, treatment procedures, infertility and no treatment. Certain worries were experienced to different degrees based on the stage of illness. Fear of death and testicular loss decreased significantly from the time of diagnosis to the time of interview, while fear of relapse increased from diagnosis to interview. The perception of emotional support during diagnosis and treatment was conveyed by 92% of patients. Significantly, less felt that they had equivalent support at the time of interview and over 60% of men interviewed would have liked formal counseling. In another mixed methods study, it was found that although no relationship existed between perceived social support and mood, testicular cancer patients, including those on surveillance, felt they would benefit from contact with another individual who had gone through a similar experience (Ord-Lawson and Fitch 1997). The findings of Moynihan's research indicate that the psychological impact of surveillance is somewhat ambiguous. On one hand, having this option is an indication and confirmation of a very good prognosis. On the other hand, uncertainty and fear with respect to recurrence and the perception that more aggressive upfront therapy would have provided more psychological closure are apparent concerns of surveillance patients, even several years after diagnosis.

Arai et al. conducted a cross-sectional survey of long-term survivors of testicular cancer comparing psychosocial well-being and quality of life across treatment modalities (Arai et al. 1996). Surveillance patients reported significantly more sleep disturbance, less ability to work and less overall satisfaction with life than patients who had received radiotherapy or chemotherapy. Limitations of this study include a small sample size (seven surveillance patients), and some baseline differences between groups, such as age, stage and prognosis at diagnosis. It is conceivable that perspective and outlook on life is different for those patients who have overcome higher-risk illness and may be more appreciative of cure. In spite of its limitations, this study sheds light on the potential adverse psychosocial impact of surveillance and corroborates Moynihan's evidence that aggressive treatment may in itself have a therapeutic effect (Moynihan 1987).

A study by Fossa et al. identified and prioritized issues of psychological and physical morbidity in long-term testicular cancer survivors (Fossa et al. 1996). Overall, results demonstrated that overall long-term morbidity was relatively low and did not differ based on management. Furthermore, physicians' perceptions of morbidity in this population were compared to those of patients. The findings highlighted the important realization that discordance exists between patients' and doctors' perception of quality of life. Overall satisfaction with treatment and health care provision was of utmost importance to patients' quality of life but was not sufficiently appreciated by doctors. In general, physicians tended to underestimate long-term somatic symptoms and overestimate psychological sequelae in testicular cancer survivors. Discrepancies between doctors' and patients' perceptions were most abundant with respect to the surveillance population.

Health-related quality of life in long-term testicular cancer survivors was examined by Rudberg using validated survey instruments (Rudberg et al. 2000). The participants included survivors who were managed by various treatments at various stages; however, 22 of the 277 respondents (8%) had been managed by surveillance alone. Overall, testicular cancer survivors rated equivalent or better than age-matched healthy controls in terms of quality of life. In this sample, surveillance patients scored significantly higher on health-related quality of life measures than those who received more aggressive therapy. In another case-control study by Joly et al., validated quality of life questionnaires yielded statistically similar results overall for long-term testicular cancer survivors and age-matched controls (Joly et al. 2002). Seventy-one cases included seven NSGCT surveillance patients and no significant differences in quality of life domains existed according to treatment type. Cases did report significantly lower sexual satisfaction and performance than controls, but it should be noted that the majority of NSGCT patients were treated with chemotherapy, RPLND or both, and there were no seminoma patients in the study managed with surveillance. Fossa demonstrated in a comparative study that long-term testicular cancer survivors have higher rates of anxiety and chronic fatigue than the general population but lower rates compared to survivors of Hodgkin's disease (Fossa et al. 2003). Ten percent of cases in this study were surveillance patients, and treatment type was not a significant predictor of anxiety or chronic fatigue. A direct comparison of health-related quality of life of testicular cancer patients according to treatment modality was made by Miyake et al. (2004). The previously validated SF-36 questionnaire was administered to patients who had undergone chemotherapy, RPLND or surveillance for testicular cancer, all of whom had been disease-free for at least 6 months. Overall, all the groups achieved satisfactory health-related quality of life scores with no significant differences in the type of management.

Because of the young age of onset and excellent cure rates, testicular cancer patients epitomize the "long-term survivor." This implores understanding on the part of health care providers of psychosocial issues and quality of life in this population. Up to this point, these issues have been addressed primarily in the allied health literature. Given the multidisciplinary nature of testicular cancer care, more research is warranted to provide further understanding of the psychological impact of the disease and health-related determinants of quality of life so that management and support may be tailored accordingly.

### 10.6.3 Cost Analysis

With comparable excellent survival outcomes for all the accepted management strategies, relative costs are important. Cost analyses, however, are fraught with assumptions and questionable generalizability, given the variable health economics and policies that govern different institutions and regions. Munro and Warde designed a Markov decision process to assess the cost-effectiveness of a variety of existing and hypothetical surveillance protocols for stage I NSGCT (Munro and Warde 1991). Their model demonstrates no significant differences in surveillance policy effectiveness, but wide variability in costs. The authors acknowledge several limitations of their analysis such as the restriction to the detection of abdominal recurrence, the assumption that each patient could only have one relapse and the fact that 100% patient compliance was assumed.

A sophisticated cost- and risk-benefit analysis comparing primary nerve-sparing RPLND and surveillance for clinical stage I NSGCT was reported by Baniel et al. (1996). Cumulative costs based on the actual local charges were calculated for 100 hypothetical patients in each treatment arm using anticipated outcomes from institutional data and literature. The costs of surgery and surveillance over a 5-year period were determined to be equal so that cost was not important for treatment decision making. Overall, RPLND demonstrated superiority in terms of fertility, toxicity and late relapse although it is noted that the authors incorporated a relatively high relapse rate (34%) into their nonrisk-adapted surveillance algorithm. In a subsequent review paper from the same institution, it was estimated that the cumulative charges incurred from a 5-year surveillance policy would not compare favorably with RPLND for clinical stage I NSGCT; however, the charges of treatment for recurrence following either management strategy were not considered (Koch 1998). Lashley and Lowe demonstrated a financial advantage to surveillance for stage I NSGCT compared to primary RPLND or adjuvant chemotherapy, especially when surveillance was selected for low-risk patients based on prognostic features (Lashley and Lowe 1998).

More recently, Link et al. published results of a detailed mathematical decision analysis model developed to compare costs of management for stage I NSGCT (Link et al. 2005). This decision tree model, based on a meta-analysis of the literature and incorporating an exhaustive list of variables and potential clinical outcomes, was developed to account for the limitations of previous cost analyses such as a lack of generalizability and the absence of laparoscopic RPLND as a treatment option. The authors aimed to derive a model that could be used to test hypotheses with sensitivity analysis and impact clinical decision making. Surveillance was the least costly option by this model, followed by adjuvant chemotherapy, laparoscopic RPLND and open RPLND, in the increasing order of cost premiums. Specifically, RPLND was 1.6 times more costly than surveillance. Furthermore, a one-way sensitivity analysis varying the probability of disease recurrence demonstrated that surveillance maintains superior cost-effectiveness until the probability of retroperitoneal recurrence was >60% (more than 2 times actual relapse rates).

Francis et al. appended a cost-benefit analysis to their outcomes paper on the management of stage I testicular germ cell tumors (Francis et al. 2000). Their analysis combined both seminoma and NSGCT and consisted of a crude summation of components of various treatment modalities over a 10-year period. While surveillance was somewhat more costly than adjuvant chemotherapy for NSGCT and adjuvant radiotherapy for seminoma, the authors hypothesized that it may be the most cost-effective strategy. Nerve-sparing RPLND and associated follow-up was the most expensive treatment modality with the investigators hypothetically halving the number of clinic visits and chest X-rays but retaining the same number of markers and CT scans as in active surveillance. This policy deviates from other reports that suggest that CT scanning may be performed less frequently following primary RPLND (Baniel et al. 1996; Koch 1998). The MRC Testis Group have recently demonstrated that the number of CT scans used in stage I NSGCT can be safely reduced from five to two, which may impact cost of management (Mead et al. 2006).

Economic analyses have produced conflicting results with respect to costs of different treatment modalities for both stage I seminoma and NSGCT. The discrepancies appear to be institution-dependent and may reflect varying protocols, a lack of standardized practice patterns, and differing assumptions made in constructing hypothetical models. The one consistency observed, which seems intuitive, is that adjuvant treatments, especially surgical, bear more up-front costs whereas surveillance costs accumulate gradually over time. Overall, there is no compelling evidence that surveillance is more expensive than other treatment options for stage I testis cancer.

## References


Albers PP, Bender HH, Yilmaz HH, Schoeneich GG, Biersack HHJ, Mueller SSC (1999) Positron emission tomography in the clinical staging of patients with Stage I and II testicular germ cell tumors. Urology 53(4):808–811

Albers P, Siener R, Kliesch S, Weissbach L, Krege S, Sparwasser C et al (2003) Risk factors for relapse in clinical stage I nonseminomatous testicular germ cell tumors: results of the German Testicular Cancer Study Group trial. J Clin Oncol 21(8):1505–1512

Albers P, Albrecht W, Algaba F, Bokemeyer C, Cohn-Cedermark G, Horwich A, Klepp O, Laguna MP, Pizzocaro G. Eur Urol. 2005 Dec;48(6):885–94. Epub 2005 Jul 18. Review.

Albers P, Siener R, Krege S, Schemelz H, Dieckmann K, Heidenreich A et al (2006) One course of adjuvant PEB chemotherapy versus retroperitoneal lymph node dissection in patients with stage I non-seminomatous germ-cell tumors (NSGCT). Results of the German prospective multicenter trial (Association of Urological Oncology[AUO]/German testicular cancer study group [GTCSG] trial 01-94). J Clin Oncol 24:220S

Alexandre J, Fizazi K, Mahe C, Culine S, Droz JP, Theodore C et al (2001) Stage I non-seminomatous germ-cell tumours of the testis: identification of a subgroup of patients with a very low risk of relapse. Eur J Cancer 37(5):576–582

Amato RJ, Ro JY, Ayala AG, Swanson DA (2004) Risk-adapted treatment for patients with clinical stage I nonseminomatous germ cell tumor of the testis. Urology 63(1):144–148; discussion 48–49

Arai Y, Kawakita M, Hida S, Terachi T, Okada Y, Yoshida O (1996) Psychosocial aspects in long-term survivors of testicular cancer. J Urol 155(2):574–578

Arai Y, Kawakita M, Okada Y, Yoshida O (1997) Sexuality and fertility in long-term survivors of testicular cancer. J Clin Oncol 15(4):1444–1448

Atsu N, Eskicorapci S, Uner A, Ekici S, Gungen Y, Erkan I et al (2003) A novel surveillance protocol for stage I nonseminomatous germ cell testicular tumours. BJU Int 92(1):32–35

Baniel J, Roth BJ, Foster RS, Donohue JP (1996) Cost- and risk-benefit considerations in the management of clinical stage I nonseminomatous testicular tumors. Ann Surg Oncol 3(1):86–93

Beck SD, Peterson MD, Bihrle R, Donohue JP, Foster RS. J Urol. 2007 Aug;178(2):504-6; discussion 506. Epub 2007 Jun 11

Blackmore C (1988) The impact of orchidectomy upon the sexuality of the man with testicular cancer. Cancer Nurs 11(1):33–40

Böhlen DD, Burkhard FFC, Mills RR, Sonntag RRW, Studer UUE (2001) Fertility and sexual function following orchiectomy and 2 cycles of chemotherapy for stage I high risk nonseminomatous germ cell cancer. J Urol 165(2):441–444

Bokemeyer CC, Schmoll HHJ (1993) Secondary neoplasms following treatment of malignant germ cell tumors. J Clin Oncol 11(9):1703–1709

Bokemeyer CC, Berger CCC, Kuczyk MMA, Schmoll HHJ (1996) Evaluation of long-term toxicity after chemotherapy for testicular cancer. J Clin Oncol 14(11):2923–2932

Boyer MM, Raghavan DD (1992) Toxicity of treatment of germ cell tumors. Semin Oncol 19(2):128–142

Boyer MJ, Cox K, Tattersall MH, Findlay MP, Grygiel J, Rogers J (1997) Active surveillance after orchiectomy for nonseminomatous testicular germ cell tumors: late relapse may occur. Urology 50(4):588–592

Bussen S, Sutterlin M, Steck T, Dietl J (2004) Semen parameters in patients with unilateral testicular cancer compared to patients with other malignancies

Chevreau CC, Mazerolles CC, Soulié MM, Gaspard MHM-H, Mourey LL, Bujan LL et al (2004) Long-term efficacy of two cycles of BEP regimen in high-risk stage I nonseminomatous testicular germ cell tumors with embryonal carcinoma and/or vascular invasion. Eur Urol 46(2):209–214; discussion 14

Classen JJ, Dieckmann KK, Bamberg MM, Souchon RR, Kliesch SS, Kuehn MM et al (2003) Radiotherapy with 16 Gy may fail to eradicate testicular intraepithelial neoplasia: preliminary communication of a dose-reduction trial of the German Testicular Cancer Study Group. Br J Cancer 88(6):828–831

Colls BM, Harvey VJ, Skelton L, Frampton CM, Thompson PI, Bennett M et al (1999) Late results of surveillance of clinical stage I nonseminoma germ cell testicular tumours: 17 years' experience in a national study in New Zealand. Br J Urol Int 83(1):76–82

Corti Ortíz DD, Fonerón Burgos AA, Troncoso Schifferli LL (1997) Treatment of stage I nonseminomatous testicular cancer with one cycle of adjuvant chemotherapy. Actas Urol Esp 21(10):961–963

Cullen MH, Stenning SP, Parkinson MC, Fossa SD, Kaye SB, Horwich AH et al (1996a) Short-course adjuvant chemotherapy in high-risk stage I nonseminomatous germ cell tumors of the testis: a Medical Research Council report. J Clin Oncol 14(4):1106–1113

Cullen MH, Billingham LJ, Cook J, Woodroffe CM (1996b) Management preferences in stage I non-seminomatous germ cell tumours of the testis: an investigation among patients, controls and oncologists. Br J Cancer 74(9):1487–1491

Daugaard G, Petersen PM, Rorth M (2003) Surveillance in stage I testicular cancer. APMIS 111(1):76–83

de Bruin MJ, Oosterhof GO, Debruyne FM (1993) Nerve-sparing retroperitoneal lymphadenectomy for low stage testicular cancer. Br J Urol 71(3):336–339

Dieckmann KKP, Loy VV (1996) Prevalence of contralateral testicular intraepithelial neoplasia in patients with testicular germ cell neoplasms. J Clin Oncol 14(12):3126–3132

Donohue JP, Foster RS (1998) Retroperitoneal lymphadenectomy in staging and treatment. The development of nerve-sparing techniques. Urol Clin North Am 25(3):461–468

Donohue JP, Maynard B, Zachary M (1982) The distribution of nodal metastases in the retroperitoneum from nonseminomatous testis cancer. J Urol 128:315–320

Donohue JP, Foster RS, Rowland RG, Bihrle R, Jones J, Geier G (1990) Nerve-sparing retroperitoneal lymphadenectomy with preservation of ejaculation. J Urol 144(2 pt 1):287–291; discussion 91–92

Dunphy CH, Ayala AG, Swanson DA, Ro JY, Logothetis C (1988) Clinical stage I nonseminomatous and mixed germ cell tumors of the testis. A clinicopathologic study of 93 patients on a surveillance protocol after orchiectomy alone. Cancer 62(6):1202–1206

Duran I, Sturgeon JFG, Jewett MAS, Berthold DR, Kakiashvili D, Anson-Cartwright L et al (2007) Initial versus recent outcomes with a non-risk adapted surveillance policy in stage I non-seminomatous germ cell tumors (NSGCT). J Clin Oncol 26:200s

Elert AA, Olbert PP, Hegele AA, Barth PP, Hofmann RR, Heidenreich AA (2002) Accuracy of frozen section examination of testicular tumors of uncertain origin. Eur Urol 41(3):290–293

Ernst DS, Brasher P, Venner PM, Czaykowski P, Moore MJ, Reyno L et al (2005) Compliance and outcome of patients with stage 1 non-seminomatous germ cell tumors (NSGCT) managed with surveillance programs in seven Canadian centres. Can J Urol 12(2):2575–2580

Fossa SD, Jacobsen AB, Aass N, Heilo A, Stenwig AE, Kummen O et al (1994) How safe is surveillance in patients with histologically low-risk non-seminomatous testicular cancer in a geographically extended country with limited computerised tomographic resources? Br J Cancer 70(6):1156–1160

Fossa SD, Moynihan C, Serbouti S (1996) Patients' and doctors' perception of long-term morbidity in patients with testicular cancer clinical stage I. A descriptive pilot study [see comment]. Support Care Cancer 4(2):118–128

Fossa SD, Dahl AA, Loge JH (2003) Fatigue, anxiety, and depression in long-term survivors of testicular cancer. J Clin Oncol 21(7):1249–1254

Fossa SD, Chen J, Schonfeld SJ, McGlynn KA, McMaster ML, Gail MH et al (2005) Risk of contralateral testicular cancer: a population-based study of 29,515 U.S. men. J Natl Cancer Inst 97(14):1056–1066

Francis R, Bower M, Brunstrom G, Holden L, Newlands ES, Rustin GJ et al (2000) Surveillance for stage I testicular germ cell tumours: results and cost benefit analysis of management options. Eur J Cancer 36(15):1925–1932

Freedman LS, Jones WG, Peckham MJ (1987) Histopathology in the prediction of relapse of patients with stage I testicular teratoma treated by orchidectomy alone. Lancet 2:294–298

Gels ME, Hoekstra HJ, Sleijfer DT, Marrink J, de Bruijn HW, Molenaar WM et al (1995) Detection of recurrence in patients with clinical stage I nonseminomatous testicular germ cell tumors and consequences for further follow-up: a single-center 10-year experience. J Clin Oncol 13(5):1188–1194

Groll RJ, Warde P, Jewett MAS (2007) A comprehensive systematic review of testicular germ cell tumor surveillance. Cri Rev Oncol Hematol

Hain SSF, O'Doherty MMJ, Timothy AAR, Leslie MMD, Partridge SSE, Huddart RRA (2000) Fluorodeoxyglucose PET in the initial staging of germ cell tumours. Eur J Nucl Med 27(5):590–594

Hao D, Seidel J, Brant R, Alexander F, Ernst DS, Summers N et al (1998) Compliance of clinical stage I nonseminomatous germ cell tumor patients with surveillance. J Urol 160(3 pt 1): 768–771

Harland SSJ, Cook PPA, Fossa SSD, Horwich AA, Mead GGM, Parkinson MMC et al (1998) Intratubular germ cell neoplasia of the contralateral testis in testicular cancer: defining a high risk group. J Urol 160(4):1353–1357

Heidenreich AA, Weissbach LL, Höltl WW, Albers PP, Kliesch SS, Köhrmann KKU et al (2001) Organ sparing surgery for malignant germ cell tumor of the testis. J Urol 166

Heidenreich A, Albers P, Krege S (2006) Management of bilateral testicular germ cell tumours-experience of the German Testicular Study Group (GTCSG). Eur J Urol

Hendry WWF, Norman AA, Nicholls JJ, Dearnaley DDP, Peckham MMJ, Horwich AA (2000) Abdominal relapse in stage 1 nonseminomatous germ cell tumours of the testis managed by surveillance or with adjuvant chemotherapy. BJU Int 86(1):89–93

Hilton SS, Herr HHW, Teitcher JJB, Begg CCB, Castéllino RRA (1997) CT detection of retroperitoneal lymph node metastases in patients with clinical stage I testicular nonseminomatous germ cell cancer: assessment of size and distribution criteria. AJR 169(2):521–525

Hoei-Hansen CCE, Rajpert-De Meyts EE, Daugaard GG, Skakkebaek NNE (2005) Carcinoma in situ testis, the

progenitor of testicular germ cell tumours: a clinical review. Ann Oncol 16(6):863–868
Hoskin P, Dilly S, Easton D, Horwich A, Hendry W, Peckham MJ (1986) Prognostic factors in stage I non-seminomatous germ-cell testicular tumors managed by orchiectomy and surveillance: implications for adjuvant chemotherapy. J Clin Oncol 4(7):1031–1036
Huddart RRA, Norman AA, Shahidi MM, Horwich AA, Coward DD, Nicholls JJ et al (2003) Cardiovascular disease as a long-term complication of treatment for testicular cancer. J Clin Oncol 21(8):1513–1523
Jewett MA (1990) Nerve-sparing technique for retroperitoneal lymphadenectomy in testis cancer. Urol Clin North Am 17(2):449–456
Jewett MA, Kong YS, Goldberg SD, Sturgeon JF, Thomas GM, Alison RE et al (1988) Retroperitoneal lymphadenectomy for testis tumor with nerve sparing for ejaculation. J Urol 139(6):1220–1224
Joly F, Heron JF, Kalusinski L, Bottet P, Brune D, Allouache N et al (2002) Quality of life in long-term survivors of testicular cancer: a population-based case-control study. J Clin Oncol 20(1):73–80
Jonker-Pool G, van Basten JP, Hoekstra HJ, van Driel MF, Sleijfer DT, Koops HS et al (1997) Sexual functioning after treatment for testicular cancer: comparison of treatment modalities. Cancer 80(3):454–464
Jonker-Pool G, Hoekstra HJ, van Imhoff GW, Sonneveld DJA, Sleijfer DT, van Driel MF et al (2004) Male sexuality after cancer treatment – needs for information and support: testicular cancer compared to malignant lymphoma. Patient Educ Couns 52(2):143–150
Kakehi Y, Kamoto T, Kawakita M, Ogawa O (2002) Follow-up of clinical stage I testicular cancer patients: cost and risk benefit considerations. Int J Urol 9(3):154–160; discussion 60–61
Kimbrough JC, Cook FEJ (1953) Carcinoma of the testis. J Am Med Assoc 153:1436
Klepp O, Dahl O, Flodgren P, Stierner U, Olsson AM, Oldbring J et al (1997) Risk-adapted treatment of clinical stage 1 non-seminoma testis cancer. Eur J Cancer 33(7):1038–1044
Koch MO (1998) Cost-effective strategies for the follow-up of patients with germ cell tumors. Urol Clin North Am 25(3): 495–502
Kollmannsberger CC, Beyer JJ, Droz JJP, Harstrick AA, Hartmann JJT, Biron PP et al (1998) Secondary leukemia following high cumulative doses of etoposide in patients treated for advanced germ cell tumors. J Clin Oncol 16(10): 3386–3391
Lashley DB, Lowe BA (1998) A rational approach to managing stage I nonseminomatous germ cell cancer. Urol Clin North Am 25(3):405–423
Lassen UU, Daugaard GG, Eigtved AA, Højgaard LL, Damgaard KK, Rørth MM (2003) Whole-body FDG-PET in patients with stage I non-seminomatous germ cell tumours. Eur J Nucl Med Mol Imaging 30(3):396–402
Leibovitch II, Foster RRS, Kopecky KKK, Albers PP, Ulbright TTM, Donohue JJP (1998) Identification of clinical stage A nonseminomatous testis cancer patients at extremely low risk for metastatic disease: a combined approach using quantitive immunohistochemical, histopathologic, and radiologic assessment. J Clin Oncol 16(1):261–268
Lewis LG (1948) Testis tumor: report on 250 cases. J Urol 59:763
Liedke S, Allhoff EP, Jonas U (1990) "Wait and see" in NSGCT clinical stage I: a critical assessment after 8 years. J Urol 143(suppl):397A
Link RE, Allaf ME, Pili R, Kavoussi LR (2005) Modeling the cost of management options for stage I nonseminomatous germ cell tumors: a decision tree analysis. J Clin Oncol 23(24):5762–5773
Magelssen HH, Haugen TTB, von Düring VV, Melve KKK, Sandstad BB, Fosså SSD (2005) Twenty years experience with semen cryopreservation in testicular cancer patients: who needs it? Eur Urol 48(5):779–785
Maroto PP, García del Muro XX, Aparicio JJ, Paz-Ares LL, Arranz JJA, Guma JJ et al (2005) Multicentre risk-adapted management for stage I non-seminomatous germ cell tumours. Ann Oncol 16(12):1915–1920
Mead GM, Rustin GJ, Stenning SP, Vasey P, Aass N, Huddart RA et al (2006) Medical Research Council trial of 2 versus 5 CT scans in the surveillance of patients with stage I non-seminomatous germ cell tumours of the testis. J Clin Oncol 24(18S):4519
Meinardi MMT, Gietema JJA, van Veldhuisen DDJ, van der Graaf WWT, de Vries EEG, Sleijfer DDT (2000) Long-term chemotherapy-related cardiovascular morbidity. Cancer Treat Rev 26(6):429–447
Miyake H, Muramaki M, Eto H, Kamidono S, Hara I (2004) Health-related quality of life in patients with testicular cancer: a comparative analysis according to therapeutic modalities. Oncol Rep 12(4):867–870
Moynihan C (1987) Testicular cancer: the psychosocial problems of patients and their relatives. Cancer Surv 6(3):477–510
Munro AJ, Warde PR (1991) The use of a Markov process to simulate and assess follow-up policies for patients with malignant disease: surveillance for stage I nonseminomatous tumors of the testis. Med Decis Mak 11(2):131–139
Nicolai N, Pizzocaro G (1995) A surveillance study of clinical stage I nonseminomatous germ cell tumors of the testis: 10-year followup. J Urol 154(3):1045–1049
Nuver JJ, Smit AJAJ, van der Meer JJ, van den Berg MPMP, van der Graaf WTWTA, Meinardi MTMT et al (2005) Acute chemotherapy-induced cardiovascular changes in patients with testicular cancer. J Clin Oncol 23(36):9130–9137
Oliver RRT, Raja MMA, Ong JJ, Gallagher CCJ (1992) Pilot study to evaluate impact of a policy of adjuvant chemotherapy for high risk stage 1 malignant teratoma on overall relapse rate of stage 1 cancer patients. J Urol 148(5):1453–1455; discussion 55
Oliver RT, Ong J, Shamash J, Ravi R, Nagund V, Harper P et al (2004) Long-term follow-up of Anglian Germ Cell Cancer Group surveillance versus patients with Stage 1 nonseminoma treated with adjuvant chemotherapy. Urology 63(3): 556–561
Ondrus D, Hornak M (1994) Orchiectomy alone for clinical stage I nonseminomatous germ cell tumors of the testis (NSGCTT): a minimum follow-up period of 5 years. Tumori 80(5):362–364
Ondrus DD, Matoska JJ, Belan VV, Kausitz JJ, Goncalves FF, Hornák MM (1998) Prognostic factors in clinical stage I nonseminomatous germ cell testicular tumors: rationale for different risk-adapted treatment. Eur Urol 33(6):562–566

Ord-Lawson S, Fitch M (1997) The relationship between perceived social support and mood of testicular cancer patients. Can Oncol Nurs J 7(2):90–95

Peckham MJ, Brada M (1987) Surveillance following orchidectomy for stage I testicular cancer. Int J Androl 10(1): 247–254

Peckham MJ, Barrett A, Husband JE, Hendry WF (1982) Orchidectomy alone in testicular stage I non-seminomatous germ-cell tumours. Lancet 2(8300):678–680

Petersen PM (2002) J Clin Oncol 20:1537–1543

Petersen PMPM, Giwercman AA, Daugaard GG, Rørth MM, Petersen JHJH, Skakkeaek NENE et al (2002) Effect of graded testicular doses of radiotherapy in patients treated for carcinoma-in-situ in the testis. J Clin Oncol 20(6):1537–1543

Pont J, Holtl W, Kosak D, Machacek E, Kienzer H, Julcher H et al (1990) Risk-adapted treatment choice in stage I nonseminomatous testicular germ cell cancer by regarding vascular invasion in the primary tumor: a prospective trial. J Clin Oncol 8(1):16–20

Pont JJ, Albrecht WW, Postner GG, Sellner FF, Angel KK, Höltl WW (1996) Adjuvant chemotherapy for high-risk clinical stage I nonseminomatous testicular germ cell cancer: long-term results of a prospective trial. J Clin Oncol 14(2): 441–448

Powles TB, Bhardwa J, Shamash J, Mandalia S, Oliver T (2005) The changing presentation of germ cell tumours of the testis between 1983 and 2002. Br J Urol Int 25:1197–2000

Raghavan D, Colls B, Levi J, Fitzharris B, Tattersall MH, Atkinson C et al (1988) Surveillance for stage I non-seminomatous germ cell tumours of the testis: the optimal protocol has not yet been defined. Br J Urol 61(6):522–526

Raman JD, Nobert CF, Goldstein M (2005) Increased incidence of testicular cancer in men presenting with infertility and abnormal semen analysis [see comment]

Read G, Stenning SP, Cullen MH, Parkinson MC, Horwich A, Kaye SB et al (1992) Medical Research Council prospective study of surveillance for stage I testicular teratoma. Medical Research Council Testicular Tumors Working Party. J Clin Oncol 10:1762–1768

Rorth M, Jacobsen GK, von der Maase H, Madsen EL, Nielsen OS, Pedersen M et al (1991) Surveillance alone versus radiotherapy after orchiectomy for clinical stage I nonseminomatous testicular cancer. Danish Testicular Cancer Study Group. J Clin Oncol 9(9):1543–1548

Rudberg L, Nilsson S, Wikblad K (2000) Health-related quality of life in survivors of testicular cancer 3 to 13 years after treatment. J Psychosoc Oncol 18(3):19–31

Sagstuen HH, Aass NN, Fosså SSD, Dahl OO, Klepp OO, Wist EEA et al (2005) Blood pressure and body mass index in long-term survivors of testicular cancer. J Clin Oncol 23(22):4980–4990

Schefer H, Mattmann S, Morner M et al (2000) Single course adjuvant bleomycin, etoposide and cisplatin (BEP) for high risk stage I non-seminomatous germ cell tumors (NSGCT). Proc Am Soc Clin Oncol 19:340a

Schmoll HJ, Souchon R, Krege S, Albers P, Beyer J, Kollmannsberger C et al (2004) European consensus on diagnosis and treatment of germ cell cancer: a report of the European Germ Cell Cancer Consensus Group (EGCCCG). Ann Oncol 15(9):1377–1399

Sharir S, Jewett MA, Sturgeon JF, Moore M, Warde PR, Catton CN et al (1999) Progression detection of stage I nonseminomatous testis cancer on surveillance: implications for the followup protocol. J Urol 161(2):472–475; discussion 75–76

Sogani PC, Perrotti M, Herr HW, Fair WR, Thaler HT, Bosl G (1998) Clinical stage I testis cancer: long-term outcome of patients on surveillance [see comment]. J Urol 159(3): 855–858

Sonneveld DJ, Hoekstra HJ, van der Graff WT, Sluiter WJ, Scharaffordt Koops H, Sleijfer DT (1999) The changing distribution of stage in nonseminomatous testicular germ cell tumours from 1987 to 1996. Br J Urol Int 84:68–74

Staubitz W (1970) Survival after RPLND alone. J Urol

Stiggelbout AM, Kiebert GM, de Haes JC, Keizer HJ, Stoter G, de Wit R et al (1996) Surveillance versus adjuvant chemotherapy in stage I non-seminomatous testicular cancer: a decision analysis. Eur J Cancer 32A(13):2267–2274

Sturgeon JF, Jewett MA, Alison RE, Gospodarowicz MK, Blend R, Herman S et al (1992) Surveillance after orchidectomy for patients with clinical stage I nonseminomatous testis tumors. J Clin Oncol 10(4):564–568

Tekgul S, Ozen H, Ozgu I, Sahin A, Ergen A, Remzi D (1995) Surveillance-only policy in clinical stage-I non-seminomatous germ-cell tumors of the testis. Bull Cancer 82(2):162–166

Thompson PI, Nixon J, Harvey VJ (1988) Disease relapse in patients with stage I nonseminomatous germ cell tumor of the testis on active surveillance. J Clin Oncol 6(10):1597–1603

Travis LB, Curtis RE, Storm H, Hall P, Holowaty E, Van Leeuwen FE et al (1997) Risk of second malignant neoplasms among long-term survivors of testicular cancer. J Natl Cancer Inst 89(19):1429–1439

Travis LBLB, Fosså SDSD, Schonfeld SJSJ, McMaster MLML, Lynch CFCF, Storm HH et al (2005) Second cancers among 40,576 testicular cancer patients: focus on long-term survivors. J Natl Cancer Inst 97(18):1354–1365

Vergouwe Y, Steyerberg EW, Eijkemans MJ, Albers P, Habbema JD (2003) Predictors of occult metastasis in clinical stage I nonseminoma: a systematic review. J Clin Oncol 21(22): 4092–4099

Weissbach L (1995) Organ preserving surgery of malignant germ cell tumors. J Urol 153(1):90–93

Wishnow KI, Johnson DE, Swanson DA, Tenney DM, Babaian RJ, Dunphy CH et al (1989) Identifying patients with low-risk clinical stage I nonseminomatous testicular tumors who should be treated by surveillance. Urology 34(6):339–343

Wood L, Kollmansberger C, Jewett M, Chung P, Hotte S, O'Malley M, Sweet J, Ason-Cartwright L, Winquist E, North S, Tyldesley S, Sturgeon J, Gospodarowicz M, Segal Roanne, Cheng T, Venner P, Moore M, Albers P, Huddart R, Nichols C, Warde P Canadian Urological Association Journal (CUAJ) 2010;4:E19-38

Young BJ, Bultz BD, Russell JA, Trew MS (1991) Compliance with follow-up of patients treated for non-seminomatous testicular cancer. Br J Cancer 64(3):606–608

# Treatment: Seminoma: Stage I

# 11

Tim Oliver, Peter W.M. Chung, Tom Powles, and Michael A.S. Jewett

## 11.1 Introduction

Testicular germ cell cancer has become the paradigm of a curable malignancy over the last 30 years since the advent of cisplatin-based chemotherapy (Einhorn and Donohue 1977) as the majority of patients are now cured. This together with the recognition of the effect of long-term treatment-related toxicity, particularly in young men, has dramatically changed the goals of management of all stages and pathological subtypes of testicular germ cell cancer. This is more evident in the last 20 years since PEB chemotherapy treatment became the standard of care for all subgroups of metastatic germ cell cancer (Einhorn and Donohue 1977; Williams et al. 1987), with the possible exception of the small number of early small-volume stage II seminoma where radiation still remains the standard of care for most, though, by no means, all centers (Oliver 2007). These changes have impacted markedly on stage I tumor management particularly stage I seminoma more than any other subgroup. This chapter reviews these changes in standards of care and attempts to identify priorities for the next decade's clinical trials.

## 11.2 Changing Natural History of Stage I seminoma

In the early 1950s, seminoma was the most frequent subgroup of testicular germ cell cancer in excess of two-thirds of all tumors (Oliver et al. 1984). However, under the influence of the two main schools of pathology that developed at that time, i.e., the British Testicular Panel under Pugh (1976) and the Armed Forces under Mostofi (Mostofi and Sobin 1977), the frequency of seminomas decreased as the practice of cutting step sections became standard and revealed occult small areas of nonseminoma in a sizeable minority. By the late 1970s, just prior to the introduction of curative chemotherapy, seminomas had fallen in frequency to about 40–50% (Oliver et al. 1984). This reclassification improved the prognosis of both seminoma and nonseminoma on the basis of the "Will Rogers" effect (Feinstein et al. 1985). Over the same period of time, but extending into the early 1980s, there was a major improvement in radiological and biochemical (tumor marker) staging with lymphogram replacing IVP and then itself being replaced by CT scan. This produced a further apparent improvement in both stage I and metastatic germ cell cancer survival (Oliver et al. 1983) by a further "Will Rogers" effect and further reduced stage I seminoma as a proportion of the total group.

In the last 30 years, the situation has been totally reversed and, once again, stage I seminoma has emerged as the most frequent subgroup of germ cell cancer constituting 65–70% of all patients presenting today (Powles et al. 2005; Bhardwa et al. 2005). This may, in part, be due to an increasing awareness among men in the age group most frequently affected, i.e., 15–50 years, about the importance of early diagnosis through school- and media-led campaigns such as the "Know your balls Check 'em out" campaign of the Orchid Cancer Appeal (www.orchid-cancer.org.uk). In addition to an increasing proportion of stage I seminomas (Table 11.1), this change has been associated with a substantial reduction in tumor size at orchidectomy over the last 30 years, implying that there is earlier diagnosis (Bhardwa et al. 2005). There have been three theories proposed to explain this increased incidence of stage I seminoma.

T. Oliver (✉)
Department of Medical Oncology, Institute of Cancer Barts and The London School of Medicine, Queen Mary University of London, London, UK
e-mail: r.t.oliver@gmail.ac.uk

M.P. Laguna et al. (eds.), *Cancer of the Testis*,
DOI: 10.1007/978-1-84800-370-5_11, © Springer-Verlag London Limited 2010

**Table 11.1** Changing presentation of germ cell tumors of the testis between 1983 and 2002 (Bhardwa et al. 2005)

| | 1983–1989 ($n$=452) (%) | 1990–1995 ($n$=585) (%) | 1996–2002 ($n$=509) (%) |
|---|---|---|---|
| Stage 1 seminoma | 34 | 44 | 50 |
| Metastatic seminoma | 10 | 8 | 8 |
| Stage I nonseminoma | 25 | 25 | 27 |
| Metastatic nonseminoma | 31 | 23 | 15 |

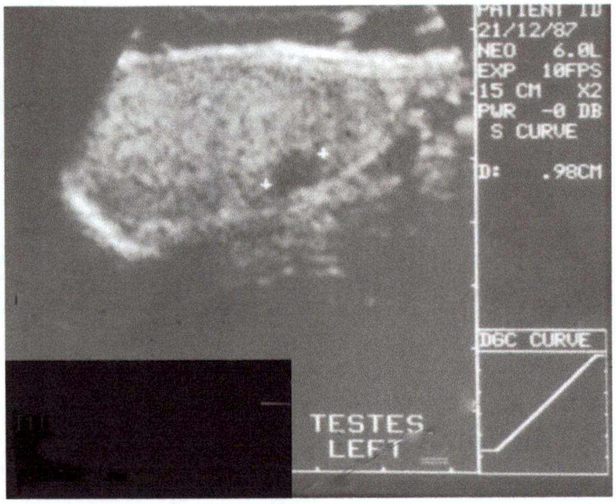


**Fig. 11.1** Testicular ultrasound on patient JC who presented without a mass detectable on palpation but with minor but persistent localized testicular discomfort described as though he had a bee sting in his testicle. At orchidectomy, this was found to be a 1-cm seminoma

The first proposes that it is a genuine change as a result of a general rise in the incidence of germ cell cancer. This has been occurring continuously since the beginning of the twentieth century, apart from the brief period between 1950 and 1980, when staging changes occurred. This general trend has been attributed to being a by-product of increasing intrauterine environmental factors (Oliver 2005a) including estrogen and xenoestrogen environmental pollution that has damaged sperm cell development in-utero, leading to declining sperm count and fertility problems, including producing the testicular dysgenesis syndrome, part of which includes testicular germ cell cancer (Carlsen et al. 1995; Sharpe 2003; Rajpert-De Meyts 2006). As seminoma appears to be the earliest manifestation of invasive malignancy (Oliver et al. 1995), the increasing testis tumor awareness and earlier diagnosis in the "at-risk" population may be producing mainly an increase in stage I seminoma. Another cofactor is the impact of an increasingly sedentary life style over the last century that records on testis cancer have been available (Kamdar et al. 1998). This is thought to be due to the established damaging effect of heat on spermatogenesis (Mieusset and Bujan 1994).

The third explanation for the increased testicular germ cell cancer is totally or at least partly an artifice of overdiagnosis. This is produced by the increasing quality and availability of testicular ultrasound that detects small "latent" seminoma that is preimmune-rejection (Fig. 11.1). These are resulting in the escalating numbers as we have seen with cervix, breast and prostate cancer screening (Peeters et al. 1989; Barry 1998). Spontaneous regression of both primary and metastatic germ cell cancer is clearly established as occurring (Oliver 1990a) and could be a factor but is unlikely to explain all of the increase that has been seen in the last 20 years but needs to be born in mind as a component of the rise in assessing the results of modern treatment.

The next section reviews the history of treatment standards of care.

## 11.3 Evolution in Management of Clinical Stage I (T1-4, N0, M0) Seminoma

### *11.3.1 The Era of Radiotherapy for All (1930–1980)*

It has long been apparent that there is differential radiosensitivity between seminoma and nonseminoma (Friedman 1944). The most recent publication reported 3,000 cGy producing 50% cure of stage II seminoma while 4,500 cGy only produced 25% cure of stage II nonseminomas (Tyrrell and Peckham 1976). As the latter had a higher propensity to metastasise and this paper does not report the in-field recurrence rate, it is not possible to precisely quantify the true differential sensitivity. As effective chemotherapy did not become available until the late 1970s, radiotherapy became standard of care for seminoma while retroperitoneal surgery remained an alternative to radiation for nonseminoma. This has meant that results from radiation based on stage do not have information on radiological staging inaccuracies that have been demonstrable in surgical studies of nonseminoma where even with today's modern scanning techniques greater than 1 in 5 patients in reports of those undergoing RPLND for stage IIa have false-positive CT scans (Stephenson et al. 2005). However, it has to be said that the only modern series of stage II seminoma cases treated by retroperitoneal lymph node dissection reported no false positives in a series of four cases (Mezvrishvili and Managadze 2006).

The first series of seminoma treated with radiation reported in 1951 achieved 80% 5-year survival for clinical stage I disease (Boden and Gibb 1951), this had changed very little by 1963 (77%) (Hope-Stone et al. 1963). Since 1979, by which time the full impact of radiological staging using lymphography played a major role, the relapse rate of patients with stage I seminoma given radiotherapy had fallen to 3% (Calman et al. 1979) where it has remained. This frequency of relapse has been confirmed by extensive literature reports with relapse free rates ranging from 95 to 96% (Table 11.2). Patients experience fatigue and mild gastrointestinal upset during therapy that is usually readily controlled with 5-hydroxytryptamine antagonists for nausea and antimotility agents for cramping and diarrhea.

If treatment is planned and delivered appropriately, follow-up imaging of the abdomen and pelvis is not required and can often be finished at 5 years. When it occurs, relapse is usually outside of the radiation field in sites such as the supraclavicular fossa, mediastinum and lung. Most relapses occur within 2 years and are salvaged with chemotherapy.

However, by the beginning of the 1980s, the first doubts about the long-term safety of radiation with more than 10 years follow-up were being aired (Hay et al. 1984) and based on similar findings in more substantial series reporting the long-term results from the use of radiation and radiation combined with chemotherapy in Hodgkin's disease (Foss Abrahamsen et al. 2002), there began two decades of search for alternative strategies for stage I seminoma.

**Table 11.2** Results of radiation therapy for stage I seminoma (Fossa et al. 1999; Classen et al. 2004; Warde et al. 2005; Santoni et al. 2003)

| Author | No. patients | % Relapse | CSS |
|---|---|---|---|
| Fossa | 242 | 3.7 | 100 |
| Warde | 283 | 5 | 100 |
| Santoni | 487 | 4.3 | 99.4 |
| Classen | 675 | 4.2 | 99.6 |

## 11.3.2 The First Decade of Surveillance Studies (1980–1990)

While good results with adjuvant radiation were being achieved in stage I seminoma, cisplatin-based chemotherapy was impacting on nonseminoma management (Einhorn and Donohue 1977) and surveillance as an alternative option began to emerge (Freedman et al. 1987). The cure of nonseminoma patients relapsing after radiation was more difficult (Anon 1985). As the same worsening of response to chemotherapy, albeit less, was seen from salvage studies of relapsed radiation-treated seminoma patients (Fossa et al. 1997), studies of surveillance in stage I seminoma began in the early 1980s (Peckham et al. 1987). This policy became widespread and, though the overall relapse rate was low (Table 11.3), there were late relapses out to 12 years albeit very rare. However, in confirmation of what has been known since the initial studies of radiation even rarer were reports of patients treated outside a major center with less than meticulous surveillance, who very occasionally presented with late relapses invading the spinal canal and causing paraplegias (Oliver 2005b).

**Table 11.3** Results of surveillance in stage I seminoma (von der Maase et al. 1993; Warde et al. 2005; Daugaard et al. 2003; Horwich et al. 1992b; Francis et al. 2000)

| Author | No. patients | Median follow-up | No. relapse (%) | CSS (%) |
|---|---|---|---|---|
| Horwich | 103 | 62 | 17 (16.5) | 100 |
| Francis | 120 | 55 | 18 (15) | 99 |
| Von der Maase | 261 | 48 | 49 (19) | 98.9 |
| Daugaard | 394 | 60 | 69 (17.5) | 100 |
| Warde | 421 | 97 | 64 (14.5) | 99.8 |

One additional problem of surveillance was the lack of a reliable serological tumor marker apart from placental alkaline phosphatase, which unfortunately gives false-positives in smokers (Tucker et al. 1985), to help with diagnosis of relapse. The result is that diagnosis of relapse relies on serial changes in lymph node size on serial scans. With improved resolution in CT scan, changing definition of pathological size criteria used and fluctuations in lymph node size even in normal individuals, confirmation of relapse may be prolonged (Oliver 1987). Patients, who choose surveillance, but are poorly compliant with follow-up, may compromise their outcome by delaying the diagnosis of recurrence until a late stage when more intensive therapy is necessary, or cure is not possible. Hao et al. (1998) described two deaths among poorly compliant patients with non-seminomatous testicular cancers on surveillance, but none among the patients who attended regularly for follow-up. Finally, at least one economic analysis has suggested that surveillance may be more costly to the health care budget than immediate radiotherapy, although the costs of managing treatment-induced second malignancies and the psychological and social costs to patients were not considered (Sharda et al. 1996).

As a consequence, by the beginning of the 1990s as longer follow-up of the old radiotherapy series was finding increased malignancy after 15 years, the world split into three camps as to what strategy to employ for stage I seminoma to diminish this potential risk. European radiation oncologists explored reducing radiation dose and field size, Canadian and Danish centers continued to enlarge their surveillance series to attempt to better define those at risk of relapse, while European surgical and medical oncologists began to explore minimum chemotherapy. Before considering these results, the next section will summarize the data on late event studies with 20–30 years follow-up.

## 11.4 Late Events Following Older Radiotherapy Schedules

While the acute side effects of radiation that develop during treatment are usually self-limiting and of minimal consequence, the side effects that arise months or years after the treatment is finished, as discussed previously, may have long-term consequences. Chronic gastrointestinal symptoms may develop and an increased incidence of peptic ulceration particularly after abdominal radiation doses in the range of 30–45 Gy has been reported, though less common with the lower doses used to treat stage I seminoma. The germinal epithelium of the testis is one of the most sensitive tissues in the body to ionizing radiation, and doses as low as 20 cGy (<1% of the dose that is usually used to treat seminoma) are sufficient to transiently elevate gonadotropins and reduce sperm counts (Hamilton et al. 1986). Even with shielding of the remaining testis, the scatter radiation dose results in a significant risk of infertility in previously fertile men, particularly at doses more than 50 cGy (Fraass et al. 1985).

Despite these concerns about late events, there was reluctance to abandon adjuvant radiation because of the late relapse rate and perceived difficulties in diagnosing it in patients with clinical stage I seminoma on surveillance. As increasing numbers of men diagnosed with testicular germ cell tumors are now being cured and survive long-term, the late effects of treatment have become ever more apparent such that any debate on the management of germ cell tumors cannot be undertaken without considering this issue. Although there were early reports suggesting that up to 10 years there was no excess mortality in seminoma patients from second nongerm cell cancer (Horwich and Bell 1994), evidence began to emerge that with longer follow-up, there was an apparent increase in second nongerm cell malignancies (Hay et al. 1984; Edmonds et al. 1993; Travis et al. 1997). The largest study of second malignant nongerm cell tumors in patients with testicular cancer (Table 11.4) was a cooperative effort involving over 40,000 patients from 16 population-based cancer registries (Travis et al. 2005). The actuarial excessive risk of developing a second malignancy increased progressively with time from diagnosis of testicular cancer, and was 18% at 25 years (relative risk RR 1.9). As well as a 2–6-fold increased risk of leukemia, there was an increased risk of solid tumors of the gastrointestinal and genitourinary tracts. This study also demonstrated that nearly 50% of the tumors that did develop did not arise within the radiation field. The mechanism of carcinogenesis in these tumors is unknown but one explanation could be that tumors may develop because of the long-term T-lymphocytopenia known to exist in a substantial minority of irradiated patients (Stjernsward et al. 1972; Fossa et al. 1989). However, as details of the exact location of some of the "out-of-field" tumors is not available, a proportion of these could be in locations that received scatter radiation.

**Table 11.4** Second non-GCT cancers in 40,576 GCT long-term survivors (Travis et al. 2005)

| | All GCT ($n$=40,576) | Seminoma ($n$=22,424) | Nonseminoma ($n$=16,776) |
|---|---|---|---|
| Radiotherapy alone ($N/n$=10,534 /1,944) | 2.0 ($n$=892) | 2.0 ($n$=700) | 2.1 ($n$=170) |
| Chemotherapy alone ($N/n$=808/3,799) | 1.8 ($n$=30) | 1.6 ($n$=6) | 1.8 ($n$=28) |
| Both ($N/n$=332/456) | 2.9 ($n$=25) | 3.8 ($n$=16) | 2.2 ($n$=9) |
| Radiotherapy alone (total $N$=4,386) (calendar year analysis) | | | |
| Year of treatment 1943–1974 | 2.0 ($n$=272) | 1.7 ($n$=192) | 2.7 ($n$=69) |
| Year of treatment 1975–2001 | 2.3 ($n$=145) | 2.5 ($n$=127) | 1.6 ($n$=18) |

*N* no of seminomas; *n* no. of nonseminoma

For men with seminoma diagnosed at age 35 years, the cumulative risk of developing a second solid cancer after 40 years (i.e., at the age of 75 years) was 36% vs. 23% for the general population.

## 11.5 Strategies to Minimize Over-Treatment of Stage I Seminoma

### 11.5.1 Minimizing Radiation Field Size and Dose

Traditionally, patients with stage I seminoma following radical orchiectomy received the so-called "dog-leg" or "hockey-stick" RT field. This encompassed the para-aortic and ipsilateral iliac lymph nodes ± inguinal lymph nodes depending on the estimated risk of inguinal involvement. The dose given was typically 25–30 Gy in 15–20 daily fractions and produced close to 100% in field control. The dose response relationship for seminoma below this level is unknown, although there are isolated reports of in-field recurrences after fractionated doses of 15 Gy and 21 Gy (Lester et al. 1986; Dosoretz et al. 1981). A report using 20 Gy in eight daily fractions with only one in-field recurrence among 263 patients (Logue et al. 2003) led the Medical Research Council in the United Kingdom (MRC UK) to organize a phase III study addressing the question of radiation dose. This compared moderate- and low-dose radiation schedules with equal fraction size (30 Gy in 15 fractions vs. 20 Gy in 10 fractions). The trial randomized 625 patients (Jones et al. 2005) and confirmed the equivalence of relapse-free survival of the lower dose (Table 11.5) in short-term follow-up (4 years). However, small-to-modest reductions in the dose of

**Table 11.5** Randomized trials of potential new standards for stage I seminoma (Jones et al. 2005; Fossa et al. 1999; Oliver et al. 2005b)

| Trial (ARM A vs. ARM B) | ARM A No. of cases | ARM A Proportion relapsing[a] | ARM B No. of cases | ARM B Proportion relapsing[a] | Median follow-up (years) |
|---|---|---|---|---|---|
| MRC TE10 (1989–1993) | 242 | 3% | 236 | 4% | 4.5 |
| Dog-leg vs. PA strip | | (0%) | | (44%) | |
| MRC TE18 (1995–1998) | 313 | 3% | 312 | 4% | 5.1 |
| 30 Gy vs. 20 Gy[b] | | (70%) | | (27%) | |
| MRC TE19 (1996–2001) | 904 | 4% | 573 | 5% | 4.0 |
| Radiation vs. carboplatin (×1) | | (38%) | | (0%) | |

Note: dog-leg field irradiation includes both PA and ipsilateral iliaclymph nodes *MRC* Medical Research Council; *PA* para-aortic
[a]Proportion of relapses in pelvic area
[b]88% of patients were given PA strip irradiation

this magnitude may not necessarily translate into a reduced risk of infertility or second malignancy, especially if treatment is administered in an otherwise conventional fashion to encompass the para-aortic and ipsilateral pelvic lymph nodes.

While para-aortic relapse accounts for 85% of recurrences in seminoma patients on surveillance, ipsilateral iliac lymph node recurrence is seen in less than 10% of patients (Horwich et al. 1992a; von der Maase et al. 1993; Warde et al. 1997). In addition, surgicopathologic series of patients with clinical stage I nonseminomatous testicular cancer have demonstrated ipsilateral common iliac nodal involvement in only about 10% of cases (Donohue et al. 1982). One of the most important factors determining the radiation dose to the remaining contralateral testis, and therefore the risk of infertility, is the distance from the inferior edge of the radiation field to the scrotum (Fraass et al. 1985). With this knowledge, several investigators have proposed limiting the radiation fields to treat only the para-aortic nodes (Sultanem et al. 1998; Kiricuta et al. 1996; Read and Johnston 1993; Fossa et al. 1999). Reducing the irradiated volume may potentially also decrease the risk of second nongerm cell malignancy. A randomized phase III study also planned by the MRCUK comparing conventional "dog-leg" RT to para-aortic RT in 478 patients was reported after a median of 4 years follow-up, and showed no difference in disease-free survival between the two arms (Fossa et al. 1999) (Table 11.5). However, unexpectedly, the relapse pattern was different with 4 of 9 recurrences in patients who received para-aortic irradiation alone occurred in the pelvis, while there were none of 9 in patients treated with "dog-leg" RT. Sperm counts after treatment were significantly higher in the para-aortic RT and recovered to normal more quickly (13 months vs. 20 months); however, at 3 years follow-up, there was no difference in sperm counts between the two groups. Despite the short follow-up, this study had an immediate significant influence on the standard of radiotherapy practice for patients with stage I seminoma, in that a greater proportion received para-aortic RT alone, mostly in the United Kingdom and Europe. However, the increased risk of iliac lymph node recurrence was not thought to have been particularly significant and the practice of minimal imaging and discharging nontrial patients after 5 years was continued (Logue et al. 2003). The observation of late relapse in the pelvis at 8 years (Classen et al. 2004) meant that some of the gain from the reduction of field size was lost, particularly in comparison to surveillance. A compromise may be to irradiate the para-aortic and ipsilateral common iliac lymph nodes by positioning the inferior border of the radiation field at the lower aspect of the sacro-iliac joints or upper level of the acetabulum (Thomas 1994), see Fig. 11.2. This encompasses the lymph nodes that are typically removed at lymphadenectomy in patients with nonseminomatous tumors (Donohue et al. 1993). The external iliac and inguinal nodes are not treated, but are unlikely to harbor occult metastases. This approach has the potential to reduce (but not eliminate) the scatter dose to the remaining testis and might help to preserve fertility without the requirement for ongoing pelvic surveillance (Schmidberger et al. 1997).

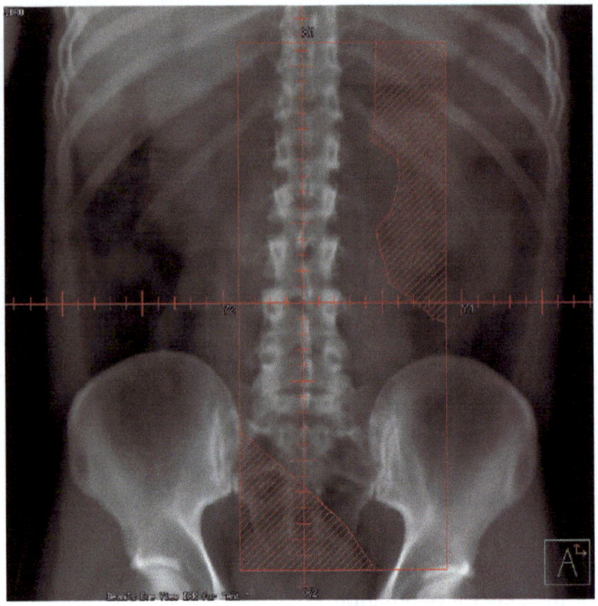

**Fig. 11.2** Adjuvant radiotherapy field for left-sided stage I seminoma

## 11.6 Carboplatin Chemotherapy

In the early 1940s, the differential radiosensitivity between seminoma and nonseminoma was demonstrated (Friedman 1944). Less has been done to clarify whether a similar degree of differential sensitivity to chemotherapy exists. Possible evidence in favor of this view was the comparative response rate to single-agent cisplatin. The initial report in 1974 showed that 10% of germ cell cancer patients achieved durable complete remission with single-agent cisplatin which included 1 out 2 seminomas and 7/68 nonseminomas (Higby et al. 1974). Ten years later, in 1984, a small study of 12 patients with metastatic seminoma reported 83% durable CR after single-agent cisplatin though only in 1 of 4 previously radiated patients (Oliver et al. 1984). This observation was subsequently confirmed by a report from Logothetis et al. (1987).

These early studies led to phase II studies of Carboplatin in metastatic and stage I disease (Table 11.6). Though it was immediately apparent that the relapse rate was somewhat higher than with cisplatin, salvage with BEP combination for the minority that relapsed was so good that the overall survival seemed to be as good as those treated with BEP as initial treatment (Horwich et al. 1992a; Oliver et al. 1990; Schmoll et al. 1993). The experience from Hodgkin's disease suggested that the worse risk of second malignancy was when radiation and chemotherapy were combined, some centers began exploring pilot studies with first two, then one course of single-agent platinum analog carboplatin at a dose of AUC×7 (approximately 530 mg/m$^2$) as adjuvant for stage I seminoma and reported 2% relapse rate (Oliver et al. 2005a). Initially, these results were not believed as there was a report of 9% relapse from Germany using one course of a lower dose of carboplatin 400 mg/m$^2$ (Dieckmann et al. 2000). In addition, these results were published just at the same time as the disappointing trial of significantly worse survival of carboplatin combination in metastatic nonseminoma (Horwich et al. 1997) and nonsignificantly worse survival of single-agent carboplatin in metastatic seminoma patients (Bokemeyer et al. 2004). Even more disappointing was a phase II study of single-agent carboplatin in early stage II a and b metastatic seminoma (Krege et al. 2006). Though not a randomized comparison, this seemed to suggest the results with carboplatin could be worse than radiation though they were similar to those seen in surveillance relapses treated with radiation (Warde et al. 1997). Also in the (Krege et al. 2006) study, the results were better in IIb clinical stage than IIa cases and the carboplatin treatment was given every 4 rather than 3 weeks with the dose calculated by Cockroft formula rather than by isotopic renal clearance. In addition, some of the centers involved in recruiting to the study were former East German centers at the time after the collapse of communism. At that time, overall long-term cure rates from other East European centers were 20–25% worse than those from the Western European countries (Sant et al. 2007).

Because of this uncertainty, despite offering a real alternative to radiation, it was nearly a decade before a

**Table 11.6** Phase II studies stage I seminoma

| | No. of cases | Relapse-free survival[a] | Overall survival (median FU in years) |
|---|---|---|---|
| *Metastatic seminoma carboplatin dose phase II studies* (Oliver et al. 2004) | | | |
| Carboplatin AUC×10 q21×3–4 | 24 | 93% | 100% |
| Carboplatin AUC×7/8 q21×4 | 17 | 88% | 94% |
| Carboplatin 450 mg/m$^2$ q21×4 | 19 | 79% | 95% |
| *Stage I seminoma* (Oliver et al. 2005a) *carboplatin dose phase II studies* | | | |
| Carboplatin 400 mg/m$^2$ q28×2 | 644 | 98.5% (NA) | 98.3% (3.8) |
| Carboplatin 400 mg/m$^2$ q28×1 | 116 | 91.4% (NA) | 99% (4) |
| Carboplatin AUC×7 (564 mg/m$^2$×1) | 274 | 98.2% (0%) | 99% (7.5) |
| *Stage I seminoma* (Logue et al. 2003) *radiation dose phase II studies* | | | |
| PA strip 20 Gy in eight fractions | 431 | 96.3% (53%) | 98% (5.2) |

*NA* not applicable; *AUC* area under curve
[a]Proportion of the relapses in the pelvic area

Fig. 11.3 Patient's diary card data from the MRC TE19 trial of Radiation verses one course of carboplatin (reproduced by kind permission of the Lancet)

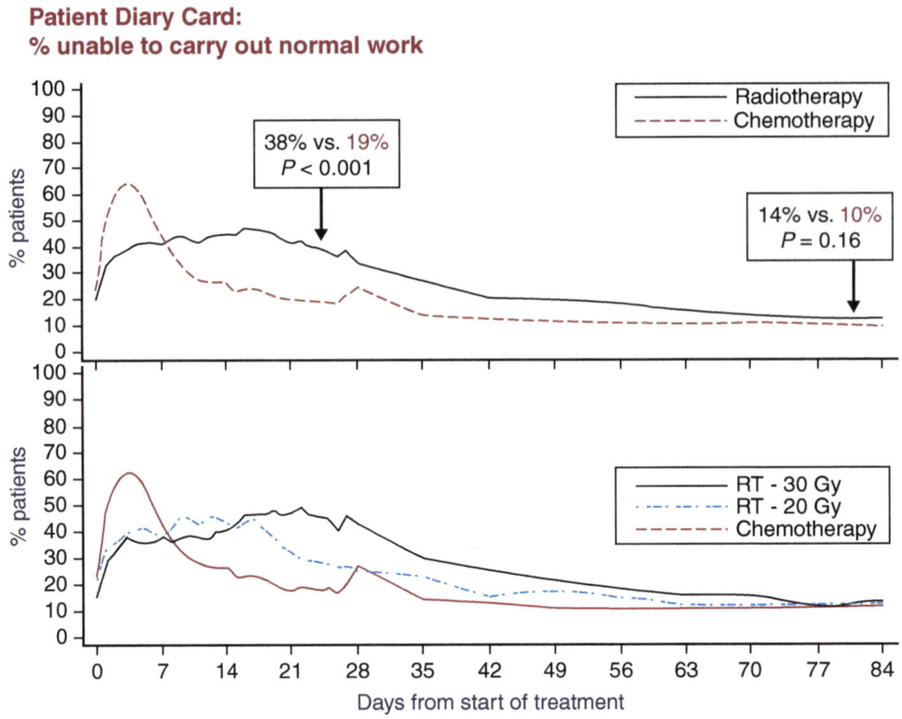


randomized trial was undertaken comparing one course carboplatin and two schedules of radiation. A similar relapse-free rate was achieved (3 years, 95% vs. 96%) (Oliver et al. 2005b). As well as showing 50% faster recovery of time to return to work in the carboplatin group (Fig. 11.3), carboplatin appeared to eliminate the increased risk of pelvic recurrence in the para-aortic field RT patients. Unexpectedly, in the carboplatin group, there was a 72% reduction of 5-year risk of second tumors in the contralateral testis compared to the para-aortic RT group, though late follow-up of the phase II studies has established that this is not durable with second GCT only being deferred and happen between 10 and 15 years (Oliver et al. 2003; Powles et al. 2008).

## 11.7 Modern Surveillance and Risk-Adapted Strategies

There was increasing awareness of the impact of early diagnosis on changing prognosis and lowered relapse rate. Recognition of the degree of overtreatment and risk of late second cancers hardened attitudes against widespread use of adjuvant treatment, whether radiation or chemotherapy. This led to a return to the use of surveillance as the primary management policy. The two largest reported series of stage I seminoma on surveillance are the Princess Margaret Hospital (PMH) and the Rigshospitalet in Copenhagen. In the PMH study of 241 patients, 5-year actuarial relapse-free survival was 86% with a median follow-up of 7.3 years (Warde and Jewett 1998). In a recent update of this study, 421 patients were followed for a median of over 8 years, with 5-year relapse-free rate of 85.5% (Warde et al. 2005). In the Rigshospitalet study (Daugaard et al. 2003), 17% of patients had failed with a median follow-up of 60 months. Other studies including those from the Royal Marsden Hospital and the Danish Testicular Cancer Study Group (DATECA) with greater than 36 month follow-up have reported similar relapse rates (Table 11.3). Site of relapse was similar in all surveillance studies with the vast majority recurring in the para-aortic and interaorto-caval nodes 33 of 37 (89%) in the PMH and 41 of 49 (82%) in the DATECA studies, respectively. While the median time to relapse ranged from 12 to 18 months, there continued to be recurrences as late as 12 years from diagnosis (Warde et al. 1997; Michael et al. 2000).

## 11.8 Prognostic Factors for Relapse in Patients on Surveillance

Prompted by cost and quality of life issues, attempts were made to identify prognostic factors for relapse. In the PMH series, only age (≤34 years) and tumor size (>6 cm) were associated with relapse (Warde et al. 1997) Among 57 patients who had no adverse prognostic factors (age > 34, tumor size < 6 cm and no lymphovascular invasion), tumor relapse was 6% at 5 years. In the DATECA study, primary tumor size was the only risk factor. Risk of relapse at 4 years was 6%, 18%, and 36% among patients with tumors <3 cm, 3–6 cm and >6 cm, respectively (von der Maase et al. 1993) In a series published by the group at Royal Marsden, only the presence of lymphovascular space involvement was associated with relapse (9% vs. 17%) (Horwich et al. 1992a).

In an attempt to develop a consensus, data from four large series was pooled (Warde et al. 2002) and two factors (tumor size >4 cm and rete testis invasion) independently predictive of relapse were identified (Table 11.7). With only one factor present, the hazard ratio (HR) for relapse was 1.7 for rete testis invasion and 2.0 for tumor size >4 cm. However, when both risk factors were present, HR was 3.4 compared to when no risk factors were present.

Surveillance has the obvious attraction that 80–85% of men will never require any further treatment and thus the threat of long-term treatment related toxicity. Therefore, it would appear to have an advantage over adjuvant therapy. However, for such a strategy to be successful, cure of the primary disease should not be compromised. In the large surveillance series reported (over 1,300 patients), there have only been four disease-related deaths and survival is equivalent to the outcome with adjuvant radiotherapy. However, although the relapse rate is only 15–20%, because of the problems of late relapse and difficulty of maintaining contact for long-term follow-up of young men at the most mobile stage in their lives, radiation has remained the standard of care for many centers (Sharda et al. 1996; Steele et al. 1999). Overall, as almost 100% of patients are cured regardless of choice of therapy postorchidectomy, it is preferable to offer patients' participation in making their choice that fits in with their particular circumstance.

For surveillance to be totally accepted for seminoma patients, efficacious management of relapse is a critical concern and particularly the ability to detect relapse as early as possible and preferably with retroperitoneal disease only at a small volume (<5 cm). For centers using radiation, such recurrences are routinely managed with RT in an attempt to do without toxic combination chemotherapy. However, patients treated in this way are at risk of secondary relapse after salvage RT and overall in the published series (Table 11.8) this was 15%. Despite this in the PMH experience overall, the need for combination chemotherapy has been similar whether the patients were managed with surveillance and radiation for first relapse (13 of 241 chemotherapy) or adjuvant RT for all (10 of 254 needed chemotherapy). However, it has to be remembered that using this radiation for first relapse strategy exposes 3–4% of the whole stage I seminoma cohort to combined chemotherapy and radiation with the worst risk of second malignancy as has been shown from studies in Hodgkin's disease (Foss Abrahamsen et al. 2002). As the data shown in Table 11.5 demonstrates (Travis et al. 2005) and more recent publications confirm (van den Belt-Dusebout et al. 2007), there is strong data suggesting that the same may be true for seminoma patients. With the reduction of number of courses of

**Table 11.7** Prognostic factors for stage I seminoma relapse on surveillance (Warde et al. 2002)

| Risk factors for relapse | No. of cases | Relapse at 5 years (%) |
|---|---|---|
| No risk factors | 176 | 12 |
| Rete testis only | 75 | 14 |
| Tumor size >4 cm only | 107 | 17 |
| Both risk factors | 95 | 31 |

**Table 11.8** Management Options for early stage I seminoma (Oliver 2007)

| | No. of cases | Relapse (%) |
|---|---|---|
| Seminoma on surveillance | 1,123 | 17 |
| Radiation for surveillance relapse | 93 | 15 |
| PEB for surveillance relapse | 33 | 3 |
| Radiation for stage IIA/B | 270 | 11 |
| Carboplatin AUC 7q28 for stage IIA/B | 108 | 13 |
| Carboplatin AUC 7-10q21 for stage IIA/B | 12 | 0 |

BEP treatment from 4 to 3 (de Wit et al. 2001) and the surprisingly good results from the use of escalated dose of Carboplatin in good-risk early metastatic seminoma (Oliver et al. 2004), which in the limited number of small-volume stage IIA and B might be as good as combination chemotherapy, it may be appropriate to use chemotherapy as first-line treatment for all relapses of seminoma on surveillance.

## 11.9 Chemotherapy as Option for Selected High-Risk Patients

Adjuvant carboplatin has the advantage of shorter duration of side effects when compared to radiotherapy and similar relapse rates with relatively short follow-up. As a consequence, one group has adopted a risk-adapted approach similar to that used in stage I nonseminoma (Aparicio et al. 2005). This involves proceeding with adjuvant treatment only in the subgroup deemed at increased risk for relapse and reserving surveillance for those at low risk of relapse, using the risk factors for relapse mentioned above. However, it has to be noted that this strategy is based on risk factors that have not yet been independently validate**d** and even in those patients with both risk factors present their recurrence risk is still less than 35%.

The main drawback of carboplatin compared to the old radiotherapy schedules is that the majority of relapses occur in the retroperitoneum and thus continued CT scan monitoring is still required. However, this is also a problem for patients treated with the newer para-aortic strip protocols, where relapse in the pelvis has been reported at 8 years. Clearly, the long-term effects of carboplatin are also as yet unknown, as although it has been in use for 20 years there are few reports of more than 10 years follow-up (Oliver et al. 2006). While it may well be relatively innocuous, only maturing data over the next decade or more will inform us as to whether this is the case.

## 11.10 New Approaches to the Late Events of Therapy

Follow-up for all the new strategies developed for reducing late events in the past decade is too short to either guarantee that they are as durable in their disease control or safer in terms of reducing nongerm cell cancer and cardiovascular risk. Equally, the optimal follow-up has not been defined though a recent review of the literature has suggested guidelines using HR for relapse as an indicator of the frequency and type of follow-up needed for the different strategies (Martin et al. 2007). With such high cure rates in men in their 30s, increasing attention is being paid to how best to gather late event information as such patients could be expected to live an extra 40–50 years. Routine follow-up in an oncology clinic is likely not feasible in men who are largely well and the purpose of this follow-up is to gather information about late events that may not be easily picked up. While cancer registry data is certainly useful, it tends to lack specific information on individual treatment that men have received. One possibility may be to obtain this sort of data through cancer survivorship networks and late effects clinics. This is starting to be recognized as important research so that men can be better informed when decision making. The increased risk of second malignancy was most clearly seen in the older radiotherapy series. The most recent report comparing radiotherapy versus chemotherapy versus both, in terms of risk of second malignancies and cardiovascular risk confirmed that these were highest in patients receiving both treatment modalities (van den Belt-Dusebout et al. 2007). There was little difference between radiotherapy and chemotherapy given alone, though most of chemotherapy patients would have been in the small numbers cured with the prolonged courses of chemotherapy given in the precisplatin era and the early series cured in the BVP era when up to six courses were given and some centers did 1 year of maintenance chemotherapy (Travis et al. 2005). There is also some preliminary evidence that patients treated in the modern era of linear accelerator radiotherapy machines which began in the early 1970s had less second nongerm cell malignancy in the first 10 years after treatment than those treated in the era of Cobalt machines (Powles et al. 2007) though this does not cover the critical period from 15 to 30 years after treatment. More worryingly, only about 50% of the excess mortality seen after irradiation of stage I seminoma was due to death from malignant disease. An equal number of excess deaths were from cardiovascular disease. Subsequent studies have suggested there may also be excess cardiac deaths which also occurred, though possibly less frequently, in men with stage I tumors treated with surveillance (Powles et al. 2007) although as with the linear accelerator data there is only reliable follow-up data to 10 years.

As surveillance patients also had an excess weight gain and elevated lipid levels indicative of the metabolic syndrome (Nuver et al. 2005) that was thought to be a reflection of the subclinical testicular atrophy present in these patients' contralateral testis which might have been made worse by the scatter radiation from the pelvic portion of the radiation. Other studies into the so-called metabolic syndrome included patients treated with surgery alone, radiotherapy or chemotherapy (patients with more advanced disease; two groups categorized as total cumulative dose of cisplatin ≤850 mg vs. >850 mg) (Haugnes et al. 2007). The syndrome existed in 40% of patients, with only those patients in the chemotherapy group who had received >850 mg of cisplatin were at increased odds of having hypertension, obesity and hypercholesterolaemia. In a similar study investigating hypertension and obesity, again only the chemotherapy group who received >850 mg of cisplatin had increased risk of both conditions. Although one or even two courses of carboplatin would be unlikely to cause the same effects as large cumulative doses of cisplatin, unfortunately, at the present time, the data on carboplatin is not yet mature enough to investigate the evolution of these potential late effects.

Increasingly, epidemiological studies are helping to understand why premature development of an "andropause" related syndrome may explain the excess metabolic syndrome (Oliver 2005a). Skakkebaek and Sharpe have long championed the view that the declining sperm count and rising testis cancer incidence is due to intrauterine exposure to excess environmental oestrogenic compounds. Such maternal factors may explain why the risk of familial germ cell cancer in sib pairs is higher than in father/son pairs and why, as mothers bearing dizygous twins have higher levels of estrogen than monozygous twins, dizygous rather than monozygous twins have a higher incidence. Though estrogen/xenoestrogens have long been the primary suspect, other factors such as radiation, smoking and genetics of inhibin control may also be involved and possibly mediate their effect via somatic mutation of genes such as c-KIT.

With this background, it is easier to understand the importance of subfertility and FSH-driven atrophy as the final common pathway of testis cancer as it is the main gonadotrophin responsible for regulating sperm production. However, such dysgenic testes also have a deficiency albeit less than sperm production of leydig cell function (Nuver et al. 2005), which may explain the increased risk of metabolic syndrome.

## 11.11 The Future

Today, more than 70% of testis cancer patients present with sperm counts in the subfertile range (Oliver 1990b) which as discussed in the previous section is probably due to subclinical intra-uterine damage to their contralateral testis. Ten percent of patients with sperm in the ejaculate at presentation become azoospermic after diagnostic orchidectomy (Petersen et al. 1999) and make it advisable that if they have not completed their family, patients should be advised to do sperm storage before orchidectomy. Given the proportion with subclinical testis atrophy, taken with the increasing longevity of society, it is clear that safe germinal and leydig epithelial preservation is the last frontier in germ cell cancer management (Oliver et al. 2003). Given that the risk of recurrence could be lifelong, such studies would not be wise as first-line treatment until a reliable noninvasive test such as semen cytology was available, or only used as short-term solutions until conceptions are no longer required.

For patients with stage I and II disease, MRI lymphography (Harisinghani et al. 2005) is offering the potential of more reliable imaging of the retroperitoneum and PET/CT offering accelerated assessment of response (Oliver et al. 2004). Laparoscopic sentinel lymph node biopsy (Satoh et al. 2005), by offering a low morbidity approach to validate the new radiological staging techniques, will accelerate their adoption but also enable surgeons to gain confidence faster to use this less-invasive laparoscopic techniques to do the smaller postchemotherapy masses seen today. It will also enable earlier use of surgery to reduce amounts of chemotherapy given.

Recent progress with salvage chemotherapy by curing 60% of primary BEP failures (Shamash et al. 2007), provides a safety net that, combined with more accurate imaging, could also enable earlier and safer testing of less-toxic and better drugs for first-line use. However, given the disappointment of the carboplatin studies in metastatic seminoma patients, only if they offered major improvement in terms of toxicity profile would the large randomized trial required to prove their safety and efficacy in stage I seminoma be justified. Based on their activities in vitro (Powles et al. 2007), there is already some evidence that the new generations of platinum drugs, including oxaliplatin and oral satraplatin, could be the first candidates though larger salvage studies of their use in salvage situations will be needed first.

## 11.12 Conclusion

"In primum non nocere" (above all else, do no harm) remains the primary priority of all healthcare, not the least for young men with a long-life expectancy and now cure can be achieved with relative ease. Nowhere is it more important and more difficult to prove than in stage I seminoma now the most frequent and curable group of germ cell cancer patients. This review has highlighted the changing management of stage I seminoma with earlier smaller tumors justifying less treatment and the short-term safety out to 5 years of an increasing number of management options including surveillance, reduced field and dose radiation and one course Carboplatin. The continuation of a low frequency of late relapse out to 10 years and lack of late information beyond 10 years for some of these alternates, does mean that for the foreseeable future efforts to get late follow-up will be a priority as will improvements in staging techniques and their verification. Until such information can be gathered, explanation of our current knowledge to patients with development of appropriate patient information leaflets will enable the techniques learnt from conducting patient preference studies in early prostate cancer (North West Uro-Oncology 2002) to benefit germ cell cancer patients. It is now apparent that virtually 100% of patients with stage I seminoma will be cured regardless of the method of postorchidectomy management. Ultimately, disease control in the adjuvant setting will be difficult to improve upon unless a robust (preferably noninvasive) method for detecting micrometastases becomes available and the emphasis for both patients and physicians will be how best to optimize management based upon individual need.

## References


Anon (1985) Prognostic factors in advanced non-seminomatous germ-cell testicular tumours: results of a multicentre study. Report from the Medical Research Council Working Party on Testicular Tumours. Lancet 1(8419):8–11

Aparicio J, Germa JR, Garcia del Muro X, Maroto P, Arranz JA, Saenz A et al (2005) Risk-adapted management for patients with clinical stage I seminoma: the Second Spanish Germ Cell Cancer Cooperative Group study. [see comment]. J Clin Oncol 23(34):8717–8723

Barry MJ (1998) PSA screening for prostate cancer: the current controversy–a viewpoint. Patient Outcomes Research Team for Prostatic Diseases. [see comment]. Ann Oncol 9(12): 1279–1282

van den Belt-Dusebout AW, de Wit R, Gietema JA, Horenblas S, Louwman MW, Ribot JG et al (2007) Treatment-specific risks of second malignancies and cardiovascular disease in 5-year survivors of testicular cancer. [see comment]. J Clin Oncol 25(28):4370–4378

Bhardwa JM, Powles T, Berney D, Baithun S, Nargund VH, Oliver RT (2005) Assessing the size and stage of testicular germ cell tumours: 1984-2003. BJU Int 96(6):819–821

Boden G, Gibb R (1951) Radiotherapy and testicular neoplasms. Lancet 2(26):1195–1197

Bokemeyer C, Kollmannsberger C, Stenning S, Hartmann JT, Horwich A, Clemm C et al (2004) Metastatic seminoma treated with either single agent carboplatin or cisplatin-based combination chemotherapy: a pooled analysis of two randomised trials. Br J Cancer 91(4):683–687

Calman FM, Peckman MJ, Hendry WF (1979) The pattern of spread and treatment of metastases in testicular seminoma. Br J Urol 51(2):154–160

Carlsen E, Giwercman A, Keiding N, Skakkebaek NE (1995) Declining semen quality and increasing incidence of testicular cancer: is there a common cause? Environ Health Perspect 103(Suppl 7):137–139

Classen J, Schmidberger H, Meisner C, Winkler C, Dunst J, Souchon R et al (2004) Para-aortic irradiation for stage I testicular seminoma: results of a prospective study in 675 patients. A trial of the German testicular cancer study group (GTCSG). Br J Cancer 90(12):2305–2311

Daugaard G, Petersen PM, Rorth M (2003) Surveillance in stage I testicular cancer. Apmis 111(1):76–83; discussion 83–85

Dieckmann KP, Bruggeboes B, Pichlmeier U, Kuster J, Mullerleile U, Bartels H (2000) Adjuvant treatment of clinical stage I seminoma: is a single course of carboplatin sufficient? Urology 55(1):102–106

Donohue JP, Zachary JM, Maynard BR (1982) Distribution of nodal metastases in nonseminomatous testis cancer. J Urol 128(2):315–320

Donohue JP, Thornhill JA, Foster RS, Rowland RG, Bihrle R (1993) Primary retroperitoneal lymph node dissection in clinical stage A non-seminomatous germ cell testis cancer. Review of the Indiana University experience 1965-1989. Br J Urol 71(3):326–335

Dosoretz DE, Shipley WU, Blitzer PH, Gilbert S, Prat J, Parkhurst E et al (1981) Megavoltage irradiation for pure testicular seminoma: results and patterns of failure. Cancer 48(10):2184–2190

Edmonds PM, Ong J, da Stavola B, Oliver RTD, Hope-Stone HF, Blandy JP (1993) Risk of a second non-testis malignancy following radiotherapy for stage 1 Seminoma. In: BAUS Annual Meeting, Harrogate, p 53

Einhorn LH, Donohue J (1977) Cis-diamminedichloroplatinum, vinblastine, and bleomycin combination chemotherapy in disseminated testicular cancer. Ann Intern Med 87(3):293–298

Feinstein AR, Sosin DM, Wells CK (1985) The Will Rogers phenomenon. Stage migration and new diagnostic techniques as a source of misleading statistics for survival in cancer. New Engl J Med 312(25):1604–1608

Foss Abrahamsen A, Andersen A, Nome O, Jacobsen AB, Holte H, Foss Abrahamsen J et al (2002) Long-term risk of second malignancy after treatment of Hodgkin's disease: the influence of treatment, age and follow-up time. Ann Oncol 13(11):1786–1791

Fossa SD, Aass N, Kaalhus O (1989) Long-term morbidity after infradiaphragmatic radiotherapy in young men with testicular cancer. Cancer 64(2):404–408

Fossa SD, Oliver RT, Stenning SP, Horwich A, Wilkinson P, Read G et al (1997) Prognostic factors for patients with advanced seminoma treated with platinum-based chemotherapy. Eur J Cancer 33(9):1380–1387

Fossa SD, Horwich A, Russell JM, Roberts JT, Cullen MH, Hodson NJ et al (1999) Optimal planning target volume for stage I testicular seminoma: a Medical Research Council randomized trial. Medical Research Council Testicular Tumor Working Group. [see comment]. J Clin Oncol 17(4):1146

Fraass BA, Kinsella TJ, Harrington FS, Glatstein E (1985) Peripheral dose to the testes: the design and clinical use of a practical and effective gonadal shield. Int J Radiat Oncol Biol Phys 11(3):609–615

Francis R, Bower M, Brunstrom G, Holden L, Newlands ES, Rustin GJ et al (2000) Surveillance for stage I testicular germ cell tumours: results and cost benefit analysis of management options. Eur J Cancer 36(15):1925–1932

Freedman LS, Parkinson MC, Jones WG, Oliver RT, Peckham MJ, Read G et al (1987) Histopathology in the prediction of relapse of patients with stage I testicular teratoma treated by orchidectomy alone. Lancet 2(8554):294–298

Friedman N (1944) Supervoltage (1 million volts) roentgen therapy at Walter Reed General Hospital. Surg Clin North Am 24:1424–1432

Hamilton C, Horwich A, Easton D, Peckham MJ (1986) Radiotherapy for stage I seminoma testis: results of treatment and complications. Radiother Oncol 6(2):115–120

Hao D, Seidel J, Brant R, Alexander F, Ernst DS, Summers N et al (1998) Compliance of clinical stage I nonseminomatous germ cell tumor patients with surveillance. J Urol 160 (3 Pt 1):768–771

Harisinghani MG, Saksena M, Ross RW, Tabatabaei S, Dahl D, McDougal S et al (2005) A pilot study of lymphotrophic nanoparticle-enhanced magnetic resonance imaging technique in early stage testicular cancer: a new method for noninvasive lymph node evaluation. Urology 66(5): 1066–1071

Haugnes HS, Aass N, Fossa SD, Dahl O, Klepp O, Wist EA et al (2007) Components of the metabolic syndrome in long-term survivors of testicular cancer. [see comment]. Ann Oncol 18(2):241–248

Hay JH, Duncan W, Kerr GR (1984) Subsequent malignancies in patients irradiated for testicular tumours. Br J Radiol 57(679):597–602

Higby DJ, Wallace HJ Jr, Albert DJ, Holland JF (1974) Diaminodichloroplatinum: a phase I study showing responses in testicular and other tumors. Cancer 33(5):1219–1225

Hope-Stone H, Blandy J, Dayan A (1963) Treatment of tumours of the testis. Br Med J 1:984–989

Horwich A, Bell J (1994) Mortality and cancer incidence following radiotherapy for seminoma of the testis. Radiother Oncol 30(3):193–198

Horwich A, Dearnaley DP, A'Hern R, Mason M, Thomas G, Jay G et al (1992a) The activity of single-agent carboplatin in advanced seminoma. Eur J Cancer 28A(8–9):1307–1310

Horwich A, Alsanjari N, A'Hern R, Nicholls J, Dearnaley DP, Fisher C (1992b) Surveillance following orchidectomy for stage I testicular seminoma. Br J Cancer 65(5):775–778

Horwich A, Sleijfer DT, Fossa SD, Kaye SB, Oliver RT, Cullen MH et al (1997) Randomized trial of bleomycin, etoposide, and cisplatin compared with bleomycin, etoposide, and carboplatin in good-prognosis metastatic nonseminomatous germ cell cancer: a Multiinstitutional Medical Research Council/European Organization for Research and Treatment of Cancer Trial. J Clin Oncol 15(5):1844–1852

Jones WG, Fossa SD, Mead GM, Roberts JT, Sokal M, Horwich A et al (2005) Randomized trial of 30 versus 20 Gy in the adjuvant treatment of stage I testicular seminoma: a report on Medical Research Council Trial TE18, European Organisation for the ResearchandTreatmentofCancerTrial30942(ISRCTN18525328). [see comment]. J Clin Oncol 23(6):1200–1208

Kamdar RH, Oliver RT, Othieno-Abinya N, Gallagher CJ, Slevin ML (1998) Geographical epidemiology of ovarian and testicular germ cell cancers. Br J Cancer 78(11):1401

Kiricuta IC, Sauer J, Bohndorf W (1996) Omission of the pelvic irradiation in stage I testicular seminoma: a study of postorchiectomy paraaortic radiotherapy. [see comment]. Int J Radiat Oncol Biol Phys 35(2):293–298

Krege S, Boergermann C, Baschek R, Hinke A, Pottek T, Kliesch S et al (2006) Single agent carboplatin for CS IIA/B testicular seminoma. A phase II study of the German Testicular Cancer Study Group (GTCSG). Ann Oncol 17(2):276–280

Lester SG, Morphis JG 2nd, Hornback NB (1986) Testicular seminoma: analysis of treatment results and failures. Int J Radiat Oncol Biol Phys 12(3):353–358

Logothetis CJ, Samuels ML, Ogden SL, Dexeus FH, Chong CD (1987) Cyclophosphamide and sequential cisplatin for advanced seminoma: long-term followup in 52 patients. J Urol 138(4):789–794

Logue JP, Harris MA, Livsey JE, Swindell R, Mobarek N, Read G (2003) Short course para-aortic radiation for stage I seminoma of the testis. Int J Radiat Oncol Biol Phys 57(5):1304–1309

von der Maase H, Specht L, Jacobsen GK, Jakobsen A, Madsen EL, Pedersen M et al (1993) Surveillance following orchidectomy for stage I seminoma of the testis. [see comment]. Eur J Cancer 29A(14):1931–1934

Martin JM, Panzarella T, Zwahlen DR, Chung P, Warde P (2007) Evidence-based guidelines for following stage 1 seminoma. Cancer 109(11):2248–2256

Mezvrishvili Z, Managadze L (2006) Retroperitoneal lymph node dissection for high-risk stage I and stage IIA seminoma. Int Urol Nephrol 38(3–4):615–619

Michael H, Lucia J, Foster RS, Ulbright TM (2000) The pathology of late recurrence of testicular germ cell tumors. Am J Surg Pathol 24(2):257–273

Mieusset R, Bujan L (1994) The potential of mild testicular heating as a safe, effective and reversible contraceptive method for men. Int J Androl 17(4):186–191

Mostofi F, Sobin L (1977) International histological classification of testicular tumors. In: International histologic classification of tumors. World Health Organisation, Geneva

North West Uro-Oncology Group (2002) A preliminary report on a patient-preference study to compare treatment options in early prostate cancer. BJU Int 90(3):253–256

Nuver J, Smit AJ, Wolffenbuttel BH, Sluiter WJ, Hoekstra HJ, Sleijfer DT et al (2005) The metabolic syndrome and disturbances in hormone levels in long-term survivors of disseminated testicular cancer. [see comment]. J Clin Oncol 23(16):3718–3725

Oliver R (2005a) Epidemiology of testis cancer. In: Vogelzang N, Shipley W, Scardino P, Debruyne F (eds) Comprehensive textbook of genitourinary oncology, 3rd edn. Lippincott Williams & Wilkins, Philadelphia, pp 547–558

Oliver T (2005b) One-dose carboplatin in seminoma.[comment]. Lancet 366(9496):1526

Oliver T (2007) Conservative management of testicular germ-cell tumors. Nat Clin Pract Urol 4(10):550–560

Oliver RT (1987) Limitations to the use of surveillance as an option in the management of stage I seminoma. Int J Androl 10(1):263–268

Oliver RT (1990a) Clues from natural history and results of treatment supporting the monoclonal origin of germ cell tumours. Cancer Surv 9(2):333–368

Oliver RT (1990b) Atrophy, hormones, genes and viruses in aetiology germ cell tumours. Cancer Surv 9(2):263–286

Oliver T, Powles T, Somasundram U, Ell PJ, Shamash J (2006) 22 year phase 1/2 study of single agent carboplatin in metastatic seminoma:could it have been accelerated by 72 hour PET scan response? J Clin Oncol 24(18S):14565

Oliver T, Dieckmann K, Steiner H, Skoneczna I (2005a) Pooled analysis of phase II reports of 2 vs. 1 course of carboplatin as adjuvant for stage 1 seminoma. In: ASCO Annual Meeting Proceedings. J Clin Oncol (abst. 4572)

Oliver T, Mead G, Mason M, Stenning S, Dieckmann K, Steiner H et al (2006) The sword of Damocles and the treatment of stage I seminoma. [comment]. J Clin Oncol 24(16):2599–2600

Oliver RT, Hope-Stone HF, Blandy JP (1983) Justification of the use of surveillance in the management of Stage I germ cell tumours of the testis. Br J Urol 55(6):760–763

Oliver RT, Hope-Stone HF, Blandy JP (1984) Possible new approaches to the management of seminoma of the testis. Br J Urol 56(6):729–733

Oliver RT, Lore S, Ong J (1990) Alternatives to radiotherapy in the management of seminoma. Br J Urol 65(1):61–67

Oliver RT, Leahy M, Ong J (1995) Combined seminoma/non-seminoma should be considered as intermediate grade germ cell cancer (GCC). Eur J Cancer 31A(9):1392–1394

Oliver RT, Ong J, Berney D, Nargund V, Badenoch D, Shamash J (2003) Testis conserving chemotherapy in germ cell cancer: its potential to increase understanding of the biology and treatment of carcinoma-in-situ. APMIS 111(1):86–91; discussion 91–92

Oliver RT, Mason MD, Mead GM, von der Maase H, Rustin GJ, Joffe JK et al (2005b) Radiotherapy versus single-dose carboplatin in adjuvant treatment of stage I seminoma: a randomised trial. Lancet 366(9482):293–300

Peckham MJ, Hamilton CR, Horwich A, Hendry WF (1987) Surveillance after orchiectomy for stage I seminoma of the testis. Br J Urol 59(4):343–347

Peeters PH, Verbeek AL, Straatman H, Holland R, Hendriks JH, Mravunac M et al (1989) Evaluation of overdiagnosis of breast cancer in screening with mammography: results of the Nijmegen programme. Int J Epidemiol 18(2):295–299

Petersen PM, Skakkebaek NE, Vistisen K, Rorth M, Giwercman A (1999) Semen quality and reproductive hormones before orchiectomy in men with testicular cancer. J Clin Oncol 17(3):941–947

Powles T, Perry J, Shamash J, Liu W, Oliver T, Joel S (2007) A comparison of the platinum analogues in bladder cancer cell lines. Urologia internationalis 79(1):67–72

Powles T, Robinson D, Shamash J, Moller H, Tranter N, Oliver T et al (2008) The long-term risks of adjuvant carboplatin treatment for stage I seminoma of the testis. Ann Oncol 19(3):443–447

Powles TB, Bhardwa J, Shamash J, Mandalia S, Oliver T (2005) The changing presentation of germ cell tumours of the testis between 1983 and 2002. BJU Int 95(9):1197–1200

Pugh R (1976) Combined tumours. In: Pathology of the testis. Blackwell Scientific, Oxford, pp 245–248

Rajpert-De Meyts E (2006) Developmental model for the pathogenesis of testicular carcinoma in situ: genetic and environmental aspects. Hum Reprod Update 12(3):303–323

Read G, Johnston RJ (1993) Short duration radiotherapy in stage I seminoma of the testis: preliminary results of a prospective study. Clin Oncol (R Coll Radiol) 5(6):364–366

Sant M, Aareleid T, Artioli ME, Berrino F, Coebergh JW, Colonna M et al (2007) Ten-year survival and risk of relapse for testicular cancer: a EUROCARE high resolution study. Eur J Cancer 43(3):585–592

Santoni R, Barbera F, Bertoni F, De Stefani A, Livi L, Paiar F et al (2003) Stage I seminoma of the testis: a bi-institutional retrospective analysis of patients treated with radiation therapy only. BJU Int 92(1):47–52; discussion 52

Satoh M, Ito A, Kaiho Y, Nakagawa H, Saito S, Endo M et al (2005) Intraoperative, radio-guided sentinel lymph node mapping in laparoscopic lymph node dissection for Stage I testicular carcinoma. Cancer 103(10):2067–2072

Schmidberger H, Bamberg M, Meisner C, Classen J, Winkler C, Hartmann M et al (1997) Radiotherapy in stage IIA and IIB testicular seminoma with reduced portals: a prospective multicenter study. Int J Radiat Oncol Biol Phys 39(2): 321–326

Schmoll HJ, Harstrick A, Bokemeyer C, Dieckmann KP, Clemm C, Berdel WE et al (1993) Single-agent carboplatinum for advanced seminoma. A phase II study. [see comment]. Cancer 72(1):237–243

Shamash J, Joel S, Irwin H, Steele J, Asterling S, Oliver R (2007) GAMEC- A novel protocol for patients with germ cell tumours (GCT) relapsing following conventional treatment or with de Novo IGCCCG for prognosis. British Journal of Cancer 97: 308–314

Sharda NN, Kinsella TJ, Ritter MA (1996) Adjuvant radiation versus observation: a cost analysis of alternate management schemes in early-stage testicular seminoma. J Clin Oncol 14(11):2933–2939

Sharpe RM (2003) The ‘oestrogen hypothesis’ – where do we stand now? Int J Androl 26(1):2–15

Steele GS, Richie JP, Stewart AK, Menck HR (1999) The National Cancer Data Base report on patterns of care for testicular carcinoma, 1985-1996. Cancer 86(10):2171–2183

Stephenson AJ, Bosl GJ, Motzer RJ, Kattan MW, Stasi J, Bajorin DF et al (2005) Retroperitoneal lymph node dissection for nonseminomatous germ cell testicular cancer: impact of patient selection factors on outcome. J Clin Oncol 23(12):2781–2788

Stjernsward J, Jondal M, Vanky F, Wigzell H, Sealy R (1972) Lymphopenia and change in distribution of human B and T lymphocytes in peripheral blood induced by irradiation for mammary carcinoma. Lancet 1(7765):1352–1356

Sultanem K, Souhami L, Benk V, Bahary JP, Roman T, Shenouda G et al (1998) Para-aortic irradiation only appears to be adequate treatment for patients with Stage I seminoma of the testis. Int J Radiat Oncol Biol Phys 40(2): 455–459

Thomas GM (1994) Alternative management options to radiation therapy for stage I and IIA testicular seminoma. [comment]. Int J Radiat Oncol Biol Phys 28(2):547–548

Travis LB, Curtis RE, Storm H, Hall P, Holowaty E, Van Leeuwen FE et al (1997) Risk of second malignant neoplasms among long-term survivors of testicular cancer. [see comment]. J Natl Cancer Inst 89(19):1429–1439

Travis LB, Fossa SD, Schonfeld SJ, McMaster ML, Lynch CF, Storm H et al (2005) Second cancers among 40, 576 testicular cancer patients: focus on long-term survivors. J Natl Cancer Inst 97(18):1354–1365

Tucker DF, Oliver RT, Travers P, Bodmer WF (1985) Serum marker potential of placental alkaline phosphatase-like activity in testicular germ cell tumours evaluated by H17E2 monoclonal antibody assay. Br J Cancer 51(5):631–639

Tyrrell CJ, Peckham MJ (1976) The response of lymph node metastases of testicular teratoma to radiation therapy. Br J Urol 48(5):363–370

Warde P, Jewett MA (1998) Surveillance for stage I testicular seminoma. Is it a good option? Urol Clin North Am 25(3): 425–433

Warde P, Gospodarowicz MK, Banerjee D, Panzarella T, Sugar L, Catton CN et al (1997) Prognostic factors for relapse in stage I testicular seminoma treated with surveillance. J Urol 157(5):1705–1709; discussion 1709–1710

Warde P, Specht L, Horwich A, Oliver T, Panzarella T, Gospodarowicz M et al (2002) Prognostic factors for relapse in stage I seminoma managed by surveillance: a pooled analysis. J Clin Oncol 20(22):4448–4452

Warde PR, Chung P, Sturgeon J, Panzarella T, Giuliani M, Tew-George B, et al (2005) Should Surveillance should be considered the standard of care in stage I seminoma? In: ASCO Annual Meeting Proceedings. J Clin Oncol (abst 4520)

Williams SD, Birch R, Einhorn LH, Irwin L, Greco FA, Loehrer PJ (1987) Treatment of disseminated germ-cell tumors with cisplatin, bleomycin, and either vinblastine or etoposide. New Engl J Med 316(23):1435–1440

de Wit R, Roberts JT, Wilkinson PM, de Mulder PH, Mead GM, Fossa SD et al (2001) Equivalence of three or four cycles of bleomycin, etoposide, and cisplatin chemotherapy and of a 3- or 5-day schedule in good-prognosis germ cell cancer: a randomized study of the European Organization for Research and Treatment of Cancer Genitourinary Tract Cancer Cooperative Group and the Medical Research Council. J Clin Oncol 19(6):1629–1640

# Part IVB

## Treatment of Advanced Stages

# Treatment of Patients with Stage II A/B and Advanced Nonseminomatous Germ Cell Tumors

# 12

Christian Kollmannsberger and Carsten Bokemeyer

## 12.1 Introduction

Since the introduction of cisplatin in the 1970s, the treatment of patients with advanced germ cell tumors has been constantly refined and improved within prospective studies (Sonneveld et al. 2001a). Unfortunately, these studies were on the basis of different prognostic models and staging systems which made the comparison of study results very difficult. In 1997, the International Germ Cell Cancer Consensus Group (IGCCCG) classification was introduced, in which patients with advanced disease are classified on the basis of their prognostic features, such as location of the primary tumor, presence of non-pulmonary visceral metastases, and serum tumor marker level (Mead 1997). Patients are grouped into a good-prognosis group, an intermediate, and a poor-prognosis group; being worldwide accepted and used, this classification has allowed the comparison of study results. Approximately 60% of all patients with advanced nonseminoma present with favorable prognostic criteria ("good prognosis"), which include a gonadal or retroperitoneal primary tumor, low tumor markers, and the presence of lung- or lymph node metastases only. For these patients, survival rates of approximately 90% are achieved using cisplatin-based combination chemotherapy. The intermediate prognosis group encompasses approximately 20–25% of patients. These patients have the same prognostic criteria as the good-prognosis patients but intermediate tumor markers. Long-term survival rates are 80% after four cycles of cisplatin-based chemotherapy. Patients with a primary mediastinal germ cell tumor, high tumor markers, or non-pulmonary visceral metastases comprise the poor-prognosis group and exhibit a much lower and very unsatisfactory long-term survival rate of only 40–50%. About 16–20% of patients with advanced disease belong to this group.

Over the past 10–15 years, various new treatment strategies have been explored in order to maintain the high cure rates while reducing toxicity for patients with good-prognosis disease and improving the cure rates for patients with intermediate or poor-prognosis disease.

C. Kollmannsberger (✉)
Division of Medical Oncology, British Columbia Cancer Agency Vancouver Cancer Centre, University of British Columbia, Vancouver, BC, Canada

## 12.2 Stage II A/B and Good Prognosis Patients

Patients with stage II A/B and/or good-prognosis disease exhibit an excellent prognosis with cure rates of 90–98%. These excellent results have not been significantly improved over the past decade (Sonneveld et al. 2001a). Because of the excellent results achieved with current standard treatment strategies, most studies performed in good-prognosis patients over the past 10 years concentrated on the reduction of treatment related toxicity while maintaining efficacy rather than improving prognosis.

### *12.2.1 Stage II A/B*

Nonseminoma patients with stage II A/B (retroperitoneal lymph nodes up to 2 cm (stage A) or 2–5 cm (stage B)) are cured in close to 98% of cases. In general, three different treatment approaches exist, all of which result in the same excellent long-term survival: a primary retroperitoneal lymphadenectomy (RLA), RLA followed by two cycles of adjuvant bleomycin, etoposide, and

M.P. Laguna et al. (eds.), *Cancer of the Testis*,
DOI: 10.1007/978-1-84800-370-5_12, 

cisplatin (BEP) chemotherapy, or primary chemotherapy with three cycles of BEP followed by resection of residual tumor masses in patients without complete remission (CR). These different strategies have been discussed for a long time without reaching an international consensus. Up front chemotherapy with three cycles of BEP induces a CR in 83–91% patients with stage II A and in 61–87% patients with stage II B (Weissbach et al. 2000; Kuczyk et al. 1999; Horwich et al. 1998). For these patients with a CR, a residual tumor resection with all its potential complications including loss of ejaculation or impotence is unnecessary. In addition, the recurrence rates after up-front chemotherapy are very low ranging from 4 to 9% for stage II A and 11 to 15% for stage II B patients (Weissbach et al. 2000; Kuczyk et al. 1999).

As a result of these advantages, today up-front chemotherapy followed by residual tumor resection represents the preferred treatment approach in most centers. This strategy was declared as the standard approach for patients with stage II A/B with elevated tumor markers by the European Interdisciplinary Consensus Conference in 2003 and again in 2006 (Schmoll et al. 2004). Patients with stage II A/B nonseminomatous germ cell tumors are therefore classified as IGCCCG "good prognosis" patients and treated accordingly.

Patients with retroperitoneal lymph nodes up to 2 cm without marker elevation (clinical stage IIA), represent a particular problem. Two options can be considered: a nerve sparing staging-RPLND or surveillance. A nerve-sparing laparoscopic RPLND is considered an alternative to an open RPLND, when performed in an experienced center. With RPLND the pathological stage can be verified immediately; if surveillance is chosen, follow up at short intervals, e.g., 6 weeks, is indicated to document changes in the lesion. If tumor growth is observed, indicating malignant retroperitoneal disease, treatment should be initiated.

### 12.2.2 Treatment of Patients with Good Prognosis Criteria According to the IGCCCG Classification

Until the end of the 1980s, four cycles of cisplatin, vinblastine, and bleomycin (PVB) were considered the standard of care for patients with advanced disease (Donohue et al. 1978). With the results of cisplatin, etoposide and bleomycin (PEB) in patients with disseminated disease published by Williams et al. (1987) in 1987, PEB became the standard for all patients with metastatic germ cell tumors. In 1989, a study of the South East Cancer Study Group demonstrated that three cycles of BEP were equally effective to but less toxic than four cycles of BEP in patients with a favorable risk profile (Einhorn et al. 1989; Saxman et al. 1998). These results were subsequently confirmed by an European Organization of Research and Treatment of Cancer (EORTC) study which randomized 812 patients with good-prognosis criteria according to the IGCCCG classification to either three cycles of BEP based on the Indiana protocol (Cisplatin 20 mg/m², Etoposide 100 mg/m² day 1–5, Bleomycin 30 IU day 1, 8, 15) or three cycles of BEP plus one cycle of PE (Etoposide/Cisplatin) (de Wit et al. 2001). In addition, patients were randomized to a 5-day and a 3-day BEP regimen in a 2×2 factorial design as in particular in the UK and Australia a 3 day BEP regimen was increasingly used. The cumulative drug doses were equal in both regimens. The relapse-free survival rates were similar for both regimens with 90.4% after three cycles of BEP and 89.4% after 3 × BEP plus one PE. There was also no survival difference between the 5-day and the 3-day regimen. However, BEP given over 3 days has increased long-term toxicity including ototoxicity, peripheral neurotoxicity, or Raynaud syndrome when four cycles are applied (Fossa et al. 2003). On the basis of the results of these randomized studies, three cycles of BEP according to the Indiana protocol represent the standard of care for patients with IGCCCG good prognosis criteria (Table 12.1).

Replacing cisplatin with the less nephro- and neurotoxic carboplatin in patients with good-prognosis nonseminomas results in an approximately 10% deterioration in relapse-free survival and a modest but significant decrease in overall survival (Bajorin et al. 1993; Bokemeyer et al. 1996a; Horwich et al. 1997). The largest of the three published randomized studies allocated patients to either four cycles of BEP or four cycles of CEB (carboplatin, etoposide, bleomycin) (Horwich et al. 1997). Treatment with CEB resulted in a 14% decrease in failure-free survival (3-year failure free survival 77% vs. 91%; $p<0.05$) which eventually resulted in a 7% reduction in overall survival (90% vs. 97%; $p<0.05$). Similar results were reported for the comparison of four cycles of PE and four cycles of CE (Bajorin et al. 1993). A German study compared three cycles of BEP to four cycles of CEB in patients with

**Table 12.1** Selected randomized studies in patients with good-prognosis nonseminoma

| Author | Classification | Regime | Study objective | CR/ PR-rate% | Continuous CR/PR-rate | Conclusion |
|---|---|---|---|---|---|---|
| Einhorn et al. (1989) and | Indiana | PEB × 4 | Reduction of number of cycles | 97 | 88 | BEP × 3 equally effective to BEP × 4 |
| Saxman et al. (1998) | | PEB × 3 | | 98 | 87 | |
| Bosl et al. (1988) | MSKCC | PE × 4 | Testing of a new 2-drug combination | 93 | 82 | PE × 4 equally effective to 3 × VAB-6 × 3 |
| | | VAB-6 × 3 | | 96 | 85 | |
| de Wit et al. (1997) | EORTC | $PE_{360}B \times 4$ | Evasion of bleomycin | 95 | 91 | PE × 4 inferior to BEP × 4 |
| | | $PE_{360} \times 4$ | | 87 | 83 | |
| Loehrer et al. (1995) | Indiana | PEB × 3 | Evasion of bleomycin | 94 | 86 | PE × 3 inferior to 3 × BEP |
| | | PE × 3 | | 88 | 69 | |
| de Wit et al. (2001) | IGCCCG | PEB × 3 + 1 PE | Reduction of number of cycles | 73 | 91 | PEB × 3 equally effective to BEP × 3 + 1 PE |
| | | PEB × 3 | | 71 | 89 | |
| Culine et al. (2003) | IGCCCG | PEB × 3 | Evasion of bleomycin | 92 | 90 | Similar high response rates, study too small to comment on relapse-free or overall survival |
| | | PE × 4 | | 91 | 84 | |
| Bajorin et al. (1993) | MSKCC | PE × 4 | Carboplatin vs. Cisplatin | 88 | 87 | CE × 4 inferior to PE × 4 |
| | | CE × 4 | | 80 | 76 | |
| Horwich et al. (1997) | MRC/EORTC | PEB × 4 | Carboplatin vs. Cisplatin | 94 | 91 | CEB × 4 inferior to BEP × 4 |
| | | CEB × 4 | | 87 | 77 | |
| Bokemeyer et al. (1996a) | Indiana | PEB × 3 | Carboplatin vs. Cisplatin | 97 | 86 | CEB inferior to BEP |
| | | CEB × 4 | | 96 | 68 | |

metastatic nonseminoma. Despite similar high complete response rates (96% CEB vs. 97% PEB), significantly more relapses were observed in the CEB arm (32% CEB vs. 13% PEB) (Bokemeyer et al. 1996a). These results clearly indicate the inferiority of carboplatin as compared to cisplatin. This is in line with the inferior results of carboplatin single agent therapy in patients with advanced seminoma (Bokemeyer et al. 2002; Horwich et al. 2000). Cisplatin cannot be replaced by carboplatin without a significant impairment of efficacy in patients with advanced disease.

Because of its significant pulmonary toxicity, the role and value of bleomycin within the BEP regimen was also investigated in three randomized trials. An ECOG study randomized patients to either three cycles of BEP or three cycles of EP both with etoposide at 500 mg/m$^2$ per cycle. Response rate as well as progression-free and overall survival was significantly inferior after three cycles of EP clearly demonstrating that three cycles of EP are inadequate treatment for patients with good-prognosis disease.

Two randomized trials have compared the efficacy of four cycles of EP to BEP in good-risk GCT therapy. One randomized trial performed by the European Organization for the Research and Treatment of Cancer (EORTC) compared four cycles of BEP vs. four cycles of EP chemotherapy. In this trial, the CR rate was lower in the EP arm, but there were no differences in relapses, time to progression, or survival after long-term follow-up. However, the dose of the etoposide in this EORTC trial was 360 mg/m$^2$ per cycle. In addition, doses of etoposide were further reduced for thrombocytopenia. In the EP regimen used in randomized trials in the United States, 500 mg/m$^2$ of etoposide is used and it is administered without dose reductions. A randomized trial comparing two BEP regimens in patients with good prognosis GCT based on modified MSKCC criteria, one with 120 mg/m$^2$ of etoposide days 1–3 and bleomycin only on day1 and the other with 100 mg/m$^2$ etoposide days 1–5 and bleomycin on days 1, 8, and 15 demonstrated a substantial better outcome for patients on the $BE_{500}P$ regimen (Indiana BEP) (Toner et al. 2001). The higher dose of etoposide and the higher cumulative bleomycin dose are likely to have contributed to the better outcome in that arm. Hence, the lower CR rate in the EORTC trial is likely due to an inadequate etoposide dose. The $BE_{360}P$ arm in the EORTC trial was also more toxic, with resulting pulmonary toxicity and Raynaud's phenomenon.

A French randomized trial compared three cycles of BEP chemotherapy vs. four cycles of EP chemotherapy. The outcome was equivalent for the primary endpoint favorable response rate (complete and marker-negative response rate). However, the trial was underpowered to detect superiority or noninferiority in progression-free or overall survival, which makes the interpretation of this trial very difficult (Culine et al. 2003).

On the basis of a retrospective analysis, four cycles of cisplatin/etoposide appear to be equally effective as three cycles of BEP. Investigators at the Memorial Sloan Kettering Cancer Center identified 289 patients with IGCCCG good prognosis criteria from previously conducted randomized trials (Kondagunta et al. 2005). Two hundred and eighty-two of the 289 patients (98%) achieved a complete response; 93% responded to chemotherapy alone and 5% responded to chemotherapy plus surgical resection of viable disease (GCT other than mature teratoma). Seventeen patients (6%) experienced relapse, and nine (3%) died as a result of disease at a long median follow-up of 7.7 years. Treatment was well tolerated.

Therefore, four cycles of EP followed by resection of residual masses remain an alternative treatment option to three cycles of BEP for patients with IGCCCG good-prognosis patients and may be the preferred treatment option for patients at risk for pulmonary toxicity.

### 12.2.3 Treatment of Patients with Intermediate Prognosis

The optimal treatment of patients with intermediate prognosis has not yet been defined, as this prognostic group only emerged from the IGCCCG meta-analysis in 1995 (Mead 1997). Only very few studies are available to date for patients with intermediate prognosis and no complete prospective randomized studies have yet been published for this subgroup. A randomized study comparing etoposide and cisplatin plus either bleomycin (EB) or ifosfamide (etoposide, ifosfamide, cisplatin (VIP)) in an intermediate prognosis patient group found comparable response rates as well as similar long-term survival rates of 83% in the PEB and 85% in the VIP arm (de Wit et al. 1998). The VIP regimen was more toxic with regard to bone marrow function. The sample size in this study was small as the study was prematurely discontinued when data became available from a competing study that showed no improved effectiveness of VIP compared with BEP in patients with poor-prognosis disease (Nichols et al. 1998). Strategies to improve the outcome of this patient group include the incorporation of new drugs as well as dose-intensified regimens. On the basis of results in relapsed or cisplatin-refractory patients, paclitaxel was added to the BEP regimen (T-BEP) within an EORTC randomized phase II/III study (Bokemeyer et al. 1996b; Motzer et al. 1994; de Wit et al. 1999). Results from this study comparing four cycles of BEP to four cycles of T-BEP are not yet available.

Four cycles of BEP with etopside at 500 mg/m$^2$ per cycle therefore remain the standard treatment for patients with intermediate prognosis achieving a long-term cure rate of approximately 80%. In case of contraindications for bleomycin, four cycles of VIP can be used. Whenever possible, treatment should be given within clinical studies in order to improve the outcome for this patient group.

### 12.2.4 Treatment of Patients with Poor-Prognosis Disease

The small group of patients presenting with poor prognostic features at initial diagnosis (approximately 16% of all metastatic patients) remains a therapeutic challenge. Improvement in outcomes for patients with advanced disseminated disease has been incremental subsequent to the initial breakthrough of cisplatin-based combinations of the 1970s (Sonneveld et al. 2001b). The first demonstration of improved outcome in this group of patients came in the randomized trial of cisplatin, bleomycin, and either vinblastine or etoposide (Williams et al. 1987). In this trial, not only was

**Table 12.2** PEB-regime (Indiana-PEB) and VIP regimen BEP regimen (Williams et al. 1987; Einhorn et al. 1989):

| Agent | Doses | Application | Application days |
|---|---|---|---|
| Cisplatin | 20 mg/m² | 30 min-infusion | Days 1–5 |
| Etoposide | 100 mg/m² | 1 h-infusion | Days 1–5 |
| Bleomycin | 30 IU | Bolus | days 1, 8, 15 |

Repeat day 22:

Repeat day 22 regardless of neutrophil count. Daily blood counts are recommended. If still neutropenic on day 4 of cycle, avoid etoposide on day 5

Delay only if neutropenic fever present or platelets <100,000/μl on day 22

There is no indication for routine prophylactic application of hematopoietic growth factors, such as granulocyte colony stimulating factor (G-CSF). However, if serious infectious complications or prolonged neutropenia has occurred during one preceding chemotherapy cycle, prophylactic administration of G-CSF is recommended in subsequent cycles

**Table 12.3** VIP regimen (Nichols et al. 1998)

| Agent | Doses (mg/m²) | Application | Application days |
|---|---|---|---|
| Cisplatin | 20 | 30 min-Infusion | Days 1–5 |
| Etoposide | 75 | 1 h-Infusion | Days 1–5 |
| Ifosfamide | 1,200 | 1 h-Infusion | Days 1–5 |
| Mesna | 400 | Bolus | Hours 0, 4, 8 days 1–5 |

Repeat day 22:

Repeat day 22 regardless of neutrophil count. Daily blood counts, if still neutropenic on day 4, avoid etoposide and ifosfamide on day 5

Delay only if neutropenic fever or platelets <100,000/μl on day 22

Dose reductions of etoposide and ifosfamide (no dose reduction for cisplatin) in the subsequent cycles only if neutropenic fever or thrombocytic bleeding developed in the previous course

G-CSF prophylaxis is recommended with the VIP regimen

Mesna prophylaxis mandatory

the etoposide-based treatment better tolerated, but BEP was also significantly more effective in the unfavorable group of patients. Unfortunately, this trial reported in 1987 was the last significant therapeutic advance to be documented in mature phase III trials for patients who presented with poor-risk features. Since then, four cycles of BEP have served as the standard of care for patients with poor prognostic features resulting in an unsatisfactory cure rate of only approximately 45–50%. A number of different treatment strategies have been tested in the past decade in order to improve these results (Tables 12.2–12.4).

The impact of high-dose cisplatin therapy in disseminated germ cell cancer was tested in a trial of the South Eastern Cancer Study Group (SECSG) and the Southwest Oncology Group (SWOG) (Nichols et al. 1991). This trial randomized patients with advanced disease according to the Indiana classification to either standard BEP with a cumulative cisplatin dose of 100 mg/m² per cycle or BEP with a cumulative cisplatin dose of 200 mg/m² per cycle. There was no survival advantage for high-dose cisplatin with regard to event-free and overall survival rates and, as expected, treatment with high-dose cisplatin combinations was significantly more toxic. In a subsequent trial to the SECSG study, the ECOG tested the substitution of ifosfamide for bleomycin (Nichols et al. 1998). Three-hundred and four patients with Indiana classification advanced disease were randomly allocated to either four cycles of BEP or four cycles of VIP. The results were strikingly similar to the SECSG study with 74% of patients alive and 64% failure-free in the VIP arm after 2 years as compared to 71% of patients being alive and 60% failure-free in the BEP arm. This study was reported a second time with long-term follow-up and with patients being re-classified according to the IGCCCG criteria (Hinton et al. 2003). Again, no difference was observed for patients with IGCCCG poor prognostic features. A significant higher myelotoxicity rate with approximately 90% grade 3/4 toxicity was observed in the VIP group for which granulocyte colony stimulating factor (G-CSF) was added when it became available in 1991. On the basis of this trial, four cycles of VIP are considered an accepted alternative to four cycles of BEP for patients with intermediate or poor prognostic criteria according to the IGCCCG classification.

Alternating regimens have also been investigated. In an EORTC/MRC trial, BEP as standard therapy was compared to a schedule-dense combination of bleomycin, oncovin (vincristine), and cisplatin followed by etoposide, ifosfamide, cisplatin, and bleomycin (BOP-VIP-B) (Kaye et al. 1998). The toxicity of the experimental arm was substantial, and, again, no improvement in survival was shown compared with standard BEP.

In recent years, dose-intensified therapy has increasingly been explored in patients with poor-prognosis criteria, in particular high-dose chemotherapy with autologous stem cell transplantation (ASCT). The rationale for high-dose chemotherapy is on the basis of the hypothesis of a dose–response relationship, in particular of carboplatin, etoposide, and cyclophosphamide/ifosfamide (Elias et al. 1991; Wolff et al. 1984). In addition, early dose intensification within sequential high-dose

**Table 12.4** Selected randomized studies in patients with poor-prognosis nonseminoma

| Author | Classification | Regime | Study objective | Continuous CR/PR- rate | Conclusion |
|---|---|---|---|---|---|
| Williams et al. (1987) | Indiana | PVB × 4<br>BEP × 4 | Substitution of vinblastin for etoposide | 38<br>63 | BEP × 4 superior to PVB × 4 |
| Ozols et al. (1988) | NCI | PVB × 4 | Increase cisplatin dose intensity | 67 | PVB inferior |
| | | P(200)EBV × 4 | Addition of etoposide | 88 | |
| Nichols et al. (1991) | Indiana | BEP × 4<br>BEP(200) × 4 | Increase cisplatin dose intensity | 73<br>68 | Equally effective |
| Wozniak et al. (1991) | SWOG | PVB × 4<br>PEV × 4 | Substitution of bleomycin for etoposide | 77<br>73 | Equally effective |
| de Wit et al. (1995) | EORTC | BEP × 4<br>PVB/BEP × 2 | Alternating regimen | 72<br>76 | Equally effective |
| Kaye et al. (1998) | MRC/EORTC | BEP × 6<br>BOP/VIP-B × 3 | Increased number of cycles, alternating regimen | 57<br>54 | Equally effective |
| Nichols et al. (1998)<br>Hinton et al. (2003) | Indiana (IGCCCG) | BEP × 4<br>VIP × 4 | Substitution of bleomycin for ifosfamide | 58 (49)<br>64 (56) | Equally effective |
| Motzer et al. (2007) | IGCCCG | BEP × 4<br>BEP × 2 + HD-CEC × 2 | Increase in dose intensity using high-dose chemotherapy with ASCT | 48<br>52 | Equally effective (possible advantage for patients with unsatisfactory marker decrease) |

*CISCA/VB* cyclophosphamide, doxorubicin, cisplatin, vinblastin, bleomycin; *P* cisplatin; *V* vinblastin; *B* bleomycin; *E* etoposide; *I* ifosfamide; *O* vincristin; *BOP-VIP-B* cisplatin, oncovin (vincristine), bleomycin – etoposide, ifosfamide, cisplatin, bleomycin; *CR* complete remission; *PR* partial remission; *Indiana* Classification System of the Indiana University, Indianapolis, USA; *EORTC* European Organization on Research and Treatment of Cancer; *MRC* Medical Research Council, UK; *NCI* National Cancer Institute, USA; *SWOG* Southwest Oncology Group, USA; *IGCCCG* International Germ Cell Cancer Consensus Group; *HD-CEC* high dose carboplatin, etoposide, cyclophosphamide; *ASCT* autologous stem cell transplantation

regimens may prevent the development of drug resistance, in particular in patients with extensive disease. Within a phase I/II study investigating a regimen consisting of one standard VIP cycle followed by three consecutive high-dose cycles of carboplatin, etoposide, and ifosfamide, the German Testicular Cancer Study Group reported very promising results with long-term cure rates of approximately 75% among poor-prognosis patients (Schmoll et al. 2003). In a retrospective matched pair analysis including patients from the afore mentioned phase I/II study as well as patients from two US randomized trials, the benefit of sequential high-dose chemotherapy was estimated to be in the range of 10–15% (Bokemeyer et al. 1999). Motzer et al. (1993) also reported very favorable results for tandem high dose chemotherapy in patients with poor prognostic features within a phase II study. Two randomized studies have been initiated. An EORTC study randomizes patients to either four cycles of standard VIP or one standard VIP cycle followed by three consecutive high-dose VIP cycles. No results have yet been reported. An US Intergroup study allocated patients to four cycles of standard BEP or two cycles of standard BEP followed by two cycles of high-dose carboplatin, etoposide, and cyclophosphamide. No difference was observed in the whole group of patients with respect to the 1-year durable CR rates of 49 and 56% in the standard BEP and experimental high-dose chemotherapy group, respectively (Motzer et al. 2007). Patients with an unsatisfactory marker decline during days 7–49 appeared to have a significantly worse outcome compared to patients with a timely marker decrease. Within a subgroup analysis, high-dose chemotherapy seemed to improve the outcome for patients with unsatisfactory marker decrease.

In summary, neither an increased dose-intensity nor high-dose chemotherapy with autologous stem cell support has yet demonstrated superiority over four cycles of BEP in a randomized trial. In addition, the toxicity of most of these regimens was significantly higher as compared to that of BEP. Four cycles of BEP therefore remain the standard of care for IGCCCG poor-prognosis patients with four cycles of VIP being an accepted alternative, in particular in patients with pre-existing lung problems or extensive lung disease and the expectancy of extensive surgery for residual lesions. Alternating chemotherapy regimens as new agents are currently tested, but no results from larger studies are yet available.

## 12.3 Practical Aspects of Chemotherapy for Metastatic Testicular Cancer

Chemotherapy should be given without dose reductions in 21-day intervals. Courses are to begin on schedule regardless of the degree of neutropenia noted on the day of scheduled treatment. If granulocytopenia was present on day 1 of a scheduled BEP course, complete blood cell counts should be obtained on day 4 to ensure adequate granulocyte recovery. If this does not occur, the fifth day of VP-16 should be deleted and single-agent cisplatin only administered on day 5. Postponing treatment, i.e. maximal of 3 days for each decision, should only be considered in cases of existing fever, or platelets <100,000/μl at day 1 of a subsequent cycle. There is no indication for routine prophylactic application of hematopoietic growth factors, such as G-CSF. However, if serious infectious complications or prolonged neutropenia has occurred during one preceding chemotherapy cycle, prophylactic administration of G-CSF is recommended in subsequent cycles (Tables 12.2 and 12.3).

In patients with poor performance status, extensive and symptomatic liver, or lung metastases, a dose reduced introduction cycle e.g., 3 day BEP, prior to four cycles of full dose BEP or VIP, is often used in order to decrease the risk of severe complications. It is important to emphasize that both the BEP and VIP regimen are continued on day 22 irrespective of blood counts. Only in case of neutropenic fever or severe thrombocytopenia, a treatment delay may be discussed.

It is essential to note, that all patients with advanced germ cell cancer must be treated by experts in experienced centers. Several studies have clearly demonstrated a significant relationship between survival and the experience of the treating institution/treating expert. Within the EORTC/MRC 30985/TE13 study, patients treated at less experienced centers had a doubled mortality risk as compared to patients treated at experienced centers (Collette et al. 1999). This was confirmed by similar study results from the Memorial Sloan Kettering Cancer Center as well as from Scandinavia (Feuer et al. 1999).

### 12.3.1 Management of Patients with Brain Metastases

The CNS is a rare site of metastatic disease in patients with germ-cell tumors. While only 2–3% of all patients with metastatic germ-cell tumor have brain metastases at initial diagnosis, approximately 10–15% of patients with advanced disease are metastasized to the brain (Spears et al. 1992; Clemm et al. 1993). A screening brain CT scan is therefore justified in these patients prior to treatment start. Despite initial brain metastases, a long-term cure rate of up to 40% can be achieved with multimodality therapy. The best prognostic group consists of patients with a solitary brain lesion detected at initial presentation (Mead 1997; Bokemeyer et al. 1997; Fossa et al. 1999). Those patients who develop brain metastases during or at relapse after initial cisplatin-based chemotherapy display a particularly dismal prognosis and very few will achieve long-term survival.

The best sequence of all three treatment modalities, chemotherapy, radiation, and surgery, has not been conclusively defined. If patients are asymptomatic, chemotherapy should be initiated and radiation therapy should be added after completion of chemotherapy. Standard chemotherapy consists of four cycles of either BEP or VIP. It has been shown that cisplatin, etoposide, cyclophosphamide, and ifosfamide are able to penetrate the blood-brain-barrier in the presence of brain lesions (Ginsberg et al. 1981; Kobayashi et al. 1989; Stewart et al. 1983). Partial and complete responses in the brain can be achieved with chemotherapy alone in these patients. To date several studies have investigated the activity of chemotherapy in patients with GCT brain metastases at initial diagnosis. Rustin treated ten patients with brain metastases of nonseminomatous GCT with a combination of vincristine, methotrexate, bleomycin, cisplatin, dactinomycin, cyclophosphamide, and etoposide (POMB/ACE) accompanied by intrathecal therapy with methotrexate (Rustin et al. 1989). Eight of the ten patients responded and five of them stayed in CR for more than 18 months. Radiation therapy has been regarded an essential part of the treatment for brain metastases from germ cell tumors (Spears et al. 1992; Bokemeyer et al. 1997; Raghavan et al. 1987). Radiation therapy is usually given as whole brain radiation with 40–45 Gy, with a tumor boost up to 50 Gy if indicated. It is currently unclear whether consolidating radiation is necessary in patients with a CR to chemotherapy in the brain. Within a large multinational study including 56 newly diagnosed patients with primary CNS involvement, radiation therapy showed no significant impact on survival of these patients in a multivariate analysis (Fossa et al. 1999). In contrast, a retrospective analysis from Germany suggested a benefit from additional radiation (Hartmann et al. 2003). Cranial irradiation can cause permanent neurologic impairment such as worsening of cognitive function, which is a major concern in young patients (van Dam et al. 1998; Crossen et al. 1994). Patients with symptomatic brain metastases should undergo combined chemo- and radiation therapy. Primary surgical resection should be restricted to those patients, who are unable to receive chemotherapy because of symptoms caused by their brain metastases.

In patients with good response to chemotherapy and a limited number of brain metastases, resection of residual lesions without radiation can be considered, but subsequent close observation is mandatory (Spears et al. 1992; Bokemeyer et al. 1997; Logothetis et al. 1982). Radiosurgery may represent another potentially valuable treatment option for patients with a limited number of brain metastases.

For patients with a CNS only relapse, who represent a prognostically unfavorable group, radiation and four cycles of salvage chemotherapy should be given in order to achieve the maximum treatment effect.

### 12.3.2 Residual Tumor Resection After Chemotherapy for Metastatic Disease in Patients with Nonseminomatous Germ Cell Tumors

Depending on the initial stage of the disease, 20–50% of patients with disseminated germ cell cancer will have postchemotherapy residual masses. Resection of residual masses should be considered in all patients with normalized serum tumor markers AFP and HCG in order to remove residual teratoma or viable cancer (Toner et al. 1990; Stephenson et al. 2005). Complete resection of residual teratomas is important because persistent teratomas may progress to invade adjacent structures and are associated with the risk for malignant transformation in non-germ cell malignancies such as sarcomas or carcinomas. Persistent teratoma has also been associated with an increased risk for late relapse (Stephenson et al. 2005). Postchemotherapy surgery should be performed 6–8 weeks after the end of their last cycle. Prior to surgery, repeat imaging should be performed as continued involution of residual masses may occur and make resection unnecessary. Patients who have received bleomycin during induction chemotherapy need special management. They may have subtle pulmonary changes as well as a diminished carbon monoxide diffusion capacity. Overhydration should be avoided during anesthesia and colloid fluids should be used for fluid replacement rather than crystalloid fluids. Of most importance, inspired oxygen concentration should not exceed 25% in the intraoperative and the postoperative phase in order to avoid lung injury. Patients with complete remission (complete resolution of lesions or residual lesion < 1 cm) can be safely observed (Kollmannsberger et al. 2010)

Pathology of residual masses after first-line chemotherapy will reveal necrosis, mature teratoma, and vital cancer in about 60%, 30%, and 10–15% of patients, respectively. If technically feasible, all residual masses should be resected. In patients with residual masses at multiples sites, an individual decision should be made regarding the number and extent of resections (Oldenburg et al. 2003). Decisions on the extent of surgery should be on the basis of the risk of relapse of an individual patient and of quality-of-life issues (Steyerberg et al. 1999; Herr 1997).

The pathological findings of the surgical specimen help to guide additional treatment decisions. Resection of residual tumors outside the abdomen or lung should also be considered on an individual basis, as discordance in histology is found in 35–50% of patients (Hendry et al. 1980; Hartmann et al. 1997). If the histology of the primarily resected mass is only necrosis, both, surveillance of the remaining residual lesions and their complete resection are acceptable therapeutic options. Because of the high treatment-related acute morbidity, surgery of residual masses should be performed at specialized centers (Schmoll et al. 2004; Nichols 2001).

After resection of necrosis or mature teratoma, no further treatment is required. In cases of vital carcinoma or immature teratoma, the role of further consolidation chemotherapy is equivocal. A retrospective analysis demonstrated an improved progression-free survival with adjuvant chemotherapy, but failed to show an improvement in overall survival (Fizazi et al. 2001). Therefore a "wait-and watch" strategy may also be justified. Patients in the "good" prognosis group, according to the IGCCCG classification, with complete resection of residual masses and with <10% vital tumor cells in the resected specimens have a favorable outcome even without adjuvant chemotherapy (Fizazi et al. 2001). If the completely resected mass contains >10% of viable cancer, or if completeness of the resection is in doubt, consolidation chemotherapy might be justified. If additional chemotherapy is given, the cumulative dose of bleomycin has to be considered. Usually, two more cycles of cisplatin-based chemotherapy, preferably a different regimen than the initially used regimen, should be administered.

Liver metastases present a particular problem. A high portion of teratoma and vital carcinoma have been reported in resected liver lesions. In addition, a significant number of patients appear to have varying histological results, mostly more unfavorable histologies, in the liver as compared with that in other localizations such as the retroperitoneum (Hahn et al. 1999; Rivoire et al. 2001).

A number of investigators have attempted to develop models for the prediction of the presence of necrosis in an effort to obviate surgery (Steyerberg et al. 1999; Albers et al. 2004). A number of variables predictive of necrosis have been identified and tested prospectively, including degree of tumor shrinkage, size of pre- and post-treatment mass(es), prechemotherapy markers, and teratomatous components in the orchiectomy specimen. However, the risk for a false-negative prediction remains approximately 20%, and thus, these risk factors are not discriminative enough for clinical use (Sheinfeld 2002).

## References

Albers P, Weissbach L, Krege S et al (2004) Predictions of necrosis after chemotherapy of advanced germ cell tumors: results of a prospective multicenter trial of the German Testicular Cancer Study Group. J Urol 171:1835–1838

Bajorin DF, Sarosdy MF, Pfister DG et al (1993) Randomized trial of etoposide and cisplatin versus etoposide and carboplatin in patients with good-risk germ cell tumors: a multiinstitutional study. J Clin Oncol 11:598–606

Bokemeyer C, Beyer J, Metzner B et al (1996a) Phase II study of paclitaxel in patients with relapsed or cisplatin-refractory testicular cancer. Ann Oncol 7:31–34

Bokemeyer C, Kohrmann O, Tischler J et al (1996b) A randomized trial of cisplatin, etoposide and bleomycin (PEB) versus carboplatin, etoposide and bleomycin (CEB) for patients with 'good-risk' metastatic non-seminomatous germ cell tumors. Ann Oncol 7:1015–1021

Bokemeyer C, Nowak P, Haupt A et al (1997) Treatment of brain metastases in patients with testicular cancer. J Clin Oncol 15:1449–1454

Bokemeyer C, Kollmannsberger C, Meisner C et al (1999) First-line high-dose chemotherapy compared to standard-dose PEB/VIP chemotherapy in patients with advanced germ cell tumors: a multivariate and matched pair analysis. J Clin Oncol 17:3450–3456

Bokemeyer C, Kollmannsberger C, Flechon A et al (2002) Prognostic factors in patients (pts) with advanced seminoma (SEM) treated with either single agent carboplatin (CP) or cisplatin-based (DDP) combination chemotherapy (CTX): a meta-analysis of prospective European trials. Proc Am Soc Clin Oncol 21:186a (abstract 740)

Bosl GJ, Geller NL, Bajorin D et al (1988) A randomized trial of etoposide + cisplatin versus vinblastine + bleomycin + cisplatin + cyclophosphamide + dactinomycin in patients with good-prognosis germ cell tumors. J Clin Oncol 6: 1231–1238

Clemm C, Gerl A, Wendt TG et al (1993) Current status of therapy of CNS metastases of germ cell tumors. Urologe A 32: 217–224

Collette L, Sylvester RJ, Stenning SP et al; European Organization for Research and Treatment of Cancer Genito-Urinary Tract Cancer Collaborative Group and the Medical Research Council Testicular Cancer Working Party (1999) Impact of the treating institution on survival of patients with "poor-prognosis" metastatic nonseminoma [see comments]. J Natl Cancer Inst 91:839–846

Crossen JR, Garwood D, Glatstein E, Neuwelt EA (1994) Neurobehavioral sequelae of cranial irradiation in adults: a review of radiation-induced encephalopathy. J Clin Oncol 12:627–642

Culine S, Kerbrat P, Kramar A et al (2007) Refining the optimal chemotherapy regimen for good-risk metastatic non-seminomatous germ cell tumors: a randomized trial of the Genito-Urinary Group of the French Federations of Cancer Centers (GETUG T93BP). Ann Oncol 18:917–924

Donohue J, Einhorn L, Perez JM (1978) Improved management of nonseminomatous testis tumors. Cancer 42:2903–2908

Einhorn LH, Williams SD, Loehrer PJ et al (1989) Evaluation of optimal duration of chemotherapy in favorable-prognosis

disseminated germ cell tumors: a Southeastern Cancer Study Group protocol. J Clin Oncol 7:387–391
Elias A, Ayash L, Eder JP et al (1991) A phase-I study of high-dose ifosfamide and escalating doses of carboplatin with autologous bone marrow support. J Clin Oncol 9:320–327
Feuer EJ, Sheinfeld J, Bosl G (1999) Does size matter? Association between number of patients treated and patient outcome in metastatic testicular cancer. J Natl Cancer Inst 91: 816–818
Fizazi K, Tjulandin S, Salvioni R et al (2001) Viable malignant cells after primary chemotherapy for disseminated nonseminomatous germ cell tumors: prognostic factors and role of postsurgery chemotherapy – results from an International Study Group. J Clin Oncol 19:2647–2657
Fossa SD, Bokemeyer C, Gerl A et al (1999) Treatment outcome of patients with brain metastases from malignant germ cell tumors. Cancer 85:988–997
Fossa SD, De Wit R, Roberts JT et al (2003) Quality of life in good prognosis patients with metastatic germ cell cancer: a Prospective Study of the European Organization for Research and Treatment of Cancer Genitourinary Group/Medical Research Council Testicular Cancer Study Group (30941/TE20). J Clin Oncol 21:1107–1118
Ginsberg S, Kirshner J, Reich S et al (1981) Systemic chemotherapy for a primary germ cell tumor of the brain: a pharmacokinetic study. Cancer Treat Rep 65:477–483
Hahn TL, Jacobson L, Einhorn LH et al (1999) Hepatic resection of metastatic testicular carcinoma: a further update. Ann Surg Oncol 6:640–644
Hartmann JT, Candelaria M, Kuczyk MA et al (1997) Comparison of histological results from the resection of residual masses at different sites after chemotherapy for metastatic non-seminomatous germ cell tumours. Eur J Cancer 33:843–847
Hartmann JT, Bamberg M, Albers P et al (2003) Multidisciplinary treatment and prognosis of patients (pts) with central nervous system metastases (CNS) from testicular germ cell tumor (GCT) origin. Proc Am Soc Clin Oncol 22:abstract 1607
Hendry WF, Barrett A, McElwain TJ et al (1980) The role of surgery in the combined management of metastases from malignant teratomas of testis. Br J Urol 52:38–44
Herr HW (1997) Does necrosis on frozen-section analysis of a mass after chemotherapy justify a limited retroperitoneal resection in patients with advanced testis cancer? Br J Urol 80:653–657
Hinton S, Catalano PJ, Einhorn L et al (2003) Cisplatin, etoposide and either bleomycin or ifosfamide in the treatment of disseminated germ cell tumors. Cancer 97:1869–1875
Horwich A, Sleijfer DT, Fossa SD et al (1997) Randomized trial of bleomycin, etoposide, and cisplatin compared with bleomycin, etoposide, and carboplatin in good-prognosis metastatic nonseminomatous germ cell cancer: a Multiinstitutional Medical Research Council/European Organization for Research and Treatment of Cancer Trial. J Clin Oncol 15:1844–1852
Horwich A, Huddart R, Dearnaley D (1998) Markers and management of germ-cell tumours of the testes. Lancet 352: 1535–1538
Horwich A, Oliver RT, Wilkinson PM et al; MRC Testicular Tumour Working Party (2000) A medical research council randomized trial of single agent carboplatin versus etoposide and cisplatin for advanced metastatic seminoma. Br J Cancer 83:1623–1629
Kaye SB, Mead GM, Fossa SD et al (1998) Intensive induction-sequential chemotherapy with BOP/VIP-B compared with treatment with BEP/EP for poor prognosis metastatic nonseminomatous germ cell tumor: a randomized Medical Research Council/European Organization for Research and Treatment of Cancer study. J Clin Oncol 16:692–701
Kobayashi T, Yoshida J, Ishiyama J (1989) Combination chemotherapy with cisplatin and etoposide for malignant intracranial germ cell tumors. J Neurosurg 70:676–681
Kollmannsberger C, Daneshmand S, So A et al (2010) Management of disseminated nonseminomatous germ cell tumors with risk-based chemotherapy followed by response guided postchemotherapy surgery. J Clin Oncol 28:537–542
Kondagunta VG, Bacik J, Bajorin D et al (2005) Etoposide and cisplatin chemotherapy for metastatic good-risk germ cell tumors. J Clin Oncol 23:9290–9294
Kuczyk M, Machtens S, Stief C, Jonas U (1999) Management of the post-chemotherapy residual mass in patients with advanced stage non-seminomatous germ cell tumors (NSGCT). Int J Cancer 83:852–855
Loehrer-PJ S, Johnson D, Elson P et al (1995) Importance of bleomycin in favorable-prognosis disseminated germ cell tumors: an Eastern Cooperative Oncology Group trial. J Clin Oncol 13:470–476
Logothetis C, Samuels ML, Trindade A (1982) The management of brain metastases in germ cell tumors. Cancer 49:12–18
Mead G; International Germ Cell Cancer Collaborative Group (1997) International Germ Cell Consensus Classification: a prognostic factor-based staging system for metastatic germ cell cancers. J Clin Oncol 15:594–603
Motzer RJ, Mazumdar M, Gulati SC et al (1993) Phase II trial of high-dose carboplatin and etoposide with autologous bone marrow transplantation in first-line therapy for patients with poor-risk germ cell tumors. J Natl Cancer Inst 85: 1828–1835
Motzer RJ, Bajorin D, Schwartz LH et al (1994) Phase II trial of paclitaxel shows antitumor activity in patients with previously treated germ cell tumors. J Clin Oncol 12: 2277–2283
Motzer RJ, Nichols C, Margolin KA et al (2007) Phase III randomized trial of conventional-dose chemotherapy with or without high-dose chemotherapy and autologous hematopoietic stem-cell rescue as first-line treatment for patients with poor-prognosis metastatic germ cell tumors. J Clin Oncol 25:247–256
Nichols C (2001) Chemotherapy of disseminated germ cell tumors. World J Urol 19:82–89
Nichols CR, Williams SD, Loehrer PJ et al (1991) Randomized study of cisplatin dose intensity in poor-risk germ cell tumors: a Southeastern Cancer Study Group and Southwest Oncology Group protocol. J Clin Oncol 9:1163–1172
Nichols CR, Catalano PJ, Crawford ED et al (1998) Randomized comparison of cisplatin and etoposide and either bleomycin or ifosfamide in treatment of advanced disseminated germ cell tumors: an Eastern Cooperative Oncology Group, Southwest Oncology Group, and Cancer and Leukemia Group B Study. J Clin Oncol 16:1287–1293
Oldenburg J, Alfsen GC, Lien HH et al (2003) Postchemotherapy retroperitoneal surgery remains necessary in patients with nonseminomatous testicular cancer and minimal residual tumor masses. J Clin Oncol 21:3310–3317

Ozols RF, Ihde DC, Linehan WM et al (1988) A randomized trial of standard chemotherapy versus a high-dose chemotherapy regimen in the treatment of poor prognosis nonseminomatous germ-cell tumors. J Clin Oncol 6:1031–1040

Raghavan D, Mackintosh JF, Fox RM et al (1987) Improved survival after brain metastases in non-seminomatous germ cell tumours with combined modality treatment. Br J Urol 60:364–367

Rivoire M, Elias D, De Cian F et al (2001) Multimodality treatment of patients with liver metastases from germ cell tumors: the role of surgery. Cancer 92:578–587

Rustin GJ, Newlands ES, Begent RH et al (1989) Weekly alternating etoposide, methotrexate, and actinomycin/vincristine and cyclophosphamide chemotherapy for the treatment of CNS metastases of chorioncarcinoma. J Clin Oncol 7:900–903

Saxman SB, Finch D, Gonin R, Einhorn LH (1998) Long-term follow-up of a phase III study of three versus four cycles of bleomycin, etoposide, and cisplatin in favorable-prognosis germ-cell tumors: the Indiana University experience. J Clin Oncol 16:702–706

Schmoll H-J, Kollmannsberger C, Metzner B et al (2003) Long-term results of first-line sequential high-dose etoposide, ifosfamide, and cisplatin chemotherapy plus autologous stem cell support for patients with advanced metastatic germ cell cancer: an Extended Phase I/II Study of the German Testicular Cancer Study Group. J Clin Oncol 21:4083–4091

Schmoll HJ, Souchon R, Krege S et al (2004) European consensus on diagnosis and treatment of germ cell cancer: a report of the European Germ Cell Cancer Consensus Group (EGCCCG). Ann Oncol 15:1377–1399

Sheinfeld J (2002) The role of adjunctive postchemotherapy surgery for nonseminomatous germ-cell tumors: current concepts and controversies. Semin Urol Oncol 20:262–271

Sonneveld DJ, Hoekstra HJ, van der GW et al (2001a) Improved long term survival of patients with metastatic nonseminomatous testicular germ cell carcinoma in relation to prognostic classification systems during the cisplatin era. Cancer 91: 1304–1315

Sonneveld DJ, Hoekstra HJ, van der Graaf WT et al (2001b) Improved long term survival of patients with metastatic nonseminomatous testicular germ cell carcinoma in relation to prognostic classification systems during the cisplatin era. Cancer 91:1304–1315

Spears WT, Morphis JG, Lester SG et al (1992) Brain metastases and testicular tumors: long-term survival. Int J Radiat Oncol Biol Phys 22:17–22

Stephenson AJ, Bosl G, Motzer R et al (2005) Retroperitoneal lymph node dissection for nonseminomatous germ cell testicular cancer: impact of patient selection factors on outcome. J Clin Oncol 23:2781–2788

Stewart OJ, Richard M, Hugenholtz H, Dennery J (1983) VP-16 (VP) and VM-26 (VM) penetration into human brain tumors (BT). Proc Am Assoc Cancer Res 24:133

Steyerberg EW, Keizer HJ, Habbema JD; ReHiT Study Group (1999) Prediction models for the histology of residual masses after chemotherapy for metastatic testicular cancer. Int J Cancer 83:856–859

Toner GC, Panicek DM, Heelan RT et al (1990) Adjunctive surgery after chemotherapy for nonseminomatous germ cell tumors: recommendations for patient selection. J Clin Oncol 8:1683–1694

Toner GC, Stockler MR, Boyer MJ et al; Australian and New Zealand Germ Cell Trial Group (2001) Comparison of two standard chemotherapy regimens for good-prognosis germ-cell tumours: a randomised trial. Lancet 357:739–745

van Dam FS, Schlagen SB, Muller MJ et al (1998) Impairment of cognitive function in women receiving adjuvant treatment for high-risk breast cancer: high-dose versus standard-dose chemotherapy. J Natl Cancer Inst 90:210–218

Weissbach L, Bussar MR, Flechtner H et al (2000) RPLND or primary chemotherapy in clinical stage IIA/B nonseminomatous germ cell tumors? Results of a prospective multicenter trial including quality of life assessment. Eur Urol 37: 582–594

Williams SD, Birch R, Einhorn LH et al (1987) Treatment of disseminated germ-cell tumors with cisplatin, bleomycin, and either vinblastine or etoposide. N Engl J Med 316: 1435–1440

de Wit R, Stoter G, Sleijfer DT et al (1995) Four cycles of BEP versus an alternating regime of PVB and BEP in patients with poor-prognosis metastatic testicular non-seminoma; a randomised study of the EORTC Genitourinary Tract Cancer Cooperative Group. Br J Cancer 71:1311–1314

de Wit R, Stoter G, Kaye SB et al (1997) Importance of bleomycin in combination chemotherapy for good-prognosis testicular nonseminoma: a randomized study of the European Organization for Research and Treatment of Cancer Genitourinary Tract Cancer Cooperative Group. J Clin Oncol 15:1837–1843

de Wit R, Stoter G, Sleijfer DT et al (1998) Four cycles of BEP vs four cycles of VIP in patients with intermediate-prognosis metastatic testicular non-seminoma: a randomized study of the EORTC Genitourinary Tract Cancer Cooperative Group. European Organization for Research and Treatment of Cancer. Br J Cancer 78:828–832

de Wit R, Louwerens M, de Mulder PHM et al (1999) Management of intermediate prognosis germ cell cancer: results of a phase I/II study of taxol-BEP. Int J Cancer 83:831–833

de Wit R, Roberts JT, Wilkinson P et al (2001) Equivalence of three or four cycles of bleomycin, etoposide, and cisplatin chemotherapy and of a 3- or 5-day schedule in good-prognosis germ cell cancer: a randomized study of the European Organization for Research and Treatment of Cancer Genitourinary Tract Cancer Cooperative Group and the Medical Research Council. J Clin Oncol 19:1629–1640

Wolff SN, Johnson DH, Hainsworth JD, Greco FA (1984) High-dose VP-16-213 monotherapy for refractory germinal malignancies: a phase II study. J Clin Oncol 2:271–274

Wozniak AJ, Samson MK, Shah NT et al (1991) A randomized trial of cisplatin, vinblastine, and bleomycin versus vinblastine, cisplatin, and etoposide in the treatment of advanced germ cell tumors of the testis: a Southwest Oncology Group study. J Clin Oncol 9:70–76

# Stage II Seminoma and Advanced Disease

13

Padraig R. Warde and Alan Horwich

## 13.1 Introduction

The vast majority patients with testicular seminoma present with early stage disease (Stage I) and are managed successfully by adjuvant radiotherapy, carboplatin or by surveillance. Fifteen to twenty percent of patients have infradiaphragmatic lymph node involvement on radiologic investigation at diagnosis (Stage II disease) and less than 5% of patients present with distant metastatic disease.

Postorchidectomy treatment options in patients with Stage II seminoma include RT, chemotherapy and in rare cases retroperiteonal node dissection. RT is the treatment of choice in patients with low bulk disease (most patients with Stage IIA/B disease) and cisplatin-based chemotherapy regimens is used in patients with more advanced disease. Cure rates in modern series are in excess of 95% and as in Stage I disease, minimizing toxicity of treatment while not compromising cure is the main current challenge for physicians dealing with these patients. Since relapses from Stage I and Stage IIA/B are rare and presentation of seminoma with disseminated metastases is also uncommon, the chemotherapy of seminoma has developed mainly in parallel with that for non seminomatous germ cell tumors. However, there are important differences including the extreme sensitivity of seminoma to platinum drugs, the lack of clear evidence of benefit from incorporation of bleomycin, and the assessment and management of residual masses.

Radiation therapy has a small role in patients with more advanced disease, very occasionally for salvage after failure of chemotherapy but mostly in palliative management of metastatic disease. In patients with brain metastases RT can be curative in a small proportion of cases.

## 13.2 Staging

The American Joint Committee on Cancer and International Union against Cancer staging classification for testicular tumors is shown in Table 13.1 (Greene et al. 2002; Sobin and Wittekind 2002). Stage II patients (retroperiteonal lymph node involvement) are subdivided into three substages based on the maximum transverse diameter of the largest lymph node mass: Stage IIA ≤2 cm, Stage IIB >2–5 cm, Stage IIC >5 cm. Routine staging investigations following orchidectomy include abdominopelvic computed tomography (CT) scan, chest CT and serum tumor markers (α-fetoprotein (AFP), beta human chorionic gonadotrophin (β-HCG)). There is no proven role for the use of positron emission tomography (PET) in the initial assessment of patients with seminoma but it may be useful in staging patients with Stage II disease after treatment with chemotherapy (Becherer et al. 2005; Cremerius et al. 1998; Ganjoo et al. 1999; Spermon et al. 2002).

## 13.3 Stage II Disease

Approximately 70% of Stage II patients have Stage IIA/B disease at presentation with lymph nodes that are less than 5 cm in greatest transverse diameter. The vast majority of these have low bulk disease with nodal

P.R. Warde (✉)
Department of Radiation Oncology, Princess Margaret Hospital, Toronto, ON, Canada

M.P. Laguna et al. (eds.), *Cancer of the Testis*,
DOI: 10.1007/978-1-84800-370-5_13, © Springer-Verlag London Limited 2010

**Table 13.1** UICC/AJCC staging of testis cancer 2003

| | |
|---|---|
| *Primary tumor* | |
| The extent of primary tumor is classified after radical orchidectomy | |
| pTX | Primary tumor cannot be assessed (if no radical orchidectomy has been performed, Tx is used) |
| pT0 | No evidence of primary tumor (e.g., histologic scar in testis) |
| pTis | Intratubular germ cell neoplasia (carcinoma in situ) |
| pT1 | Tumor limited to the testis and epididymis without vascular/lymphatic invasion. Tumor may invade into the tunica albuginea but not the tunica vaginalis |
| pT2 | Tumor limited to the testis and epididymis with vascular/lymphatic invasion, or tumor extending through the tunica albuginea with involvement of the tunica vaginalis |
| pT3 | Tumor invades the spermatic cord with or without vascular/lymphatic invasion |
| pT4 | Tumor invades the scrotum with or without vascular/lymphatic invasion |
| *Regional lymph nodes (N)* | |
| Clinical | |
| NX | Regional lymph nodes cannot be assessed |
| N0 | No regional lymph node metastasis |
| N1 | Metastasis with a lymph node mass 2 cm or less in greatest dimension; or multiple lymph nodes, none more than 2 cm in greatest dimension |
| N2 | Metastasis with a lymph node mass, more than 2 cm but not more than 5 cm in greatest dimension; or multiple lymph nodes, any one mass greater than 2 cm but not more than 5 cm in greatest dimension |
| N3 | Metastasis with a lymph node mass more than 5 cm in greatest dimension |
| *Pathologic lymph nodes (pN)* | |
| pNX | Regional lymph nodes cannot be assessed |
| pN0 | No regional lymph node metastasis |
| pN1 | Metastasis with a lymph node mass, 2 cm or less in greatest dimension and less than or equal to five nodes positive, none more than 2 cm in greatest dimension |
| pN2 | Metastasis with a lymph node mass, more than 2 cm but not more than 5 cm in greatest dimension; or more than five nodes positive, none more than 5 cm; or evidence of extranodal extension of tumor |
| pN3 | Metastasis with a lymph node mass more than 5 cm in greatest dimension |
| *Distant metastasis (M)* | |
| MX | Distant metastasis cannot be assessed |
| M0 | No distant metastasis |
| M1 | Distant metastasis |
| M1a | Nonregional nodal or pulmonary metastasis |
| M1b | Nonpulmonary visceral metastasis |
| *Serum tumor markers (S)* | |
| SX | Marker studies not available or not performed |
| S0 | Marker study levels within normal limits |

**Table 13.1** (continued)

| | | | | |
|---|---|---|---|---|
| S1 | LDH < 1.5 × N and | | | |
| | HCG (mIu/mL) < 5,000 and | | | |
| | AFP (ng/mL) < 1,000 | | | |
| S2 | LDH 1.5–10 × N or | | | |
| | HCG (mIu/mL) 5,000–50,000 or | | | |
| | AFP (ng/mL) 1,000–10,000 | | | |
| S3 | LDH > 10 × N or | | | |
| | HCG (mIu/mL) >50,000 or | | | |
| | AFP (ng/mL) >10,000 | | | |
| N indicates the upper limit of normal for the LDH assay | | | | |
| *Stage grouping* | | | | |
| Stage 0 | pTis | N0 | M0 | S0 |
| Stage I | pT1-4 | N0 | M0 | SX |
| Stage IA | pT1 | N0 | M0 | S0 |
| Stage 1B | pT2 | N0 | M0 | S0 |
| | pT3 | N0 | M0 | S0 |
| | pT4 | N0 | M0 | S0 |
| Stage IS | Any T | N0 | M0 | S1–3 |
| Stage II | Any T | N1-3 | M0 | SX |
| Stage IIA | Any T | N1 | M0 | S0 |
| | Any T | N1 | M0 | S1 |
| Stage IIB | Any T | N2 | M0 | S0 |
| | Any T | N2 | M0 | S1 |
| Stage IIC | Any T | N3 | M0 | S0 |
| | Any T | N3 | M0 | S1 |
| Stage III | Any T | Any N | M1 | SX |
| Stage IIIA | Any T | Any N | M1a | S0 |
| | Any T | Any N | M1a | S1 |
| Stage IIIB | Any T | N1–3 | M0 | S2 |
| | Any T | Any N | M1a | S2 |
| Stage IIIC | Any T | N1-3 | M0 | S3 |
| | Any T | Any N | M1a | S3 |
| | Any T | Any N | M1B | Any S |

involvement extending over only 1–2 vertebral bodies. The incidence of Stage II disease is too small to mount phase III studies of management, and treatment decisions are mostly based on reports from single institutions where patients have been treated in a uniform fashion.

The most important prognostic factor in Stage II seminoma is the bulk of retroperitoneal tumor, measured as the transverse diameter of the largest lymph node or lymph node mass visible on CT scan. Lymph node size was the only factor that predicted recurrence in 95 patients with Stage II seminoma treated with radiotherapy at the PMH between 1981 and 1999 (Chung et al. 2004). The 5-year relapse-free rate in 79 patients with nodal disease of 5 cm (IIA/B) was 91% (7 of 79 patients), as compared to 44% (9 of 16 patients) in patients with bulkier disease (IIC). Recurrence occurred most commonly in mediastinal or supraclavicular lymph nodes, lung or bone. Thirteen patients were treated with chemotherapy at relapse, and nine were free of the disease at last follow-up. Two patients had salvage RT in the early 1980s (would now be treated with salvage chemotherapy) and 1 was free of disease on follow-up. These five patients plus one additional patient who refused salvage died of progressive seminoma. Thirty one patients (23 with nodal disease >5 cm) received initial chemotherapy for Stage II disease with two relapses, one of whom was salvaged by second line chemotherapy. These results are similar to other series in the literature (Table 13.2) and support the continued use of primary radiotherapy in Stage II patients with small bulk lymphadenopathy (Chung et al. 2004; Zagars and Pollack 2001; Vallis et al. 1995; Classen et al. 2003; Bayens et al. 1992). However, the high failure rate following radiotherapy in patients with bulky retroperitoneal disease, the fact that not all patients with recurrence were salvaged, and the apparently better outcome of similar patients who were treated with chemotherapy at diagnosis mandates primary chemotherapy instead of radiation in this population. In addition, RT to patients with retroperiteonal disease >5 cm in diameter may well compromise renal function as it may be necessary to treat substantial portions of the kidney to beyond renal parenchymal tolerance.

Staging should not be the only parameter used to decide on treatment of retroperitoneal disease in patients with Stage II seminoma. Tumor bulk must also be considered e.g., a patient with nodal disease extending 8–9 cm from L1 to L5 in the retroperitoneum with a maximum transverse diameter of 3.5 cm would be classified as having IIB disease. Patients with bulky disease such as this should be treated with chemotherapy rather than with RT. Other patient and tumor-related factors should also be taken into account. Lymph node masses that are situated laterally may necessitate irradiating a large volume of one or both kidneys or the liver in order to adequately encompass the tumor. The same situation may arise in cases of abnormal anatomy, such as with horseshoe or pelvic kidney. These patients are better treated with chemotherapy because of an unacceptably high risk of radiation toxicity. Those rare patients in whom radiotherapy and chemotherapy are contraindicated or in whom the diagnosis is uncertain should be considered for retroperitoneal lymph node dissection.

The technique of radiation in Stage II seminoma is similar to that used in Stage I disease. The treatment volume includes the gross tumor as well as the paraaortic and ipsilateral common and external iliac lymph nodes. The radiation dose is typically 25–30 Gy plus a boost of a further 5–10 Gy to the gross lymphadenopathy. At PMH, this boost is given concurrently with the large field treatment (25 Gy in 20 fractions + 10 Gy/20 fractions as boost). A CT scan with the patient in treatment position is used to ensure that the gross tumor is

**Table 13.2** Results of retroperitoneal RT in Stage II A/B seminoma

| References | Number of patients | Years of study | Number of relapse (%) | Cause-specific survival (%) |
|---|---|---|---|---|
| Bayens et al. (1992) | 29 | 1975–1985 | 7 (24%) | 93 |
| Chung et al. (2004) | 79 | 1981–1999 | 7 (8.8%) | 97.5 |
| Classen et al. (2003) | 87 | 1991–1994 | 4(4.6%) | 100 |
| Vallis et al. (1995) | 48 | 1974–1989 | 3 (6%) | 98 |
| Zagars and Pollack (2001) | 37 | 1984–1999 | 5(13.5%) | 100 |

adequately encompassed by the radiation fields and that the minimal possible volume of kidney and liver are irradiated. The contralateral iliac lymph nodes may also be treated in cases where lymphadenopathy in the low paraaortic area is deemed to increase the risk of these nodes being involved by tumor. However, this is probably of most concern in patients with bulky retroperitoneal lymphadenopathy who are better treated with primary chemotherapy as discussed previously. A recent study from Germany has suggested that lower radiation doses (30 Gy) may be sufficient for Stage IIA disease and that the lower border of the field may be set at the cranial rim of the acetabulum (Classen et al. 2003).

Adjuvant radiation of supraclavicular lymph nodes in patients with Stage II disease has been recommended by some although is not justified on a routine basis in view of the low risk of isolated supraclavicular recurrence (2/79 patients of patients with IIA/B disease in the PMH series) (Zagars and Pollack 2001; Chung et al. 2003). The ease with which supraclavicular lymph nodes can be followed clinically, the availability of effective salvage chemotherapy for these cases, the possibility of compromising bone marrow reserve for subsequent chemotherapy should it be necessary, as well as the potential for radiation-induced cardiac toxicity must be considered.

The use of combination carboplatin and radiation therapy in Stage IIA/B seminoma has been suggested by Patterson et al. (2001). This Royal Marsden study described a series of 30 patients treated with one course of carboplatin 4–6 weeks prior to radiation therapy. They reported a 5 year relapse survival rate of 96.9% as compared to 80.7% in a historical cohort (largely treated in the 1980s) treated with radiation alone. A major problem with interpreting the result is the possibility of stage migration improving the results in the combined therapy group suggested by the relatively low control rate with RT alone. This approach should not be accepted as routine practice without further data. A pilot study of 3–4 cycles of single agent carboplatin in 106 patients with Stage IIA/B seminoma concluded that this did not safely eradicate disease (Krege et al. 2006).

The commonest sites of recurrence following radiotherapy in Stage II patients are mediastinal or supraclavicular nodes, lung and bone. Most relapsing patients are cured with chemotherapy, which underscores the importance of regular follow-up with clinical examination and chest X-ray after radiation. CT imaging of the abdomen and pelvis is not necessary after complete resolution of abdominal disease. In the PMH series, 2 of the 7 patients who recurred after RT had bone metastases, and both presented with spinal cord compression as the first sign of recurrence. Therefore, all patients with unexplained back pain require a bone scan to exclude metastases, and those with new onset neurologic deficits require urgent imaging of the spine with magnetic resonance imaging.

## 13.4 Advanced Disease

Patients with supradiaphragmatic metastases and patients with extranodal metastases should all be treated with chemotherapy. Patients presenting with extragonadal disease appear to have the same chemosensitivity as testicular presentations and since these tumors usually present with bulky disease in the retroperitoneum or mediastinum, they should also be treated with chemotherapy.

## 13.5 Prognosis After Chemotherapy

In a prognostic factor analysis of chemotherapy results in germ cell tumors, the International Germ Cell Cancer Cooperative Group (IGCCCG) reviewed 637 patients treated for advanced seminoma. The 3-year survival was 82% (International Germ Cell Cancer Collaborative 1997). However, the majority of patients were in a good prognostic subgroup with metastasis confined to either lymph nodes or lung fields and in this group, the 5-year survival was 86%. Those with non pulmonary visceral metastases had a 5-year survival of 72%. In an analysis of a subset of 236 of these patients treated with cisplatin-based chemotherapy at ten European oncology units, a very good prognosis (GP) group was identified comprising patients who had not had previous radiotherapy and who had either abdominal node metastases with any level of serum lactate dehydrogenase or alternatively Stage C patients without non pulmonary visceral metastases whose serum LDH was less than twice the upper limit of normal (Fossa et al. 1997). These patients had a 94% 3-year progression-free survival whereas the remainder of patients comprising a poor prognostic group had a 56% 3-year progression-free survival. A retrospective, single institution analysis of 142 patients treated in New York was consistent with these prognostic conclusions but also suggested that an elevated pretreatment HCG may indicate a poorer outcome (Mencel et al. 1994).

## 13.6 Combination Chemotherapy of Seminoma

There are relatively few prospective randomized trials of different chemotherapy regimens in advanced seminoma and in interpreting reports of uncontrolled trials it should be noted that over the last two decades there have been considerable changes in staging patients, in the use of radiotherapy for metastatic seminoma and in the response definition. The modern era of successful chemotherapy for seminoma was heralded by the introduction of cisplatin in 1974 (Higby et al. 1974). It was recognized rapidly that a combination of cisplatin, vinblastine and bleomycin, so successful in the treatment of patients with non seminomatous germ cell tumors, was also effective in the treatment of seminoma (Einhorn and Williams 1980). This observation from Indiana was soon complemented by a large multicentre collaborative report from Europe and by a report from the Memorial Sloan Kettering Cancer Center of the efficacy of the VAB6 regimen (vinblastine/actinomycinD/bleomycin/cisplatin/cyclophosphamide)(Stanton et al. 1985).

More recently, most centers have replaced vinblastine in the PVB schedule with etoposide in an attempt to reduce toxicity, creating the current standard regimen BEP. The seminal prospective randomized trial comparing these regimens in patients with metastatic germ cell tumors contained only a small number of patients with pure seminoma (Williams et al. 1987). However, results appeared equivalent or better with BEP and toxicity was reduced. A further question is over the role of bleomycin. The convention at MSKCC was to treat patients with the combination of etoposide and cisplatin (EP). In a report on 60 patients, 55 achieved long-term progression-free survival (Mencel et al. 1994). The durable response rates were 79% for 43 patients treated with VAB-6, 92% of 62 patients treated with EP and 83% of 35 patients treated with etoposide, carboplatin (EC).an alternative approach to reducing the risk of lung toxicity and improve efficacy against seminoma, an alkylating agent has been introduced in the VIP combination of cisplatin, ifosphamide and vinblastin (Clemm et al. 1986). Subsequently, vinblastine was replaced by etoposide in this regimen. Fossa et al. reported a multicentre experience of the HOP combination of ifosphamide, cisplatin and vincristine which revealed 90% long-term disease-free survival in 42% of patients (Fossa et al. 1995). These combination chemotherapy approaches are summarized in Table 13.3 where it can be seen that cisplatin-based combination chemotherapy achieves long-term progression-free survival of between 80 and 90% in the majority of represented series (Clemm et al. 1986; Fossa et al. 1995; Arranz Arija et al. 2001; Peckham et al. 1985; Logothetis et al. 1987; Horwich et al. 2000).

Attempts have also been made to avoid the renal and neurotoxicity of cisplatinum by replacing it with carboplatin, following demonstration of the efficacy of this drug as a single agent (Horwich et al. 1989) (see below). Amato and colleagues have conducted a study at the MD Anderson Hospital of the combination of carboplatin

**Table 13.3** Cisplatin-based combination chemotherapy for advanced seminoma

| Series | Regimen | Patients | Continuous DFS (%) |
|---|---|---|---|
| Peckham et al. (1985) | PVB or BEP | 39 | 90 |
| Logothetis et al. (1987) | CyP | 42 | 92 |
| Clemm et al. (1986) | VIP | 24 | 83 |
| Mencel et al. (1994) | EP | 60 | 92 |
| Fossa et al. (1995) | HOP | 42 | 90 |
| Horwich et al. (2000) | EP | 66 | 81 |
| Arranz Arija et al. (2001) | EP | 64 GP | 89 |

*GP* good prognosis; *P* cisplatinum; *V* vinblasstine; *B* bleomycin; *A* doxorubicin; *Cy* cyclophosphamide; *I* ifosfamide; *O* vincristine; *E* etoposide and cyclophosphamide, given in a 28 day cycle with myelosuppression supported by haemopioetic growth factor (Amato et al. 2000). Forty six patients were treated, 30 with chemotherapy alone and the remainder with some consolidation to a residual mass (usually radiotherapy). The long-term continuous disease-free survival was 93%.

With regard to the number of chemotherapy cycles, the standard approach with EP has been 4 cycles, with E at 360–500 mg/m$^2$ per cycle and cisplatin at 100 mg/m$^2$ per cycle. For BEP, a trial in 812 patients with all histologies of testicular GCT compared 2 vs. 4 cycles and showed no significant differences in outcomes; 23% of patients had pure seminoma, 93 randomized to 3 cycles and 89 to 4 cycles (de Wit et al. 2001). Patients with seminoma were stratified at randomization. It can be concluded that for B at 30 i.u. per week, E at 500 mg/m$^2$ and P at 100 mg/m$^2$ per cycle, 3 cycles of BEP is sufficient for patients with GP seminoma.

## 13.7 Single Agent Platinum Drugs in Seminoma

The pilot study of single agent carboplatin from RMH was supported by a phase II study from Germany. These results led to the launch of a prospective randomized trial by the UK Medical Research Council (Horwich et al. 2000). A total of 130 patients with advanced seminoma were randomized between single agent carboplatin or the combination of etoposide + cisplatinum. The estimated progression-free survival rate at 3 years was 71% in those randomized to carboplatin and 81% in those randomized to EP (Horwich et al. 2000). The difference was not statistically significant and there was also no significant difference in overall survival. However, it was recognized that this may be a consequence of the relatively small size of the trial and it was therefore concluded that the standard approach should continue to be with the combination of etoposide and cisplatinum. A similar concept was evaluated in multicentre trial in 251 patients in Germany with the control arm being the combination of platinum, etoposide and ifosphamide (PEI), and the results were similar, with carboplatin achieving a nonsignificantly inferior progression-free survival (Bokemeyer et al. 2004). A combined analysis of the two trials included 361 patients and confirmed inferior results from single agent carboplatin for both progression-free and overall survival (Bokemeyer et al. 2004).

## 13.8 Salvage Chemotherapy

In patients failing BEP-type chemotherapy there is good evidence for the benefit of salvage with an ifosphamide-containing regimen. Miller et al., reported on 24 patients with seminoma recurring after cisplatin-based chemotherapy. After VeIP (vinblastine, ifosphamide, cisplatin) 54% were long-term survivors. There is some evidence that this approach is as effective as high dose chemotherapy.

## 13.9 Residual Mass Following RT or Chemotherapy

Following treatment, patients with Stage II disease require follow-up imaging of the abdomen until complete regression of disease has occurred. Residual retroperitoneal masses that may either regress slowly over time or remain stable are frequently seen. A stable persistent mass often represents fibrosis or necrosis and only the minority contain active tumor. However, the possibility of a nonseminomatous component to explain the residual mass needs to be kept in mind even in patients whose primary tumors show pure seminoma. In addition, surgical extirpation of retroperitoneal nodes in the setting of seminoma is technically challenging and associated with a higher acute morbidity.

Therapeutic options for patients with residual masses after treatment include observation, surgical removal or, occasionally after chemotherapy, RT can be considered. PET scanning has been reported to be of little value in this setting by some authors but others have reported it is a clinically useful predictor of tumor, especially in residual masses after chemotherapy, and particularly if the mass is greater than 3 cm in diameter. A small number of centers have reviewed their experience with surgery for residual masses in the setting of seminoma. The MSKCC group published their data in 55 of 104 patients who demonstrated residual masses post chemotherapy (Herr et al. 1997). Of these 55 patients, 32 (58%) had a formal RPLND and 23 (42%) had multiple intraoperative biopsies performed, as the residual mass was deemed unresectable. Among patients with a mass >3 cm ($n = 27$), 8 (30%) had residual viable tumor. Interestingly 2 of the 8 recurrences were teratoma and 6 were seminoma. No patients with tumors <3 cm had viable tumor at final pathology. Among the 8 patients with preoperative tumor masses >3 cm and positive pathological findings 6 remained NED at 47 months follow up. Two patients both with poorly defined masses on CT died of disease. Given this high proportion of persistent malignancy, MSKCC investigators have recommended resection or biopsy of masses of 3 cm or larger. In contrast, Culine et al. have suggested that as long as the retroperitoneal mass continues to decrease in size after treatment, then continued observation is a reasonable strategy (Culine and Droz 1996).

The use of RT in patients with post chemotherapy masses is often mentioned as a therapeutic option. Horwich and colleagues published their experience with both observation and radiotherapy for these masses and found that the recurrence rate was similar whether RT or observation was performed (Horwich et al. 1997). The MRC Testicular Tumor Working Party published a retrospective pooled analysis assessing the role of RT for post chemotherapy residual mass among men with seminoma (Duchesne et al. 1997). Among the 123 patients with a residual abdominal residual mass 56% received consolidative radiotherapy. There was no significant difference in outcome among patients who did or did not receive RT. Given these data it was concluded that routine RT is not indicated for a post chemotherapy residual mass.

It is clear that patients with a residual mass of 3 cm or less can safely be observed. For patients with bulkier disease up front surgery or observation can be instituted with therapy reserved for masses that increase in size. Using this approach at PMH, only 6 patients have required surgery over the past 15 years.

## 13.10 Summary

Advanced seminoma is extremely sensitive to modern combination chemotherapy. The high cure rates and relatively young age of patients make it important to consider long-term toxicity issues in constructing a treatment plan. In Stage IIA/B seminoma, radiation therapy is the treatment of choice for low volume disease cases with combination chemotherapy being preferred for more advanced disease.

## References


Amato RJ, Millikan R, Daliani D, Wood L, Logothetis C, Pollack A (2000) Cyclophosphamide and carboplatin and selective consolidation in advanced seminoma. Clin Cancer Res 6(1):72–77

Arranz Arija JA, Garcia del Muro X, Guma J, Aparicio J, Salazar R, Saenz A, Carles J, Sanchez M, Germa-Lluch JR. E400P in advanced seminoma of good prognosis according to the international germ cell cancer collaborative group (IGCCCG) classification: the Spanish Germ Cell Cancer Group experience. *Ann Oncol* 2001;12(4):487–491

Bayens YC, Helle PA, Van PW, Mali SP (1992) Orchidectomy followed by radiotherapy in 176 stage I and II testicular seminoma patients: benefits of a 10-year follow-up study. Radiother Oncol 25(2):97–102

Becherer A, De Santis M, Karanikas G, Szabo M, Bokemeyer C, Dohmen BM, Pont J, Dudczak R, Dittrich C, Kletter K (2005) FDG PET is superior to CT in the prediction of viable tumour in post-chemotherapy seminoma residuals. Eur J Radiol 54(2):284–288

Bokemeyer C, Kollmannsberger C, Stenning S, Hartmann JT, Horwich A, Clemm C, Gerl A, Meisner C, Ruckerl CP, Schmoll HJ, Kanz L, Oliver T (2004) Metastatic seminoma treated with either single agent carboplatin or cisplatin-based combination chemotherapy: a pooled analysis of two randomised trials. Br J Cancer 91(4):683–687

Chung PW, Warde PR, Panzarella T, Bayley AJ, Catton CN, Milosevic MF, Jewett MA, Sturgeon JF, Moore M, Gospodarowicz MK (2003) Appropriate radiation volume for stage IIA/B testicular seminoma. Int J Radiat Oncol Biol Phys 56(3):746–748

Chung PW, Gospodarowicz MK, Panzarella T, Jewett MA, Sturgeon JF, Tew-George B, Bayley AJ, Catton CN, Milosevic MF, Moore M, Warde PR (2004) Stage II testicular seminoma: patterns of recurrence and outcome of treatment. Eur Urol 45(6):754–759; discussion 759–760

Classen J, Schmidberger H, Meisner C, Souchon R, Sautter-Bihl ML, Sauer R, Weinknecht S, Kohrmann KU, Bamberg M (2003) Radiotherapy for stages IIA/B testicular seminoma: final report of a prospective multicenter clinical trial. J Clin Oncol 21(6):1101–1106

Clemm C, Hartenstein R, Willich N, Boening L, Wilmanns W (1986) Vinblastine-ifosfamide-cisplatin treatment of bulky seminoma. Cancer 58(10):2203–2207

Cremerius U, Effert PJ, Adam G, Sabri O, Zimmy M, Wagenknecht G, Jakse G, Buell U (1998) FDG PET for detection and therapy control of metastatic germ cell tumor. J Nucl Med 39(5):815–822

Culine S, Droz JP (1996) Optimal management of residual mass after chemotherapy in advanced seminoma: there is time for everything. J Clin Oncol 14(10):2884–2885

Duchesne GM, Stenning SP, Aass N, Mead GM, Fossa SD, Oliver RT, Horwich A, Read G, Roberts IT, Rustin G, Cullen

MH, Kaye SB, Harland SJ, Cook PA (1997) Radiotherapy after chemotherapy for metastatic seminoma–a diminishing role. MRC Testicular Tumour Working Party. Eur J Cancer 33(6):829–835

Einhorn LH, Williams SD (1980) Chemotherapy of disseminated seminoma. Cancer Clin Trials 3(4):307–313

Fossa SD, Droz JP, Stoter G, Kaye SB, Vermeylen K, Sylvester R (1995) Cisplatin, vincristine and ifosphamide combination chemotherapy of metastatic seminoma: results of EORTC trial 30874. EORTC GU Group. Br J Cancer 71(3): 619–624

Fossa SD, Oliver RT, Stenning SP, Horwich A, Wilkinson P, Read G, Mead GM, Roberts JT, Rustin G, Cullen MH, Kaye SB, Harland SJ, Cook P (1997) Prognostic factors for patients with advanced seminoma treated with platinum-based chemotherapy. Eur J Cancer 33(9):1380–1387

Ganjoo KN, Chan RJ, Sharma M, Einhorn LH (1999) Positron emission tomography scans in the evaluation of postchemotherapy residual masses in patients with seminoma. J Clin Oncol 17(11):3457–3460

Greene FL, Page DL, Fleming ID, Fritz AG, Balch CM, Haller DG, Morrow M (eds) (2002) AJCC cancer staging manual, 6th edn. Springer, New York

Herr HW, Sheinfeld J, Puc HS, Heelan R, Bajorin DF, Mencel P, Bosl GJ, Motzer RJ (1997) Surgery for a post-chemotherapy residual mass in seminoma. J Urol 157(3):860–862

Higby DJ, Wallace HJ Jr, Albert D, Holland JF (1974) Diamminodichloroplatinum in the chemotherapy of testicular tumors. J Urol 112(1):100–104

Horwich A, Dearnaley DP, Duchesne GM, Williams M, Brada M, Peckham MJ (1989) Simple nontoxic treatment of advanced metastatic seminoma with carboplatin. J Clin Oncol 7(8):1150–1156

Horwich A, Paluchowska B, Norman A, Huddart R, Nicholls J, Fisher C, Husband J, Dearnaley DP (1997) Residual mass following chemotherapy of seminoma. Ann Oncol 8(1):37–40

Horwich A, Oliver RT, Wilkinson PM, Mead GM, Harland SJ, Cullen MH, Roberts JT, Fossa SD, Dearnaley DP, Lallemand E, Stenning SP (2000) A medical research council randomized trial of single agent carboplatin versus etoposide and cisplatin for advanced metastatic seminoma. MRC Testicular Tumour Working Party. Br J Cancer 83(12):1623–1629

International Germ Cell Cancer Collaborative Group (1997) International Germ Cell Consensus Classification: a prognostic factor-based staging system for metastatic germ cell cancers. J Clin Oncol 15:594–603

Krege S, Boergermann C, Baschek R, Hinke A, Pottek T, Kliesch S, Dieckmann KP, Albers P, Knutzen B, Weinknecht S, Schmoll HJ, Beyer J, Ruebben H (2006) Single agent carboplatin for CS IIA/B testicular seminoma. A phase II study of the German Testicular Cancer Study Group (GTCSG). Ann Oncol 17(2):276–280

Logothetis CJ, Samuels ML, Ogden SL, Dexeus FH, Chong CD (1987) Cyclophosphamide and sequential cisplatin for advanced seminoma: long-term followup in 52 patients. J Urol 138(4):789–794

Mencel PJ, Motzer RJ, Mazumdar M, Vlamis V, Bajorin DF, Bosl GJ (1994) Advanced seminoma: treatment results, survival, and prognostic factors in 142 patients. J Clin Oncol 12(1):120–126

Patterson H, Norman AR, Mitra SS, Nicholls J, Fisher C, Dearnaley DP, Horwich A, Mason MD, Huddart RA (2001) Combination carboplatin and radiotherapy in the management of stage II testicular seminoma: comparison with radiotherapy treatment alone. Radiother Oncol 59(1):5–11

Peckham MJ, Horwich A, Hendry WF (1985) Advanced seminoma: treatment with cis-platinum-based combination chemotherapy or carboplatin (JM8). Br J Cancer 52(1):7–13

Sobin LH, Wittekind CL (eds) (2002) International Union Against Cancer (UICC): TNM classification of malignant tumors, 6th edn. Wiley, New York

Spermon JR, De Geus-Oei LF, Kiemeney LA, Witjes JA, Oyen WJ (2002) The role of (18)fluoro-2-deoxyglucose positron emission tomography in initial staging and re-staging after chemotherapy for testicular germ cell tumours. BJU Int 89(6): 549–556

Stanton GF, Bosl GJ, Whitmore WF Jr, Herr H, Sogani P, Morse M, Golbey RB (1985) VAB-6 as initial treatment of patients with advanced seminoma. J Clin Oncol 3(3):336–339

Vallis KA, Howard GC, Duncan W, Cornbleet MA, Kerr GR (1995) Radiotherapy for stages I and II testicular seminoma: results and morbidity in 238 patients. Br J Radiol 68(808): 400–405

Williams SD, Birch R, Einhorn LH, Irwin L, Greco FA, Loehrer PJ (1987) Treatment of disseminated germ-cell tumors with cisplatin, bleomycin, and either vinblastine or etoposide. N Engl J Med 316(23):1435–1440

de Wit R, Roberts JT, Wilkinson PM, de Mulder PH, Mead GM, Fossa SD, Cook P, de Prijck L, Stenning S, Collette L (2001) Equivalence of three or four cycles of bleomycin, etoposide, and cisplatin chemotherapy and of a 3- or 5-day schedule in good-prognosis germ cell cancer: a randomized study of the European Organization for Research and Treatment of Cancer Genitourinary Tract Cancer Cooperative Group and the Medical Research Council. J Clin Oncol 19(6):1629–1640

Zagars GK, Pollack A (2001) Radiotherapy for stage II testicular seminoma. Int J Radiat Oncol Biol Phys 51(3):643–649

# 14 Treatment of Relapse

Aude Fléchon and Jean-Pierre Droz

## 14.1 Relapse and Failure of First-Line Treatment

### 14.1.1 Failure of First-Line Treatment

Few studies have focused specifically on the evolution during follow-up of patients after chemotherapy with or without resection of residual disease, apart from the overall survival and continuously CR rates. The most important investigations performed in patients with GCT have reported the incidence of favorable responses: e.g., CR to chemotherapy only, necrosis and/or fibrosis and CR response after surgical resection of either teratoma, necrosis or fibrosis (pCR or pathological CR) or active residual disease (sCR or surgical CR). They have also stated the rate of unfavorable responses, the definition of which varies among the different investigator groups (Bosl et al. 2007; Einhorn 1990). A review of these studies shows that the rate of unfavorable responses is different between the good-risk and intermediate- or poor-risk groups. In the good-risk group, the initial failure rate is never above 3–5%, except when patients are undertreated, as demonstrated in trials studying bleomycin deletion in the 3-BEP-cycle schedule (Loehrer et al. 1995) or replacement of cisplatin by carboplatin (Bajorin et al. 1993) where the initial failure rate may be as high as 10–12%. In the intermediate-risk and, more importantly, the poor-risk groups, the initial failure rate is as high as 20% and 50%, respectively (Nichols et al. 1991; Nichols et al. 1998; Motzer et al. 2007). Nevertheless, relapse rates are always less than 20%: 5–10% (Einhorn et al. 1989; de Wit et al. 2001) in patients with good prognosis factors and 10–15% (Nichols et al. 1991, 1998; Motzer et al. 2007) in patients with poor prognosis. Only patients with sCR may have a slightly higher relapse rate – 35% in the international study published in 2001 (Fizazi et al. 2001), whereas several individual randomized trials have reported rates of 20–50% in this situation.

A. Fléchon (✉)
Medical Oncology Department, Centre Léon-Bérard,
28 Rue LAENNEC, Lyon, France
e-mail: flechon@lyon-fnclec.fr

### 14.1.2 Patient Follow-Up After Complete Response to First-Line Treatment

On the basis of our results (Flechon et al. 2005) and a review of the literature (National Cancer Centre Network 2007; Schmoll et al. 2004), we observe that patients in CR after first-line treatment should undergo careful follow-up with physical examination and determination of serum marker levels (AFP and hCG) every month in the first year, every 2 months in the second year, every 3 months in the third year, every 4 months in the fourth year, every 6 months in the fifth year, and annually thereafter. This follow-up will also include thoraco-abdominal CT scans every 6 months in the first 2 years, then yearly during the following years. The inclusion of a CT-scan of the thorax is debatable. The NNCN (2007) recommendation is to perform a chest-x-ray and abdomen CT-scan, but two studies have demonstrated that a CT-scan of the thorax is more sensitive than chest-X-ray to detect thoracic recurrence (Gietema et al. 2002; White et al. 1999). This recommendation is supported by the American Society of Clinical Oncology (ASCO) (Kondagunta et al. 2003).

M.P. Laguna et al. (eds.), *Cancer of the Testis*,
DOI: 10.1007/978-1-84800-370-5_14, © Springer-Verlag London Limited 2010

### 14.1.3 Characteristics of Relapse

One must consider separately relapsing patients and those who fail to respond to first-line treatment.

On the one hand, it is well established that a majority of relapsing patients will do so within the first 2 years after the end of treatment (Kondagunta et al. 2003). The median time to relapse, in a specific study of patients with relapses, was 6 months (Flechon et al. 2005). This period was slightly shorter than usually reported, but the date of onset of surveillance reported in the literature is sometimes doubtful (surveillance either includes the treatment period or not). Several studies have reported a trend in favor of shorter median relapse intervals in patients with poor-risk characteristics. In the randomized trial that compared four cycles of BEP with or without double-dose cisplatin, all patients but one relapsed within 9 months (Nichols et al. 1991). Characteristics of relapse are rarely described. In a retrospective study of 96 relapsing patients, we were able to show the major characteristics that can be drawn (Flechon et al. 2005). It is noteworthy that STM were found elevated in only 65% of the cases, whereas relapse was seen on the thoraco-abdominal CT-scan in 85%. However, the only sign of relapse was confirmed STM elevation in 7% of cases, abnormal clinical examination (supra clavicular lymph-node) in one case, and neurological signs and abnormal CNS MRI in five cases. Finally, the most frequent sites of relapse were the retroperitoneum (50% of cases), the thorax (15%), the thorax and abdomen (15%), and the CNS (8%). Sites of relapse and of primary tumor were identical in only 43% of the patients.

On the other hand, patients with incomplete or unfavorable response during first-line chemotherapy have a specific fundamental characteristic: primarily cisplatin-refractory disease, which is a very poor prognosis factor; a study of high-dose chemotherapy (HDCT) in the salvage setting has described cisplatin refractoriness as the worst prognostic factor for survival (Beyer et al. 1996). Unfavorable response is clearly a potentially serious problem which is almost only observed in poor-risk patients. Its mechanism is not clear. Defects in the mismatch repair pathway may cause microsatellite instability. Cell resistance may be the direct consequence of a failure to detect DNA damage and to initiate the apoptotic cascade, or it may be only the indirect consequence of an accumulation of mutations possibly affecting apoptosis. Overexpression of the MDR (multidrug resistance) protein or GST (glutathion-*S*-transferase) enzyme does not seem frequent in the setting of refractory GCT (Mayer et al. 2003).

### 14.1.4 Prognostic Factors of Relapse

Investigators at the Memorial Sloan-Kettering Cancer Center (MSKCC) have performed a unique study on the specific risk of relapse after chemotherapy followed or not by surgical resection of residual disease (Geller et al. 1989). They have observed 38 relapses in 216 patients treated by cisplatin-based chemotherapy who entered complete remission, and analyzed prognostic factors for time to relapse using the Cox proportional hazards model. They concluded that patients who require surgery for residual active disease are at much higher risk for relapse, as well as those who have high lactate dehydrogenase (LDH) and hCG levels at the time of initial chemotherapy. Baseline STM values at initial diagnosis reflect the initial prognostic group determined according to the IGCCC (Anon 1997). The presence of active residual disease has been extensively studied (Fizazi et al. 2001). A retrospective analysis of more than 300 patients after surgical removal of residual active germ cell disease has shown that the most important risk factors of relapse are incomplete surgery and a proportion of residual active disease superior to 10% of the residual volume. No difference in recurrence rates has been observed between patients receiving two additional cycles of chemotherapy and those who did not. One can conclude from this study that patients undergoing complete resection of residual disease must be carefully followed, whatever be the proportion of active disease.

## 14.2 Standard Salvage Chemotherapy

### 14.2.1 Activity of Ifosfamide

The first drugs with demonstrated activity in GCT of the testis were vinblastine and bleomycin (Samuels et al. 1975), and then cisplatin (Higby et al. 1974); the three drugs were then used in combination (PVB regimen) (Einhorn and Donohue 1977). Patients who failed to respond to PVB received etoposide, which induced a 30% response rate (Lederman et al. 1983). The drug was then tested in the first-line setting. The seminal study in the field, conducted at Indiana University (IU), compared PVB to BEP (Williams et al. 1987). Four cycles of each chemotherapy regimen were administered to an unselected population of patients with advanced disease. The IU study demonstrated that the BEP regimen is less toxic than PVB (mainly in terms of hematological and neurological toxicities) and achieves similar survival rates. It was then necessary to develop alternative chemotherapy regimens to use in the salvage setting. Ifosfamide is an old drug developed in Germany for the treatment of GCT before the introduction of cisplatin (Schmoll 1989). It is a prodrug from the family of alkylating agents. It is metabolized in the liver, and inactive metabolites are excreted in the urine. The administration of mesna at a dose corresponding to 120% of the dose of ifosfamide is required to circumvent urinary tract toxicity. Ifosfamide induces 50–70% response in nonpretreated patients and in patients not receiving cisplatin, vs. only 20% in cisplatin-refractory patients (Schmoll 1989). The experience of pretreatment by PVB has led to combining ifosfamide to etoposide, with addition of cisplatin (VIP regimen of chemotherapy), as a proportion of patients are not refractory to the drug but suffer from relapse, and then may have retained some sensitivity to cisplatin. However, the further substitution of etoposide by vinblatine has led to include the combination of vinblastine, ifosfamide, and cisplatin in the second-line treatment of GCT after BEP failure.

### 14.2.2 Ifosfamide-Based Salvage Chemotherapy Regimens

The first published studies of Ifosfamide-containing salvage chemotherapy generally included etoposide (Loehrer et al. 1988; Ghosn et al. 1988) and patients were treated in second, third, or further line. Interestingly, these studies suggested several preliminary conclusions: the rate of long-term CR and nonevolutive disease (NED) was around 30%; initial bulky disease and absence of CR to first-line chemotherapy were predictive of failure; after adjustment for other variables, etoposide appeared likely to induce treatment response; double-dose cisplatin (Ghosn et al. 1988) did not appear more active than standard-dose cisplatin. However, the universal use of etoposide in the first-line chemotherapy setting almost systematically led to using vinblastine (0.11 mg/kg/ day on days 1 and 2 of each cycle) in combination with ifosfamide and cisplatin (VeIP protocol).

The bulk of results from ifosfamide-based chemotherapy regimens were obtained using the VeIP protocol. A summary of these results is given in Table 14.1. Studies are characterized by their great heterogeneity. For example, around 25% of the patients have

**Table 14.1** Conventional salvage chemotherapy regimens

| Reference | Protocol | Nb pts | CR (%) | cCR (%) | NED (%) | Poor-risk* (%) |
|---|---|---|---|---|---|---|
| IU (Loehrer et al.1998) | VeIP | 135 | 50 | 24 | 30 | 59 |
| MSKCC (McCaffrey et al. 1997) | VIP/VeIP | 56 | 36 | 23 | 34 | 30 |
| Milan (Pizzocaroet al. 1992) | Modified VIP/VeIP | 36 | 56 | 42 | 40 | 30 |
| IGR (Farhat et al.1996) | VIP/VeIP | 54 | 31 | 20 | 30 | 39 |
| MSKCC (Motzeret al. 2000a) | TIP | 30 | 80 | 73 | 80 | 0 |
| MRC (Mead et al.2005) | TIP | 43 | 10 | ? | 70 | 40 |
| Mardiak et al.(2005) | TIP | 17 | 41 | ? | 47 | ? |

*IU* Indiana university; *MSKCC* Memorial Sloan-Kettering Cancer Center; *IGR* Institut Gustave-Roussy; *MRC* Medical Research Council; *VeIP* vinblastine+ifosfamide+cisplatin; *VIP* etoposide+ifosfamide+cisplatin; *TIP* paclitaxel+ifosfamide+cisplatin; *Nb pts* patients number; *CR* complete response; *cCR* continuous CR; *NED* long-term nonevolutive disease

*According to MSKCC prognostic factor classification (McCaffrey et al. 1997)

extragonadal GCT, the majority of which being of mediastinal origin which is known to have very unfavorable prognostic significance. However, it is quite impossible to delineate the results obtained in primary testis tumors, which are our focus of interest. Another problem arises from the publication of partial reports of the same studies which makes the interpretation or results confusing; it is thus important to consider only the latest results available. All studies were conducted in the first salvage setting. The most important series published by the IU group included 135 patients treated by VeIP only after they had received etoposide in first line; 59% of the patients had poor prognosis characteristics (Loehrer et al. 1998). The CR rate, continuous CR rate, and NED rate were 50%, 24%, and 30%, respectively. The MSKCC series was more heterogeneous: 56 patients received either VIP (etoposide) or VeIP (vinblastine) because only 68% of them had received etoposide in first line; around 30% of the patients had poor-risk baseline characteristics (McCaffrey et al. 1997). The CR rate, continuous CR rate, and NED rate were 36%, 23%, and 34%, respectively. Thirty-six patients from the National Cancer Institute in Milan received a slightly modified VeIP/VIP regimen; 60% had received prior etoposide and 75% had good prognosis initial characteristics (Pizzocaro et al. 1992). The CR rate, continuous CR rate, and NED rate were 56%, 42%, and 40%, respectively. Fifty-four patients were treated at the Institut Gustave-Roussy (IGR); only 46% received etoposide, and 11 received HDCT as consolidation treatment (Farhat et al. 1996). At baseline, 39% of the patients had poor-risk factors. The CR rate, continuous CR rate, and NED rate were 31%, 20%, and 30%, respectively. However, these results were obtained in the 1990s and did include patients initially not treated by BEP or treated by other regimens not containing etoposide; prognostic assessment was not based on the IGCCC, but on previous prognostic classifications (Droz et al. 1992). Nevertheless, these results are the basis of our knowledge of prognostic factors in patients undergoing salvage chemotherapy and have provided the background for tailoring salvage treatments to prognostic factors. Additionally, a randomized study has shown that using hematopoietic growth factor may decrease the incidence of grade 4 neutropenia and the rate of neutropenic fever (Bajorin et al. 1995).

### 14.2.3 Prognostic Factors Studies in Patients Receiving Ifosfamide-Based Chemotherapy

Three prognostic factor studies must be considered. The primary analysis published by the German group (Gerl et al. 1995) was further integrated into the European Study (Fossa et al. 1999a) for validation of the model. The European study is particularly interesting because it includes a population of 164 patients, of whom only five had a primary tumor located in the mediastinum. However, there are many concerns about this study, mainly because information is available only for 103 patients, of whom only 15 received Ifosfamide-based chemotherapy, whereas 89 received various undetermined cisplatin-based chemotherapy regimens; seven patients had no salvage treatment. The authors observed 53 CR, 48 PRm(−) (partial response with normalization of STM, e.g., 61.5% response rate), 52 incomplete responses, and 11 disease progressions (38.5% failures). Prognostic factors were determined using a multivariate analysis based on the Cox model (Fossa et al. 1999a). Three factors retained prognostic value: (1) time (from the beginning of first-line chemotherapy) to progression less than 2 years; (2) absence of CR after first-line treatment; and (3) either serum AFP > 100 kU/L or serum hCG > 100 IU/L. Patients with at most two adverse prognostic factors were classified in the good-risk group (75% of patients) with a 47% five-year overall survival rate. Patients with poor-risk characteristics had 0% long-term survival. Within the group of patients included in the good-risk group, those with a time to progression >2 years had a 61% five-year survival rate. The model was validated in an independent population of 66 patients. Two problems must be mentioned: the redundancy between time to progression and the presence or not of a CR to first-line treatment; the fact that STM level is very dependent on time. This model is certainly methodologically valid, but it is not really clinically significant.

The other two models based on IU (Loehrer et al. 1998) and MSKCC (McCaffrey et al. 1997) studies are clinically valid. The IU study included a multivariate analysis of factors (Cox regression model), but the study population included 32 patients with extragonadal GCT, none of whom survived (Loehrer et al. 1998). The multivariate analysis found three favorable prognostic factors: CR after initial treatment ($P=0.0067$), good-risk group at initial diagnosis ($P=0.0371$), and testis primary ($P=0.0242$). No prognostic classification has been proposed by the authors; nevertheless, the relative prognostic weight of each factor shows that CR status after first-line treatment is the most powerful predictor of prognosis. This is confirmed by the MSKCC study where 17 patients with testis primary and CR to initial treatment had a 60% two-year survival rate, whereas 39 patients with either extragonadal primary (10 patients) and/or incomplete response to initial treatment had a 30% two-year survival rate (McCaffrey et al. 1997). It is therefore reasonable to consider that patients in the first salvage setting may expect favorable outcome if they have testis primary and have experienced CR to first-line treatment; contrariwise, they may expect poor outcome if they have extra gonadal primary and no CR after initial treatment. The role of the prognostic group classification at diagnosis is less clear: as stated earlier, it may influence the lack of response to initial chemotherapy. A classification based on these pragmatic factors is currently used in trials and in routine clinical practice.

## 14.3 High-Dose Chemotherapy in the Salvage Setting

Patients with relapsed GCT treated with the standard chemotherapy regimen VeIP have a poor prognosis: only 25% remain NED in the long term. New approaches, such as HDCT, have been developed to improve the NED rate and decrease the relapse rate. Many phase I–II trials have focused on the salvage treatment of patients with relapsing or refractory disease. Only two recently published randomized trials have explored the treatment of patients in first relapse.

### 14.3.1 *Phase I Feasibility Trials*

Thirty years ago, there was no clear rationale for the use of HDCT in GCT. Active drugs in this disease were cisplatin, bleomycin, etoposide, and ifosfamide. Only few phase II studies have tested single drugs. Combination chemotherapy has rapidly become the treatment most studied in trials, when the activity of a single drug was suspected. So far, only few trials have addressed the role of drug dosage. Complete studies have only been performed with cisplatin-based regimens. Samson has demonstrated that a cisplatin dose-intensity of 18.75 mg/m²/week is less active than a 30-mg/m²/week dose-intensity (Samson et al. 1984). Conversely, Nichols has shown that increasing the cisplatin dose-intensity (66 mg/m²/week) does not increase the cure rate (Nichols et al. 1991). No other randomized study has addressed the question of drug dose-intensity. In 1984, investigators in Europe and in the USA began to study HDCT with autologous bone-marrow transplantation (ABMT). The first reports concerned protocols with high-dose cyclophosphamide, etoposide (Postmus et al. 1984), etoposide + cyclophosphamide (Blijham et al. 1981), and etoposide + cyclophosphamide + cisplatin (Droz et al. 1991). The observation of carboplatin activity in GCT (O'Reilly et al. 1992) shortly led to introducing this drug in HDCT regimens: its toxicity is mainly hematologic and can be circumvented by hematopoietic stem cell support. Different phase I studies have identified the best combinations of drugs to be used in this setting: etoposide and carboplatin (Nichols et al. 1989), etoposide+cyclophosphamide+carboplatin (Ibrahim et al. 1993; Motzer et al. 1993), or etoposide+ifosfamide+carboplatin (Lotz et al. 1991; Siegert et al. 1994).

All trials performed between 1986 and 1990 used ABMT with or without hematopoietic growth factors. Since 1990, patients have received peripheral blood stem cell (PBSC) support. The use of growth factors and PBSC shortens the duration of neutropenia and thrombocytopenia and decreases hospitalization duration (Siegert et al. 1994; van der WE et al. 1994). It is noteworthy that no trial has studied the problem of hematologic support specifically in GCT. The answers to questions on the role of hematologic support technologies have been given in other specific phase I and feasibility trials in patients with different tumor types. However, Motzer studied prognostic factors of toxicity in a retrospective series of 58 patients and showed that the use of G-CSF is an independently predictive factor associated with a more rapid neutrophil count recovery and a smaller number of days of hospitalization (Motzer et al. 1996). PBSC are mobilized either by a cycle of standard salvage chemotherapy plus G-CSF or by G-CSF only if upfront HDCT is scheduled. Generally, the minimal total number of CD34+ cells required for HDCT is $2 \times 10^6$ CD34+ cells/kg body weight. A study of circulating malignant cells during PBSC procedure demonstrated the presence of malignant cells but was not practically conclusive (Hildebrandt et al. 1998).

### 14.3.2 Prognostic Factors of Response to Salvage High-Dose Chemotherapy

A multi-institutional retrospective study of 310 patients treated by HDCT has identified prognostic factors of response to HDCT and of failure-free survival (FFS) in patients with relapsed or cisplatin-refractory GCT (Beyer et al. 1996). It is noteworthy that the assessment of prognostic factors was performed immediately before the administration of HDCT, thus taking into account patient response to the conventional chemotherapy that had just been administered, even if given for stem cell recruitment. This study has identified five prognostic factors: absolute refractory disease (scored 2 points), hCG level greater than 1,000 IU/L (2 points), refractory disease before HDCT (1 point), mediastinal nonseminomatous primary germ-cell tumor (1 point), and progressive disease before HDCT (1 point). The total score of each patient was calculated by adding the scores of each item. Three prognostic groups were defined: good-risk (no adverse prognostic factor), intermediate risk (1 or 2 factors), and poor-risk (>2 factors). The 2-year FFS was 51%, 27%, and 5% for good, intermediate, and poor-risk groups, respectively. Rick et al. prospectively tested this model in 46 patients (1998); the 2 year FFS rate in their population study was slightly worse than estimated by the model. Two major criticisms can be raised: the model is statistically significant but not really clinically significant (scoring system), and the difference between absolute refractory disease, refractory disease before HDCT, and progressive disease before HDCT is not clear. There are actually three different settings: patients who never achieve response to first-line treatment (absolute refractory), patients with refractoriness to conventional salvage regimen (refractory disease before HDCT), and patients responding or not to prior chemotherapy but who have disease progression during induction chemotherapy immediately before HDCT.

### 14.3.3 Phase II Studies of First Salvage Chemotherapy

Recently updated results of first salvage HDCT have become available. We have identified five series with a total of 233 patients treated by HDCT as part of their first salvage chemotherapy. The different studies are summarized in Table 14.2. Some studies were performed very early (Flechon et al. 1999; Horwich et al. 1993; Barnett et al. 1993). Several studies were published successively by IU research groups. In the first step, 25 patients were treated with 1 or 2 cycles of VeIP or VIP regimen plus one (6 patients) or two (19 patients) courses of HDCT (carboplatin and etoposide: CE regimen) with hematological stem-cell support (Broun et al. 1997). Sixteen of 25 patients were in CR, seven of whom after surgery. Thirteen of the 25 patients treated were NED after a median follow-up of 26 months. Secondly, results of this preliminary study were updated with the inclusion of 65 patients (Bhatia et al. 2000). It is noteworthy that several patients received two cycles of upfront HDCT without any initial standard chemotherapy. Finally, 135 patients were treated between 1996 and 2004. Seventy percent of the patients treated in this setting are NED (Einhorn et al. 2007). In conclusion it appears that HDCT may have a positive impact on survival.

Beyer et al. have performed a matched pair analysis in order to assess the role of HDCT as first salvage treatment for patients with relapsed or refractory disease (2002). Their conclusion is that HDCT may improve survival by 10%, which is lower than the benefit previously expected.

### 14.3.4 Randomized First-Line Salvage Studies

Only two published randomized trials have explored the role of HDCT in the first-line salvage treatment of GCT (Pico et al. 2005; Lorch et al. 2007). The IT94 trial is an international study performed in Europe which compared the standard salvage regimens VeIP/VIP or PEI (four cycles) to the experimental combination of the same chemotherapy regimen for three cycles plus one cycle of high-dose carboplatin, etoposide, and

**Table 14.2** High-dose chemotherapy trials in the firs-line salvage treatment

| Reference | Protocol | Nb pts | CR | NED |
|---|---|---|---|---|
| CLB (Flechon et al. 1999) | VIC | 7 | 3 | 4 |
| RMH (Horwich et al. 1993) | ICE | 11 | 7 | 7 |
| Barnett et al. (1993) | ICE/CEC | 15 | ? | 11 |
| IU(1992–1998) (Bhatia et al. 2000) | CE×2 | 65 | 42 (65%) | 40 (62%) |
| IU(1996–2004) (Einhorn et al. 2007) | CE×2 | 135 | ? | 94 (70%) |
| MSKCC (Motzer et al. 2000b) | TICE | 29 | 17 | 13 |
| Randomized trials | | | | |
| IT94 (Pico et al. 2005) | Standard | 136 | 42% | 47% |
| | Experimental | 138 | 43% | 47% |
| GTCSG (Lorch et al. 2007) | Sequential | 111 | 47% | 48% |
| | IT94 | 105 | 45% | 46% |

*CLB* Center Léon-Bérard; *RMH* Royal Marsden Hospital; *IU* Indiana university; *MSKCC* Memorial Sloan-Kettering Cancer Center; *IT94* International Trial 94; *GTCSG* German testicular cancer study group; *VIC* high-dose etoposide+ifosfamide+double-dose cisplatin; *ICE* ifosfamide+carboplatin+etoposide; *CE* carboplatin+etoposide; *TICE* two cycles of paclitaxel and ifosfamide followed by three cycles of high-dose CE; *Nb pts* patients number; *CR* complete response; *cCR* continuous CR; *NED* long-tern non-evolutive disease

cyclophosphamide (CEC or CarboPEC) (Pico et al. 2005). All 280 patients included were in the first-line salvage setting; they were not primarily cisplatin-refractory; they were stratified according to three factors: CR after first-line treatment, presence of lung metastases, and primary site. The statistical hypothesis was a 1-year event-free survival of 25% and 40% in the standard and experimental treatment arms, respectively, with a two-sided $\alpha=5\%$ and $\beta=20\%$, assuming 20% refractory patients after two cycles. There was neither a difference in CR and PR rates nor in overall survival between treatment arms. The toxic death rate was 3% and 7% in the standard and experimental treatment arms, respectively. The rate of 3-year overall survival was 53% in both arms. The results of standard chemotherapy were consistent with published results of patients treated by VeIP/VIP, and the toxic death rate was acceptable. It was concluded that one cycle of HDCT in nonrefractory patients adds no benefit over standard VeIP. Another randomized trial published in 2007 by the German group (Lorch et al. 2007) compared the experimental treatment arm of the IT94 to sequential HDCT which consisted of one cycle of VIP followed by three cycles of the HDCT CE regimen (carboplatin 1,500 mg/m$^2$ and etoposide 1,500 mg/m$^2$). In this trial, 15% of the patients had received at least one previous line of salvage chemotherapy, and 25% had cisplatin-refractory or absolute refractory disease. The trial was stopped prematurely after recruitment of 216 patients because of a 16% toxic death rate observed in the IT94 arm (vs. 4% in the sequential HDCT arm). There was neither a difference in CR and PR rates nor in overall survival between treatment arms. The 3-year overall survival rate was 47% in both arms (Lorch et al. 2007). However, no firm conclusion can be drawn from this study as it was prematurely closed and did not fit the initial statistical hypothesis, i.e., the detection of a 15% increase in event-free survival with $\alpha=5\%$ and $\beta=20\%$; besides, there is no indication of whether the study was one- or two-sided. The practical conclusion is that the toxicity of the IT94 experimental arm is excessive in this setting and there is no trend in favor of sequential HDCT. The standard first-line salvage treatment of GCT remains the standard VeIP regimen of chemotherapy.

### 14.3.5 Further Lines of Salvage High-Dose Chemotherapy

Many trials with different combinations of drugs have been performed in this setting. In the early eighty, HDCT regimens did not include platinum derivates (Postmus et al. 1984; Mulder et al. 1988), then double-dose cisplatin was added (Droz et al. 1991; Flechon et al. 1999) and, since 1990, HDCT regimens have been based on the association of carboplatin and etoposide (CE regimen) alone or combined with cyclophosphamide (CEC or CarboPEC regimens) or ifosfamide (ICE regimen).

The largest experience with the CE regimen has been accumulated at IU (Nichols et al. 1989, 1992; Bhatia et al. 2000; Einhorn et al. 2007; Broun et al. 1995). Between 1986 and 1988, 33 patients with refractory disease received two cycles of carboplatin (900–2,000 mg/m²) and etoposide (1,200 mg/m²) in a phase I/II trial (Nichols et al. 1989). The maximum tolerated dose (MTD) of carboplatin was 1,500–1,800 mg/m². Then a multicenter phase II trial was performed in 40 patients with relapsing or refractory disease treated with carboplatin (1,500 mg/m²) and etoposide (1,200 mg/m²) followed by ABMT: Autologous Bone narow Transformation (Nichols et al. 1992). Broun et al. have reported a trial with dose escalation of carboplatin (1,650–2,100 mg/m²) and etoposide (1,200–2,250 mg/m²) in the same group of patients (1995). The MTDs of etoposide and carboplatin were 2,250 mg/m² and 2,100 mg/m² respectively. Einhorn et al. have reported the evolution of patients with relapsed or refractory germ-cell tumors treated with the CE regimen between 1996 and 2006 at IU (2007). Forty-nine patients received third-line or subsequent-line treatment: 45% are NED. The line of treatment has been identified as a prognostic factor of poor outcome, as well as cisplatin refractoriness and IGCCC poor-risk group at initial diagnosis.

To improve the results of treatments combining high-dose etoposide plus carboplatin, the addition of cyclophosphamide has been assessed. Buckner has demonstrated the efficacy of high-dose cyclophosphamide for the first-line treatment of germ-cell tumors before the cisplatin era (Buckner et al. 1974). Ibrahim et al. have conducted a phase I trial testing the association of etoposide and cyclophosphamide at fixed doses with escalated dose of carboplatin (800–1,600 mg/m²) and ABMT (1993). At the MSKCC, 58 patients with relapsing or refractory disease received the CEC regimen and ABMT (Motzer et al. 1996). Twenty-seven received two cycles of HDCT. CR and NED rates were 40% (23 patients) and 21% (12 patients), respectively. Eleven of the 25 patients with relapsed disease and 6 of the 33 patients with refractory disease were alive after a median follow-up of 24 months. Linkesch et al. have undertaken a study of 42 refractory patients treated with a combination of etoposide (1,500 mg/m²), carboplatin (1,500 mg/m²), and cyclophosphamide (120 mg/kg) plus ABMT. Eleven patients had CR, of whom nine were long-term NED (1993).

Ifosfamide has also been tested in combination with etoposide and carboplatin. Broun et al. have reported the experience at IU, but the study had to be stopped prematurely because of renal toxicity (1991). Elias et al. have treated 18 patients with GCT in a phase I trial, testing the association of carboplatin (1,200–1,800 mg/m²), ifosfamide (12–16 g/m²), and etoposide (0–1,200 mg/m²) (1994). The MTDs were 16 g/m² for ifosfamide, 1,800 mg/m² for carboplatin, and 1,200 mg/m² for etoposide. Lotz et al. have included 20 patients in a phase I–II trial (1991); 14 patients received two cycles of HDCT; the MDTs were 7.5 g/m² for ifosfamide, 1,000 mg/m² for carboplatin, and 1,250 mg/m² for etoposide. Margolin et al. (1996) have evaluated the efficacy of two cycles of the ICE regimen with hematological support for the treatment of patients with GCT in sensitive relapse. The most important experience with the ICE regimen has been reported by the German group in Berlin (Siegert et al. 1994; Rick et al. 1998; Beyer et al. 1997a). As a whole, 150 patients with relapsed or refractory GCT have received ICE plus hematological stem-cell support after conventional salvage treatment (Rick et al. 1998). Sixty-seven percent of the patients were sensitive to cisplatin, 25% were refractory to cisplatin, and 8% were absolute refractory. No refractory or absolute refractory and 11/101 nonrefractory patients were in CR after HDCT. Fifty-one patients (34%) had NED after a median follow-up of 55 months (range 21–88 months). The NED rate was just a little greater than that with conventional salvage treatment. Results of this study demonstrate that ifosfamide increases the renal toxicity of HDCT, especially in heavily pretreated patients. Rodenhuis et al. have treated patients with relapsed or refractory GCT with a high-dose regimen including two courses of CE without autologous stem-cell transfusion and one course of the association of carboplatin, etoposide, and thiotepa (CTC regimen) (1999).

No randomized trial has been performed in this group of patients. In summary, the overall NED rate in these patients is between 10 and 30%, depending on the cisplatin response status, disease extension at salvage treatment, and initial IGCCC risk group. An interesting study has been conducted by the IU group in patients with adverse prognostic factors (Vaena et al. 2003). Eighty patients were treated with two cycles of HDCT plus EC. The 13 patients with primary mediastinum GCT died of disease progression. Patients with a Beyer's score greater than two still had a 2-year FFS of 25–35%, apart from those with AFP >1,000 ng/mL whose 2-year FFS was only 18%. This means that HDCT still has a role to play in the treatment of a small proportion of selected poor-risk patients in relapse.

## 14.4 New Drugs and Old Drugs in the Salvage Setting

### *14.4.1 Paclitaxel Activity and Paclitaxel Combination Chemotherapy Regimens*

Paclitaxel is a potent cytotoxic drug in in vitro germ-cell models (Droz and Culine 1998) that has been investigated in three phase II trials (Motzer et al. 1994; Bokemeyer et al. 1996; Sandler et al. 1998). All patients had been heavily pretreated by standard chemotherapy regimens. A great proportion of patients had cisplatin-refractory disease. At a dose of 225 mg/m$^2$ (3-h infusion) (Bokemeyer et al. 1996) – 250 mg/m$^2$ (24-h infusion) (Motzer et al. 1994), paclitaxel induced an objective response in 12/51 patients (23%). The response rate was only 2/18 (11%) with a dose of 170–200 mg/m$^2$ (24-h infusion) (Sandler et al. 1998). These studies provided interesting results and sufficient background to include paclitaxel in both first-line (de Wit et al. 1999) and salvage treatments. Paclitaxel was then studied in the standard salvage chemotherapy setting (TIP = paclitaxel plus ifosfamide plus cisplatin) (Motzer et al. 2000a) and in the sequential HDCT setting. The TIP regimen and other paclitaxel-containing regimens consist of different dosages or modes of administration of paclitaxel and ifosfamide, depending on institutions. At the MSKCC, paclitaxel is given at a dose of 200 mg/m$^2$ administered as a 24-h continuous infusion on day 1 of the cycle (Motzer et al. 2000a; Motzer et al. 2000b). In the German group, paclitaxel is given on day 1 at a dose of 175 mg/m$^2$ administered as a 3-h infusion (Rick et al. 2001), as well as in the Medical research Council (MRC) (Mead et al. 2005) and in Mardiak et al. (2005) trials. In the French group, the dose of paclitaxel is 250 mg/m$^2$ administered as a 3-h infusion (Lotz et al. 2005).

At the MSKCC, the TIP regimen (Motzer et al. 2000a) was administered as first-line salvage therapy in good-risk patients. Four cycles of chemotherapy were administered at 21-day intervals with G-CSF. Thirty patients were treated: the CR rate, continuous CR rate, and NED rate were 80%, 73%, and 80% respectively. The same TIP protocol induces a CR rate of 60% in 43 patients (73% in the MSKCC good-risk group) in the MRC trial (Mead et al. 2005) and a 65% CR rate in Mardiak et al. study (2005). The German group developed a protocol with three cycles of TIP followed by one cycle of high-dose etoposide, carboplatin, and thiotepa (Rick et al. 2001). Eighty patients were treated: 67% were in the first-line salvage setting, 76% were cisplatin sensitive, and 35% only had achieved prior CR status. One patient experienced a toxic death, and 18 patients did not receive HDCT. The CR rate, continuous CR rate, and NED rate were 35%, 26%, and 33% respectively. The French group developed a protocol with two cycles of the combination of epirubicin and paclitaxel followed by one cycle of high-dose cyclophosphamide and thiotepa and two cycles of high-dose CE (Lotz et al. 2005). Forty-five patients were included in the trial. The prognostic score according to Beyer's classification (Beyer et al. 1996) was 0, 1–2, and >2 in 20%, 55%, and 25% of the patients respectively. Fifteen percent of the patients were in the first-line salvage setting (refractory disease). Only 33 patients received HDCT, of whom 22 completed the whole program. There were five treatment-related deaths. The CR rate, continuous CR rate, and NED rate were 22%, 19%, and 23% respectively. The 3-year overall survival of patients with Beyer's score of 1–2 was 13% only. The MSKCC group also developed a sequential dose-intensive protocol of chemotherapy, TICE (Motzer et al. 2000b). TICE consists of two cycles of paclitaxel and ifosfamide followed by three cycles of high-dose CE. Thirty-seven patients were included in the trial: all had unfavorable characteristics (incomplete response in 84% of the patients, extragonadal primary, and more than one line of treatment). There were no toxicity-related deaths. The CR rate, continuous CR rate, and NED rate were 62%, 41%, and 49% respectively. Conversely, the introduction of low dose (McNeish et al. 2004) or high dose (Margolin et al. 2005) of paclitaxel in the HDCT regimen itself has not proven higher evident efficiency.

### 14.4.2 Prognostic Factor-Based Salvage Strategy

If one considers tailoring salvage treatment to the prognostic profile of each patient, results obtained with the VeIP and TIP regimens on the one hand and results of HDCT trials on the other hand may help decision making. Patients in the good-risk group have testis primary with CR after first-line treatment. Their expected overall survival rate is 65% with the VeIP regimen (McCaffrey et al. 1997) and 80% with the TIP regimen (Motzer et al. 2000a). However, it is impossible to compare these protocols because prognostic assessment was performed retrospectively in the former and prospectively in the later, and the number of patients in each trial is too small.

Patients in the poor-risk group have mediastinum primary, but for the purpose of this chapter it is more important to focus on those with testis primary with IR to first-line treatment, failure to first-line salvage therapy, or cisplatin refractoriness. Their expected overall survival rate is 30% with the VeIP regimen (McCaffrey et al. 1997; Motzer et al. 2000b), and 49% with the TICE regimen (Motzer et al. 2000b). However, no firm conclusion can be drawn because the patient population in the two trials was heterogeneous, regardless of best response to prior chemotherapy, cisplatin refractoriness, and line of treatment. The treatment of patients in this poor-risk group requires the inclusion of new chemotherapeutic drugs, a careful definition of patient characteristics, and possibly a comparison of experimental treatments with standard chemotherapy, of experimental treatments with one another, and of experimental treatments with HDCT regimens.

### 14.4.3 Other Conventional-Dose Chemotherapy Regimens

This aspect will be developed in a specific chapter. Recently published reviews (Kollmannsberger et al. 2006; Sonpavde et al. 2007) show that apart from paclitaxel, other drugs (gemcitabine, oxaliplatin, and irinotecan) have also been studied alone or in diverse combinations. The interpretation of the results of the different studies published is difficult because of the heterogeneity of patients characteristics (proportion of cisplatin-refractory patients, of patients pretreated by HDCT, and of late relapses), of drug dosage, and of the schedule of combined treatments (Kollmannsberger et al. 2006). The response rate is generally 10–25% with one drug (whatever the drug) and 20–50% when drugs are combined two by two. However, the long-term NED rate is marginal, with only 5–15% when using a combination of drugs. An old drug, epirubicin, was recently re-evaluated in combination with cisplatin (Bedano et al. 2006). Doxorubicin and epirubicin had been extensively studied in the past (Droz and Culine 1998). Thirty patients received epirubicin 90 mg/m$^2$ plus cisplatin 100 mg/m$^2$ for four cycles. It is noteworthy that 70% of these patients experienced late relapses. Nevertheless, nine achieved a CR, seven of which were long-lasting (more than 2 years). This is an interesting observation for the treatment of late relapses, which will be developed in another chapter.

## 14.5 Salvage Surgery. Surgical Exeresis of Postchemotherapy Residual Disease. The Case of Growing Teratoma

Salvage surgery has been reported in different series (Murphy et al. 1993; Eastham et al. 1994; Coogan et al. 1997; Albers et al. 2000; Ravi et al. 1998). All patients with detectable, refractory disease, even with elevated STM, are candidates for surgical resection of their tumors ("desperation surgery"). The long-term NED rate reported in the literature is around 25%. However, patients must be strictly selected: only those with only one tumor site, a limited number of metastases, and a possibility of complete resection are eligible for salvage surgery. Results of the published studies must be interpreted with caution, keeping in mind that patients have been strictly selected, that several of them have experienced late relapses with very specific biological pattern, and that other patients actually had a growing teratoma. Moreover, none of these studies has analyzed the role of fluorodeoxyglucose-tomography emission positron (FDG-TEP) scan in the selection of patients for surgery.

A particular point to consider is the role of complete surgical resection of residual disease after

**Table 14.3** Role of the complete surgical exeresis of active residual disease

| Reference | Regimen | Result of surgery | NED |
|---|---|---|---|
| Conventional treatment | | | |
| Fossa (1999a) | Various regimens | Surgical CR: 31 pts,<br>PRm(−): 32 pts | |
| IT94 (Pico et al. 2005) | Standard | sCR: 5% | sCR: 66%, IR: 30% |
| HDCT | | | |
| IT94 | Experimental | sCR: 8% | |
| GTCSG (Lorch et al.2007) | Sequential<br>IT94 | sCR: 10%, sCR: 9% | ? |
| Rick et al. (2004) | Sequential | Viable tumor: 22 pts,<br>Nonviable tumor : 33 pts | 42%, 84% |
| IU. Bhatia et al. (2000) | CE×2 | sCR: 4 pts | 1 pt |

*IU* Indiana university; *IT94* International Trial 94; *GTCSG* German testicular cancer study group; *CE* carboplatin+etoposide; *pts* patients; *CR* complete response; *sCR* surgical CR (complete exeresis of active viable residual tumor); *NED* long-tern nonevolutive disease; *PRm*(−) partial response with nomalized STM

conventional salvage chemotherapy and after HDCT in the salvage setting (e.g., importance of sCR). The different studies are summarized in Table 14.3. After conventional salvage treatment, the question has been well studied by Fossa et al. (Fossa et al. 1999a): the 3-year survival, of patients in whom residual disease was completely removed (31 patients) or not (32 patients) was 52% and 31% respectively. After HDCT, in the IT94 trial (Pico et al. 2005) and in the German randomized trial (Lorch et al. 2007) respectively, 5 and 8% and 10 and 9% of the patients in both arms of the protocols had sCR. In the IT94 trial, the 3-year overall survival of patients with sCR and IR with viable GCT was 66% and 30%, respectively. Similar information is not available for the German randomized trial. However, extensive experience has been acquired from phase II HDCT salvage studies of the German group (Rick et al. 2004). Fifty-seven patients had a resection of residual disease after HDCT. The characteristics were: completeness of resection in 52 patients, disease limited to one site in 39 patients, or involving several sites in 18. Necrosis with or without mature teratoma was observed in 33 cases, and viable tumor (with other components or not) in 22 patients. Four patients had transformation of teratoma in non-GCT histological pattern. The 5-year overall survival of patients with resection of viable tumor or nonviable residual disease was 42% and 84%, respectively (Table 14.4).

Another important indication of salvage surgery is the management of growing teratoma. It is thus very important to obtain a complete resection of all residual disease, even after HDCT. The definition of growing teratoma is an increase of mature teratoma without other germ-cell components and with normal serum marker level during or after chemotherapy (Logothetis et al. 1982). The incidence of growing teratoma is 2–12% (Logothetis et al. 1982; Jeffery et al. 1991; Andre et al. 2000), but 80% of the patients have mature teratoma at the primary site. Treatment should be complete surgical excision, which is all the more easy as the volume is small. Recurrence may occur when resection is incomplete and the development of secondary malignancies with nongerm-cell elements may be observed.

**Table 14.4** Role of surgery in the salvage treatment after failure to HDCT

| Reference | IU (Porcu et al. 2000) | Pont et al. (Pont et al. 1997) | CLB (Flechon et al. 2001) |
|---|---|---|---|
| Nb pts | 101 | 48 | 32 |
| No treatment | 35 | 0 | 3 |
| Response to treatment | 12 | 8 | 12 |
| NED pts | 5 | 1 | 6 |
| Of whom by surgery | 5 | 0 | 6 |

*CLB* Centre Léon-Bérard; *IU* Indiana university; *Nb pts* patients number; *NED* long-tern nonevolutive disease

## 14.6 Miscellaneous Settings

### 14.6.1 The Case of Seminoma

The case of seminoma is particular: the different salvage studies published to date have either included 10–20% of patients with seminoma (conventional chemotherapy or HDCT studies), or excluded seminoma patients (Loehrer et al. 1998). Only one study has focused on the question of salvage treatment for seminoma patients (Vuky et al. 2002). Vuky et al. have reported on 27 patients with relapsing progressive seminoma, 15 of whom received standard chemotherapy and 12 were entered in different HDCT trials. In total, the CR rate, continuous CR rate, and NED rate were 56%, 48%, and 52% respectively after a median follow-up of 72 months. It is noteworthy that the histological pattern of tumors biopsied before salvage treatment showed some cytologic atypia, and that all patients undergoing surgical resection of active residual disease relapsed and eventually died of disease. Thus, it is concluded that salvage chemotherapy is as active in seminoma patients as in nonseminoma patients, but that relapsing seminoma may have a particular biological profile which requires specific studies. Nevertheless, it is not clear whether HDCT is more active in these patients than standard chemotherapy regimens.

### 14.6.2 Do Patients with Complete Surgical Response to First-Line Treatment Require Additional Salvage Chemotherapy?

The tumor must be considered chemoresistant; therefore, complete surgical removal is the most effective treatment (Fox et al. 1993). The outcome of patients with postchemotherapy residual active disease has been studied. The general treatment recommendation for these patients is to administer two additional cycles of the same chemotherapy. A retrospective analysis of more than 300 patients after surgical removal of residual active germ cell disease has shown that the most important risk factors of relapse are incomplete surgery and a proportion of residual active disease superior to 10% of the residual volume (Fizazi et al. 2001). No difference in the recurrence rate has been observed between the patients receiving two additional cycles of chemotherapy and others. One can conclude from this study that patients undergoing complete resection of residual disease must be carefully followed up, whatever be the proportion of active disease. Conversely, patients with incomplete resection of residual disease may be switched to salvage treatment. It is therefore essential to perform complete resection of all residual disease.

### 14.6.3 Do Patients with Very High hCG Levels Require Additional Salvage Chemotherapy?

In the first-line treatment of GCT, a particular subgroup of poor-risk patients, those with very high serum hCG levels (e.g., >50,000 U/L) (Zon et al. 1998), requires a specific management. These patients are unlikely to recover normal serum hCG levels after the fourth cycle of BEP. Before deciding to switch to salvage chemotherapy or surgical resection of residual disease, careful follow-up must be proposed, with serial weekly determination of serum hCG levels. Half of the patients may recover normal serum hCG levels with complete regression of residual disease (mainly lung metastases) and remain NED. The other 50% will have increased serum hCG levels requiring salvage chemotherapy (Zon et al. 1998).

### 14.6.4 CNS Relapses

In the study by Fossa et al. (1999b) of 83 patients with brain metastases, relapses occurred after a median interval of 9 months; 21 patients had no symptoms and brain metastases were diagnosed by systematic CT-scan. They recommend to perform systematic cerebral MRI when patients have pure choriocarcinoma, elevated serum hCG level, and/or clinical symptoms. Relapses with cerebral localizations occur early, in the first 2 years after first-line chemotherapy. The prognosis of patients is usually poor, although it is better when patients have less than two cerebral lesions and no other metastatic site involved. The 5-year overall survival is 12% when patients have multiple lesions and 39% when patients have solitary cerebral metastases. It is unlikely to observe patients with asymptomatic metastases, normal tumor marker level, and no other relapse site, the only situation likely to justify systematic brain imaging. Therefore, our opinion is to perform this examination only in the case of neurological symptoms or evident relapse.

### 14.6.5 Treatment After Relapse from HDCT

Three studies of the treatment of relapse after HDCT have been published (Pont et al. 1997; Porcu et al. 2000; Flechon et al. 2001), including 181 patients in total. Thirty-two patients did not receive any treatment and more than 50% received various chemotherapy regimens. The overall response rate was 32/181 (18%); the drugs which induced the best response rates were oral etoposide (Porcu et al. 2000) and the combination of paclitaxel and ifosfamide (Pont et al. 1997). However, only 12 patients (7%) were long-term NED. It is noteworthy that 11 of them had had a complete resection of active residual disease combined with different chemotherapy regimens. Thus, the surgical resection of operable lesions remains a valuable option for patients with refractory disease. The activity of oral etoposide after HDCT led investigators at the IU to propose adjuvant oral etoposide after HDCT for a 3-months period (Cooper and Einhorn 1995). This option has never been validated.

### 14.6.6 Late Complications of Salvage Chemotherapy

Few studies have focused on the long-term effects of salvage chemotherapy and particularly of HDCT. A specific study of secondary leukemia after HDCT in GCT patients (Kollmannsberger et al. 1998) enrolled a total of 302 patients treated with a median cumulative dose of etoposide of 5 g/m$^2$ (range, 2.4–14 g/m$^2$). Four cases of secondary acute myeloid leukemia (AML) were observed, which resulted in a cumulative incidence of 1.3% (95% confidence interval [CI], 0.38–3.59%) at 52 months of median follow-up (range, 12–198 months). Based on these four cases of AML, which are most likely etoposide-related, it was concluded that the risk for developing this disease is significantly increased in comparison to the age-matched general population. The German group studied long-term complications in 28 patients after a median follow-up of 4 years (range, 3.2–5.6 years) (Beyer et al. 1997b). The most important toxicities reported were grade 2/3 peripheral nervous toxicity in eight patients, grade 2 hearing loss in five patients, and renal toxicity (creatinine clearance impairment) grade 1 in five patients, whereas one patient required hemodialysis for chronic renal failure. This issue will be developed in another chapter.

## 14.7 Standard Treatment Recommendations

The NCCN (2007) and the European Consensus group (EGCCCG) (Schmoll et al. 2004) have produced recommendations for the treatment of GCT, specifically for salvage treatment. Both recommendations are based on an assessment of prognosis according to histological status and on a strategy combining salvage chemotherapy and complete resection of all residual disease whenever possible.

The NNCN recommends distinguishing patients with initial good-risk characteristics from those with poor-risk features. Good-risk patients would receive standard VeIP chemotherapy or the TIP regimen. In the case of IR or relapse, they would be offered treatment with HDCT. The poor-risk group would be proposed HDCT, preferably in the setting of a clinical trial. In the case of failure, they would be offered experimental treatment.

The European Consensus recommends ifosfamide-based salvage chemotherapy regimens such as VIP, or more commonly VeIP and more recently TIP. As no evidence of a benefit of HDCT has yet been demonstrated in these patients; it is recommended to enroll them in prospective clinical trials. Anyhow, surgical resection of residual disease should be proposed whenever possible.

**Acknowledgments** The authors thank Marie-Dominique Reynaud for editing the manuscript.

## References

Albers P, Ganz A, Hannig E, Miersch WD, Muller SC (2000) Salvage surgery of chemorefractory germ cell tumors with elevated tumor markers. J Urol 164(2):381–384

Andre F, Fizazi K, Culine S et al (2000) The growing teratoma syndrome: results of therapy and long-term follow-up of 33 patients. Eur J Cancer 36(11):1389–1394

Anon (1997) International Germ Cell Consensus Classification: a prognostic factor-based staging system for metastatic germ cell cancers. International Germ Cell Cancer Collaborative Group. J Clin Oncol 15(2):594–603

Bajorin DF, Sarosdy MF, Pfister DG et al (1993) Randomized trial of etoposide and cisplatin versus etoposide and carboplatin in patients with good-risk germ cell tumors: a multiinstitutional study. J Clin Oncol 11(4):598–606

Bajorin DF, Nichols CR, Schmoll HJ et al (1995) Recombinant human granulocyte-macrophage colony-stimulating factor as an adjunct to conventional-dose ifosfamide-based chemotherapy for patients with advanced or relapsed germ cell tumors: a randomized trial. J Clin Oncol 13(1):79–86

Barnett MJ, Coppin CM, Murray N et al (1993) High-dose chemotherapy and autologous bone marrow transplantation for patients with poor prognosis nonseminomatous germ cell tumours. Br J Cancer 68(3):594–598

Bedano PM, Brames MJ, Williams SD, Juliar BE, Einhorn LH (2006) Phase II study of cisplatin plus epirubicin salvage chemotherapy in refractory germ cell tumors. J Clin Oncol 24(34):5403–5407

Beyer J, Kramar A, Mandanas R et al (1996) High-dose chemotherapy as salvage treatment in germ cell tumors: a multivariate analysis of prognostic variables. J Clin Oncol 14(10): 2638–2645

Beyer J, Kingreen D, Krause M et al (1997) Long-term survival of patients with recurrent or refractory germ cell tumors after high dose chemotherapy. Cancer 79(1):161–168

Beyer J, Stenning S, Gerl A, Fossa S, Siegert W (2002) High-dose versus conventional-dose chemotherapy as first-salvage treatment in patients with non-seminomatous germ-cell tumors: a matched-pair analysis. Ann Oncol 13(4):599–605

Bhatia S, Abonour R, Porcu P et al (2000) High-dose chemotherapy as initial salvage chemotherapy in patients with relapsed testicular cancer. J Clin Oncol 18(19):3346–3351

Blijham G, Spitzer G, Litam J et al (1981) The treatment of advanced testicular carcinoma with high dose chemotherapy and autologous marrow support. Eur J Cancer 17(4):433–441

Bokemeyer C, Beyer J, Metzner B et al (1996) Phase II study of paclitaxel in patients with relapsed or cisplatin-refractory testicular cancer. Ann Oncol 7(1):31–34

Bosl GJ, Motzer RJ (1997) Testicular germ-cell cancer. N Engl J Med 337(4):242–253

Bosl GJ, Bajorin DF, Sheinfeld J, Motzer RJ, Chaganti RSK (2007) Cancer of the testis. In: DeVita VT, Hellman S, Rosenberg SA (eds) Cancer. Principles and practice of oncology, 7th edn. Lippincott Williams & Wilkins, Philadelphia, 1269–1293

Broun ER, Nichols CR, Tricot G, Loehrer PJ, Williams SD, Einhorn LH (1991) High dose carboplatin/VP-16 plus ifosfamide with autologous bone marrow support in the treatment of refractory germ cell tumors. Bone Marrow Transplant 7(1):53–56

Broun ER, Nichols CR, Mandanas R et al (1995) Dose escalation study of high-dose carboplatin and etoposide with autologous bone marrow support in patients with recurrent and refractory germ cell tumors. Bone Marrow Transplant 16(3):353–358

Broun ER, Nichols CR, Gize G et al (1997) Tandem high dose chemotherapy with autologous bone marrow transplantation for initial relapse of testicular germ cell cancer. Cancer 79(8):1605–1610

Buckner CD, Clift RA, Fefer A et al (1974) High-dose cyclophosphamide (NSC-26271) for the treatment of metastatic testicular neoplasms. Cancer Chemother Rep 58(5 Pt 1):709–714

Coogan CL, Foster RS, Rowland RG et al (1997) Postchemotherapy retroperitoneal lymph node dissection is effective therapy in selected patients with elevated tumor markers after primary chemotherapy alone. Urology 50(6):957–962

Cooper MA, Einhorn LH (1995) Maintenance chemotherapy with daily oral etoposide following salvage therapy in patients with germ cell tumors. J Clin Oncol 13(5):1167–1169

de Wit R, Louwerens M, de Mulder PH, Verweij J, Rodenhuis S, Schornagel J (1999) Management of intermediate-prognosis germ-cell cancer: results of a phase I/II study of Taxol-BEP. Int J Cancer 83(6):831–833

de Wit R, Roberts JT, Wilkinson PM et al (2001) Equivalence of three or four cycles of bleomycin, etoposide, and cisplatin chemotherapy and of a 3- or 5-day schedule in good-prognosis germ cell cancer: a randomized study of the European Organization for Research and Treatment of Cancer Genitourinary Tract Cancer Cooperative Group and the Medical Research Council. J Clin Oncol 19(6):1629–1640

Dieckmann KP, Albers P, Classen J et al (2005) Late relapse of testicular germ cell neoplasms: a descriptive analysis of 122 cases. J Urol 173(3):824–829

Droz JP, Culine S (1998) New prospects for the treatment of germ-cell tumours. Expert Opin Investig Drugs 7(7):1139–1157

Droz JP, Pico JL, Ghosn M et al (1991) Long-term survivors after salvage high dose chemotherapy with bone marrow rescue in refractory germ cell cancer. Eur J Cancer 27(7):831–835

Droz JP, Kramar A, Rey A (1992) Prognostic factors in metastatic disease. Semin Oncol 19(2):181–189

Eastham JA, Wilson TG, Russell C, Ahlering TE, Skinner DG (1994) Surgical resection in patients with nonseminomatous germ cell tumor who fail to normalize serum tumor markers after chemotherapy. Urology 43(1):74–80

Einhorn LH (1990) Treatment of testicular cancer: a new and improved model. J Clin Oncol 8(11):1777–1781

Einhorn LH, Donohue J (1977) Cis-diamminedichloroplatinum, vinblastine, and bleomycin combination chemotherapy in disseminated testicular cancer. Ann Intern Med 87(3):293–298

Einhorn LH, Williams SD, Loehrer PJ et al (1989) Evaluation of optimal duration of chemotherapy in favorable-prognosis disseminated germ cell tumors: a Southeastern Cancer Study Group protocol. J Clin Oncol 7(3):387–391

Einhorn LH, Williams SD, Chamness A, Brames MJ, Perkins SM, Abonour R (2007) High-dose chemotherapy and stem-cell rescue for metastatic germ-cell tumors. N Engl J Med 357(4):340–348

Elias AD, Ayash LJ, Wheeler C et al (1994) High-dose ifosfamide/carboplatin/etoposide with autologous hematopoietic stem cell support: safety and future directions. Semin Oncol 21(5 suppl 12):83–85

Farhat F, Culine S, Theodore C, Bekradda M, Terrier-Lacombe MJ, Droz JP (1996) Cisplatin and ifosfamide with either vinblastine or etoposide as salvage therapy for refractory or relapsing germ cell tumor patients: the Institut Gustave Roussy experience. Cancer 77(6):1193–1197

Fizazi K, Tjulandin S, Salvioni R et al (2001) Viable malignant cells after primary chemotherapy for disseminated nonseminomatous germ cell tumors: prognostic factors and role of postsurgery chemotherapy–results from an international study group. J Clin Oncol 19(10):2647–2657

Flechon A, Biron P, Droz JP (1999) High-dose chemotherapy with hematopoietic stem-cell support in germ-cell tumor patient treatment: the French experience. Int J Cancer 83(6):844–847

Flechon A, Rivoire M, Biron P, Droz JP (2001) Importance of surgery as salvage treatment after high dose chemotherapy failure in germ cell tumors. J Urol 165(6 Pt 1):1920–1926

Flechon A, Culine S, Theodore C, Droz JP (2005) Pattern of relapse after first line treatment of advanced stage germ-cell tumors. Eur Urol 48(6):957–963

Fossa SD, Stenning SP, Gerl A et al (1999a) Prognostic factors in patients progressing after cisplatin-based chemotherapy for malignant non-seminomatous germ cell tumours. Br J Cancer 80(9):1392–1399

Fossa SD, Bokemeyer C, Gerl A et al (1999b) Treatment outcome of patients with brain metastases from malignant germ cell tumors. Cancer 85(4):988–997

Fox EP, Weathers TD, Williams SD et al (1993) Outcome analysis for patients with persistent nonteratomatous germ cell tumor in postchemotherapy retroperitoneal lymph node dissections. J Clin Oncol 11(7):1294–1299

Geller NL, Bosl GJ, Chan EY (1989) Prognostic factors for relapse after complete response in patients with metastatic germ cell tumors. Cancer 63(3):440–445

Gerl A, Clemm C, Schmeller N, Hartenstein R, Lamerz R, Wilmanns W (1995) Prognosis after salvage treatment for unselected male patients with germ cell tumours. Br J Cancer 72(4):1026–1032

Ghosn M, Droz JP, Theodore C et al (1988) Salvage chemotherapy in refractory germ cell tumors with etoposide (VP-16) plus ifosfamide plus high-dose cisplatin. A VIhP regimen. Cancer 62(1):24–27

Gietema JA, Meinardi MT, Sleijfer DT, Hoekstra HJ, van der Graaf WT (2002) Routine chest X-rays have no additional value in the detection of relapse during routine follow-up of patients treated with chemotherapy for disseminated non-seminomatous testicular cancer. Ann Oncol 13(10):1616–1620

Greene FL (2002) Testis cancer. In: Page DL, Fleming IDFA et al (eds) AJCC cancer staging handbook. Springer, New York, p 469

Higby DJ, Wallace HJ Jr, Albert D, Holland JF (1974) Diamminodichloroplatinum in the chemotherapy of testicular tumors. J Urol 112(1):100–104

Hildebrandt MO, Blaser F, Beyer J et al (1998) Detection of tumor cells in peripheral blood samples from patients with germ cell tumors using immunocytochemical and reverse transcriptase-polymerase chain reaction techniques. Bone Marrow Transplant 22(8):771–775

Horwich A, Wilson C, Cornes P, Gildersleve J, Dearnaley D (1993) Increasing the dose intensity of chemotherapy in poor-prognosis metastatic non-seminoma. Eur Urol 23(1):219–222

Ibrahim A, Zambon E, Bourhis JH et al (1993) High-dose chemotherapy with etoposide, cyclophosphamide and escalating dose of carboplatin followed by autologous bone marrow transplantation in cancer patients. A pilot study. Eur J Cancer 29A(10):1398–1403

Jeffery GM, Theaker JM, Lee AH, Blaquiere RM, Smart CJ, Mead GM (1991) The growing teratoma syndrome. Br J Urol 67(2):195–202

Kollmannsberger C, Beyer J, Droz JP et al (1998) Secondary leukemia following high cumulative doses of etoposide in patients treated for advanced germ cell tumors. J Clin Oncol 16(10):3386–3391

Kollmannsberger C, Nichols C, Bokemeyer C (2006) Recent advances in management of patients with platinum-refractory testicular germ cell tumors. Cancer 106(6):1217–1226

Kondagunta GV, Sheinfeld J, Motzer RJ (2003) Recommendations of follow-up after treatment of germ cell tumors. Semin Oncol 30(3):382–389

Lederman GS, Garnick MB, Canellos GP, Richie JP (1983) Chemotherapy of refractory germ cell cancer with Etoposide. J Clin Oncol 1(11):706–709

Linkesch W, Greinix A, Hocker P, Krainer M, Wagner A (1993) Long-term follow-up of a phase I/II trial ultra-high dose carboplatin, VP-16, Cyclophosphamide with ABMT in refractory or relapsed NSCGCT.(Abstract). Proc Am Assoc Cancer Res 34:232

Loehrer PJ Sr, Lauer R, Roth BJ, Williams SD, Kalasinski LA, Einhorn LH (1988) Salvage therapy in recurrent germ cell cancer: ifosfamide and cisplatin plus either vinblastine or etoposide. Ann Intern Med 109(7):540–546

Loehrer PJ Sr, Johnson D, Elson P, Einhorn LH, Trump D (1995) Importance of bleomycin in favorable-prognosis disseminated germ cell tumors: an Eastern Cooperative Oncology Group trial. J Clin Oncol 13(2):470–476

Loehrer PJ Sr, Gonin R, Nichols CR, Weathers T, Einhorn LH (1998) Vinblastine plus ifosfamide plus cisplatin as initial salvage therapy in recurrent germ cell tumor. J Clin Oncol 16(7):2500–2504

Logothetis CJ, Samuels ML, Trindade A, Johnson DE (1982) The growing teratoma syndrome. Cancer 50(8):1629–1635

Lorch A, Kollmannsberger C, Hartmann JT et al (2007) Single versus sequential high-dose chemotherapy in patients with relapsed or refractory germ cell tumors: a prospective randomized multicenter trial of the German Testicular Cancer Study Group. J Clin Oncol 25(19):2778–2784

Lotz JP, Machover D, Malassagne B et al (1991) Phase I-II study of two consecutive courses of high-dose epipodophyllotoxin, ifosfamide, and carboplatin with autologous bone marrow transplantation for treatment of adult patients with solid tumors. J Clin Oncol 9(10):1860–1870

Lotz JP, Bui B, Gomez F et al (2005) Sequential high-dose chemotherapy protocol for relapsed poor prognosis germ cell tumors combining two mobilization and cytoreductive treatments followed by three high-dose chemotherapy regimens supported by autologous stem cell transplantation. Results of the phase II multicentric TAXIF trial. Ann Oncol 16(3):411–418

Mardiak J, Salek T, Sycova-Mila Z et al (2005) Paclitaxel plus ifosfamide and cisplatin in second-line treatment of germ cell tumors: a phase II study. Neoplasma 52(6):497–501

Margolin K, Doroshow JH, Ahn C et al (1996) Treatment of germ cell cancer with two cycles of high-dose ifosfamide, carboplatin, and etoposide with autologous stem-cell support. J Clin Oncol 14(10):2631–2637

Margolin KA, Doroshow JH, Frankel P et al (2005) Paclitaxel-based high-dose chemotherapy with autologous stem cell rescue for relapsed germ cell cancer. Biol Blood Marrow Transplant 11(11):903–911

Mayer F, Honecker F, Looijenga LH, Bokemeyer C (2003) Towards an understanding of the biological basis of response to cisplatin-based chemotherapy in germ-cell tumors. Ann Oncol 14(6):825–832

McCaffrey JA, Mazumdar M, Bajorin DF, Bosl GJ, Vlamis V, Motzer RJ (1997) Ifosfamide- and cisplatin-containing chemotherapy as first-line salvage therapy in germ cell tumors: response and survival. J Clin Oncol 15(7):2559–2563

McNeish IA, Kanfer EJ, Haynes R et al (2004) Paclitaxel-containing high-dose chemotherapy for relapsed or refractory testicular germ cell tumours. Br J Cancer 90(6):1169–1175

Mead GM, Cullen MH, Huddart R et al (2005) A phase II trial of TIP (paclitaxel, ifosfamide and cisplatin) given as second-line (post-BEP) salvage chemotherapy for patients with metastatic germ cell cancer: a medical research council trial. Br J Cancer 93(2):178–184

Mostofi FK, Sesterhen IA (1994) Revised international classification of testicular tumors. In: Jones WG, Harnden P, Appleyard I (eds) Germ cell tumors III. Oxford Pergamon, London, p 153

Motzer RJ, Gulati SC, Tong WP et al (1993) Phase I trial with pharmacokinetic analyses of high-dose carboplatin, etoposide, and cyclophosphamide with autologous bone marrow transplantation in patients with refractory germ cell tumors. Cancer Res 53(16):3730–3735

Motzer RJ, Bajorin DF, Schwartz LH et al (1994) Phase II trial of paclitaxel shows antitumor activity in patients with previously treated germ cell tumors. J Clin Oncol 12(11):2277–2283

Motzer RJ, Mazumdar M, Bosl GJ, Bajorin DF, Amsterdam A, Vlamis V (1996) High-dose carboplatin, etoposide, and cyclophosphamide for patients with refractory germ cell tumors: treatment results and prognostic factors for survival and toxicity. J Clin Oncol 14(4):1098–1105

Motzer RJ, Sheinfeld J, Mazumdar M et al (2000a) Paclitaxel, ifosfamide, and cisplatin second-line therapy for patients with relapsed testicular germ cell cancer. J Clin Oncol 18(12):2413–2418

Motzer RJ, Mazumdar M, Sheinfeld J et al (2000b) Sequential dose-intensive paclitaxel, ifosfamide, carboplatin, and etoposide salvage therapy for germ cell tumor patients. J Clin Oncol 18(6):1173–1180

Motzer RJ, Nichols CJ, Margolin KA et al (2007) Phase III randomized trial of conventional-dose chemotherapy with or without high-dose chemotherapy and autologous hematopoietic stem-cell rescue as first-line treatment for patients with poor-prognosis metastatic germ cell tumors. J Clin Oncol 25(3):247–256

Mulder PO, de Vries EG, Koops HS et al (1988) Chemotherapy with maximally tolerable doses of VP 16-213 and cyclophosphamide followed by autologous bone marrow transplantation for the treatment of relapsed or refractory germ cell tumors. Eur J Cancer Clin Oncol 24(4):675–679

Murphy BR, Breeden ES, Donohue JP et al (1993) Surgical salvage of chemorefractory germ cell tumors. J Clin Oncol 11(2):324–329

National Cancer Centre Network (NCCN) (2007) http://www.nccn.org/professionals/physician_gls/PDF/testicular.pdf. . Ref Type: Internet Communication

Nichols CR, Tricot G, Williams SD et al (1989) Dose-intensive chemotherapy in refractory germ cell cancer–a phase I/II trial of high-dose carboplatin and etoposide with autologous bone marrow transplantation. J Clin Oncol 7(7):932–939

Nichols CR, Williams SD, Loehrer PJ et al (1991) Randomized study of cisplatin dose intensity in poor-risk germ cell tumors: a Southeastern Cancer Study Group and Southwest Oncology Group protocol. J Clin Oncol 9(7):1163–1172

Nichols CR, Andersen J, Lazarus HM et al (1992) High-dose carboplatin and etoposide with autologous bone marrow transplantation in refractory germ cell cancer: an Eastern Cooperative Oncology Group protocol. J Clin Oncol 10(4):558–563

Nichols CR, Catalano PJ, Crawford ED, Vogelzang NJ, Einhorn LH, Loehrer PJ (1998) Randomized comparison of cisplatin and etoposide and either bleomycin or ifosfamide in treatment of advanced disseminated germ cell tumors: an Eastern Cooperative Oncology Group, Southwest Oncology Group, and Cancer and Leukemia Group B Study. J Clin Oncol 16(4):1287–1293

O'Reilly SM, Rustin GJ, Smith DB, Newlands ES (1992) Single agent activity of carboplatin in patients with previously untreated non-seminomatous germ cell tumours. Ann Oncol 3(2):163–164

Pico JL, Rosti G, Kramar A et al (2005) A randomised trial of high-dose chemotherapy in the salvage treatment of patients failing first-line platinum chemotherapy for advanced germ cell tumours. Ann Oncol 16(7):1152–1159

Pizzocaro G, Salvioni R, Piva L, Faustini M, Nicolai N, Gianni L (1992) Modified cisplatin, etoposide (or vinblastine) and ifosfamide salvage therapy for male germ-cell tumors. Long-term results. Ann Oncol 3(3):211–216

Pont J, Bokemeyer C, Harstrick A, Sellner F, Greinix H, Stoiber F (1997) Chemotherapy for germ cell tumors relapsing after high-dose chemotherapy and stem cell support: a retrospective multicenter study of the Austrian Study Group on Urologic Oncology. Ann Oncol 8(12):1229–1234

Porcu P, Bhatia S, Sharma M, Einhorn LH (2000) Results of treatment after relapse from high-dose chemotherapy in germ cell tumors. J Clin Oncol 18(6):1181–1186

Postmus PE, Mulder NH, Sleijfer DT, Meinesz AF, Vriesendorp R, de Vries EG (1984) High-dose etoposide for refractory malignancies: a phase I study. Cancer Treat Rep 68(12):1471–1474

Ravi R, Ong J, Oliver RT, Badenoch DF, Fowler CG, Hendry WF (1998) Surgery as salvage therapy in chemotherapy-resistant nonseminomatous germ cell tumours. Br J Urol 81(6):884–888

Rick O, Beyer J, Kingreen D et al (1998) High-dose chemotherapy in germ cell tumours: a large single centre experience. Eur J Cancer 34(12):1883–1888

Rick O, Bokemeyer C, Beyer J et al (2001) Salvage treatment with paclitaxel, ifosfamide, and cisplatin plus high-dose carboplatin, etoposide, and thiotepa followed by autologous stem-cell rescue in patients with relapsed or refractory germ cell cancer. J Clin Oncol 19(1):81–88

Rick O, Bokemeyer C, Weinknecht S et al (2004) Residual tumor resection after high-dose chemotherapy in patients with relapsed or refractory germ cell cancer. J Clin Oncol 22(18):3713–3719

Rodenhuis S, de Wit R, de Mulder PH et al (1999) A multicenter prospective phase II study of high-dose chemotherapy in germ-cell cancer patients relapsing from complete remission. Ann Oncol 10(12):1467–1473

Samson MK, Rivkin SE, Jones SE et al (1984) Dose-response and dose-survival advantage for high versus low-dose cisplatin combined with vinblastine and bleomycin in disseminated testicular cancer. A Southwest Oncology Group study. Cancer 53(5):1029–1035

Samuels ML, Johnson DE, Holoye PY (1975) Continuous intravenous bleomycin (NSC-125066) therapy with vinblastine (NSC-49842) in stage III testicular neoplasia. Cancer Chemother Rep 59(3):563–570

Sandler AB, Cristou A, Fox S et al (1998) A phase II trial of paclitaxel in refractory germ cell tumors. Cancer 82(7):1381–1386

Schmoll HJ (1989) The role of ifosfamide in testicular cancer. Semin Oncol 16(1 suppl 3):82–95

Schmoll HJ, Souchon R, Krege S et al (2004) European consensus on diagnosis and treatment of germ cell cancer: a report of the European Germ Cell Cancer Consensus Group (EGCCCG). Ann Oncol 15(9):1377–1399

Siegert W, Beyer J, Strohscheer I et al (1994) High-dose treatment with carboplatin, etoposide, and ifosfamide followed by autologous stem-cell transplantation in relapsed or refractory germ cell cancer: a phase I/II study. The German Testicular Cancer Cooperative Study Group. J Clin Oncol 12(6):1223–1231

Sonpavde G, Hutson TE, Roth BJ (2007) Management of recurrent testicular germ cell tumors. Oncologist 12(1):51–61

Vaena DA, Abonour R, Einhorn LH (2003) Long-term survival after high-dose salvage chemotherapy for germ cell malignancies with adverse prognostic variables. J Clin Oncol 21(22):4100–4104

van der WE, Richel DJ, Holtkamp MJ et al (1994) Bone marrow reconstitution after high-dose chemotherapy and autologous peripheral blood progenitor cell transplantation: effect of graft size. Ann Oncol 5(9):795–802

Vuky J, Tickoo SK, Sheinfeld J et al (2002) Salvage chemotherapy for patients with advanced pure seminoma. J Clin Oncol 20(1):297–301

White PM, Adamson DJ, Howard GC, Wright AR (1999) Imaging of the thorax in the management of germ cell testicular tumours. Clin Radiol 54(4):207–211

Williams SD, Birch R, Einhorn LH, Irwin L, Greco FA, Loehrer PJ (1987) Treatment of disseminated germ-cell tumors with cisplatin, bleomycin, and either vinblastine or etoposide. N Engl J Med 316(23):1435–1440

Zon RT, Nichols C, Einhorn LH (1998) Management strategies and outcomes of germ cell tumor patients with very high human chorionic gonadotropin levels. J Clin Oncol 16(4):1294–1297

# 15 Postchemotherapy Retroperitoneal Lymph Node Dissection

Jay D. Raman, Peter Albers, and Joel Sheinfeld

## 15.1 Background

Postchemotherapy surgery for the management of advanced germ cell tumors (GCT) has evolved significantly over the past 25 years (Sheinfeld et al. 1997; Bajorin et al. 1992; Sheinfeld 2002). Prior to the utilization of platinum-based regimens, surgical debulking was followed by ineffective chemotherapy resulting in high relapse rates and poor overall survival (Merrin et al. 1977; Donohue et al. 1980). Improvements in radiographic staging, a better understanding of the role of serum tumor markers, and the introduction of cisplatin-based chemotherapy have all contributed to postchemotherapy surgery assuming a more central role in the management of patients with advanced GCT (Bosl et al. 2005; Donohue et al. 1982; Einhorn 1981; Donohue and Rowland 1984). This multimodal approach has resulted in survival rates approaching 80% in patients with advanced GCT (Sheinfeld et al. 1997; Einhorn 1981; Bosl et al. 1986).

With improvements in cure rates for advanced GCT, increasing emphasis has been placed on reducing treatment related toxicities. Examples of this include clinical trials supporting the safety and efficacy of surveillance for select patients with clinical stage I nonseminomatous germ cell tumors (NSGCTs) as well as a reduction in the duration and toxicity of chemotherapeutic agents necessary for effective systemic therapy (Bosl et al. 1988; Einhorn et al. 1981a, 1989; Peckham 1985). Investigators have further attempted to identify those patients with postchemotherapy residual masses in the retroperitoneum which contain only necrosis or fibrosis. Theoretically, this would identify a subset of patients who would not benefit therapeutically from surgical resection and, thus, could avoid adjunctive surgery with its associated risks and morbidity (Sheinfeld et al. 1997; Sheinfeld 2002).

The vast majority of patients with a residual retroperitoneal mass and elevated tumor markers following primary cisplatin-based chemotherapy are considered to have unresectable, viable GCT. Second-line or "salvage" chemotherapy is recommended in these incomplete or nonresponders. On the other hand, the recommendations for adjunctive surgery in patients with a residual mass and normalized tumor markers following chemotherapy are variable and often contradictory (Sheinfeld et al. 1997; Bajorin et al. 1992; Sheinfeld 2002). These recommendations have ranged from observation of patients irrespective of residual radiographic findings to surgical exploration of all patients following chemotherapy (Fossa et al. 1989a; Levitt et al. 1985).

Most clinicians favor surgical exploration for patients with normalized tumor markers and residual radiographic abnormalities following chemotherapy. There are no standardized guidelines, however, to identify which patients can safely avoid adjunctive postchemotherapy surgery. Reported variables for patients who can safely be managed by observation rather than adjunctive surgery include a "normal" postchemotherapy CT scan, small residual retroperitoneal masses (less than 1.5 cm in diameter and/or less than 20 mL in volume), or significant volume reduction following chemotherapy (greater than 90% volume reduction of the prechemotherapy mass without teratoma in the orchiectomy specimen) (Carter et al. 1987; Donohue et al. 1987; Gelderman et al.

J. Sheinfeld (✉)
Department of Urology, Memorial Sloan-Kettering Cancer Center, New York, NY, 10021 USA

M.P. Laguna et al. (eds.), *Cancer of the Testis*,
DOI: 10.1007/978-1-84800-370-5_15, © Springer-Verlag London Limited 2010

1988; Stomper et al. 1985). With such inconsistent criteria, the proportion of patients undergoing surgery following chemotherapy varies significantly and has ranged from 28 to 73% (Bosl et al. 1988; Levi et al. 1988; Wozniak et al. 1991; Ozols et al. 1988; Williams et al. 1987).

## 15.2 Postchemotherapy RPLND (PC-RPLND): Management Controversies

The early reports of pathologic findings at the time of PC-RPLND indicated that necrosis, teratoma, and persistent viable germ cell tumor were each present in approximately one-third of cases (Donohue et al. 1980). More recently, however, investigators have reported a decrease in the proportion of patients with viable carcinoma with a corresponding increase in the percentage of patients with necrosis (Sheinfeld 2002; Donohue et al. 1987; Fossa et al. 1992). This trend is attributable to the stage migration of testis cancer as well as the improved efficacy of chemotherapy regimens. As such, the reported histologic distribution following primary chemotherapy in the contemporary era notes necrosis/fibrosis in approximately 50% of resected specimens, teratoma in approximately 40%, and viable GCT in the remaining 10% (Donohue et al. 1982; Fossa et al. 1992; Tait et al. 1984; Freiha et al. 1984; Steyerberg et al. 1995; Steyerberg et al. 2001; Stenning et al. 1998). Following second-line or "salvage" chemotherapy, the pathologic distribution has historically been more ominous with viable GCT comprising 50% of resected specimens, teratoma in 40% of cases, and necrosis only in 10% (Sheinfeld et al. 2002; Fox et al. 1993). Of note, Eggener et al. recently have demonstrated that patients receiving taxane-based chemotherapy regimens as salvage therapy had lower rates of viable GCT at the time of PC-RPLND (2007).

Almost 50% of resected retroperitoneal specimens following primary chemotherapy contain only necrosis or fibrotic tissue. Multiple studies have attempted to reliably predict their presence thus identifying a subset of patients who could safely avoid the morbidity of postchemotherapy surgery.

### *15.2.1 Predicting Necrosis*

#### 15.2.1.1 Computed Tomography (CT) Criteria

Observation has been recommended in patients whose tumor markers have normalized and in whom the postchemotherapy CT is "normal." The definition of a "normal" CT scan in the reported literature, however, is inconsistent ranging from no visible masses to retroperitoneal lymph node diameters of less than 10, 15, or 20 mm (Stomper et al. 1985; Fossa et al. 1992; Richie et al. 1982; Mead et al. 1992). Despite these strict CT scan criteria, several studies have demonstrated that a significant percentage of patients will have teratoma or viable GCT in the resected specimen (Bosl et al. 2005; Fossa et al. 1989a). Fossa et al. (1989a) reported that 12 of 37 patients (32%) with normal markers and a normal CT scan (residual nodes ≤10 mm) following chemotherapy had teratoma and one patient had viable germ cell tumor in resected specimens. In a subsequent study from the same institution, Oldenberg et al. (2003) noted that despite contemporary refinements in chemotherapy regimens and CT imaging, 16 of 38 patients (42%) with residual masses ≤10 mm had teratoma or viable GCT in the resected specimen. Similarly, Richie (1984) reported viable GCT in 4 of 38 patients with a normal CT scan following four cycles of cisplatin, vinblastine, and bleomycin, and Toner et al. (1990) noted that 8 of 39 (21%) patients with residual masses of ≤15 mm had viable GCT or teratoma resected.

Beyond radiographic size criteria, attenuation values of residual masses have also been inconsistent in predicting necrosis (Donohue et al. 1987; Stomper et al. 1985; Husband et al. 1982). While Husband et al. (1982) reported that postchemotherapy masses with low attenuation values were more likely to represent necrosis, neither Stomper et al. (1985) nor Donohue et al. (1987) were able to confirm these findings.

As such, there are presently no CT criteria that can reliably distinguish necrosis from teratoma or viable carcinoma in the postchemotherapy setting.

#### 15.2.1.2 Teratoma in the Primary Specimen

Teratoma in the orchiectomy specimen predicts the presence of teratoma or viable GCT in the retroperitoneum following chemotherapy (Beck et al. 2002; Carver et al. 2006a). Conversely, several studies have found that the absence of teratomatous elements in the orchiectomy specimen does not imply absence in the retroperitoneum following chemotherapy. Donohue et al. (1987) reported in 1987 on 80 patients with sequential CT scans before and after chemotherapy. Among 15 of these patients without teratoma in the orchiectomy specimen and a 90% or greater decrease in retroperitoneal tumor volume (formula $v=0.52d$ (Bajorin et al. 1992)), none had viable GCT or teratoma in the final resected specimen. These data suggested that PC-RPLND could be avoided in patients without teratoma in the primary specimen and a significant volume reduction in the postchemotherapy retroperitoneal mass. In a follow-up study from Indiana University, however, Debono et al. (1997) found that only 74% of patients with these same criteria were still free of disease. Other investigators have reported similar findings. Toner et al. (1990) reported that 25 of 75 patients (33%) without teratoma in the primary tumor had teratomatous elements resected from metastatic sites. Loehrer et al. (1986) noted that of 51 patients with teratomatous elements in postchemotherapy resections, 28% of the orchiectomy specimens failed to contain teratoma. In an updated study from the same institution, Beck et al. (2002) reported that almost 50% of patients without teratoma in the primary specimen had teratoma in the retroperitoneum.

In summary, although the presence of teratoma in the orchiectomy specimen predicts for teratoma in the retroperitoneum, its absence does not preclude its presence in the retroperitoneum.

#### 15.2.1.3 Predictive Models

Over the past 15 years, several statistical models have been generated in an attempt to accurately predict the presence of necrosis in resected retroperitoneal specimens. Toner et al. (1990) identified 4 independent predictors of necrosis in the RPLND specimen: residual mass <1.5 cm, ≥90% shrinkage postchemotherapy, and pretreatment alpha-fetoprotein (AFP) and lactate dehydrogenase (LDH) serum tumor marker levels. Multivariate regression analysis with these variables was able to accurately predict necrosis in 83% of patients. The false negative rate, however, was 20%. Fossa et al. (1989b) evaluated 101 patients with residual masses following platinum-based chemotherapy and reported that the absence of teratoma in the primary specimen, complete radiographic resolution, and normalized markers following chemotherapy predicted necrosis. Recently, Steyerberg et al. (1998) utilized an international data set comprised of over 550 patients from 6 different study groups. Statistical modeling identified 6 variables as predictors of necrosis including the absence of teratoma in the orchiectomy specimen, normal pretreatment AFP and human chorionic gonadotropin (HCG) levels, elevated prechemotherapy LDH levels, a small pre- or postchemotherapy mass, and a large volume reduction following treatment. The predictive model reliably distinguished necrosis from viable GCT or teratoma (area under the receiver operating curve [ROC] curve 0.84), but was much less sensitive in distinguishing viable GCT from teratoma (area under ROC curve 0.66). The Steyerberg model's performance was also poor in patients treated with chemotherapy regimens including bleomycin, etoposide, and cisplatin. A subsequent update of this model with more than 1,000 patients was unable to improve on the ability to predict necrosis across the cohort of patients (Vergouwe et al. 2007). Finally, in an effort to improve on the Steyerberg model, the German Testicular Cancer Study Group (GTCSG) recently reported on 261 patients who underwent a PC-RPLND (8% after second-line chemotherapy). Prechemotherapy AFP levels <20 ng/mL and a tumor volume shrinkage following chemotherapy of >90% predicted patients with necrosis in the retroperitoneum. However, in ROC analysis the accuracy for predicting necrosis across the cohort was only 75% rendering this model clinically irrelevant (Albers et al. 2004).

#### 15.2.1.4 Summary

Patient selection for observation following induction chemotherapy is controversial. Multiple studies demonstrate that approximately 20% of patients predicted to have necrosis/fibrosis will harbor either teratoma or viable GCT in the resected retroperitoneal specimen (Steyerberg et al. 1995; Toner et al. 1990). CT criteria alone are not sufficiently reliable to distinguish viable tumor or teratoma from necrosis. PET scanning has been studied as an adjunctive radiographic modality especially for seminoma following chemotherapy where it proved to be a valuable tool to predict viable germ cell tumor (Becherer et al. 2005). However, the inability to distinguish teratoma from fibrosis confounds its utility in the management of NSGCT (Spermon et al. 2002; Cremerius et al. 1999). Currently, no combination of criteria can predict a negative retroperitoneal pathology with sufficient accuracy to obviate the need for PC-RPLND (Sheinfeld et al. 1997; Bosl et al. 2005). If viable GCT is present, it will be at least partially chemo-resistant with the potential for progression if left untreated. In fact, the cure rates for recurrent GCT with ifosfamide-based salvage regimens are only 25% (Motzer et al. 1992). Further, unresected teratoma has the potential for growth ("growing teratoma syndrome"), local invasion, or malignant transformation. These data collectively suggest that the undertreatment of patients with advanced GCT after chemotherapy may result in inferior outcomes compared with those who have immediate retroperitoneal surgery.

## 15.3 Timing of Postchemotherapy RPLND

It is generally recommended to perform PC-RPLND as early after chemotherapy as possible. The timing of surgery is dependent on the recovery of white blood cell and platelet counts which typically occurs 3 weeks after first line chemotherapy and sometimes longer following second-line or high-dose chemotherapy regimens. Hendry et al. (2002) noted that if surgery is performed within 3 months of completion of chemotherapy an overall 5-year survival rate of 83% can be achieved. However, if surgery is delayed until progression of a lesion under surveillance, they noted that the 5-year survival rate dropped to 62%.

## 15.4 Postchemotherapy RPLND: Technique

The recommended limits of PC-RPLND vary widely in the literature ranging from excision of the residual mass only to modified template dissections and full bilateral RPLND (Sheinfeld et al. 2002; Hendry et al. 1993). Simple excision of masses is not an acceptable therapeutic modality given the high probability of incomplete resection. Modified templates, initially developed for patients with low stage disease in an effort to preserve ejaculatory function, have traditionally not been recommended because patients with advanced disease are at a higher risk of disease outside of the template. Wood et al. (1992a) reported on 113 patients who underwent a PC-RPLND and noted that nonpalpable viable tumor or teratoma was located outside the limits of the modified template in 9 of 113 (8%) of cases. A follow-up study from the same institution by Carver et al. (2006b) noted 32% of patients had disease outside of the borders of the modified template and found no difference in the pathologic distribution of specimens resected within or outside of the modified template. Two recent series from Germany have suggested that a template resection is feasible in select patients (Wittenhuhn et al. 2007; Pfister et al. 2007). The resected template is defined as the region where the initial metastatic lesion is detected and, thus, is not always identical to the unilateral templates commonly described for primary RPLND. By limiting the field of resection, the two series collectively with 159 patients noted no in-field relapses with preservation of ejaculatory function in 85% of these patients who underwent PC-RPLND. The authors concluded that for small unilateral tumors, ipsilateral nerve-sparing techniques were feasible and enhanced the postoperative ejaculation rate. They acknowledged, however, that the follow-up period of about 2 years is still too short to recommend this as standard practice (Wittenhuhn et al. 2007; Pfister et al. 2007). For bilateral PC-RPLND, in a select subset of patients with small-volume residual masses and minimal postchemotherapy desmoplastic reaction, prospective nerve-sparing techniques may be feasible with preservation of the sympathetic chains, postganglionic sympathetic fibers (L2, L3, and L4), and the hypogastric plexus (Coogan et al. 1996; Wahle et al. 1994). Pettus et al. (2007) recently reported on over 130 patients with an 80% successful antegrade ejaculation rate underscoring that the functional return of antegrade ejaculation is feasible following chemotherapy without compromising the oncologic efficacy of the operation. The 5-year relapse-free survival in this study was 98%.

Many of the same surgical techniques and principles described for primary RPLND are applicable when performing a postchemotherapy lymphadenectomy.

Large retroperitoneal masses with associated desmoplastic reaction make the PC-RPLND one of the most difficult and technically demanding operations performed by urologists. As such, this operation should be performed by experienced surgeons comfortable with complex vascular anatomy in referral centers (Sheinfeld 2002).

The choice of incision is based on tumor size and location. In general, a transabdominal incision will provide adequate exposure to the retroperitoneum. Large masses that are located high in the retroperitoneum may require a thoracoabdominal approach or costal extension of the midline incision. Large left-sided tumors with suprahilar extension may require a "visceral roll" which can provide good exposure to the para-aortic area cephalad to the left renal artery. Extension into the retrocrural or posterior mediastinal areas is occasionally necessary to achieve a complete resection. The margins of resection involve removing all nodal tissue between both ureters from the level of the renal hilum down to the bifurcation of the common iliac arteries.

The falciform ligament is divided between silk ties or excised *en bloc* with the preperitoneal fat. The wound edges are separated with self retaining retractors and the abdomen, retroperitoneum, and pelvis are explored. The transverse colon, stomach, and omentum are placed on the chest of the patient, and the posterior parietal peritoneum is incised from the ligament of Treitz, around the cecum, and up the right paracolic gutter. The duodenum is kocherized allowing for cephalad mobilization of the small bowel, cecum, and right colon. Attachments between the pancreas and duodenum and the anterior surface of the left renal vein and great vessels are divided to avoid traction injuries. A self-retaining retractor (Bookwalter, Omni, Gallagher) is then used.

Additional exposure of the left distal para-aortic and left para-iliac regions can be accomplished by further extending the left leaf of the peritoneum inferiorly and sacrificing the IMA (inferior mesenteric artery) as needed. The left colon can be reflected medially by incising the left white line of Toldt and developing the plane between the colonic mesentery and Gerota's fascia. The IMV can be double ligated and divided to get more access to the left renal hilum. Wide excision of the spermatic cord is necessary to avoid potential paracolic recurrences within the retroperitoneal surgical field (Chang et al. 2002).

The "split and roll" technique is then used to perform the lymphadenectomy (Bosl et al. 2005; Sheinfeld et al. 2002; Donohue 1977). Separating the mass or lymph nodes from the great vessels requires great care to avoid subadventitial dissection along the aorta (Melchior et al. 2003). Stripping of the aortic wall adventitia is often not amenable to suture repair and may result in delayed rupture. Direct invasion of the aorta or vena cava may require resection of that portion of the great vessel with graft interposition (Beck et al. 2001; Kelly et al. 1995). Adjunctive procedures such as nephrectomy are sometimes necessary to achieve a complete resection (Nash et al. 1998). Stephenson et al. (2006) reported on almost 650 PC-RPLNDs and noted that adjunctive nephrectomy was necessary in 5% of cases. Many of these adjunctive nephrectomies were performed in high-risk scenarios such as postsalvage chemotherapy, desperation RPLND, late relapses, and re-operative RPLND. Extensive serosal injuries or enterotomies predispose patients to life-threatening fistulas, and omental interposition is advisable. Tumor involvement of the SMA, celiac axis, or porta hepatic often precludes surgical extirpation.

## 15.5 Postchemotherapy Laparoscopic RPLND

Laparoscopic RPLND (L-RPLND) is a technically demanding procedure that should be undertaken by experienced laparoscopic surgeons familiar with retroperitoneal anatomy and adept with vascular techniques in the event of an open conversion. Primary L-RPLND is a reasonable staging tool for clinical stage I patients with long-term oncologic data continuing to mature (Neyer et al. 2007; Abdel-Aziz et al. 2006). In the postchemotherapy setting, L-RPLND have been limited to unifocal small-volume masses with initial reports describing significant intraoperative and postoperative morbidities. Rassweiler et al. (1996) converted 7 of 9 postchemotherapy stage II patients from laparoscopic to open RPLND, while Palese et al. (2002) reported that 2 of 7 patients in the Johns Hopkins experience required open conversion. Further, several of the reported complications included significant vascular injuries including transection of the external iliac artery, renal artery hematoma, and renal artery thrombosis. Permongkosol et al. (2007) recently updated the Johns Hopkins experience noting a decreased complication rate with no retroperitoneal recurrences at a mean follow-up of 3 years. At this time, postchemotherapy L-RPLND requires continued prospective analysis to determine durable oncologic outcomes.

## 15.6 Clinical Prognosis After Postchemotherapy RPLND

Following PC-RPLND, the patient's prognosis and subsequent management is dependent upon tumor marker levels at the time of surgery, prior treatment burden, pathology of the resected specimens, and the completeness of resection (Sheinfeld et al. 2002; Donohue et al. 1998). The risk for relapse in patients with necrosis or teratoma in the retroperitoneal specimen is approximately 5–10%; therefore additional chemotherapy is not required (Sheinfeld et al. 1997; Bajorin et al. 1992; Bosl et al. 2005; Toner et al. 1990).

The finding of viable GCT, however, is associated with a higher risk for relapse and decreased survival rates (Fox et al. 1993; Einhorn et al. 1981b; Geller et al. 1989; Logothetis and Samuels 1984). Fox et al. (1993) noted that if viable GCT is present in the retroperitoneal specimen but is entirely resected, two additional cycles of adjuvant chemotherapy confers a survival benefit. They reported that 18 of 27 (70%) patients who underwent complete postchemotherapy resection of viable GCT were disease-free with two additional cycles of adjuvant chemotherapy compared to 0 of 7 without additional chemotherapy. Geller et al. (1989) and Logothetis et al.(Logothetis and Samuels 1984) reported 66% (12 of 18) and 53% (9 of 17) long-term survivors, respectively, in patients receiving adjuvant chemotherapy following complete resection of viable GCT. The use of two adjuvant cycles of chemotherapy, however, has recently been challenged by Fizzazi et al. (2001) who identified three independent prognostic variables for survival (complete resection, good risk IGCCCG classification, and <10% viable malignant cells) in a retrospective, multicenter study of 146 patients. They concluded that adjuvant chemotherapy only benefited patients with one risk factor, but not those without risk factors or those with two or more risk factors.

Of note, while the probability of viable GCT is higher following salvage chemotherapy and the likelihood of achieving complete resection is lower, Fox et al. (1993) noted that two additional cycles of chemotherapy do not confer any therapeutic advantage in this setting.

### 15.6.1 *Implications of Teratoma*

While teratoma is histologically benign, its biologic potential is unpredictable. Teratoma may grow, invade local structures, and become unresectable; hence, operative intervention for complete resection is ideal when the volume of disease is low (Logothetis et al. 1982; Morgentaler et al. 1988). There is also a 6–8% risk of malignant transformation of teratoma to non-germ cell elements such as adenocarcinoma or sarcoma (Motzer et al. 1998; Ahmed et al. 1985; Ulbright et al. 1984). Transformed elements are often resistant to standard chemotherapy regimens with poor overall prognosis if complete resection is not achieved (Donadio et al. 2003). Finally, unresected teratoma may result in late recurrence (Dieckmann et al. 2005; Borge et al. 1988; Gerl et al. 1997; George et al. 2003; Baniel et al. 1995).

### 15.6.2 *High-Risk Postchemotherapy RPLND for Advanced NSGCT*

Experience with PC-RPLND has identified a subset of patients with higher relapse rates and poorer overall survival. Donohue et al. (1998) reviewed data on over 800 men who underwent PC-RPLND and identified four unfavorable characteristics: (1) salvage chemotherapy; (2) postchemotherapy patients with elevated tumor markers ("desperation RPLND"); (3) unresectable patients; and (4) patients requiring re-operative surgery. Patients with one or more of these risk factors had a relapse rate of 45% compared with a relapse rate of 11.8% in patients without any risk factors.

Patients undergoing PC-RPLND following salvage chemotherapy regimens are characterized by lower rates of complete resection and at least a 50% incidence of viable GCT in the resected specimen

(Fox et al. 1993). In a German series of 57 patients who underwent a PC-RPLND after high-dose salvage chemotherapy, the incidence of viable germ cell tumor or sarcoma was 47%, and 16% were found with teratoma. The long-term disease free survival of patients undergoing complete resection with viable cancer and teratoma was 44% and 77%, respectively (Rick et al. 2004). Complete surgical resection is critical as additional chemotherapy cycles fail to benefit patients in this setting (Fox et al. 1993).

Historically, surgical intervention has been avoided in patients with persistently elevated tumor markers following chemotherapy, as most were considered to have unresectable GCT (Sheinfeld et al. 1997). More recently, however, a number of investigators have shown that carefully selected patients with elevated tumor markers may achieve a 20–50% cure rate with complete resection (Melchior et al. 2003; Wood et al. 1992b; Murphy et al. 1993; Eastham et al. 1994). In this scenario, an elevated AFP compared to HCG tumor marker level and the presence of retroperitoneal disease vs. visceral metastases have been associated with a more favorable prognosis (Wood et al. 1992b).

The third group of high-risk patients is those with disease deemed unresectable. In a study by Donohue et al. (1998), patients with unresectable disease did very poorly with 90% experiencing relapse and overall survival rate of 21%. Stenning et al. (1998) similarly showed that the 2-year progression-free survival rates were 88% for patients with complete resection compared with 60% for those patients with incomplete resection.

The final high-risk group encompasses patients who have undergone a prior PC-RPLND with relapse in the operative field necessitating a redo-RPLND. Re-operative retroperitoneal surgery is a technically demanding procedure due to extensive adhesions and significant desmoplastic reaction from prior surgery, chemotherapy, and extravasated blood and/or lymphatic fluid (Sheinfeld 2007). Intraoperative and postoperative complication rates are high ranging between 20 and 40% in most contemporary series (Donohue et al. 1998; Sexton et al. 2003; McKiernan et al. 2003). Data from Indiana University and the Memorial Sloan-Kettering Cancer Center (MSKCC) show that patients undergoing redo-RPLND are severely compromised regardless of other risk factors (Donohue et al. 1998; McKiernan et al. 2003). Donohue et al. (1998) reported a decrease in survival rate from 84.1% in the primary postchemotherapy group to 55.3% in the redo group. Similarly, McKiernian et al. (2003) reported a 56% disease-specific survival rate for patients requiring re-operation compared with 90% for those undergoing primary PC-RPLND.

## 15.7 Complications

The complication rate for PC-RPLND is higher than that of primary RPLND. In 1995, Baniel and Sella (1999) reported 38 (8%) major complications in 478 patients who underwent a primary RPLND compared with 106 (18%) of 603 patients after PC-RPLND. Furthermore, there were five deaths in the postchemotherapy group and none in the primary group. Large-volume residual disease, postchemotherapy desmoplastic reaction, and prior exposure to chemotherapeutic agents (particularly bleomycin) have all contributed to higher morbidity rates. Fortunately, the morbidity appears to decreasing with time.

Meticulous technique, knowledge of the retroperitoneal anatomy, and improved peri-operative management has resulted in better clinical outcomes. Mosharafa et al. (2004) reported, a lower operative complication rate and hospital duration in patients who underwent a PC-RPLND between 2000 and 2002 vs. 1990–1992. Careful monitoring of peri-operative oxygen concentrations and strict fluid management with emphasis on the use of colloid has further improved morbidity postoperatively (Donat and Levy 1998). Finally, retrospective data suggests that clinical care pathways has benefited the postoperative convalescence (Chang et al. 2002).

### 15.7.1 Lymphatic

Postoperative chylous ascites occurs in 2–3% of cases, with predisposing factors including suprahilar dissection, resection of the IVC, or hepatic resections. The clinical presentation may include abdominal distension, a prolonged ileus, or an abdominal fluid wave. The diagnosis can be confirmed by CT or ultrasound guided aspiration with characteristic fat and protein content of chyle. Management is typically conservative with diuretics, low fat/medium-chain triglyceride diet, or total parenteral nutrition as needed (Sheinfeld et al. 2002).

### 15.7.2 Pulmonary

Atelectasis is the most common pulmonary complication. Pneumonia requires antibiotic therapy. Adult respiratory distress syndrome (ARDS) in bleomycin treated patients may be lethal and requires mechanical ventilation and steroid therapy.

### 15.7.3 Infectious

Superficial wound infections comprise the majority of infectious complications. Urinary tract infections are rare. *Clostridium difficile* infections require appropriate antibiotic therapy. Routine appendectomy at the time of RPLND is associated with a higher rate of infectious complications and is no longer performed (Leibovitch et al. 1995).

### 15.7.4 Neurologic

Careful positioning has minimized peripheral nerve injuries. The more serious complication of spinal cord ischemia is very rare and is associated with older age, simultaneous mediastinal and retroperitoneal dissections, prior radiation therapy, and intraoperative hypotension. The anterior spinal artery (usually at the T8 level) should be identified if dissection occurs in this region (Leibovitch et al. 1996).

### 15.7.5 Vascular

Renovascular injury seen in 2–3% of cases may result in partial or total loss of a renal unit and possibly hypertension. To minimize injury, it is important to note that approximately 20% of patients have accessory renal arteries (Sheinfeld et al. 2002). Minor injuries to the great vessels can be repaired with 4-0 or 5-0 vascular suture, while major vascular injury may require graft interposition. Intravenous mannitol as well as topical papavarine can be used to minimize arterial vasospasm during dissection.

### 15.7.6 Gastrointestinal

Paralytic ileus is often self-limiting but an underlying cause such as retroperitoneal hematoma, mesenteric hematoma, pancreatitis, urinary extravasation, and bowel infarction should be considered. Small bowel obstruction occurs in 2–3% of patients and can be managed conservatively. Re-exploration is reserved for signs of toxicity or failure to respond to prolonged nasogastric tube decompression. Pancreatitis, usually due to traction during RPLND, presents as a prolonged ileus with hyperamylasemia and can usually be managed conservatively.

## 15.8 Conclusions

Postchemotherapy retroperitoneal surgical resection is necessary when tumor markers have normalized and residual radiographic abnormalities are present. The need for a PC-RPLND in the face of a normal CT scan is controversial. No combination of variables can predict negative retroperitoneal pathology with sufficient accuracy following induction chemotherapy to eliminate the risk of unresected teratoma or viable germ cell tumor. Approximately 20% of patients predicted to have necrosis will have viable GCT or teratoma. The biology of residual teratoma is unpredictable with growth, malignant transformation, and/or late recurrence all reported outcomes. Unresected viable GCT is at least partially chemorefractory and, if untreated, will progress. Surgical margins should not be compromised in an attempt to preserve ejaculation, although nerve-sparing dissections are possible in appropriately selected cases.

Completeness of resection is an independent and consistent predictive variable of clinical outcome. Patients who are resected incompletely and require re-operative surgery are severely compromised. The size and location of residual masses coupled with the retroperitoneal desmoplastic reaction makes PC-RPLND a technically demanding procedure that should be performed by experienced surgeons in dedicated referral centers.

## References


Abdel-Aziz KF, Anderson JK, Svatek R, Margulis V, Sagalowsky AI, Cadeddu JA (2006) Laparoscopic and open retroperitoneal lymph-node dissection for clinical stage I nonseminomatous germ-cell testis tumors. J Endourol 20:627

Ahmed T, Bosl GJ, Hajdu SI (1985) Teratoma with malignant transformation in germ cell tumors in men. Cancer 56:860

Albers P, Weissbach L, Krege S, Kliesch S, Hartmann M, Heidenreich A, Walz P, Kuczyk M, Fimmers R (2004) Prediction of necrosis after chemotherapy of advanced germ cell tumors: results of a prospective multicenter trial of the German Testicular Cancer Study Group. J Urol 171:1835

Bajorin DF, Herr H, Motzer RJ, Bosl GJ (1992) Current perspectives on the role of adjunctive surgery in combined modality treatment for patients with germ cell tumors. Semin Oncol 19:148

Baniel J, Sella A (1999) Complications of retroperitoneal lymph node dissection in testicular cancer: primary and post-chemotherapy. Semin Surg Oncol 17:263

Baniel J, Foster RS, Einhorn LH, Donohue JP (1995) Late relapse of clinical stage I testicular cancer. J Urol 154:1370

Becherer A, De Santis M, Karanikas G, Szabo M, Bokemeyer C, Dohmen BM, Pont J, Dudczak R, Dittrich C, Kletter K (2005) FDG PET is superior to CT in the prediction of viable tumour in post-chemotherapy seminoma residuals. Eur J Radiol 54:284

Beck SD, Foster RS, Bihrle R, Koch MO, Wahle GR, Donohue JP (2001) Aortic replacement during post-chemotherapy retroperitoneal lymph node dissection. J Urol 165:1517

Beck SD, Foster RS, Bihrle R, Ulbright T, Koch MO, Wahle GR, Einhorn LH, Donohue JP (2002) Teratoma in the orchiectomy specimen and volume of metastasis are predictors of retroperitoneal teratoma in post-chemotherapy nonseminomatous testis cancer. J Urol 168:1402

Borge N, Fossa SD, Ous S, Stenwig AE, Lien HH (1988) Late recurrence of testicular cancer. J Clin Oncol 6:1248

Bosl GJ, Gluckman R, Geller NL, Golbey RB, Whitmore WF Jr, Herr H, Sogani P, Morse M, Martini N, Bains M et al (1986) VAB-6: an effective chemotherapy regimen for patients with germ-cell tumors. J Clin Oncol 4:1493

Bosl GJ, Geller NL, Bajorin D, Leitner SP, Yagoda A, Golbey RB, Scher H, Vogelzang NJ, Auman J, Carey R et al (1988) A randomized trial of etoposide + cisplatin versus vinblastine + bleomycin + cisplatin + cyclophosphamide + dactinomycin in patients with good-prognosis germ cell tumors. J Clin Oncol 6:1231

Bosl G, Bajorin D, Sheinfeld J (2005) Cancer of the testis. In: De Vita VT, Hellman S, Rosenberg SA (eds) Cancer: principles and practice of oncology, 7th edn. Lippincott, Williams, & Wilkins, Philadelphia, pp. 1269–1290

Carter GE, Lieskovsky G, Skinner DG, Daniels JR (1987) Reassessment of the role of adjunctive surgical therapy in the treatment of advanced germ cell tumors. J Urol 138:1397

Carver BS, Bianco FJ Jr, Shayegan B, Vickers A, Motzer RJ, Bosl GJ, Sheinfeld J (2006a) Predicting teratoma in the retroperitoneum in men undergoing post-chemotherapy retroperitoneal lymph node dissection. J Urol 176:100

Carver BS, Shayegan B, Motzer RJ, Stasi J, Bajorin D, Bosl GJ, Sheinfeld J (2006b) The incidence and implications of disease outside a modified template in men undergoing post-chemotherapy retroperitoneal lymph node dissection (PC-RPLND) for metastatic non-seminomatous germ cell tumors (NSGCT). J Urol 175:192

Chang SS, Mohseni HF, Leon A, Sheinfeld J (2002) Paracolic recurrence: the importance of wide excision of the spermatic cord at retroperitoneal lymph node dissection. J Urol 167:94

Coogan CL, Hejase MJ, Wahle GR, Foster RS, Rowland RG, Bihrle R, Donohue JP (1996) Nerve sparing post-chemotherapy retroperitoneal lymph node dissection for advanced testicular cancer. J Urol 156:1656

Cremerius U, Wildberger JE, Borchers H, Zimny M, Jakse G, Gunther RW, Buell U (1999) Does positron emission tomography using 18-fluoro-2-deoxyglucose improve clinical staging of testicular cancer?–results of a study in 50 patients. Urology 54:900

Debono DJ, Heilman DK, Einhorn LH, Donohue JP (1997) Decision analysis for avoiding postchemotherapy surgery in patients with disseminated nonseminomatous germ cell tumors. J Clin Oncol 15:1455

Dieckmann KP, Albers P, Classen J, De Wit M, Pichlmeier U, Rick O, Mullerleile U, Kuczyk M (2005) Late relapse of testicular germ cell neoplasms: a descriptive analysis of 122 cases. J Urol 173:824

Donadio AC, Motzer RJ, Bajorin DF, Kantoff PW, Sheinfeld J, Houldsworth J, Chaganti RS, Bosl GJ (2003) Chemotherapy for teratoma with malignant transformation. J Clin Oncol 21:4285

Donat SM, Levy DA (1998) Bleomycin associated pulmonary toxicity: is perioperative oxygen restriction necessary? J Urol 160:1347

Donohue JP (1977) Retroperitoneal lymphadenectomy: the anterior approach including bilateral suprarenal-hilar dissection. Urol Clin North Am 4:509

Donohue JP, Rowland RG (1984) The role of surgery in advanced testicular cancer. Cancer 54:2716

Donohue JP, Einhorn LH, Williams SD (1980) Cytoreductive surgery for metastatic testis cancer: considerations of timing and extent. J Urol 123:876

Donohue JP, Roth LM, Zachary JM, Rowland RG, Einhorn LH, Williams SG (1982) Cytoreductive surgery for metastatic testis cancer: tissue analysis of retroperitoneal masses after chemotherapy. J Urol 127:1111

Donohue JP, Rowland RG, Kopecky K, Steidle CP, Geier G, Ney KG, Einhorn L, Williams S, Loehrer P (1987) Correlation of computerized tomographic changes and histological findings in 80 patients having radical retroperitoneal lymph node dissection after chemotherapy for testis cancer. J Urol 137:1176

Donohue JP, Leviovitch I, Foster RS, Baniel J, Tognoni P (1998) Integration of surgery and systemic therapy: results and principles of integration. Semin Urol Oncol 16:65

Eastham JA, Wilson TG, Russell C, Ahlering TE, Skinner DG (1994) Surgical resection in patients with nonseminomatous germ cell tumor who fail to normalize serum tumor markers after chemotherapy. Urology 43:74

Eggener SE, Carver BS, Loeb S, Kondagunta GV, Bosl GJ, Sheinfeld J (2007) Pathologic findings and clinical outcome of patients undergoing retroperitoneal lymph node dissection after multiple chemotherapy regimens for metastatic testicular germ cell tumors. Cancer 109:528

Einhorn LH (1981) Testicular cancer as a model for a curable neoplasm: The Richard and Hinda Rosenthal Foundation Award Lecture. Cancer Res 41:3275

Einhorn LH, Williams SD, Troner M, Birch R, Greco FA (1981a) The role of maintenance therapy in disseminated testicular cancer. N Engl J Med 305:727

Einhorn LH, Williams SD, Mandelbaum I, Donohue JP (1981b) Surgical resection in disseminated testicular cancer following chemotherapeutic cytoreduction. Cancer 48:904

Einhorn LH, Williams SD, Loehrer PJ, Birch R, Drasga R, Omura G, Greco FA (1989) Evaluation of optimal duration of chemotherapy in favorable-prognosis disseminated germ cell tumors: a Southeastern Cancer Study Group protocol. J Clin Oncol 7:387

Fizazi K, Tjulandin S, Salvioni R, Germa-Lluch JR, Bouzy J, Ragan D, Bokemeyer C, Gerl A, Flechon A, de Bono JS, Stenning S, Horwich A, Pont J, Albers P, De Giorgi U, Bower M, Bulanov A, Pizzocaro G, Aparicio J, Nichols CR, Theodore C, Hartmann JT, Schmoll HJ, Kaye SB, Culine S, Droz JP, Mahe C (2001) Viable malignant cells after primary chemotherapy for disseminated nonseminomatous germ cell tumors: prognostic factors and role of postsurgery chemotherapy–results from an international study group. J Clin Oncol 19:2647

Fossa SD, Ous S, Lien HH, Stenwig AE (1989a) Post-chemotherapy lymph node histology in radiologically normal patients with metastatic nonseminomatous testicular cancer. J Urol 141:557

Fossa SD, Aass N, Ous S, Hoie J, Stenwig AE, Lien HH, Paus E, Kaalhus O (1989b) Histology of tumor residuals following chemotherapy in patients with advanced nonseminomatous testicular cancer. J Urol 142:1239

Fossa SD, Qvist H, Stenwig AE, Lien HH, Ous S, Giercksky KE (1992) Is postchemotherapy retroperitoneal surgery necessary in patients with nonseminomatous testicular cancer and minimal residual tumor masses? J Clin Oncol 10:569

Fox EP, Weathers TD, Williams SD, Loehrer PJ, Ulbright TM, Donohue JP, Einhorn LH (1993) Outcome analysis for patients with persistent nonteratomatous germ cell tumor in postchemotherapy retroperitoneal lymph node dissections. J Clin Oncol 11:1294

Freiha FS, Shortliffe LD, Rouse RV, Mark JB, Hannigan JF Jr, Aston D, Spaulding JT, Williams RD, Torti FM (1984) The extent of surgery after chemotherapy for advanced germ cell tumors. J Urol 132:915

Gelderman WA, Schraffordt Koops H, Sleijfer DT, Oosterhuis JW, Van der Heide JN, Mulder NH, Marrink J, De Bruyn HW, Oldhoff J (1988) Results of adjuvant surgery in patients with stage III and IV nonseminomatous testicular tumors after cisplatin-vinblastine-bleomycin chemotherapy. J Surg Oncol 38:227

Geller NL, Bosl GJ, Chan EY (1989) Prognostic factors for relapse after complete response in patients with metastatic germ cell tumors. Cancer 63:440

George DW, Foster RS, Hromas RA, Robertson KA, Vance GH, Ulbright TM, Gobbett TA, Heiber DJ, Heerema NA, Ramsey HC, Thurston VC, Jung SH, Shen J, Finch DE, Kelley MR, Einhorn LH (2003) Update on late relapse of germ cell tumor: a clinical and molecular analysis. J Clin Oncol 21:113

Gerl A, Clemm C, Schmeller N, Hentrich M, Lamerz R, Wilmanns W (1997) Late relapse of germ cell tumors after cisplatin-based chemotherapy. Ann Oncol 8:41

Hendry WF, A'Hern RP, Hetherington JW, Peckham MJ, Dearnaley DP, Horwich A (1993) Para-aortic lymphadenectomy after chemotherapy for metastatic non-seminomatous germ cell tumours: prognostic value and therapeutic benefit. Br J Urol 71:208

Hendry WF, Norman AR, Dearnaley DP, Fisher C, Nicholls J, Huddart RA, Horwich A (2002) Metastatic nonseminomatous germ cell tumors of the testis: results of elective and salvage surgery for patients with residual retroperitoneal masses. Cancer 94:1668

Husband JE, Hawkes DJ, Peckham MJ (1982) CT estimations of mean attenuation values and volume in testicular tumors: a comparison with surgical and histologic findings. Radiology 144:553

Kelly R, Skinner D, Yellin AE, Weaver FA (1995) En bloc aortic resection for bulky metastatic germ cell tumors. J Urol 153:1849

Leibovitch I, Rowland RG, Goldwasser B, Donohue JP (1995) Incidental appendectomy during urological surgery. J Urol 154:1110

Leibovitch I, Nash PA, Little JS Jr, Foster RS, Donohue JP (1996) Spinal cord ischemia after post-chemotherapy retroperitoneal lymph node dissection for nonseminomatous germ cell cancer. J Urol 155:947

Levi JA, Thomson D, Sandeman T, Tattersall M, Raghavan D, Byrne M, Gill G, Harvey V, Burns I, Snyder R (1988) A prospective study of cisplatin-based combination chemotherapy in advanced germ cell malignancy: role of maintenance and long-term follow-up. J Clin Oncol 6:1154

Levitt MD, Reynolds PM, Sheiner HJ, Byrne MJ (1985) Non-seminomatous germ cell testicular tumours: residual masses after chemotherapy. Br J Surg 72:19

Loehrer PJ Sr, Hui S, Clark S, Seal M, Einhorn LH, Williams SD, Ulbright T, Mandelbaum I, Rowland R, Donohue JP (1986) Teratoma following cisplatin-based combination chemotherapy for nonseminomatous germ cell tumors: a clinicopathological correlation. J Urol 135:1183

Logothetis CJ, Samuels ML (1984) Surgery in the management of stage III germinal cell tumors. Observations on the M.D. Anderson Hospital experience, 1971-1979. Cancer Treat Rev 11:27

Logothetis CJ, Samuels ML, Trindade A, Johnson DE (1982) The growing teratoma syndrome. Cancer 50:1629

McKiernan JM, Motzer RJ, Bajorin DF, Bacik J, Bosl GJ, Sheinfeld J (2003) Reoperative retroperitoneal surgery for nonseminomatous germ cell tumor: clinical presentation, patterns of recurrence, and outcome. Urology 62:732

Mead GM, Stenning SP, Parkinson MC, Horwich A, Fossa SD, Wilkinson PM, Kaye SB, Newlands ES, Cook PA (1992) The Second Medical Research Council study of prognostic factors in nonseminomatous germ cell tumors. Medical Research Council Testicular Tumour Working Party. J Clin Oncol 10:85

Melchior D, Muller SC, Albers P (2003) Extensive surgery in metastatic testicular cancer. Aktuelle Urol 34:214

Merrin C, Takita H, Beckley S, Kassis J (1977) Treatment of recurrent and widespread testicular tumor by radical reductive surgery and multiple sequential chemotherapy. J Urol 117:291

Morgentaler A, Garnick MB, Richie JP (1988) Metastatic testicular teratoma invading the inferior vena cava. J Urol 140:149
Mosharafa AA, Foster RS, Koch MO, Bihrle R, Donohue JP (2004) Complications of post-chemotherapy retroperitoneal lymph node dissection for testis cancer. J Urol 171:1839
Motzer RJ, Bajorin DF, Vlamis V, Weisen S, Bosl GJ (1992) Ifosfamide-based chemotherapy for patients with resistant germ cell tumors: the Memorial Sloan-Kettering Cancer Center experience. Semin Oncol 19:8
Motzer RJ, Amsterdam A, Prieto V, Sheinfeld J, Murty VV, Mazumdar M, Bosl GJ, Chaganti RS, Reuter VE (1998) Teratoma with malignant transformation: diverse malignant histologies arising in men with germ cell tumors. J Urol 159:133
Murphy BR, Breeden ES, Donohue JP, Messemer J, Walsh W, Roth BJ, Einhorn LH (1993) Surgical salvage of chemorefractory germ cell tumors. J Clin Oncol 11:324
Nash PA, Leibovitch I, Foster RS, Bihrle R, Rowland RG, Donohue JP (1998) En bloc nephrectomy in patients undergoing post-chemotherapy retroperitoneal lymph node dissection for nonseminomatous testis cancer: indications, implications and outcomes. J Urol 159:707
Neyer M, Peschel R, Akkad T, Springer-Stohr B, Berger A, Bartsch G, Steiner H (2007) Long-term results of laparoscopic retroperitoneal lymph-node dissection for clinical stage I nonseminomatous germ-cell testicular cancer. J Endourol 21:180
Oldenburg J, Alfsen GC, Lien HH, Aass N, Waehre H, Fossa SD (2003) Postchemotherapy retroperitoneal surgery remains necessary in patients with nonseminomatous testicular cancer and minimal residual tumor masses. J Clin Oncol 21:3310
Ozols RF, Ihde DC, Linehan WM, Jacob J, Ostchega Y, Young RC (1988) A randomized trial of standard chemotherapy v a high-dose chemotherapy regimen in the treatment of poor prognosis nonseminomatous germ-cell tumors. J Clin Oncol 6:1031
Palese MA, Su LM, Kavoussi LR (2002) Laparoscopic retroperitoneal lymph node dissection after chemotherapy. Urology 60:130
Peckham MJ (1985) Surveillance following orchiectomy for clinical stage I testicular germ-cell malignancy. Prog Clin Biol Res 203:523
Permpongkosol S, Lima GC, Warlick CA, Allaf ME, Varkarakis IM, Bagga HS, Kohanim S, Kavoussi LR (2007) Postchemotherapy laparoscopic retroperitoneal lymph node dissection: evaluation of complications. Urology 69:361
Pettus JA, Carver BS, Stasi J, Sheinfeld J (2007) Preservation of ejaculation in patients in undergoing nerve-sparing postchemotherapy retroperitoneal lymph node dissection for advanced testicular cancer. J Urol 177:278
Pfister D, Ohlmann CH, Thuer D, Sahi D, Heidenreich A (2007) Post-chemotherapy retroperitoneal resection of residual masses in germ cell cancer with modified template resection. J Urol 177:330
Rassweiler JJ, Henkel TO, Stock C, Seemann O, Frede T, Alken P (1996) Retroperitoneal laparoscopic lymph node dissection for staging non-seminomatous germ cell tumors before and after chemotherapy. Lymphology 29:36
Richie JP (1984) The surgical management of advanced abdominal disease. Semin Urol 2:238
Richie JP, Garnick MB, Finberg H (1982) Computerized tomography: how accurate for abdominal staging of testis tumors? J Urol 127:715
Rick O, Bokemeyer C, Weinknecht S, Schirren J, Pottek T, Hartmann JT, Braun T, Rachud B, Weissbach L, Hartmann M, Siegert W, Beyer J (2004) Residual tumor resection after high-dose chemotherapy in patients with relapsed or refractory germ cell cancer. J Clin Oncol 22:3713
Sexton WJ, Wood CG, Kim R, Pisters LL (2003) Repeat retroperitoneal lymph node dissection for metastatic testis cancer. J Urol 169:1353
Sheinfeld J (2002) The role of adjunctive postchemotherapy surgery for nonseminomatous germ-cell tumors: current concepts and controversies. Semin Urol Oncol 20:262
Sheinfeld J, Sogani P. (2007) Re-operative retroperitoneal surgery in testicular cancer. Urol Clin North Am 34(2):227-233
Sheinfeld J, Bajorin D, Solomon M (1997) Management of postchemotherapy residual masses in advanced germ cell tumors. AUA Update Series 17:18
Sheinfeld J, McKernian J, Bosl GJ (2002) Surgery of testicular tumors. In: Walsh PC, Retick AB, Vaughan ED Jr, Wein AJ (eds) Campbell's urology, 8th edn. W.B. Saunders, Philadelphia, pp 2920–2944
Spermon JR, De Geus-Oei LF, Kiemeney LA, Witjes JA, Oyen WJ (2002) The role of (18)fluoro-2-deoxyglucose positron emission tomography in initial staging and re-staging after chemotherapy for testicular germ cell tumours. BJU Int 89:549
Stenning SP, Parkinson MC, Fisher C, Mead GM, Cook PA, Fossa SD, Horwich A, Jones WG, Newlands ES, Oliver RT, Stenwig AE, Wilkinson PM (1998) Postchemotherapy residual masses in germ cell tumor patients: content, clinical features, and prognosis. Medical Research Council Testicular Tumour Working Party. Cancer 83:1409
Stephenson AJ, Tal R, Sheinfeld J (2006) Adjunctive nephrectomy at post-chemotherapy retroperitoneal lymph node dissection for nonseminomatous germ cell testicular cancer. J Urol 176:1996
Steyerberg EW, Keizer HJ, Fossa SD, Sleijfer DT, Toner GC, Schraffordt Koops H, Mulders PF, Messemer JE, Ney K, Donohue JP et al (1995) Prediction of residual retroperitoneal mass histology after chemotherapy for metastatic nonseminomatous germ cell tumor: multivariate analysis of individual patient data from six study groups. J Clin Oncol 13:1177
Steyerberg EW, Gerl A, Fossa SD, Sleijfer DT, de Wit R, Kirkels WJ, Schmeller N, Clemm C, Habbema JD, Keizer HJ (1998) Validity of predictions of residual retroperitoneal mass histology in nonseminomatous testicular cancer. J Clin Oncol 16:269
Steyerberg EW, Vergouwe Y, Keizer HJ, Habbema JD (2001) Residual mass histology in testicular cancer: development and validation of a clinical prediction rule. Stat Med 20:3847
Stomper PC, Jochelson MS, Garnick MB, Richie JP (1985) Residual abdominal masses after chemotherapy for nonseminomatous testicular cancer: correlation of CT and histology. AJR Am J Roentgenol 145:743
Tait D, Peckham MJ, Hendry WF, Goldstraw P (1984) Post-chemotherapy surgery in advanced non-seminomatous germ-cell testicular tumours: the significance of histology with particular reference to differentiated (mature) teratoma. Br J Cancer 50:601

Toner GC, Panicek DM, Heelan RT, Geller NL, Lin SY, Bajorin D, Motzer RJ, Scher HI, Herr HW, Morse MJ et al (1990) Adjunctive surgery after chemotherapy for nonseminomatous germ cell tumors: recommendations for patient selection. J Clin Oncol 8:1683

Ulbright TM, Loehrer PJ, Roth LM, Einhorn LH, Williams SD, Clark SA (1984) The development of non-germ cell malignancies within germ cell tumors. A clinicopathologic study of 11 cases. Cancer 54:1824

Vergouwe Y, Steyerberg EW, Foster RS, Sleijfer DT, Fossa SD, Gerl A, de Wit R, Roberts JT, Habbema JD (2007) Predicting retroperitoneal histology in postchemotherapy testicular germ cell cancer: a model update and multicentre validation with more than 1000 patients. Eur Urol 51:424

Wahle GR, Foster RS, Bihrle R, Rowland RG, Bennett RM, Donohue JP (1994) Nerve sparing retroperitoneal lymphadenectomy after primary chemotherapy for metastatic testicular carcinoma. J Urol 152:428

Williams SD, Birch R, Einhorn LH, Irwin L, Greco FA, Loehrer PJ (1987) Treatment of disseminated germ-cell tumors with cisplatin, bleomycin, and either vinblastine or etoposide. N Engl J Med 316:1435

Wittenhuhn R, De Geeter P, Albers P (2007) Retroperitoneal residual tumor resection for testicular cancer – template instead of full bilateral resection. J Urol 177:331

Wood DP Jr, Herr HW, Heller G, Vlamis V, Sogani PC, Motzer RJ, Fair WR, Bosl GJ (1992a) Distribution of retroperitoneal metastases after chemotherapy in patients with nonseminomatous germ cell tumors. J Urol 148:1812

Wood DP Jr, Herr HW, Motzer RJ, Reuter V, Sogani PC, Morse MJ, Bosl GJ (1992b) Surgical resection of solitary metastases after chemotherapy in patients with nonseminomatous germ cell tumors and elevated serum tumor markers. Cancer 70:2354

Wozniak AJ, Samson MK, Shah NT, Crawford ED, Ford CD, Altman SJ, Stephens RL, Natale RB, Bouroncle BA, Blumenstein BA et al (1991) A randomized trial of cisplatin, vinblastine, and bleomycin versus vinblastine, cisplatin, and etoposide in the treatment of advanced germ cell tumors of the testis: a Southwest Oncology Group study. J Clin Oncol 9:70

# 16 Surgical Resection at Other Sites

Kenneth A. Kesler and Stephen D.W. Beck

## 16.1 Introduction

Nonseminomatous germ cell tumors (NSGCTs) of testicular origin are the most common neoplasm in males under the age of 40 years (Bosl and Motzer 1997). It is estimated that 8,000 new cases will be diagnosed in the United States each year, with the worldwide incidence doubling over the past 40 years. Despite the increasing incidence of testicular NSGCT, mortality rates have dramatically fallen by an estimated 70% since the advent of cisplatin-based chemotherapy regimens in the 1970s (Levi et al. 2001; McKiernan et al. 1999). The paradigm of cisplatin-based chemotherapy followed by surgery to remove residual disease is currently viewed as the most successful multimodality cancer treatment model against which other solid cancer treatments are compared.

NSGCT most frequently metastasizes to the retroperitoneum following a very predictable pattern of spread. Resection of residual retroperitoneal masses after systemic chemotherapy in NSGCT is uniformly accepted worldwide. The rationale for resection is the inability to accurately predict histology. Surgery is an accurate staging procedure identifying patients harboring necrosis and is therapeutic with the removal of residual teratoma. Resection of active cancer can be therapeutic and identifies patients that may benefit from adjuvant chemotherapy. The histology of residual retroperitoneal tumors, predictors of histology and long-term outcome for each histologic subtype has been widely reported. Similar data for non-retroperitoneal sites of disease are limited. In the this chapter, we will address the epidemiology, patterns of dissemination, predictors of histology, and survival as it relates to non-retroperitoneal masses.

Although hematogenous metastases to the lung, bone, or brain may occur, testicular NSGCT most frequently metastasizes via lymphatics to the retroperitoneum and may subsequently metastasize to contiguous mediastinal lymphatics. Cisplatin-based chemotherapy alone will cure the majority of patients with supradiaphragmatic metastases. Approximately 10–20% of testicular NSGCT cases that present with or subsequently develop supradiaphragmatic metastases will require at least one thoracic surgical procedure in the form of either mediastinal dissection and/or pulmonary metastasectomy to remove persistent radiographic abnormalities following chemotherapy (Kesler and Donohue 1999).

## 16.2 Mediastinal Disease

### 16.2.1 Incidence and Patterns of Spread

Metastatic NSGCT to the thorax presents in the lungs from hematogenous spread in 80% of cases, mediastinum from lymphatic spread in 10%, or disease in both lungs and mediastinum in 10%. Unlike primary mediastinal germ cell tumors, which originate in the anterior mediastinal thymic tissue, mediastinal metastases from NSGCTs of a testicular origin follow a predictable pattern of dissemination mainly along the distribution of the thoracic duct and its major lymphatic tributaries. At Indiana University, we favor using the mediastinal compartments described by Shields who designates the middle mediastinum as consisting of the

K.A. Kesler (✉)
Cardiothoracic Surgery Department, Indiana University School of Medicine, Indianapolis, IN, USA

M.P. Laguna et al. (eds.), *Cancer of the Testis*,
DOI: 10.1007/978-1-84800-370-5_16, 

"visceral" mediastinum from the thoracic inlet to the diaphragmatic cura (Shields 1999). In this designation, the middle mediastinum includes not only the ascending and aortic arch, brachiocephalic vessels, and esophagus superiorly but also the descending thoracic aorta, adjacent azygous vein, and esophagus to the diaphragmatic crura inferiorly. This designation is more logical from embryologic, anatomic, and pathologic standpoints with respect to keeping all the major lymphatic vessels within the middle mediastinum as compared to the more frequently utilized designation where major arteries and adjacent lymphatics course through at least two of the mediastinal compartments with somewhat arbitrary boundaries. Moreover, subdividing the middle or "visceral" mediastinum into roughly equal thirds (i.e., upper, mid, and lower) dictates optimal surgical approaches to remove residual intrathoracic disease (Strollo et al. 1997). Although the residual disease appears to rather uniformly disseminate throughout the major lymphatics of the middle or "visceral" mediastinum, occasionally metastases will additionally present in the anterior compartment and paravertebral sulcus, presumably as a result of branch lymphatic spread likely contributed by malignant obstruction of more cephalic lymphatic vessels. However, we found no case of isolated metastases in the anterior mediastinal compartment or paravertebral sulcus without middle mediastinal metastases. Nonseminomatous germ cell cancer isolated to the anterior compartment in a patient with a history of testicular NSGCT should therefore be considered a second primary neoplasm.

### 16.2.2 Indications for Surgery

The indications to remove residual mediastinal disease after cisplatin-based chemotherapy are on based on multiple factors, including disease stage at presentation, the serologic and radiographic response to chemotherapy, and if performed, the pathologic findings of postchemotherapy retroperitoneal lymph node dissection (RPLND). In general, following completion of cisplatin-based chemotherapy, patients are restaged with serum tumor markers (STMs) and CT body scans. The majority of patients normalize previously elevated STMs and achieve either a significant reduction or resolution of all radiographic evidence of disease in the retroperitoneum and chest. Patients who demonstrate progression of disease during or soon after first-line chemotherapy are given second-line cisplatin-based chemotherapy.

If significant radiographic abnormalities remain in the retroperitoneum and chest, then RPLND is typically performed first. As there is a high correlation between the pathological findings of tumor necrosis in residual retroperitoneal and intrathoracic masses following successful first-line chemotherapy, radiographic observation of persistent mediastinal abnormalities is usually indicated if only necrosis is pathologically demonstrated in the RPLND specimen and especially if the major bulk of disease mass was in the retroperitoneum (Steyerberg et al. 1997a). If more extensive residual mediastinal disease is present following second-line chemotherapy, then mediastinal dissection in general is indicated even if RPLND pathology demonstrates tumor necrosis. Bulky areas of residual "necrosis" may contain viable cells with future growth and/or malignant degeneration potential in these higher risk cases. Bulky residual mediastinal masses suspected of containing tumor necrosis not infrequently represent situations where dissection is technically difficult secondary to obscured tissue planes. Adjacent and even adherent intrathoracic organs such as the great arteries, trachea, and esophagus can typically be spared, however, to avoid morbidity.

In our reported series of 268 patients undergoing thoracic surgery to remove residual mediastinal disease following either first or second-line cisplatin-based chemotherapy, 59% of residual masses contained mature teratoma, with only 15% demonstrating tumor necrosis, as many patients with suspected tumor necrosis did not undergo mediastinal surgery after successful first-line chemotherapy and RPLND (Kesler et al. 2003). Therefore, thoracic surgery is mainly performed for residual low-density cystic masses in the mediastinum suspected of containing teratoma. Given the high potential for cure as well as the ability to more readily dissect teratomatous masses from major intrathoracic organs and nerves without sacrifice, surgery is indicated regardless of the extent of residual mediastinal disease in this setting. Finally, as our institution is a referral center for NSGCT, 25–30% of our patients undergoing mediastinal surgery have either persistent NSGCT or degeneration into nongerm cell cancer pathologically demonstrated in resected specimens. This is higher than the anticipated 10–15% incidence of these types of chemotherapy refractory cases.

"Salvage" thoracic surgery is performed for limited mediastinal disease in select patients with masses containing either persistent NSGCT (usually signified by significant STM elevation following second-line chemotherapy or late relapse) or degenerative nongerm cell cancer. Moreover, a more aggressive surgical approach is sometimes necessary, removing adherent or frankly involved adjacent organs or great vessels in these "salvage" thoracic surgery cases.

### 16.2.3 Surgical Techniques

Specific surgical approaches for all mediastinal compartments harboring radiographic evidence of residual disease is based on minimizing the overall number of thoracic procedures necessary while optimizing exposure. In addition to the level(s) and location (left and/or right side) of residual mediastinal disease, other variables which need to be considered when determining the optimal thoracic surgical approach and/or sequence of all surgical approaches include the presence of contiguous or noncontiguous retroperitoneal or neck disease and the need to perform anatomic pulmonary resection and/or pulmonary metastasectomy. Surgical strategies to remove all residual disease following chemotherapy are therefore individualized for each patient. For example, a patient with residual noncontiguous mediastinal disease involving the upper and lower middle mediastinum isolated to either hemithorax can usually undergo complete extirpation of residual disease through an extended posterolateral thoracotomy with sixth rib resection thus gaining adequate exposure to both compartments. We would also attempt to reduce the overall number of surgical procedures. One thoracic surgical procedure can usually be performed in conjunction with RPLND and/or modified neck dissection (MND) particularly when contiguous disease is present in the retroperitoneum and thoracic inlet, respectively. The decision to sequentially stage or combine surgical procedures is dependent on the location and volume of residual disease in the chest, neck, and retroperitoneum.

As the majority of NSGCT patients receive bleomycin therapy preoperatively, to minimize the potential for operative morbidity, we believe that surgical procedures lasting more than 10–12 h or combination procedures requiring anatomic pulmonary resection (such as lobectomy or pneumonectomy) should be avoided. In addition, a planned mediastinal dissection under the same anesthetic should be deferred if there has been excessive blood loss and/or cardiorespiratory instability during RPLND. Patients otherwise undergoing routine RPLND typically can undergo mediastinal dissection to remove noncontiguous and nonbulky disease under the same anesthetic. If bilateral mediastinal disease is present, then the mediastinal side containing the least amount of disease would be operated under the same anesthetic deferring surgery for the more extensive side until satisfactory recovery has occurred, which is usually 6–8 weeks later.

#### 16.2.3.1 Outcome and Morbidity

The largest series evaluating outcome in patients undergoing resection of residual mediastinal disease after chemotherapy was reported at Indiana University (Kesler et al. 2003). This study included 268 patients with metastatic testicular cancer. All patients had a component of NSGCT in their testicular pathology with the majority (69.4%) demonstrating embryonal cell carcinoma, while 21.3% demonstrated elements of teratoma and 24.2% seminomatous germ cell cancer. Most patients ($n=170$, 65.9%) presented with supradiaphragmatic (III) disease; however, the other 98 patients, manifested mediastinal disease either during or subsequent to receiving cisplatin-based chemotherapy. Ninety-four (35.1%) patients received second-line chemotherapy prior to removing residual intrathoracic disease. The overall 5 and 10-year survival was $86 \pm 2\%$ and $74 \pm 4\%$, respectively. The "worst" pathology of residual mediastinal disease was necrosis in 14.9% ($n=39$), teratoma in 58.8% ($n=154$), persistent NSGCT in 15.6% ($n=41$), and nongerm cell cancer in 10.7% ($n=28$). In a Cox regression model, older age at diagnosis ($P=0.005$), elevated beta human chorionic gonadotropin (bHCG) at surgery ($P=0.028$), and persistent or degenerative germ cell cancer in residual mediastinal disease ($P=0.006$) were the only variables found to be independently predictive of poorer long-term survival.

In the above series, there were three operative deaths (1.1% of patients). Two patients died of acute respiratory distress syndrome (ARDS) following lobectomy and pneumonectomy for extensive residual middle mediastinal and hilar disease. Both of these patients had only necrosis in the resected specimens. One patient died of complications secondary to gastric perforation following a combined thoracoabdominal approach to remove residual teratoma. Thirty-two (11.9%) patients developed nonfatal postoperative complications including pneumonia, significant atelectasis and/or >48 h mechanical ventilation ($n=9$), persistent chylothorax >10 days ($n=8$), prolonged air leak >10 days ($n=8$), bleeding requiring reoperation ($n=4$), atrial dysrhythmias ($n=3$), pleural space infection ($n=3$), recurrent nerve palsy ($n=2$), and pulmonary embolism ($n=2$). Of significant note, six patients manifested postoperative lower extremity paresis/paraplegia following circumferential lower descending thoracic aorta dissection to remove residual masses containing teratoma. Four patients demonstrated significant improvement of neurologic function and two did not.

A follow-up study from Indiana University evaluated the outcome of 134 patients undergoing 186 surgical procedures to remove residual malignant intrathoracic metastases of germ-cell origin (Kesler et al. 2005). Fifty-nine patients had removal of pulmonary metastases, 49 had removal of mediastinal metastases, and 26 had removal both pulmonary and mediastinal metastases. Surgical pathology demonstrated 84 patients with persistent NSGCT, 38 with degeneration into nongerm cell cancer, and 12 with both malignant pathologic categories. The overall survival was 5.6 years, with 55 (42.3%) alive after a mean follow-up of 5.1 years. Seventeen variables were analyzed by using Cox regression. Of these, older age, pulmonary metastases (vs. mediastinal metastases), and 4 or more (vs. 1) total intrathoracic metastases were significantly ($P \leq 0.01$) predictive of inferior long-term survival.

Although many patients diagnosed with NSGCT of testicular origin present with stage III disease, only a minority will ultimately require surgical removal of residual mediastinal disease following cisplatin-based chemotherapy. Patients who do undergo mediastinal dissection have residual disease distributed throughout the lower, mid, and/or upper middle or "visceral" mediastinum from the thoracic inlet to the diaphragmatic crura, with residual disease in the mid middle mediastinum being most common. Residual disease in the paravertebral sulcus and anterior mediastinal compartment occurs much less frequently. Long-term survival of patients who demonstrate either necrosis or teratoma in residual mediastinal disease is excellent, which clearly justifies an aggressive surgical approach, even when extensive mediastinal or circumferential descending thoracic aortic involvement is present. Bilateral and/or multiple thoracic surgical procedures are not infrequently necessary. Operative morbidity and mortality are low as attempts to spare adjacent organs and nerves are usually possible particularly with residual teratomatous disease. At this referral center for testicular NSGCT cases, we continue to evaluate an increasing number of patients with chemotherapy refractory disease. Salvage surgery to remove mediastinal disease in these cases, represent situations where significantly poorer long-term survival is anticipated; however, an aggressive surgical approach is justified in select patients.

## 16.3 Pulmonary Disease

### 16.3.1 Incidence and Pattern of Spread

Of patients presenting with supradiaphragmatic disease, approximately 10% will undergo pulmonary resection for residual disease after platinum-based chemotherapy. Hematogenous spread from the testicle to the lung occurs directly from the testicle or indirectly through lymphatic spread into the thoracic duct, draining into the subclavian vein and then to the lung.

### 16.3.2 Predictors of Pulmonary Pathology

Selection of patients for pulmonary resection typically includes patients with residual lung nodules and normal STMs after chemotherapy. Resection of residual teratoma or active cancer can be therapeutic and therefore the morbidity of thoracotomy is justified. Conversely, resection of residual necrosis is a staging procedure only. Efforts have been made to predict pulmonary histology on the basis of retroperitoneal pathology, testicular pathology, and serum tumor levels in an attempt to avoid the morbidity of thoracotomy in patients predictive to harbor necrosis only.

Excluding series with less than 100 patients, there are only two retrospective studies identifying variables predictive of pulmonary histology. Tognini et al. reviewed 143 post chemotherapy patients who underwent resection of residual retroperitoneal and chest disease under the same anesthetic (Tognoni et al. 1998). Concordance existed in 77.5% of patients with necrosis, 70% with teratoma, and 69% with cancer of the abdomen. Categorizing patients as uncomplicated (first-line chemotherapy, normalization of STMs, and no previous RPLND) revealed a concordance of 86% for patients with necrosis in the retroperitoneum and in the chest.

An international, multicenter, retrospective review evaluated the concordance of retroperitoneal and pulmonary histology in 215 patients (Steyerberg et al. 1997b). The pulmonary mass histology was necrosis in 116 (54%), mature teratoma in 70 (33%), and cancer in 29 (13%). The strongest predictor of pulmonary histology was the histology found at RPLND. If RPLND histology revealed necrosis, the probability of necrosis at thoracotomy was 89%. When the RPLND histology was necrosis and the primary tumor was teratoma negative, the predictive probability of necrosis at thoracotomy was as high as 93%. For patients with a teratoma positive tumor, the probability was slightly lower at 87%.

With the above data as well as other studies, a cogent argument can be made to observe pulmonary nodules in order to avoid the morbidity of thoracotomy in a subgroup of patients. In subgroups with necrosis in the retroperitoneum, observation of pulmonary nodules would spare more than 90% of patients from surgery. Arguably, with observation strategies with chest imaging every 2 months for the first year and every 4 months for the second year, the small portion of patients with residual teratoma (5%) or active cancer (1–4%) will be identified and treated early with no detriment in cancer survival. Proponents of observation state the risk of growing teratoma syndrome or malignant transformation for residual teratoma and the risk of disease progression in the small population with active cancer. There are no data comparing immediate resection of residual pulmonary nodules/masses vs. delayed resection upon progression. At Indiana University, it is our clinical experience that appropriate observation protocols in select patients avoid unnecessary surgery in a large population of patients with residual pulmonary nodules without compromising survival. Decision-making with regard to residual mass resection must take in account technical feasibility, patient morbidity and potential benefit, access to health care, and patient preference.

### 16.3.3 Surgical Technique

The two primary goals of removing metastatic NSCGT pulmonary disease are to minimize both removal of normal parenchyma and the morbidity of large thoracotomy incisions. We believe because of the relatively benign nature of residual teratoma that utilizing minimally invasive thoracoscopic techniques will not compromise a chance of cure. Furthermore in our experience, smaller areas of parenchymal abnormality, identifiable only by lung palpation, most frequently represent residual scar tissue only and therefore do not require resection. We therefore utilize this minimally invasive approach as the procedure of choice for removing 2–3 small and peripheral pulmonary metastases. In "Combination but Separate" procedures we would choose to operate the lung where metastatectomy is amenable to thoracoscopy and delay the lung requiring an open thoracotomy for 2–4 weeks allowing recovery. For nonroutine cases where active NSCGT, sarcomatous, or carcinomatous transformation are suspected, we have a lower threshold to perform open thoracotomy which allows wide resection and careful palpation of the remaining lung. For cases with multiple peripheral pulmonary masses, we have found that using endostaplers for wedge resections through a muscle sparing thoracotomy approach is helpful in minimizing postoperative pain. A muscle sparing open thoracotomy approach is also used for large or more central teratoma in the lung parenchyma. Using electrocautery, a pneumotomy is made to literally "shell out" teratomatous masses deep in the parenchyma, followed by suture closure which is appropriate for parenchymal sparing purposes. The very small incidence of local recurrence justifies this parenchymal preserving technique particularly when total pneumonectomy can be avoided. For larger central lesions, however, we would perform anatomic resections including formal lobar resections in 13% of pulmonary resection cases, and superior segmentectomies of bilateral lower lobes in 6% of cases. In our experience, pneumonectomy is only rarely required in routine teratoma cases. In cases where multiple (>10–20) wedge resections are required, or complete pneumonectomy is anticipated, thoracotomy would be delayed to allow full recovery following RPLND.

### 16.3.4 Morbidity and Survival

Bleomycin induced pulmonary fibrosis can decrease pulmonary compliance and therefore contribute to atelectasis and bronchopleural fistulae from parenchymal suture/staple lines. In addition, the potential for underlying compromise in oxygen diffusing capacity underscores our policy of judicious intraoperative and postoperative fluid administration as well as avoiding large retroperitoneal/thoracic surgery combination procedures in patients requiring multiple wedge or large anatomic resections. For more extensive retroperitoneal/thoracic surgery procedures, we observe a conservative extubation policy, allowing excellent oxygenation and lung expansion by continuing mechanical ventilation through the evening of surgery, with extubation early on the first postoperative morning. Epidural narcotic infusions for the first 48–72 postoperative hours allow the patients to emerge from general anesthesia comfortably, and they are more capable of cooperating with pulmonary physiotherapy exercises that greatly reduce pulmonary morbidity. ICU transfer is usually accomplished by the first postoperative evening and oral alimentation resumed after return of bowel function following RPLND. Prolonged chyle leakage through chest tubes may occur after extensive mediastinal dissection but is usually self limiting or successfully treated by dietary modifications and/or parenteral nutrition, rarely requiring reoperation.

## 16.4 Brain

Germ cell metastasis to the brain is rare. The International Germ Cell Cancer Collaborative Group (IGCCCG) evaluated 5,862 patients with germ-cell cancer to identify prognostic variables.[12] Brain metastases was present in 70 patients (1.2%) with a 5 year overall survival of 33% for patient with non seminomatous germ cell tumor (NSGCT) and 57% for patients with pure seminoma. A European multicenter study evaluated 56 patients with brain metastases at diagnosis (Group 1) and 83 patients with brain metastases after cisplatin-based chemotherapy (Group 2).[13] The 5-year cause specific survival rate in Group 1 was 45%. Neurosurgery and the absence of extracerebral, nonpulmonary visceral disease were independent predictors of a good prognosis. The 5-year cause specific survival rate in Group 2 was 12%, but was 39% in patients with an isolated brain recurrence. In a series of 68 patients with brain involvement, Balmaceda et al reported a 57% complete response rate with chemotherapy alone.[14]

Currently, for patients presenting with CNS metastases, we advocate treating with chemotherapy alone in the case of most CNS metastases and then reevaluate with brain imaging. If complete remission is achieved, no additional treatment is required and close follow-up is recommended. However, if residual CNS disease is small or a single lesion, we recommend subsequent surgical excision or stereotactic radiosurgery. Due to the potential of significant neurologic toxicity, at Indiana University, we now reserve whole brain radiotherapy for patients with large CNS metastases, highly symptomatic patients, or those with persistent or recurrent metastases. (Azar, Schneider, Einhorn: Int J Rad Oncol Biol Phys, 69:163-166, 2007).

## 16.5 Liver

The initial presence of liver metastases represents an independent poor prognostic variable in patients with germ-cell cancer. The IGCCC reported an incidence of liver involvement in 6% of 5,202 patients presenting with NSGCT and in 26 (4%) of 595 patients with pure seminoma (Anon 1997). In this study, the 5-year overall survival was 49% and 54% for NSGCT and seminoma, respectively.

A multicenter European study reported on 43 patients undergoing hepatic resection after platinum based chemotherapy (Hartmann et al. 2005). Histology revealed necrosis in 67%, teratoma in 12%, and viable cancer in 21%. Twelve (39%) of the 31 patients who underwent liver surgery and resection of additional sites showed dissimilar histologic findings in hepatic and extrahepatic tumor masses. Indiana University recently evaluated the concordance of histology in patients undergoing liver resection and RPLND (Jacobsen et al. 2006). In 58 patients, liver histology revealed necrosis in 73%, teratoma in 17%, and cancer in 10%. The histologic concordance between retroperitoneal histology and liver histology was 94.4% for necrosis, 25.9% for teratoma, and 38.5% for active cancer.

In a previous report from Indiana, Hahn reported an 89% survival at a median follow-up of 47 months for patients with necrosis in the liver vs. 29% for patients with active cancer (Hahn et al. 1999). Observation of liver metastases should be considered when retroperitoneal histology reveals necrosis or when the volume and/or location of the hepatic involvement necessitate a significant surgical undertaking. If on follow-up, the mass enlarges then surgery or second-line chemotherapy should be considered.

## 16.6 Conclusion

Although many patients diagnosed with NSGCT of testicular origin present with advanced disease, there is an anticipated 80–90% chance of cure following successful first-line chemotherapy. Residual retroperitoneal disease requires surgical resection as there is no accurate means to predict histology and the morbidity of surgery is generally low. The management of patients with residual supradiaphragmatic and liver tumors must be individualized to select those patients most likely to benefit from surgery and avoid unnecessary morbidity in those not benefiting from surgery, without decreasing survival. Appropriate patient selection requires a multidisciplinary team including medical oncologists, urologists, and thoracic and general surgeons.

## References


Anon (1997) International germ cell consensus classification: a prognostic factor-based staging system for metastatic germ cell cancers. International Germ Cell Cancer Collaborative Group. J Clin Oncol 15:594

Balmaceda C, Heller G, Rosenblum M, Diez B, Villablanca JG, Kellie S et al (1996) Chemotherapy without irradiation–a novel approach for newly diagnosed CNS germ cell tumors: results of an international cooperative trial. The First International Central Nervous System Germ Cell Tumor Study. J Clin Oncol 14:2908

Bosl GJ, Motzer RJ (1997) Testicular germ-cell cancer. N Engl J Med 337:242

Fossa SD, Bokemeyer C, Gerl A, Culine S, Jones WG, Mead GM et al (1999) Treatment outcome of patients with brain metastases from malignant germ cell tumors. Cancer 85: 988

Hahn TL, Jacobson L, Einhorn LH, Foster R, Goulet RJ Jr (1999) Hepatic resection of metastatic testicular carcinoma: a further update. Ann Surg Oncol 6:640

Hartmann JT, Rick O, Oechsle K, Kuczyk M, Gauler T, Schoffski P et al (2005) Role of postchemotherapy surgery in the management of patients with liver metastases from germ cell tumors. Ann Surg 242:260

Jacobsen NB, Foster RS, Beck SDW, Bihrle R, Einhorn L, Donohue JP (2006) Is retroperitoneal histology predictive of liver histology at the time of concurrent post chemotherapy retroperitoneal lymph node dissection. J Urol 175:191 (Abstract)

Kesler K, Donohue JP (1999) Combined urologic and thoracic approaches for advanced or disseminated testis cancer. Atlas Urol Clin North Am 7:79–94

Kesler KA, Brooks JA, Rieger KM, Fineberg NS, Einhorn LH, Brown JW (2003) Mediastinal metastases from testicular nonseminomatous germ cell tumors: patterns of dissemination and predictors of long-term survival with surgery. J Thorac Cardiovasc Surg 125:913

Kesler KA, Wilson JL, Cosgrove JA, Brooks JA, Messiha A, Fineberg NS et al (2005) Surgical salvage therapy for malignant intrathoracic metastases from nonseminomatous germ cell cancer of testicular origin: analysis of a single-institution experience. J Thorac Cardiovasc Surg 130:408

Levi F, La Vecchia C, Boyle P, Lucchini F, Negri E (2001) Western and eastern European trends in testicular cancer mortality. Lancet 357:1853

McKiernan JM, Goluboff ET, Liberson GL, Golden R, Fisch H (1999) Rising risk of testicular cancer by birth cohort in the United States from 1973 to 1995. J Urol 162:361

Shields T (1999) The mediastinum, its compartments, and the mediastinal lymph nodes. In: Shields TW, LoCicero J III, Ponn RB (eds) General thoracic surgery, 5th edn. Lippincott Williams and Wilkins, Philadelphia, pp 1983–1986

Steyerberg EW, Donohue JP, Gerl A, Toner GC, Schraffordt Koops H, Fossa SD et al (1997a) Residual masses after chemotherapy for metastatic testicular cancer: the clinical implications of the association between retroperitoneal and pulmonary histology. Re-analysis of Histology in Testicular Cancer (ReHiT) Study Group. J Urol 158:474

Steyerberg EW, Keizer HJ, Messemer JE, Toner GC, Schraffordt Koops H, Fossa SD et al (1997b) Residual pulmonary masses after chemotherapy for metastatic nonseminomatous germ cell tumor. Prediction of histology. ReHiT Study Group. Cancer 79:345

Strollo DC, Rosado de Christenson ML, Jett JR (1997) Primary mediastinal tumors. Part 1: tumors of the anterior mediastinum. Chest 112:511

Tognoni PG, Foster RS, McGraw P, Heilman D, Bihrle R, Rowland RG et al (1998) Combined post-chemotherapy retroperitoneal lymph node dissection and resection of chest tumor under the same anesthetic is appropriate based on morbidity and tumor pathology. J Urol 159:1833

# 17 Extra-Gonadal Germ Cell Tumors

Ton A. Roeleveld and Simon Horenblas

## 17.1 Extragonadal Germ Cell Tumors

Extragonadal germ cell tumors (EGCTs) are rare tumors that predominantly affect young males. They are located in the body midline. The most common sites of EGCTs are the mediastinum (50–70%), the retroperitoneum (25–40%), the pineal gland (5%), and the sacrococcygeal area (less than 5%) (Goss et al. 1994). However, less common sites from suprasellar region to prostate have been reported. The only known risk factor for EGCTs is the Klinefelter syndrome (47XXY) that is associated with mediastinal nonseminomatous germ cell tumors (NSGCTs) (Hasle et al. 1995).

The exact incidence of EGCTs is unknown, but about 2–5% of GCTs are considered to be of extragonadal origin (Collins and Puch 1964). A Norwegian study estimated the yearly incidence of EGCTs to be 0.5/100,000 (Dueland et al. 1998). An EGCT is characterized by the absence of a palpable or radiologically visible lesion in the testis. The incidence of EGCTs may be overestimated by the existence of the "burned-out " phenomenon. It has been shown that a considerable proportion of presumed EGCTs have in fact a scrotal scar that represents a regressed primary testicular cancer (Comiter et al. 1996; Scholz et al. 2002a). Especially presumed retroperitoneal EGCTs may represent metastases from a testicular cancer, with spontaneous necrosis of the primary tumor.

T.A. Roeleveld (✉)
Urology Department, Medical Centre Alkmaaar, Alkmaar, The Netherlands

## 17.2 Sex and Age

About 90% of malignant EGCTs occur in men. Sacrococcygeal lesions are predominantly found in women. Teratomas ("benign" EGCTs) are equally distributed in both men and women. In children, both benign and malignant EGGCTs occur equally in both sexes. More than 60% of childhood GCTs are extragonadal. EGCTs account for approximately 3% of all childhood cancers.

## 17.3 Pathophysiology

Considering cytogenetics and the pathology of GCTs and teratomas, five subtypes can be classified (Oosterhuis and Looijenga 2005):

I: Teratoma/yolk sac tumors of infancy
II: Seminoma and nonseminoma of young adults
III: Spermatocytic seminoma of elderly men, exclusively in the testis
IV: Dermoid cyst, almost exclusively in the ovary
V: Gestational trophoblastic tumor

Only type I and II GCTs occur both in the gonads and in extragonadal localizations. Furthermore, type I tumors are seen even more frequently extragonadally than in the gonads.

Germ cells can be derived from embryonic stem cells. There are good explanations for the distribution of EGCTs (Oosterhuis et al. 2007). The anatomical distribution of EGCTs might be explained by the migration of primordial germ cells from the yolk sac

M.P. Laguna et al. (eds.), *Cancer of the Testis*,
DOI: 10.1007/978-1-84800-370-5_17, © Springer-Verlag London Limited 2010

(proximal epiblast) along the hindgut and its mesentery to the bilateral genital ridges.

Malignant transformation of germ cells is the result of a multistep process of genetic changes. One of the earliest events is the increased copy number of 12p, either as one or more copies of i(12p) or as duplications of chromosome arm 12p. Genomic imprinting of body cells means that the expression of certain genes depends on their parental origin. The biparental pattern of genomic imprinting of somatic cells is erased in the early stages of germ lineage. In primordial germ cells and gonocytes, genomic imprinting is erased. Maternal and paternal imprinting is restored during oogenesis and spermatogenesis (Oosterhuis et al. 2007). It has been shown that all type II GCTs have an erased imprinting (Szabo and Mann 1995). The type I GCTs in contrast are only partially erased, regardless of histology and anatomical site. This suggests that they originate developmentally closer to the embryonic stem cell than a primordial germ cell of which the type II tumors originate. The precursor cells of type I GCTs do not form tumors of neoplastic germ cells, and they lack the totipotency of the type II tumors.

Germ cells and therefore GCTs are derived from embryonal stem cells. Extragonadal GCTs are considered to develop from pluripotent embryonal stem cells that because of conditions in the midline of the embryo have undergone germ cell differentiation. Thus, precursor cells of GCTs could have differentiated from embryonal stem cells in extragonadal localizations. For the derivation of GCTs it seems impossible to discriminate between embryonic stem cells and primitive germ cells. Type II GCTs have a more limited anatomical distribution than type I GCTs. This might be explained by a more differentiated state of the germ cells from which they are derived. These cells probably have a more limited survival potential outside the gonads. Site specific features like presence of Y-chromosomal material (like testis specific protein, Y encoded) and stem cell factor production probably explain why type II EGCTs survive in limited anatomical locations (Oosterhuis et al. 2007).

There is a remarkable association between mediastinal EGCTs and hematologic malignancies (Downie et al. 1994; Hartmann et al. 2000). Although it is unknown why they are associated with only mediastinal tumors, genetic studies have shown that both the GCT and hematopoietic components are clonally related (Downie et al. 1994; Ladanyi et al. 1990). The germ cell component involved is typically yolk sac tumor but other nonseminomatous GCTs have also been reported. In about half of the cases of associated hematopoietic malignancy, acute myeloid leukemia with megakaryocytic or monocytic differentiation is found. Various other concommitant hematopoietic malignancies and myeloproliferative disorders have however also been described. Genetically, the relationship between the mediastinal EGCT and hematologic malignancy is frequently shown by an isochromosome 12p abnormality (Downie et al. 1994).

## 17.4 Clinical Presentation

EGCTs often reach a considerable size before becoming symptomatic. They frequently arise in body parts where considerable growth can occur without compromising vital functions. Therefore, presentation is often in an advanced local stage and with distant metastases. Metastatic sites are predominantly regional lymph nodes, lung, liver, and bone. The best data on clinical presentation of this infrequent tumor come from a pooled analysis of 635 patients treated at 11 institutions (Bokemeyer et al. 2002).

### *17.4.1 Mediastial Germ Cell Tumors*

The mediastinum is the most common anatomic site, harboring 50–70% of all EGCTs.

Histology of GCTs in the mediastinum is similar to the one in the gonads. Mature teratomas, however, are seen more frequently and they account for 60% of all mediastinal GCTs. Malignant mediastinal GCTs show seminoma in 40% and nonseminomatous GCTs in 60%.

The majority of mediastinal GCTs present with symptoms. Dyspnoe (25%) is often seen, followed by chest pain (23%), cough (17%), fever (13%), weight loss (11%), vena cava superior syndrome (6%), fatigue/weakness (6%), and other pain complaints (5%) (Bokemeyer et al. 2002).

Metastases are present in 40–50% at diagnosis. Seminomatous tumors show merely lymph node metastases, whereas in nonseminomatous tumors especially lung metastases are seen.

In about 70% of nonseminomatous mediastinal GCTs alpha-fetoprotein (AFP) was elevated, in 40% beta-human chorionic gonadotropin (β-HCG).

On physical examination mediastinal germ cell tumors may be silent; sometimes airway obstruction or pleural effusion is present.

### 17.4.2 Retroperitoneal Germ Cell Tumors

Between 25 and 40% of all EGCTs occur in the retroperitoneum. Often tumors reach a considerable size before they become symptomatic. Abdominal pain (29%) and back pain (14%) are the most encountered symptoms. Less frequent symptoms are weight loss (9%), fever/night sweats (8%), venous thrombosis (9%), palpable mass (10%), scrotal edema/hydrocele (5%), and gynaecomastia (5%). AFP is elevated in about 50% and β-HCG in 75%. They are metastasized in 50% and metastasized more often to multiple locations than mediastinal EGCTs (48 vs. 26%) (Bokemeyer et al. 2002).

On examination often a large abdominal mass can be palpated.

### 17.4.3 Intracranial Germ Cell Tumors

These are rare tumors of adolescents and young adults. They are preferentially localized in the pineal and suprasellar regions. The age distribution of afflicted patients is unimodal, centering with an abrupt surge in frequency in the early pubertal years. Nongerminomatous GCTs demonstrate an earlier age of onset than do germinomas.

Germinoma is the most frequently found intracranial GCT. It is histologically identical to the ovarian dysgerminoma and testicular seminoma. Germinomas (or seminomas) account for 60–70% of intracranial GCTs and have a predilection for the suprasellar region. Embryonal carcinomas, yolk sac tumors, and choriocarcinomas mainly occur in the pineal region. A Canadian national retrospective study showed a mean annual incidence of CNS GCT of 1.06 per million children (0.7 per million for germinoma and 0.3 per million for non-germinomatous GCT) (Keene et al. 2007). The majority of germinomas arise in the suprasellar cistern, while most non-germinomatous GCTs preferentially involve the pineal gland.

Pineal tumors present with headache, nausea, and vomiting because of increased intracranial pressure. Deterioration of intellectual functions, gait abnormalities with frequent falls, and sphincteric incontinence are common. Choreic movements and ataxia of the limbs with spastic weakness appear in later stages.

Suprasellar tumors may show precocious pseudopuberty, diabetes insipidus with or without anterior pituitary dysfunctions, hypothyroidism, growth hormone deficiency, and hypogonadism. Decreased visual acuity, visual field defect, diplopia, obesity, psychosis, and obsessive-compulsive symptoms have also been reported.

These tumors require a neurologic and endocrine workup.

## 17.5 Diagnostic Work up

A complete physical examination is warranted. The testes should be examined thoroughly followed by an ultrasound examination. If there is any suggestion of testicular abnormalities on scrotal ultrasound, a primary testicular tumor must be considered. All testicular abnormalities revealed by testicular ultrasound must be treated adequately with orchiectomy because they may show primary malignancy and can act as a sanctuary site. Especially in retroperitoneal EGCTs there is a high frequency of minor pathological ultrasound findings. When these testes are removed up to 76% may show viable cancer or scar tissue (Scholz et al. 2002b).

Tumor markers AFP and β-HCG are elevated in many EGCTs. AFP elevations are seen in yolk-sac tumors and embryonal carcinoma but never in pure seminomatous tumors. Choriocarcinoma, embryonal carcinoma, and a minority of seminomas (<10%) produce β-HCG. Lactate dehydrogenase (LDH) is a non-specific marker but its level correlates well with tumor burden. Levels of tumor markers should be known before treatment starts, and during and after treatment they must be checked at regular intervals. These tumor markers provide diagnostic, staging, and prognostic information. There are some exceptional cases of intracranial GCTs that show elevations of tumor markers AFP and β-HCG in the serum or cerebrospinal fluid.

The extent of the disease is best established by CT scan. Because of the metastatic properties of GCTs, CT scanning of pelvis, abdomen, chest, and supraclavicular region is indicated.

Intracranial EGCTs are best visualized by CT or MRI. In primary staging of GCTs, fluorodeoxyglucose positron emission tomography (FDG-PET) has no benefit over CT. In restaging, a negative FDG-PET result predicts fibrotic residual mass in seminomatous GCT. Moreover, it could be useful to predict fibrotic residual mass in NSGCT in those patients with no teratoma component in their primary tumor (Spermon et al. 2002).

Before starting treatment, pathology of the tumor should be obtained. A choice has to be made between a fine needle aspiration (FNA) or a biopsy. A FNA study is certainly of diagnostic value (Chao et al. 1997; Ustün et al. 2002). Each subtype of EGCT has its own morphological characteristics. Seminomatous tumors with large and noncohesive cells, showing one to several distinct nucleoli are often well recognizable. Nonseminomatous aspirates, however, can be pluriform and especially in mixed GCT two or more subtypes of tumor cells can be observed in the FNA, which makes diagnosis more difficult. Immunochemistry can help to confirm the cytologic impression (Chao et al. 1997). Often a biopsy is required to establish the diagnosis. Depending on size, localization, extent, and spread of tumor, a core biopsy, incisional biopsy, or excisional biopsy can be chosen. The diagnosis of an intracranial germinoma is also possible with a FNA; the features on neuroimaging are similar to other tumors. Modern neurosurgical navigation techniques have made tissue sampling by stereotactic biopsy a safe and rapid method of determining tumor histology.

Pathology determines the histologic subtype. The histologic features do not differ from their gonadal counterparts.

## 17.6 "Burned-Out" Testicular Primary Tumor

By definition, in EGCTs a testicular primary tumor must be excluded. In all cases of EGCTs, a testicular primary has to be ruled out by all means. Especially in retroperitoneal EGCTs, this is important because the retroperitoneum is the primary metastatic landing zone for testicular GCTs.

Nowadays, the use of high resolution ultrasonography has shown a considerable proportion of presumed retroperitoneal EGCT to be of testicular origin (Saltzman et al. 1986). It has even been stated that primary EGCTs in the retroperitoneum are a rare or nonexisting entity and should be considered as metastases of a viable or burned-out testicular cancer. In a retrospective study of 26 patients treated as having primary EGCTs, all histologically examined testes had pathological findings. In 76%, either viable tumor or scar tissue was found (Scholz et al. 2002a). Two other groups found the same pathological evidence of a burned-out testicular carcinoma, each in 5 patients with presumed EGCTs (Comiter et al. 1996; Fabre et al. 2004).

Patients with EGCTs, particularly those with retroperitoneal or nonseminomatous tumors, and also those with primary mediastinal EGCTs are at an increased risk of metachronous testicular cancer. The cumulative risk of developing a metachronous testicular cancer 10 years after a diagnosis of EGCT was 10.3% in 635 patients (Hartmann et al. 2001b).

In a series of 68 patients with EGCTs, systematic bilateral biopsies of the testis showed testicular carcinoma in situ (CIS) in 21 patients (31%) (Fosså et al. 2003). Predominantly, this was found in those with a retroperitoneal tumor and also in 3 out of 15 mediastinal EGCTs. Patients in this study also had a considerable risk of metachronous testicular cancer development (7%) despite chemotherapeutic treatment.

The mechanism of spontaneous histopathologic regression of cancer remains unclear. It has been described in other forms of cancer like melanoma, renal cell cancer, and breast carcinoma. It is thought that cell mediated immune responses are responsible for this phenomenon. Testicular tumor regression could also be associated with immune mediated surveillance but this has not been investigated yet. An EGCT and especially a retroperitoneal EGCT should always be considered to be a possible metastasis of a "burned-out" testicular primary. In case of any suspicious testicular abnormality the testis must be removed.

## 17.7 Treatment

Treatment decisions in EGCTs are based on localization, histology type, extent of disease, and risk stratification. The International Germ Cell Consensus Classification also takes into account extragonadal tumors (International Germ Cell Cancer Collaborative Group 1997).

### 17.7.1 Mediastial Germ Cell Tumors

In a multicenter study with pooled data from 11 centers, a disease-free survival (DFS) of 88% in patients with extragonadal mediastinal seminoma at 5 years was achieved with cisplatin-based chemotherapy (Bokemeyer et al. 2001 1). No survival difference was found between patients with primary retroperitoneal or mediastinal seminoma. Primary radiotherapy was associated with a significantly higher rate of disease recurrence. Currently four cycles of bleomycine, etoposide, and cisplatin (BEP) is standard of care for mediastinal seminoma. In the case of bulky disease, radiotherapy can be considered afterward.

For nonseminomatous mediastinal GCTs, chemotherapeutic treatment with four cycles of BEP is the first choice. If tumor markers do not normalize, second line or salvage chemotherapy is warranted. In the case of residual lesions after chemotherapy, surgical resection should be prompted. When pathology of residual lesions shows vital tumor, adjuvant chemotherapy should be considered. In 287 patients of 11 institutions with primary mediastinal nonseminomatous EGCTs, a 5-year DFS was 44% (Bokemeyer et al. 2002). A single institution study of Fizzazi et al. described 29 patients with mediastinal EGCTs of which 11 (39%) had metastasis (Fizzazi et al. 1998). A complete response (CR) was obtained in 19 of 29 patients (66%) after chemotherapy and surgery. Only ten patients (34.5%) remained free of disease after a median follow-up of 89 months. In a German multicenter trial, first line high dose VIP in mediastinal EGCTs yielded a 2-year DFS of 64% (Bokemeyer et al. 2003). This result seems promising but is at the cost of higher treatment related morbidity. In postchemotherapy surgery for mediastinal nonseminomatous EGCTs, up to 57% of resected specimens show vital tumor (Kang et al. 2008). Of 143 patients in the study of Bokemeyer et al. that underwent surgery for residual tumor 35% had vital tumor at pathology (Bokemeyer et al. 2001).

In a multivariate analysis of 158 patients at Indiana University who underwent surgery after chemotherapy for primary mediastinal EGCTs, it was shown that persistent germ cell or non-germ cell cancer, and elevated serum tumor markers after operation were independently predictive of survival (Kesler et al. 2008). In patients with operable residual lesions after chemotherapy, 5-year DFS of 60% was achieved (Kang et al. 2008). Patients pathologically demonstrating persistent germ cell or non-germ cell cancer have poor but possible long-term survival; surgery therefore should be considered if residual lesions are operable. If disease relapses after or progresses on first-line chemotherapy and surgery, prognosis is very poor. In salvage therapy with high dose chemotherapy, with or without autologous bone marrow transplant, a long-term disease free survival of only 11–14% was achieved for primary mediastinal nonseminomatous EGCTs (Hartmann et al. 2001a; De Giorgi et al. 2005). In children with malignant mediastinal GCTs, treatment is not different from that in adults. A survival rate of about 70% can be achieved with chemotherapy and aggressive surgical approach of the residual tumor (Billmire et al. 2001). Older age (>12 years) gives a higher risk of mortality from tumor progression.

### 17.7.2 Retroperitoneal Germ Cell Tumors

For retroperitoneal EGCTs also, primary chemotherapy with four cycles of BEP is recommended for both seminomas and nonseminomas. An analysis of 52 retroperitoneal seminomatous EGCTs shows a 5-year DFS of 77% (Spermon et al. 2002). This is somewhat lower than for mediastinal primaries although not significantly. Seminomatous tumors are also very sensitive to radiotherapy. Radiotherapy has been proposed as primary treatment for small volume seminomatous retroperitoneal EGCTs (Nichols and Fox 1991). Treatment for these tumors with radiotherapy alone however has been shown inferior to chemotherapy (Bokemeyer et al. 2001).

Overall 5-year survival for non-seminomatous retroperitoneal EGCTs is better than for their mediastinal counterparts (62 vs. 45%). DFS however is comparable (45 vs. 44%) (Bokemeyer et al. 2002). In a Greek study, 9 of 11 patients with nonseminomatous retroperitoneal EGCTs were alive without disease at 5 years (Pectasides et al. 1999). Residual lesions after chemotherapy for non seminomatous retroperitoneal tumors should be removed. In 101 resected residual tumor masses, vital tumor was found in 25% of cases and mature teratoma in 16% (Bokemeyer et al. 2002).

### 17.7.3 Sacrococcygeal Germ Cell Tumors

Sacrococcygeal GCTs are a relatively uncommon tumor affecting neonates, infants, and children. Sacrococcygeal teratoma is the most common solid tumor in neonates. Malignant sacrococcygeal GCTs also occur in infants and children. Prompt diagnosis is essential because the frequency of malignant transformation increases from 10 to 20% in neonates to 67% in patients over 2 months of age. Diagnostic imaging studies help confirm the diagnosis of a clinically palpable sacrococcygeal mass, determine its relationship to other structures, and detect metastases. In a retrospective study of 79 sacrococcygeal GCTs, 62 (78%) were benign, whereas 17 (22%) contained malignant yolk sac tumor elements. The median age at examination in cases with malignant elements present was significantly greater than in those with benign sacrococcygeal teratoma only (Sebire et al. 2004). In children with sacrococcygeal teratomas, survival rate reaches 90% (Rescorla et al. 1998). Surgery is primary treatment in these patients and is performed by sacral or abdominosacral approach. Surgical resection alone is adequate therapy for those non-metastatic malignant tumors (Rescorla et al. 1998; Collins and Puch 1964). Benign teratomas have a significant recurrence rate mandating close follow-up for several years. Survival for malignant lesions with metastases is excellent with modern chemotherapy.

### 17.7.4 Intracranial Germ Cell Tumors

The management of patients with central nervous system GCTs is evolving. Radiotherapy alone results in long-term relapse free survival rates of about 90% in patients with germinoma. But although curative, radiation can cause significant neurological sequelae. Preirradiation chemotherapy reduces the total radiation exposure and may increase the cure rate. Various prospective trials evaluated the results of combinations of chemotherapy and reduced dose and/or volume of radiotherapy. Beside the delayed injury induced by radiotherapy, the late injury induced by chemotherapy is becoming increasingly evident. The challenge lies in curing these patients while avoiding late and permanent sequelae of radiation and/or chemotherapy. A combined chemoradiotherapy approach is associated with minimal endocrinopathy and minimal neurocognitive dysfunction.

Five-year survival rates are 96% for germinomas, 100% for mature teratomas, 67% for immature teratomas, and for β-HCG secreting germinomas the rate is only 38%. Patients with choriocarcinoma, embryonal carcinoma, or yolk sac tumor have the lowest survival (Brandes et al. 2000).

For intracranial germinoma, excellent treatment results with >90% survival are achieved with radiotherapy alone at the cost of doses at the primary site of about 50 Gy (Maity et al. 2004). A review of radiation therapies for intracranial germinoma since 1988 concluded that reduced-volume radiotherapy plus boost should replace craniospinal radiotherapy when a radiotherapy-only approach is used (Rogers et al. 2005).

In Japan, a consistent policy of surgical removal with histological verification followed by radiation therapy with or without chemotherapy yielded excellent 10-year survival rates of 93% for primary intracranial germinoma as well as teratoma. However, patients with pure malignant GCTs (embryonal carcinoma, yolk sac tumor, or choriocarcinoma) had a 3-year survival rate of only 27% (Matsutani et al. 1997). Treatment with etoposide and cisplatin for pure germinomas, and ifosfamide, cisplatin, and etoposide for other GCTs followed by low-dose involved-field radiotherapy gives a 93% 5-year overall survival for intracranial GCT (Aoyama et al. 2002). No change in intelligence quotient was found at 4 years with this treatment. The optimum therapy for intracranial nongerminomatous GCT remains controversial; different combinations of chemotherapy, radiotherapy, and surgery are proposed. Intensive cisplatin and cyclophosphamide-based combination chemotherapy as monotherapy were effective in one-third of nongerminomatous GCTs (Kellie et al. 2004). Salvage therapy, including irradiation, was feasible in patients with recurrent disease leading to a 5-year overall survival of 75%. Another option is neoadjuvant therapy consisting of combined chemo- and radiotherapy which are performed before complete excision of residual tumor (Kochi et al. 2003). Only two out of 11 had a CR on neoadjuvant therapy. However, after surgical resection of residual lesions in nine patients only one patient died after median follow-up of 8 years.

## 17.8 Surgery in Extragonadal Germ Cell Tumors

In nonseminomatous EGCTs, it is standard of care to remove residual masses after chemotherapeutic treatment. To date, there are still no well defined factors that can predict histology of residual lesions. Therefore, all radiologically visible residual lesions must be considered for removal. The surgical resection should include all gross disease with en bloc resection of all involved structures that can be sacrificed. Mediastinal GCTs are often best approached by midline sternotomy; sometimes a thoracotomy is chosen. Resection often includes pericardium and thymus because of their relation to the tumor. Sometimes aortic involvement necessitates an aortic prosthesis. A midline laparotomy is normally performed in case of residual retroperitoneal GCTs. They are treated like testicular primary tumors.

Pineal tumors are treated by an occipital transtentorial approach or supracerebellar infratentorial approach.

It is important to note that teratomas in fact can be effectively treated by surgery only. Therefore, surgery should be the primary treatment when teratoma is diagnosed.

## References


Aoyama H, Shirato H, Ikeda J, Fujieda K, Miyasaka K, Sawamura Y (2002) Induction chemotherapy followed by low-dose involved-field radiotherapy for intracranial germ cell tumors. J Clin Oncol 20(3):857–865

Billmire D, Vinocur C, Rescorla F, Colombani P, Cushing B, Hawkins E, London WB, Giller R, Lauer S (2001) Malignant mediastinal germ cell tumors: an intergroup study. J Pediatr Surg 36(1):18–24

Bokemeyer C, Droz JP, Horwich A, Gerl A, Fossa SD, Beyer J, Pont J, Schmoll HJ, Kanz L, Einhorn L, Nichols CR, Hartmann JT (2001) Extragonadal seminoma: an international multicenter analysis of prognostic factors and long term treatment outcome. Cancer 91(7):1394–1401

Bokemeyer C, Nichols CR, Droz JP, Schmoll HJ, Horwich A, Gerl A, Fossa SD, Beyer J, Pont J, Kanz L, Einhorn L, Hartmann JT (2002) Extragonadal germ cell tumors of the mediastinum and retroperitoneum: results from an international analysis. J Clin Oncol 20(7):1864–1873

Bokemeyer C, Schleucher N, Metzner B, Thomas M, Rick O, Schmoll HJ, Kollmannsberger C, Boehlke I, Kanz L, Hartmann JT (2003) First-line sequential high-dose VIP chemotherapy with autologous transplantation for patients with primary mediastinal nonseminomatous germ cell tumours: a prospective trial. Br J Cancer 89(1):29–35

Brandes AA, Pasetto LM, Monfardini S (2000) The treatment of cranial germ cell tumours. Cancer Treat Rev 26(4):233–242

Chao TY, Nieh S, Huang SH, Lee WH (1997) Cytology of fine needle aspirates of primary extragonadal germ cell tumors. Acta Cytol 41(2):497–503

Collins DH, Puch RC (1964) Classification and frequency of testicular tumours. Br J Urol 36(suppl):1–11

Comiter CV, Renshaw AA, Benson CB, Loughlin KR (1996) Burned-out primary testicular cancer: sonographic and pathological characteristics. J Urol 156(1):85–88

De Giorgi U, Demirer T, Wandt H, Taverna C, Siegert W, Bornhauser M, Kozak T, Papiani G, Ballardini M, Rosti G; Solid Tumor Working Party of the European Group for Blood and Marrow Transplantation (2005) Second-line high-dose chemotherapy in patients with mediastinal and retroperitoneal primary non-seminomatous germ cell tumors: the EBMT experience. Ann Oncol 16(1):146–151

Downie PA, Vogelzang NJ, Moldwin RL, Le Beau MM, Anastasi J, Allen RJ, Myers SE, Larson RA, Smith SD (1994) Establishment of a leukemia cell line with i(12p) from a patient with a mediastinal germ cell tumor and acute lymphoblastic leukemia. Cancer Res 54(18):4999–5004

Dueland S, Stenwig AE, Heilo A et al (1998) Treatment and outcome of patients with extragonadal germ cell tumours–the Norwegian Radium Hospital's experience 1979–94. Br J Cancer 77(2):329–335

Fabre E, Jira H, Izard V, Ferlicot S, Hammoudi Y, Theodore C, Di Palma M, Benoit G, Droupy S (2004) "Burned-out" primary testicular cancer. BJU Int 94(1):74–78

Fizzazi K, Culine S, Droz JP, Kramar A, Théodore C, Ruffié P, Le Chevalier T (1998) Primary mediastinal nonseminomatous germ cell tumors: results of modern therapy including cisplatin-based chemotherapy. J Clin Oncol 16(2): 725–732

Fosså SD, Aass N, Heilo A, Daugaard G, E Skakkebaek N, Stenwig AE, Nesland JM, Looijenga LH, Oosterhuis JW (2003) Testicular carcinoma in situ in patients with extragonadal germ-cell tumours: the clinical role of pretreatment biopsy. Ann Oncol 14(9):1412–1418

Goss PE, Schwertfeger L, Blackstein ME et al (1994) Extragonadal germ cell tumors – a 14-year Toronto experience. Cancer 73:1971–1979

Hartmann JT, Nichols CR, Droz JP, Horwich A, Gerl A, Fossa SD, Beyer J, Pont J, Fizazi K, Einhorn L, Kanz L, Bokemeyer C (2000) Hematologic disorders associated with primary mediastinal nonseminomatous germ cell tumors. J Natl Cancer Inst 92(1):54–61

Hartmann JT, Fossa SD, Nichols CR, Droz JP, Horwich A, Gerl A, Beyer J, Pont J, Fizazi K, Hecker H, Kanz L, Einhorn L, Bokemeyer C (2001a) Incidence of metachronous testicular cancer in patients with extragonadal germ cell tumors. J Natl Cancer Inst 93(22):1733–1738

Hartmann JT, Einhorn L, Nichols CR, Droz JP, Horwich A, Gerl A, Fossa SD, Beyer J, Pont J, Schmoll HJ, Kanz L, Bokemeyer C (2001b) Second-line chemotherapy in patients with relapsed extragonadal nonseminomatous germ cell tumors: results of an international multicenter analysis. J Clin Oncol 19(6): 1641–1648

Hasle H, Mellemgaard A, Nielsen J et al (1995) Cancer incidence in men with Klinefelter syndrome. Br J Cancer 71(2): 416–420

International Germ Cell Cancer Collaborative Group (1997) International Germ Cell Consensus Classification: a prognostic factor-based staging system for metastatic germ cell cancers. J Clin Oncol 15(2):594–603

Kang CH, Kim YT, Jheon SH, Sung SW, Kim JH (2008) Surgical treatment of malignant mediastinal nonseminomatous germ cell tumor. Ann Thorac Surg 85(2):379–384

Keene D, Johnston D, Strother D, Fryer C, Carret AS, Crooks B, Eisenstat D, Moghrabi A, Wilson B, Brossard J, Mpofu C, Odame I, Zelcer S, Silva M, Samson Y, Hand J, Bouffet E; Canadian Pediatric Brain Tumor Consortium (2007) Epidemiological survey of central nervous system germ cell tumors in Canadian children. J Neurooncol 82(3):289–295

Kellie SJ, Boyce H, Dunkel IJ, Diez B, Rosenblum M, Brualdi L, Finlay JL (2004) Primary chemotherapy for intracranial nongerminomatous germ cell tumors: results of the second international CNS germ cell study group protocol. J Clin Oncol 22(5):846–853

Kesler KA, Rieger KM, Hammoud ZT, Kruter LE, Perkins SM, Turrentine MW, Schneider BP, Einhorn LH, Brown JW (2008) A 25-year single institution experience with surgery for primary mediastinal nonseminomatous germ cell tumors. Ann Thorac Surg 85(2):371–378

Kochi M, Itoyama Y, Shiraishi S, Kitamura I, Marubayashi T, Ushio Y (2003) Successful treatment of intracranial nongerminomatous malignant germ cell tumors by administering neoadjuvant chemotherapy and radiotherapy before excision of residual tumors. J Neurosurg 99(1):106–114

Ladanyi M, Samaniego F, Reuter VE, Motzer RJ, Jhanwar SC, Bosl GJ, Chaganti RS (1990) Cytogenetic and immunohistochemical evidence for the germ cell origin of a subset of acute leukemias associated with mediastinal germ cell tumors. J Natl Cancer Inst 82(3):221–227

Maity A, Shu HK, Janss A, Belasco JB, Rorke L, Phillips PC, Sutton LN, Goldwein JW (2004) Craniospinal radiation in the treatment of biopsy-proven intracranial germinomas: twenty-five years' experience in a single center. Int J Radiat Oncol Biol Phys 58(4):1165–1170

Matsutani M, Sano K, Takakura K, Fujimaki T, Nakamura O, Funata N, Seto T (1997) Primary intracranial germ cell tumors: a clinical analysis of 153 histologically verified cases. J Neurosurg 86(3):446–455

Nichols CR, Fox EP (1991) Extragonadal and pediatric germ cell tumors. Hematol Oncol Clin North Am 5(6):1189–1209

Oosterhuis JW, Looijenga LH (2005) Testicular germ-cell tumours in a broader perspective. Nat Rev Cancer 5(3): 210–222

Oosterhuis JW, Stoop H, Honecker F, Looijenga LH (2007) Why human extragonadal germ cell tumours occur in the midline of the body: old concepts, new perspectives. Int J Androl 30(4):256–263

Pectasides D, Aravantinos G, Visvikis A, Bakoyiannis C, Halikia A, Kalofonos C, Kosmidis P, Skarlos D, Fountzilas G (1999) Platinum-based chemotherapy of primary extragonadal germ cell tumours: the Hellenic Cooperative Oncology Group experience. Oncology 57(1):1–9

Rescorla FJ, Sawin RS, Coran AG, Dillon PW, Azizkhan RG (1998) Long-term outcome for infants and children with sacrococcygeal teratoma: a report from the Childrens Cancer Group. J Pediatr Surg 33(2):171–176

Rogers SJ, Mosleh-Shirazi MA, Saran FH (2005) Radiotherapy of localised intracranial germinoma: time to sever historical ties? Lancet Oncol 6(7):509–519

Saltzman B, Pitts WR, Vaughan ED Jr (1986) Extragonadal retroperitoneal germ cell tumors without apparent testicular involvement. A search for the source. Urology 27(6):504–507

Scholz M, Zehender M, Thalmann GN, Borner M, Thöni H, Studer UE (2002) Extragonadal retroperitoneal germ cell tumor: evidence of origin in the testis. Ann Oncol 13(1): 121–124

Sebire NJ, Fowler D, Ramsay AD (2004) Sacrococcygeal tumors in infancy and childhood; a retrospective histopathological review of 85 cases. Fetal Pediatr Pathol 23(5–6): 295–303

Spermon JR, De Geus-Oei LF, Kiemeney LA, Witjes JA, Oyen WJ (2002) The role of (18)fluoro-2-deoxyglucose positron emission tomography in initial staging and re-staging after chemotherapy for testicular germ cell tumours. BJU 89(6): 549–556

Szabo PE, Mann JR (1995) Biallelic expression of imprinted genes in the mouse germ line: implications for erasure, establishment, and mechanisms of genomic imprinting. Genes Dev 9(15):1857–1868

Ustün M, Heilo A, Fosså S, Aass N, Berner A (2002) Ultrasound-guided fine needle cytology of retroperitoneal masses in patients with malignant germ cell tumours: diagnosis and therapeutic impact. Eur Urol 42(3):221–228

# New Systemic Therapies for Refractory Tumors

# 18

Gedske Daugaard and Martin H. Fenner

## 18.1 Introduction

In 1987, Williams et al. published data on the combination of cisplatin, etoposide, and bleomycin (BEP) for the treatment of metastatic germ cell tumors (GCTs). No prospective trial in the last 20 years has shown any advantage for other chemotherapy regimens in good, intermediate, or poor prognostic group. There has been a general improvement of survival in the poor prognostic group over these years from around 40% to 60% and this can mainly be attributed to improvements in supportive care.

Despite the high cure rate for most patients with metastatic GCTs, 20–30% of patients treated with cisplatin-based chemotherapy will relapse and these patients have a less favorable prognosis. A criterion for a poor prognosis in this setting includes an absolute refractoriness to cisplatin, incomplete remission, visceral metastases, and mediastinal nonseminomas.

No standard second line treatment exists and data for the treatment of relapsed patients are mostly derived from small retrospective studies. Prospective studies are needed in order to define the most effective treatment and we have to look for new systemic treatment in poor risk and refractory GCTs. At present, two kinds of strategies are being pursued: high-dose chemotherapy (HD-CT) and the introduction of novel cancer drugs including paclitaxel, gemcitabine, oxaliplatin, irinotecan, and targeted therapies. Clinicians treating GCTs with salvage chemotherapy tend to choose conventional dose chemotherapy in patients with good prognostic features and HD-CT in patients with poor prognostic criteria. However, we have no data from randomized studies to support this strategy.

The development of standard second or third line therapy in germ cell cancer is difficult because of the small number of patients eligible for clinical trials; therefore, international collaboration is needed. An increased knowledge about the biology in platinum refractory patients could foster the development of biological therapies and lead to new therapeutic options and thereby increase the number of cured patients with GCTs.

## 18.2 Relapse Treatment

As previously mentioned, there is no standard treatment for relapsed GCTs. Often patients are offered cisplatin and ifosfamide-based therapy combined with a third drug, which can be etoposide, vinblastine, or paclitaxel (Table 18.1) at their first relapse. Ifosfamide in combination with vinblastine plus cisplatin in the VeIP regimen results in 25–35% long-term remissions. With a combination of cisplatin, ifosfamide, and paclitaxel (TIP), 36–63% of patients obtained durable remissions, depending on prognostic factors. Details concerning these regimens have recently been discussed by Sonpavde et al. (2007).

Patients with relapses after second-line cisplatin-based therapy are usually treated with HD-CT. Patients who relapse after HD-CT, or patients not eligible for HD-CT, are usually treated with paclitaxel, gemcitabine, and oxaliplatin as single agents or in combination (Table 18.2). With single agent gemcitabine, oxaliplatin, or paclitaxel objective tumor response has been observed in 11–19% of patients,

G. Daugaard (✉)
Department of Oncology 5073, Copenhagen University Hospital, Rigshospitalet, Blegdamsvej 9, Copenhagen, Denmark

M.P. Laguna et al. (eds.), *Cancer of the Testis*,
DOI: 10.1007/978-1-84800-370-5_18, 

**Table 18.1** Second line salvage treatment for recurrent germ cell tumors

| Regimen | No. of patients | Long-term remission (%) | Reference |
|---|---|---|---|
| VeIP/VIP | 319 | 23–35 | (Loehrer et al. 1998; McCaffrey et al. 1997; Pico et al. 2005) |
| VeIP/VIP followed by HD-CT | 271 | 42–68 | (Pico et al. 2005; Einhorn et al. 2006a) |
| TIP | 106 | 36–63 | (Kondagunta et al. 2005; Mardiak et al. 2005; Mead et al. 2005) |
| TIP followed by HD-CT | 62 | 25 | (Rick et al. 1998) |

*VeIP* vinblastine, ifosfamide, and cisplatin; *VIP* etoposide, ifosfamide, and cisplatin; *TIP* paclitaxel, ifosfamide, and cisplatin, *HD-CT* high-dose chemotherapy

**Table 18.2** Third or more lines of treatment for germ cell tumors

| Regimen | No of patients | RR/CR | Reference |
|---|---|---|---|
| Paclitaxel | 24 | 25%/– | (Bokemeyer et al. 1996) |
| Gemcitabine | 51 | 15%/– | (Einhorn et al. 1999; Bokemeyer et al. 1999a) |
| Gemcitabine, paclitaxel | 60 | –/15% | (Hinton et al. 2002; Einhorn et al. 2007a) |
| Oxaliplatin | 32 | 13%/– | (Kollmannsberger et al. 2002) |
| Oxaliplatin, gemcitabine | 81 | –/10% | (Kollmannsberger et al. 2004; Pectasides et al. 2004a; Di Giorgi et al. 2006) |
| Paclitaxel, oxaliplatin | 26 | –/0% | (Theodore et al. 2004) |
| Irinotecan, cisplatin | 18 | –/9% | (Miki et al. 2002) |
| Irinotecan, oxaliplatin | 18 | –/22% | (Pectasides et al. 2004b) |
| Paclitaxel, oxaliplatin, gemcitabine | 41 | 51%/5% | (Bokemeyer et al. 2008) |

*RR* response rate; *CR* complete remission

including patients who had previously received HD-CT (Bokemeyer et al. 1996, 1999a; Einhorn et al. 1999; Kollmannsberger et al. 2002). These promising single agent activities have stimulated the development of combination chemotherapy regimens including two or three of these drugs (Table 18.2). In 41 patients who were platinum refractory or had relapse after high-dose therapy, a response rate on all 3 drugs of 51% was observed (Bokemeyer et al. 2008). Five percent obtained a complete remission on chemotherapy alone and 15% of patients were still in complete remission (CR) after chemotherapy ± surgery with a median follow-up of 5 months. However, in most published series, the median survival is only between 4 and 8 months in patients with multiple relapses or refractoriness to cisplatin (Hinton et al. 2002; Kollmannsberger et al. 2002, 2004; Pectasides et al. 2004a; Di Giorgi et al. 2006). Irinotecan has not been effective as single agent in heavily pretreated patients, but in combination with platinum, the results are more encouraging (Pectasides et al. 2004a). Responses in the different treatment series are related to whether the patients, previously treated with HD-CT, are platinum refractory or have late relapses.

A combination of cisplatin, gemcitabine, and paclitaxel is currently under investigation (www.clinicaltrials.gov).

## 18.3 High-Dose Chemotherapy

Numerous small studies with HD-CT have shown promising results in poor prognosis metastatic disease and in relapses after cisplatin-based chemotherapy. In 1999, Bokemeyer et al. (1999b) published a comparison between first-line HD-CT with autologous blood stem-cell transplantation and standard-dose chemotherapy in male patients with advanced GCTs. It was a matched-pair analysis within a homogenous group of patients classified as having either Indiana advanced disease or a poor prognosis according to International Germ Cell Cancer Consensus Group (IGCCCG) criteria. They concluded that first-line HD-CT in patients with poor-prognosis GCT might result in a significant improvement of progression-free and overall survival (OS) as compared with standard chemotherapy. A recent prospective clinical trial comparing HD-CT to conventional BEP showed no benefit for HD-CT (Motzer et al. 2007) in previously untreated patients with intermediate or poor prognosis, but the trial was underpowered to detect a 20% difference in the primary endpoint of durable complete responses at 1 year. A randomized trial comparing four cycles of BEP with one cycle of VIP followed by three sequential intensified cycles of VIP with stem-cell support has recently been closed due to slow accrual. Results will probably be available in 2010.

Einhorn et al. (2007b) performed a retrospective review of treatment results in 184 patients treated with HD-CT as second line, third line, or later therapy. The majority of patients had two cycles of HD-CT. A prognostic scoring algorithm was developed, which included timing of HD-CT (second, third, or subsequent line), platinum refractory disease, and IGCCCG poor-prognosis group. A score of 3 was given for third-line chemotherapy, 2 for platinum refractoriness, and 2 for poor-prognosis risk group. For patients in the low risk group (0 points), intermediate risk group (2–3 points), and high-risk group (4–7 points), the 5 year survival was around 80, 60, and 40%, respectively.

A retrospective matched-pair analysis comparing HD-CT to standard dose chemotherapy as first-line salvage therapy indicated a 6–12% benefit in OS and a 9–11% benefit in event free survival (EFS) after 2 years for the patients treated with HD-CT (Beyer et al. 2002). The only randomized clinical trial comparing conventional dose salvage therapy with HD-CT, the IT94 trial by the European Group for Blood and Marrow Transplantation (EBMT), failed to show an advantage for HD-CT. There were no statistically significant differences in EFS or OS after 3 years in this study (Pico et al. 2005).

The third published randomized HD-CT trial compared single dose HD-CT to sequential HD-CT in relapsed or refractory GCT patients (Lorch et al. 2007). There were no survival differences between the two treatment arms, but sequential HD-CT was better tolerated and resulted in less treatment related deaths. Treatment results for patients relapsing after HD-CT are usually poor, with only few long-term survivors (Sonpavde et al. 2007). At the moment, we have no tools to pick-up the right patients for HD-CT, but the majority of investigators agree that HD-CT is an important treatment option for patients with relapses after second-line chemotherapy.

Further progress with conventional chemotherapy or HD-CT for patients with poor prognosis metastatic or relapsed disease is probably limited. A better understanding of the molecular biology of GCTs will be important and it might lead to new therapeutic options.

## 18.4 Molecular Biology of Germ Cell Tumors and Effect of Targeted Therapy

Seminomas and nonseminomatous germ cell tumors (NSGCTs) derive from pluripotent primordial germ cells and represent about 95% of all testicular tumors (Oosterhuis and Looijenga 2005). Their biology and clinical course differ from those of spermatocytic seminomas. The latter tumors are derived from more mature germ cells, frequently have genetic changes in chromosome 9 (Looijenga et al. 2006), and almost never metastasize (Bomeisl and MacLennan 2007).

Stem cell research currently attracts a lot of public attention, but the relevant work concerning GCTs is on the basis of studies on teratocarcinomas in the 1950s (Yu and Thomson 2008). These tumors are made up of undifferentiated embryonic carcinomas and differentiated teratomas that can contain all three germ layers. GCTs show an expression profile similar to that of pluripotent stem cells. The transcription factors NANOG and OCT4 are not only highly expressed in GCTs, but can also be used for generating pluripotent stem cells (iPS) from somatic cells (Kristensen et al. 2008). Similar to pluripotent stem cells, GCTs frequently show promoter hypomethylation (Smiraglia et al. 2002). Hopefully, ongoing studies in pluripotent stem cells will result in further insights into the molecular biology of GCT.

The research concerning cisplatin resistance, isochromosome 12, and the role of receptor tyrosine kinases as potential drug targets is also highly relevant when future treatment possibilities in GCT are discussed.

## 18.5 Cisplatin Resistance

Most GCTs are sensitive to cisplatin-based chemotherapy and the majority of patients with metastatic disease can be cured. The mechanisms of cisplatin sensitivity – and cisplatin resistance in a minority of patients – are still not completely understood. Impaired DNA repair mechanisms involving XPA and ERCC1 are probably involved in cisplatin sensitivity (Houldsworth et al. 2006). Promoter hypermethylation has been associated with cisplatin-resistant GCTs (Koul et al. 2004).

In GCT's, the p53 protein is rarely mutated as in other tumors (Riou et al. 1995; Schenkman et al. 1995). Induction of apoptosis has been independent of p53 status in several GCT cell lines (Burger et al. 1999). The p53 expression levels in cisplatin-resistant tumor are similar to those in cisplatin-sensitive tumors (Kersemaekers et al. 2002). The small RNAs miR-372 and miR-373 are expressed in many GCTs and induce a phenotype similar to p53 mutations (Voorhoeve et al. 2006). Impaired p53 signaling and these microRNAs were also implicated when the gene expression profiles of testicular cancer cell lines with and without cisplatin treatment were compared (Duale et al. 2007).

## 18.6 Isochromosome 12

A gain in the short arm of chromosome 12 can be found in about 50% of seminomas and 80% of NSGCTs. This is the most frequent genetic change observed in GCTs (Horwich et al. 2006). These tumors either have an isochromosome 12, or amplification in the region 12p11.2-p12.1 (Mostert et al. 1998). It is not known which gene(s) is (are) involved in the pathogenesis of GCTs in that region. K-RAS is frequently mutated in other tumors and is located at 12p12.1, but K-RAS mutations are rare events in GCTs. Olie et al. (1995) found three K-RAS mutations in 40 seminoma samples and one K-RAS mutation in 60 NSGCT samples. All mutations were detected in exon 12. Roelofs et al. (2000) found no K-RAS mutations in 55 samples (primary tumors and metastatic sites) from 44 patients with cisplatin-refractory GCTs. The high occurrence of an extra 12p in the pathogenesis of GCT remains poorly defined and the clinical relevance is still unclear.

Another potential candidate in tumorigenesis of GCT is CCND2, the gene encoding Cyclin D2, which is located at 12p13 near the frequently amplified region. Cyclin D2 is overexpressed in 70% of GCTs, but no amplifications were detected by Southern Blot (Schmidt et al. 2001). The embryonic transcription factor NANOG also maps to 12p13. NANOG expression was detected in 20/20 seminomas, 18/18 embryonal carcinomas, 0/19 teratomas, 0/6 yolk sac tumors, and 0/5 choriocarcinomas (Santagata et al. 2007). The frequency of amplifications or mutations of NANOG in GCTs is not known.

## 18.7 c-KIT

The receptor tyrosine kinase c-KIT is a key regulator of gonadal development and spermatogenesis (Manova et al. 1990). c-KIT expression can be detected in 80–100% of seminomas and 7–32% of NSGCTs (Izquierdo et al. 1995; Madani et al. 2003). Activating c-KIT mutations are characteristic for gastrointestinal stromal tumors, and the inhibition of c-KIT signaling is the basis for the clinical activity of imatinib and sunitinib in these tumors. These mutations are uncommon events in GCTs. McIntyre et al. detected activating exon 17 mutations in 4/31 seminomas and 0/17 NSGCTs (McIntyre et al. 2005). Looijenga et al. (2003) detected the D816V c-KIT mutation in exon 17 in 3/224 unilateral and 57/61 bilateral GCTs. Biermann et al. (2007) found exon 17 mutations (Y823D, D816V, D816H and N822K) in 10/155 unilateral and 14/22 bilateral GCTs. In contrast to the last two reports, Coffey et al. (2008) found that c-KIT mutations in bilateral GCTs were uncommon. By examining mutations in exon 11 or 17 in 220 GCT samples, c-KIT mutations were found in 9/175 unitaleral and 1/38 bilateral tumors. All mutations were in seminomas and all but one mutation were in exon 17. Amplifications of c-KIT were studied in addition to activating mutations. In a series of 190 GCT samples, 21% of seminomas and 9% of NSGCTs showed c-KIT amplification, and c-KIT expression levels were higher in seminomas compared to that in normal testis and NSGCTs (McIntyre et al. 2005).

Einhorn et al. (2006b) screened 18 cisplatin-refractory patients for c-KIT expression by immunohistochemistry. Six patients had c-KIT expression, but their mutation status was not reported. Patients were treated with imatinib 600 mg daily. No objective responses were obtained, but one patient had a relevant marker decline. One case of CR for more than 24 months has been published after imatinib treatment in a patient with c-KIT overexpression, but the mutation status is unknown (Pedersini et al. 2007).

## 18.8 Epidermal Growth Factor Receptor

The receptor tyrosine kinase epidermal growth factor receptor (EGFR) is a major anticancer drug target in colorectal cancer and other solid tumors. EGFR expression in 182 GCT samples was studied by Hechelhammer et al. (2003). No EGFR expression was detected in 44 seminomas and 32 yolk sac tumors, but 20/28 teratomas and 7 choriocarcinomas showed EGFR expression. EGFR expression was detected in 16/24 GCTs in another study, with strong expression in the HCG-positive tumor cells (Moroni et al. 2001). EGFR was also expressed in 65% of GCT samples in another study (Madani et al. 2003), including 11/15 tumor samples in patients with late relapse and 4/8 transformed teratomas. HER-2/neu, successfully targeted by trastuzumab in breast cancer, was overexpressed in 3/18 GCT samples and in 7/28 GCT samples with teratomatous components (Mandoky et al. 2003).

One study targeting the epidermal growth factor (EGF) pathway with gefitinib has stopped inclusion of patients, but treatment results have not yet been published.

## 18.9 Vascular Endothelial Growth Factor

Formation of new blood vessels is required for tumor growth and metastasis, and this angiogenesis is mediated by vascular endothelial growth factor (VEGF) and other growth factors. VEGF mRNA and protein are significantly overexpressed in GCTs and correlate with microvascular density within these tumors (Fukuda et al. 1999). The VEGF receptors VEGFR1 (also known as FLT-1) and VEGFR2 (also known as KDR) are barely expressed in normal testis, but are frequently overexpressed both in GCTs and in the endothelial cells of these tumors (Olivarez et al. 1994; Viglietto et al. 1996). The expression of VEGF or the VEGF receptors was different between organ confined tumors and metastatic disease in some studies (Fukuda et al. 1999; Olivarez et al. 1994), but no difference was seen in another report (Adam et al. 2003).

One trial with thalidomide has been undertaken in cisplatin-refractory patients or relapse after HD-CT (Rick et al. 2006). Fifteen patients were included, but no objective responses were recorded. A decrease in tumor marker was observed in a few patients. Some effect of bevacizumab has been observed in two cases (Mego et al. 2007; Voigt et al. 2006).

Overall, about 90 patients with GCTs have been treated with targeted therapy (Table 18.3) (Fenner et al. 2008). Some cases of disease stabilizations have been observed together with tumor marker decline in some patients. However, only in two patients objective responses have been observed. So far, only one phase II trial with one of the newer targeting agents has been published. Studies with sunitinib as well as bevacizumab are ongoing and one study with gefitinib has finished inclusion, but is yet to be published (www.clinicaltrials.gov).

## 18.10 Single Drugs Without Activity

Patients who relapse after HD-CT or second line therapy, can only be offered palliative chemotherapy and few patients will obtain long-term remissions. New chemotherapeutic agents and targeted treatment are therefore tested in this patient population. As single drug, irinotecan, vinorelbine, mitoxantrone, mitomycin C, bendamustin, epirubicin, topotecan, and capecitabine have shown no activity (Kollmannsberger et al. 2006; Oechsle et al. 2007).

## 18.11 Prognostic Factor Analysis

The following factors are of prognostic value for patients having their first relapse after standard treatment: relapse-free interval, CR on previous treatment,

**Table 18.3** Case reports and phase 2 trials with targeted therapy in germ cell tumors

| Drug | No. of patients | Objective response | Time to progression | Reference |
|---|---|---|---|---|
| Isotretinoin | 15 | 0 | ND | (Gold et al. 1984) |
| Suramin | 14 | 0 | ND | (Motzer et al. 1993) |
| Retinoin | 16 | 0 | <3 months | (Moasser et al. 1995) |
| Trastuzumab | 1 | Decrease in AFP | 10 weeks | (Kollmannsberger et al. 1999) |
| Imatinib | 6 | 0 | 8 weeks | (Einhorn et al. 2006b) |
| Thalidomide | 15 | 0<br>Decrease in markers in 5 | 3 months | (Rick et al. 2006) |
| Arsenic trioxide | 20 | 0 | 1 months | (Beer et al. 2006) |
| Bevacizumab | 1 | SD | 6 months | (Mego et al. 2007) |
| Bevacizumab + HD-CT | 1 | PR | 5 months | (Voigt et al. 2006) |
| Imatinib | 1 | CR | Not reached | (Pedersini et al. 2007) |
| Imatinib | Recruiting completed | | | www.clinicaltrials.gov |
| Gefitinib | Recruiting completed | | | www.clinicaltrials.gov |
| Sunitinib, 2 studies | Recruiting | | | www.clinicaltrials.gov |
| Bevacizumab+oxaliplatin | Recruiting | | | www.clinicaltrials.gov |

From: Fenner et al. (2008)

and increased levels of tumor markers (AFP and hCG). In one study, it has been shown that patients did not survive 3 years if the relapse-free interval was less than 2 years, CR was not obtained on previous treatment, or the patients had increased tumor markers (Fossa et al. 1999).

In 1996, Beyer et al. (1996) published a prognostic score model based on refractoriness to platinum (progression within 4 weeks after treatment with cisplatin), absolute refractoriness to platinum (no response to initial platinum therapy), mediastinal nonseminomatous germ cell tumor, and a serum hCG level ≥1,000 IU/L. The two latter groups were assigned 2 points, whereas the other factors were assigned 1 point. Patients with a score of 0 points and 3 points or higher had a 2 years survival of 51% and 5%, respectively. Most patients in the Beyer study (Beyer et al. 1996) were only treated with one cycle of HD-CT.

The different results between this prognostic model and the one developed by Einhorn might be related to the fact that most patients in the Einhorn study (Einhorn et al. 2007b) were treated as second line, while more patients were treated with third line therapy in the Beyer study (Beyer et al. 1996) and a higher percentage was cisplatin refractory. An international analysis of prognostic factors in more than 1,000 patients with relapses after cisplatin-based chemotherapy is currently underway and results are expected in 2010. This analysis will help to define prognostic subgroups for further clinical trials in this patient population.

## 18.12 Conclusion

With the use of cisplatin-based combination chemotherapy, advanced GCTs can be cured in 70–80% of the patients; however, patients refractory to cisplatin-based chemotherapy continue to have a poor prognosis. Different drugs have been tested in this patient population and the combination of gemcitabine, oxaliplatin, and paclitaxel is currently the most active treatment regimen with CRs in selected patients. Although HD-CT has improved the outcome in some GCT patients with an acceptable toxicity profile, the exact role of HD-CT is still not clearly defined. A significant number of patients still relapse after HD-CT and these patients are usually treated with palliative intent. Surgical resection of residual tumor is an integral part of salvage therapy, and this will be discussed in details in Chaps. 15 and 16. Resection of residual tumors in patients with progressive disease and resistance to chemotherapy can result in long-term survival in around 25% and should be performed if technically feasible. Even patients with increased marker will in some cases benefit from surgery. The following factors can influence the outcome of surgery: elevated hCG levels, resection of visceral metastases, incomplete resection, and cancer in the resected specimen (Rick et al. 2004; Murphy et al. 1993; Habuchi et al. 2003; Beck et al. 2005).

The molecular mechanisms of cisplatin resistance have been studied intensively, but are still not completely understood. An increased knowledge about these mechanisms and insight into the biology of GCTs can result in the design of new drugs or new therapeutic options. Clinical trials with targeted therapies are ongoing, but siginificant clinical activity has not yet been observed. Data that can increase our knowledge and understanding of prognostic factors in patients with relapse after cisplatin-based chemotherapy are presently collected through a collaborative international effort. This could be the first step in defining relevant treatment strategies for patients with relapsed GCTs in the future.

## References


Adam M, Schmidt D, Wardelmann E, Wernert N, Albers P (2003) Angiogenetic protooncogene ets-1 induced neovascularization is involved in the metastatic process of testicular germ cell tumors. Eur Urol 44(3):329–336

Beck SD, Foster RS, Bihrle R, Einhorn LH, Donohue JP (2005) Outcome analysis for patients with elevated serum tumor markers at postchemotherapy retroperitoneal lymph node dissection. J Clin Oncol 23:6149–6156

Beer TM,Tangem CM Nichols CR et al (2006) Southwest Oncology group phase II study of arsenic trioxidein patients with refractory germ cell malignancies. Cancer 106:2624–2629

Beyer J, Kramar A, Mandanas R et al (1996) High-dose chemotherapy as salvage treatment in germ cell tumors: a multivariate analysis of prognostic variables. J Clin Oncol 14:2638–2645

Beyer J, Stenning S, Gerl A, Fossa S, Siegert W (2002) High-dose versus conventional-dose chemotherapy as first-salvage treatment in patients with non-seminomatous germ-cell tumors: a matched-pair analysis. Ann Oncol 13:599–605

Biermann K, Göke F, Nettersheim D et al (2007) c-KIT is frequently mutated in bilateral germ cell tumours and down-regulated during progression from intratubular germ cell neoplasia to seminoma. J Pathol 213(3):311–318

Bokemeyer C, Beyer J, Metzner B et al (1996) Phase II study of paclitaxel in patients with relapsed or cisplatin-refractory testicular cancer. Ann Oncol 7:31–34

Bokemeyer C, Gerl A, Schoffski P et al (1999a) Gemcitabine in patients with relapsed or cisplatin-refractory testicular cancer. J Clin Oncol 17:512–516

Bokemeyer C, Kollmannsberger C, Meisner C et al (1999b) First-line high-dose chemotherapy compared with standard-dose PEB/VIP chemotherapy in patients with advanced germ cell tumors: a multivariate and matched-pair analysis. J Clin Oncol 17:3450–3456

Bokemeyer C, Oechsle K, Honecker F et al (2008) Combination chemotherapy with gemcitabine, oxaliplatin and paclitaxel in patients with cisplatin-refractory or multiply relapsed germ-cell tumors: a study of the German Testicular Study Group. Ann Oncol 19:448–453

Bomeisl PE, MacLennan GT (2007) Spermatocytic seminoma. J Urol 177(2):734

Burger H, Nooter K, Boersma AW et al (1999) Distinct p53-independent apoptotic cell death signalling pathways in testicular germ cell tumour cell lines. Int J Cancer 81(4): 620–628

Coffey J, Linger R, Pugh J et al (2008) Somatic KIT mutations occur predominantly in seminoma germ cell tumors and are not predictive of bilateral disease: report of 220 tumors and review of literature. Genes Chromosomes Cancer 47(1): 34–42

Di Giorgi U, Rosti G, Aieta M et al (2006) Phase II study of oxaliplatin and gemcitabine salvage chemotherapy in patients with cisplatin-refractory nonseminomatous germ cell tumor. Eur Urol 50:1032–1038

Duale N, Lindeman B, Komada M et al (2007) Molecular portrait of cisplatin induced response in human testis cancer cell lines based on gene expression profiles. Mol Cancer 6:53

Einhorn LH, Stender MJ, Williams SD (1999) Phase II trial of gemcitabine in refractory germ cell tumors. J Clin Oncol 17:509–511

Einhorn LH, Williams S, Abonour R (2006a) Salvage chemotherapy with high dose carboplatin and etoposide (HDCE) and peripheral blood stem cell transplant (PBSCT) in patients with germ cell tumors (GCT). J Clin Oncol 24: 4549a

Einhorn LH, Brames MJ, Heinrich MC et al (2006b) Phase II study of imatinib mesylate in chemotherapy refractory germ cell tumors expressing KIT. Am J Clin Oncol 29:12–13

Einhorn LH, Brames MJ, Juliar B, Williams SD (2007a) Phase II study of paclitaxel plus gemcitabine salvage chemotherapy for germ cell tumors after progression following high-dose chemotherapy with tandem transplant. J Clin Oncol 25: 513–516

Einhorn LH, Williams SD, Chamness A et al (2007b) High-dose chemotherapy and stem-cell rescue for metastatic germ-cell tumors. New Engl J Med 357:340–348

Fenner MH, Beutel G, Grünwald V (2008) Targeted therapies for patients with germ cell tumors. Expert Opin Investig Drugs 17:511–522

Fossa SD, Stenning SP, Gerl A et al (1999) Prognostic factors in patients progressing after cisplatin-based chemotherapy for malignant non-seminomatous germ cell tumours. Br J Cancer 80:1392–1399

Fukuda S, Shirahama T, Imazono Y et al (1999) Expression of vascular endothelial growth factor in patients with testicular germ cell tumors as an indicator of metastatic disease. Cancer 85(6):1323–1330

Gold EJ, Bosl GJ, Itri LM (1984) Phase II trial of 13-cis-retinoic acid in patients with advanced non-seminomatous germ cell tumors. Cancer Treat Rep 68:1287–1288

Habuchi T, Kamoto T, Hara I, Kawai K, Nakao M, Nonomura N et al (2003) Factors that influence the results of salvage surgery in patients with chemorefractory germ cell carcinomas with elevated tumor markers. Cancer 98:1635–1642

Hechelhammer L, Störkel S, Odermatt B, Heitz PU, Jochum W (2003) Epidermal growth factor receptor is a marker for syncytiotrophoblastic cells in testicular germ cell tumors. Virchows Arch 443(1):28–31

Hinton S, Catalano PJ, Einhorn L et al (2002) Phase II trial of paclitaxel and gemcitabine in refractory germ cell tumors. J Clin Oncol 20:1859–1863

Horwich A, Shipley J, Huddart R (2006) Testicular germ-cell cancer. Lancet 367(9512):754–765

Houldsworth J, Korkola JE, Bosl GJ, Chaganti RS (2006) Biology and genetics of adult male germ cell tumors. J Clin Oncol 24(35):5512–5518

Izquierdo MA, Van der Valk P, Van Ark-Otte J et al (1995) Differential expression of the c-kit proto-oncogene in germ cell tumours. J Pathol 177(3):253–258

Kersemaekers AM, Mayer F, Molier M et al (2002) Role of P53 and MDM2 in treatment response of human germ cell tumors. J Clin Oncol 20(6):1551–1561

Kollmannsberger C, Pressler H, Mayer F et al (1999) Cisplatin-refractory, HER2/ neu-expressing germ-cell cancer: induction of remission by the monoclonal antibody trastuzumab. Ann Oncol 10:1393–1394

Kollmannsberger C, Rick O, Derigs HG et al (2002) Activity of oxilaplatin in patients with relapsed or cisplatin-refractory germ cell cancer: a study of the German testicular Cancer Study Group. J Clin Oncol 20:2031–2037

Kollmannsberger C, Beyer J, Lietsch R et al (2004) Combination chemotherapy with gemcitabine plus oxaliplatin in patients with intensively pretreated or refractory germ cell cancer: a study of the German Testicular Cancer Study Group. J Clin Oncol 22:108–114

Kollmannsberger C, Nichols C, Bokemeyer C (2006) Recent advances in management of patients with platinum-refractory testicular germ cell tumors. Cancer 106:1217–1226

Kondagunta GV, Bacik J, Donadio A et al (2005) Combination of paclitaxel, ifosfamide, and cisplatin is an effective second-line therapy for patients with relapsed testicular germ cell tumors. J Clin Oncol 23:6549–6555

Koul S, McKiernan JM, Narayan G et al (2004) Role of promoter hypermethylation in Cisplatin treatment response of male germ cell tumors. Mol Cancer 3:16

Kristensen DM, Sonne SB, Ottesen AM et al (2008) Origin of pluripotent germ cell tumours: the role of microenvironment during embryonic development. Mol Cell Endocrinol 288: 111–118

Loehrer PJ, Gonin R, Nichols CR et al (1998) Vinblastine plus ifosfamide plus cisplatin as initial salvage therapy in recurrent germ cell tumor. J Clin Oncol 16:2500–2504

Looijenga LH, de Leeuw H, van Oorschot M et al (2003) Stem cell factor receptor (c-KIT) codon 816 mutations predict development of bilateral testicular germ-cell tumors. Cancer Res 63(22):7674–7678

Looijenga LH, Hersmus R, Gillis AJ et al (2006) Genomic and expression profiling of human spermatocytic seminomas: primary spermatocyte as tumorigenic precursor and DMRT1 as candidate chromosome 9 gene. Cancer Res 66:290–302

Lorch A, Kollmannsberger C, Hartmann JT et al (2007) Single versus sequential high-dose chemotherapy in patients with relapsed or refractory germ cell tumors: a prospective randomized trial of the German Testicular Study Group. J Clin Oncol 25:2778–2784

Madani A, Kemmer K, Sweeney C et al (2003) Expression of KIT and epidermal growth factor receptor in chemotherapy refractory non-seminomatous germ-cell tumors. Ann Oncol 14(6):873–880

Mandoky L, Geczi L, Bodrogi I, Toth J, Bak M (2003) Expression of HER-2/neu in testicular tumors. Anticancer Res 23(4): 3447–3451

Manova K, Nocka K, Besmer P, Bachvarova RF (1990) Gonadal expression of c-kit encoded at the W locus of the mouse. Development 110(4):1057–1069

Mardiak J, Salek T, Sycova-Mila Z et al (2005) Paclitaxel plus ifosfamide and cisplatin in second-line treatment of germ cell tumors: a phase II study. Neoplasma 52:497–501

McCaffrey JA, Mazumdar M, Bajorin DF et al (1997) Ifosfamide- and cisplatin-containing chemotherapy as first-line salvage therapy in germ cell tumors: response and survival. J Clin Oncol 15:2559

McIntyre A, Summersgill B, Grygalewicz B et al (2005) Amplification and overexpression of the KIT gene is associated with progression in the seminoma subtype of testicular germ cell tumors of adolescents and adults. Cancer Res 65(18):8085–8089

Mead GM, Cullen MH, Huddart R et al (2005) A phase II trial of TIP (paclitaxel, ifosfamide and cisplatin) given as second-line (post-BEP) salvage chemotherapy for patients with metastatic germ cell cancer: a medical research council trial. Br J Cancer 93:178–184

Mego M, Reckova M, Sycova-Mila Z et al (2007) Bevacizumab in a growing teratoma syndrome. Case report. Ann Oncol 18:962–963

Miki T, Mizutani Y, Nonomura N et al (2002) Irinotecan plus cisplatin has substantial antitumor effect as salvage chemotherapy against germ cell tumours. Cancer 95:1879–1885

Moasser MM, Motzer RJ, Khoo KS et al (1995) All-trans retinoic acid for treating germ-cell tumors. In vitro activity andresults of a phase II study. Cancer 76:680–686

Moroni M, Veronese S, Schiavo R et al (2001) Epidermal growth factor receptor expression and activation in nonseminomatous germ cell tumors. Clin Cancer Res 7(9):2770–2775

Mostert MC, Verkerk AJ, van de Pol M et al (1998) Identification of the critical region of 12p over-representation in testicular germ cell tumors of adolescents and adults. Oncogene 16(20):2617–2627

Motzer RJ, Dmitrovsky E, Miller WH et al (1993) Suramin for germ cell tumors. In vitro growth inhibition and results of a phase II trial. Cancer 72:3313–3317

Motzer RJ, Nichols CJ, Margolin KA, Bacik J, Richardson PG, Vogelzang NJ, Bajorin DF, Lara PN Jr, Einhorn L, Mazumdar M, Bosl GJ (2007) Phase III randomized trial of conventional-dose chemotherapy with or without high-dose chemotherapy and autologous hematopoietic stem-cell rescue as first-line treatment for patients with poor-prognosis metastatic germ cell tumors. J Clin Oncol 25(3):247–256

Murphy BR, Breeden ES, Donohue JP, Messemer J, Walsh W, Roth BJ et al (1993) Surgical salvage of chemorefractory germ cell tumors. J Clin Oncol 11:324–329

Oechsle K, Honecker F, Kollmannsberger C et al (2007) An open label, multicenter phase II trial of capecitabine in patients with cisplatin refractory or relapsed germ cell tumors. Anticancer Drugs 18:273–276

Olie RA, Looijenga LH, Boerrigter L et al (1995) N- and KRAS mutations in primary testicular germ cell tumors: incidence and possible biological implications. Genes Chromosomes Cancer 12(2):110–116

Olivarez D, Ulbright T, DeRiese W et al (1994) Neovascularization in clinical stage A testicular germ cell tumor: prediction of metastatic disease. Cancer Res 54(10):2800–2802

Oosterhuis JW, Looijenga LH (2005) Testicular germ-cell tumours in a broader perspective. Nat Rev Cancer 5(3): 210–222

Pectasides D, Pectasides M, Farmakis D et al (2004a) Gemcitabine and oxaliplatin (GEMOX) in patients with cisplatin-refractory germ cell tumors: a phase II study. Ann Oncol 15:493–497

Pectasides D, Pectasides M, Farmakis D et al (2004b) Oxaliplatin and irinotecan plus granulocyte stimulating factor as third-line treatment in relapsed or cisplatin-refractory germ-cell tumor patients: a phase II study. Eur Urol M46:216–222

Pedersini R, Vattemi E, Mazzoleni G, Graiff C (2007) Complete response after treatment with imatinib in pretreated disseminated testicular seminoma with overexpression of c_KIT. Lancet Oncol 8:1039–1040

Pico JL, Rosti G, Kramer A et al (2005) A randomized trial of high-dose chemotherapy in the salvage treatment of patients failing first-line platinum chemotherapy for advanced germ cell tumors. Ann Oncol 16:1152–1159

Rick O, Beyer J, Kingreen D et al (1998) High-dose chemotherapy in germ cell tumours: a large single centre experience. Eur J Cancer 34:1883–1888

Rick O, Bokemeyer C, Weinknecht S, Schirren J, Pottek T, Hartmann JT et al (2004) Residual tumor resection after high-dose chemotherapy in patients with relapsed or refractory germ cell cancer. J Clin Oncol 22:3713–3719

Rick O, Braun T, Siegert W, Beyer J (2006) Activity of thalidomide in patients with platinum-refractory germ-cell tumors. Eur J Cancer 42:1775–1779

Riou G, Barrois M, Prost S, Terrier MJ, Théodore C, Levine AJ (1995) The p53 and mdm-2 genes in human testicular germ-cell tumors. Mol Carcinog 12(3):124–131

Roelofs H, Mostert MC, Pompe K et al (2000) Restricted 12p amplification and RAS mutation in human germ cell tumors of the adult testis. Am J Pathol 157(4):1155–1166

Santagata S, Ligon KL, Hornick JL (2007) Embryonic stem cell transcription factor signatures in the diagnosis of primary and metastatic germ cell tumors. Am J Surg Pathol 31(6): 836–845

Schenkman NS, Sesterhenn IA, Washington L et al (1995) Increased p53 protein does not correlate to p53 gene mutations in microdissected human testicular germ cell tumors. J Urol 154(2 Pt 1):617–621

Schmidt BA, Rose A, Steinhoff C, Strohmeyer T, Hartmann M, Ackermann R (2001) Up-regulation of cyclin-dependent kinase 4/cyclin D2 expression but down-regulation of cyclin-dependent kinase 2/cyclin E in testicular germ cell tumors. Cancer Res 61(10):4214–4221

Smiraglia DJ, Szymanska J, Kraggerud SM, Lothe RA, Peltomäki P, Plass C (2002) Distinct epigenetic phenotypes in seminomatous and nonseminomatous testicular germ cell tumors. Oncogene 21:3909–3916

Sonpavde G, Hutson TE, Roth BJ (2007) Management of recurrent testicular germ cell tumors. Oncologist 12:51–61

Theodore C, Flechon A, Fizazi K et al (2004) A phase II multicentre study of oxaliplatin (Ox) in combination with Paclitaxel (Px) in patients who failed cisplatin (CDDP) based chemotherapy for germ cell tumors. Proc Am Soc Clin Oncol 23:389

Viglietto G, Romano A, Maglione D et al (1996) Neovascularization in human germ cell tumors correlates with a marked increase in the expression of the vascular endothelial growth factor but not the placenta-derived growth factor. Oncogene 13(3):577–587

Voigt W, Kegel T, Maher G et al (2006) Bevazicumab plus high-dose ifosfamide, etoposide and carboplatin (HD-ICE) as third line salvage chemotherapy induced an unexpected dramatic response in highly platinum refratory germ cell cancer. Ann Oncol 17:531–553

Voorhoeve PM, le Sage C, Schrier M et al (2006) A genetic screen implicates miRNA-372 and miRNA-373 as oncogenes in testicular germ cell tumors. Cell 124(6):1169–1181

Williams SD, Birch R, Einhorn L et al (1987) Treatment of disseminated germ-cell tumors with cisplatin, bleomycin and either vinblastine or etoposide. N Engl J Med 316:1435–1440

Yu J, Thomson JA (2008) Pluripotent stem cell lines. Genes Dev 22:1987–1997

# 19 Management of Late Relapse

Paul D. Maroni, Friedemann U. Honecker, and Richard S. Foster

## 19.1 Introduction

Late relapse of testis cancer is defined as recurrence of disease 2 years or more after initial successful complete remission. The management of late relapse does not follow standard models developed for early recurrences, and should be so recognized by any physician managing these patients. While systemic disease at initial presentation sometimes involves chemotherapy, late relapse (LR) patients do not respond similarly to medical therapy making management more surgically based. With an incidence of approximately 4–5% (range one to ten percent), cases of LR have been observed occurring up to 35 years after successful treatment for germ cell tumor (GCT) (Borge et al. 1988; Baniel et al. 1995a; Gerl et al. 1997; Shahidi et al. 2002; Chung and Warde 2006; Oldenburg et al. 2006). Seminomatous GCT and nonseminomatous GCT (NSGCT) follow different natural histories and recurrence patterns with regard to LR. While the treatment of LR in chemotherapy naïve seminoma patients is straight forward, the management of LR for NSGCT and chemotherapy-exposed seminoma patients is more complicated.

## 19.2 Seminoma

### *19.2.1 Pattern of LR*

LR in traditionally-treated patients with pure seminoma at orchiectomy occurs with a 1% risk at 10-years (Oldenburg et al. 2006). Initial stage and treatment modality may affect the rate or pattern of recurrence (Shahidi et al. 2002). While late relapse in seminoma has been described more than 20 years after initial presentation, in general a patient destined to relapse with seminoma will do so within 36 months with the bulk of the remainder relapsing before 60 months (Shahidi et al. 2002; Oldenburg et al. 2006; Dieckmann et al. 2005). Dieckmann et al.'s evaluation of 50 seminoma LR patients with 72% recurring before 5 years contrasts with 48% of nonseminoma recurring in less than 5 years. In the Dieckmann cohort 80% were clinical stage (CS) I at initial staging (Dieckmann et al. 2005). Careful observation of Kaplan-Meier curves in seminoma patients show virtually complete flattening of curves beyond 3 years for stages 2 and higher (Shahidi et al. 2002). The exception demonstrating smoldering LR rates are CS I patients on surveillance protocols and CS II patients between 2 and 5 years (Shahidi et al. 2002; Chung and Warde 2006; Classen et al. 2003). With the frequently indolent behavior of seminoma, LR in surveillance patients has low, but significant rates. While late relapse in surveillance has not been specifically analyzed, data from surveillance studies demonstrates LR rates of up to 10% by 10 years with examples of late relapse beyond this period of time (Warde et al. 2002). This contrasts dramatically with 1% LR rates at 10 years in retrospective studies in traditionally treated patients, i.e., retroperitoneal radiotherapy (Oldenburg et al. 2006; Classen et al. 2004). While adjuvant abdominal radiation has been the recommended treatment for stage I seminoma patients for decades, numerous prospective studies suggest surveillance protocols offer equivalent survival rates with reduced potential for late side effects of therapy (Chung and Warde 2006). As surveillance becomes more commonly practiced, LR in patients with CS I seminoma will undoubtedly become more common and follow-up

P.D. Maroni (✉)
Department of Urology, Indiana University School of Medicine, Indianapolis, IN, USA

M.P. Laguna et al. (eds.), *Cancer of the Testis*,
DOI: 10.1007/978-1-84800-370-5_19, © Springer-Verlag London Limited 2010

will need to be more rigorous. Alternatively, single-dose carboplatin can be substituted for radiotherapy with equivalent efficacy in CS I patients (Oliver et al. 2005). These patients are at similar risk of LR to patients receiving radiotherapy (1–2%). Numerous factors help predict recurrence in patients on observation including the presence of rete testis invasion, primary tumor size greater than 4 cm, and lymphovascular invasion (Chung and Warde 2006).

In patients with stage II disease, LR after multi-agent chemotherapy or retroperitoneal radiotherapy appears to be rare in analysis of prospective trials (Classen et al. 2003). A retrospective study by Shahidi et al. with extended follow-up showed an LR rate of about 6% by 10 years in stage II patients (Royal Marsden staging system) treated with mixed modalities (Shahidi et al. 2002). They suggested that stage II patients receiving single-agent carboplatin might have a slightly higher risk of late relapse. A nonrandomized German trial investigating the role of carboplatin in stage IIA/B seminoma has revealed higher rates of early relapse; observation for incidence of late relapses is ongoing (Krege et al. 2006). LR in CS II patients treated with radiotherapy alone occurs at low rates (Classen et al. 2003; Chung et al. 2004). Remarkably, recurrence in patients with metastatic seminoma treated with multiagent chemotherapy virtually always occurs within 2 years with rare relapse after this period (Shahidi et al. 2002). In the two largest series examining LR in seminoma patients, 1 out of 10 and 2 out of 40 had UICC stage III disease at presentation (Oldenburg et al. 2006; Dieckmann et al. 2005). The denominator is unknown in these cohort studies, but considering about 10% of seminoma patients will present with stage III/IV disease, LR seems to be underrepresented and not directly related to initial stage. Shahidi et al. had no LR in 38 patients with stage III–IV followed for at least 5 years, and 23 patients with 10 years of follow-up (2002).

Serum tumor markers (TM) certainly play a role in detecting LR in patients initially presenting with seminoma with bHCG elevated in about a third and AFP elevated in about 10% of patients (Dieckmann et al. 2005). Other causes of TM elevation should be ruled out. If AFP is genuinely elevated or bHCG is exceptionally high, pure seminoma in the relapse should be excluded. A full review of systems and physical examination should be performed focusing on neck/supraclavicular, abdominal, or neurologic pathology. Practitioners should proceed with detailed imaging of the chest, abdomen, and pelvis. Intracranial or skeletal imaging should be performed if prompted by signs or symptoms, but LR in these areas is extremely uncommon. Historically, roughly half the patients will be detected on follow-up with the other half presenting with symptoms (Oldenburg et al. 2006; Dieckmann et al. 2005). A variety of symptoms have heralded relapse with the most common being back pain, abdominal pain, dyspnea, or fatigue. Treating physicians should have a low threshold for obtaining imaging in patients with symptoms relating to the abdomen, pelvis, or thorax as about 80–90% of patients will have relapse in these locations. Patients should also be aware of the symptoms of relapse and bring any new neck or abdominal masses to the physician's attention.

### 19.2.2 Management of LR

The management of LR in seminoma patients is uniquely different from NSGCT patients in that the tumors are commonly chemo-sensitive. In particular, relapses before 5 years in patients on surveillance protocols appear similar to patients with early relapse. As >90% patients were initially CS I or II, most have not received prior multiagent chemotherapy (Oldenburg et al. 2006; Dieckmann et al. 2005). While chemotherapy alone can be curative, a biopsy of the mass can help direct therapy. Relapse appears to always contain viable malignancy and initial chemotherapy without biopsy is tempting. However, several arguments exist for proceeding with surgical or percutaneous biopsy prior to chemotherapy in patients initially presenting with pure seminoma. While the series examining the pathology of late relapse in patients with seminoma have been small, 17–38% of patients have other histologies in addition to seminoma in their tumor specimen. Oldenburg et al. reported that in 40% of late relapses after seminoma, NSGCT or non-GCT were observed (Oldenburg et al. 2006). Furthermore, choriocarcinoma, embryonal carcinoma, yolk sac tumor, and lymphoma have all been described in LR patients with pure initial seminoma (Gerl et al. 1997; Oldenburg et al. 2006; Classen et al. 2004). A thorough review of the initial histology by a pathologist experienced in GCT is warranted as a missed mixed germ cell element can change management. Finding NSGCT would obviate radiotherapy as a salvage treatment alternative.

A questionable argument against radiotherapy for recurrent disease would be the potential for NSGCT elements in the recurrence that would not respond to salvage radiotherapy. While interesting in concept, no case reports in the literature describe this situation. If surgical resectability seems straight forward on radiographic imaging, e.g., a solitary, small mass not requiring removal of adjacent organs or major vascular reconstruction, surgical excision with or without local lymphadenectomy may be diagnostic and curative avoiding the side effects of chemotherapy. However, surgical resection can be technically challenging in LR patients with initial seminoma, especially if recurrences occur in areas that have been treated with radiotherapy at initial diagnosis. Alternatively, CT/PET scanning could help determine the nature of radiologic or serologic residual disease. Patients with PET positive lesions in multiple areas might be better treated with primary or salvage chemotherapeutic regimens prior to surgical therapy. As LR appears to be extremely rare in patients with CS I or II at initial diagnosis, the possibility of a (gonadal or extragonadal) metachronous tumor must be considered; therefore, careful examination of the contralateral testis by ultrasound is warranted (Shahidi et al. 2002; Bauman et al. 1998).

Provided pathologic analysis supports recurrent seminoma, a variety of options are available. Patients who have not received radiation therapy and have minimal retroperitoneal disease may be salvaged by surgery or radiotherapy. Bulky, systemic disease or relapse in patients previously receiving radiotherapy or single-agent carboplatin will usually require multiagent chemotherapy which will salvage the majority of patients. Prospective analyses of treatment protocols specifically for late relapse have not been performed, but late relapse in seminoma follows a relatively similar course to early relapse with favorable outcome in about 80% of patients (Dieckmann et al. 2005).

## 19.3 Nonseminomatous Germ Cell Tumors (NSGCT)

### *19.3.1 Pattern of LR*

Relapse patterns, pathology, and management in patients with NSGCT are much more complicated than in patients with seminoma. Early relapse and LR are distinct entities that require different approaches. Contrary to seminoma, LR in nonseminoma occurs more consistently over time, tends to have a higher stage at initial presentation, and responds irregularly to chemotherapy. Aggressive surgical management is the cornerstone of therapy due to the chemo-refractory nature. Overall, about 2–3% of patients with NSGCT will have LR up to 10 years (Baniel et al. 1995a; Oldenburg et al. 2006). Median time for recurrence is typically between 5 and 9 years (Borge et al. 1988; Baniel et al. 1995a; George et al. 2003). This is unfortunate, as many patients (and physicians) believe that cure has been achieved by this point and have become subject to surveillance fatigue. The retroperitoneum is the most common site of relapse with approximately 50–65% of cases, followed by the lungs (10–25%) and mediastinum (~10%) (Baniel et al. 1995a; Dieckmann et al. 2005; George et al. 2003). Disease may recur in other sites including, but not limited to, the neck and liver. Most patients will relapse in only one site, but 20–35% will relapse in two or more (George et al. 2003; Geldart et al. 2006). Oldenburg et al. mapped retroperitoneal LR in patients previously treated with RPLND (Oldenburg et al. 2006). Recurrences seem to occur in areas outside the normal RPLND template, e.g., pelvic or suprarenal. Care should be taken to examine these areas during RPLND with resection extended into any radiographically or palpably abnormal area.

Patients may present on routine follow-up with elevated markers. While both AFP and bHCG may be elevated, AFP is more likely to be the presenting tumor marker and typically heralds recurrent carcinoma. Marker elevation will be present in 30–76% of patients and will nearly always coexist with imaging abnormalities (Oldenburg et al. 2006; Dieckmann et al. 2005; George et al. 2003). Serum markers may increase without radiographic evidence of disease. In seven patients with marker-only LR, 6 had radiographic manifestations of disease at a median of 19 months after presentation (range 3–32) (George et al. 2003). While proceeding with chemotherapy in these patients is tempting, the last patient did not have radiographic progression at 79+ months, thus arguing for careful observation. Any marker elevation should prompt a thorough search for recurrent disease with body imaging. In a large cohort report by Dieckmann et al, an AFP <100 at LR inferred a positive response to therapy as 80% were cured, while only 25% of patients with AFP >100 had favorable outcomes (Dieckmann et al. 2005). LR may present symptomatically 24–60% of the time. In a series comprising more than 700 patients with NSGCT, 65% of late relapses were asymptomatic and detected by routine imaging or rising TM (Geldart et al. 2006). Common symptoms of LR are abdominal or back pain, neck mass, or chest pain. The presence of symptoms at LR indicates larger masses, but the impact on outcome is debated (Oldenburg et al. 2006; Dieckmann et al. 2005; George et al. 2003). Fortunately, more recent studies have lower proportions of patients presenting with symptoms assumedly due to increased awareness of LR.

Of the 30–35% observed CS I patients destined to relapse on surveillance, 90% do so within 2 years after initial orchiectomy (Read et al. 1992; Boyer et al. 1997; Sogani et al. 1998; Albers et al. 2003). Roughly 1–5% will have late recurrences regardless of initial treatment or surveillance. 66–92% of initial stage I NSGCT patients with LR will recur within 5 years following a similar pattern of recurrence to seminoma (Shahidi et al. 2002; Dieckmann et al. 2005). LR is slightly more common in patients on observation protocols (3–5%), but overall survival is not impaired (Read et al. 1992). Most LR for CS I will occur within 5 years of the initial diagnosis with rare exceptions after this period. As this is an extraordinarily small group of patients, ideal treatments have not been examined. Pathologic stage (PS) I patients with well performed RPLND should have LR rates less than 1% with disease recurrence more commonly in the thorax, but this may depend on the quality of the RPLND (Donohue et al. 1993). In patients referred to Indiana University for recurrence management, Baniel et al. examined 31 patients with LR after RPLND for initial CS I GCT. Nineteen patients had recurrence in the retroperitoneum, presumably indicating inadequate RPLND (Baniel et al. 1995b). This highlights the importance of removing all lymphatic tissue in designated templates. Examples of LR after two cycles of chemotherapy for CS I disease are not often reported in the literature.

Patients initially diagnosed with metastatic NSGCT follow a unique pattern with regard to LR. About 3% of stage II and 7% of stage III/IV patients will have LR up to 10 years (Shahidi et al. 2002; Ronnen et al. 2005). Forty to sixty percent of LR will occur more than 5 years after completing treatment, contrasting an earlier recurrence pattern with stage I NSGCT (Shahidi et al. 2002; Dieckmann et al. 2005). Kaplan-Meier curves do not flatten beyond 5 years in Stage III–IV NSGCT as with all seminoma LR and lower stage NSGCT. Patients with high stage NSGCT seem to be at continued risk of 2–4% per 5 years of follow-up. Recurrences may be seen over 30 years after successful therapy (Baniel et al. 1995a). The hypothesis of LR in areas of previously regressed disease is not supported by investigation as the area of recurrence at LR is frequently (60%) in an area not involved at initial presentation (Geldart et al. 2006).

### 19.3.2 Multiple Relapses

Occurence of multiple relapses is a well recognized phenomenon in patients with LR especially, but not exclusively in patients showing teratoma in tumor specimen at relapse. A series including 1,263 patients reported a total incidence of 3.5% multiple relapses; however, this indicates that 20% of all patients showing LR will have multiple relapses (Shahidi et al. 2002). In another, population-based series, total incidence of multiple relapses was lower with 0.35%; nonetheless, 36% of all patients with LR had more than one relapse (Oldenburg et al. 2006). Other analyses report rates of multiple relapses as high as 53–54% after first late relapse (Michael et al. 2000; Lipphardt and Albers 2004). At least one report indicates that the prognosis of patients with multiple relapses is worse, with approximately 70% of patients finally dying of the disease, compared to a death rate of approximately 40% in patients showing a single relapse (George et al. 2003). The biology underlying the phenomenon of multiple relapses remains to be resolved.

### 19.3.3 Pathology of LR

The stimuli for tumor growth that may occur quite suddenly after long cancer free periods are largely unknown. Metachronous disease in the contralateral testicle must always be ruled out. Malignant transformation of mature teratoma is one explanation for nongerm cell carcinomas, primitive neuroectodermal tumors (PNET), or sarcomas. Hypothetically, patients with a history of GCT may be at risk of developing extragonadal GCT (more resistant to chemotherapy similar to LR patients). The location of late relapse argues against this point. Most likely, a microscopic focus of GCT smolders subclinically until genetic events allow for malignant behavior.

In a study of 91 late relapse patients with pathology reviewed at Indiana University, teratoma was the most common element found in 60% of specimens with 22% containing teratoma-only (Michael et al. 2000). YST was the second most common malignant element observed with its presence in 43% of pathologic specimens. In LR, YST is often atypical showing glandular, parietal, clear cell or pleomorphic histology, and can occur together with non-GCT, making this entity challenging for pathologists. Non-GCT types made up a significant portion of this study with 23% containing non-GCT with or without GCT (mostly YST) or teratoma. Of the non-GCT types in LR, adenocarcinomas, PNET, and sarcomas are the most prevalent, whereas leukemias, which are associated with mediastinal NSGCTs usually occur earlier in the course of the disease, i.e., within a few months after initial diagnosis (Hartmann et al. 2001; Donadio et al. 2003). Population-based studies may offer a more representative picture of LR in general vs. the experience of Indiana University as a testis cancer referral center (Oldenburg et al. 2006; Geldart et al. 2006). Assuming comprehensive pathologic analysis, up to 57% of LR specimens will have teratoma only with YST - the second most common pathology observed at 20–30%. Lower proportions of non-GCT malignancies were observed in these studies as well. Necrosis is an uncommon finding at resection.

### 19.3.4 Molecular Aspects

Future directions for treatment of relapse in GCT may be based on biologic variables. Sugimura et al. examined 19 retroperitoneal specimens with either NSGCT (with yolk sac, embryonal carcinoma, and teratoma represented) or teratoma converting to PNET (Sugimura et al. 2004). An attempt was made to observe for differences in gene expression and chromosomal abnormalities between early and late relapse. As gene up- or downregulation seemed more strongly related to tumor histology, generalizations may be difficult except for yolk sac tumors demonstrating differential expression of numerous genes including upregulation of phospholipase A2 in early recurrence and less downregulation of *GSTT1* in late relapse. Chromosomal abnormalities were identified in almost all patients with notable gains in chromosome 12p, 6p (more in LR), and Y (more in ER). Examination of orchiectomy specimens in relation to ultimate relapse and outcome would be helpful for risk stratification. Unfortunately, obtaining initial tissue adequate for investigation is difficult as most patients have procurement at primary centers. George et al. evaluated FoxD3, Apel expression, and chromosome 12p in late relapse patients and correlated outcomes with genetic variables (George et al. 2003). While compelling, no firm conclusions could be made predicting survival due to these biologic differences. Isolated examination of molecular differences based on histology of recurrence may yield useful prognostic information.

### 19.3.5 Management of LR

Treatment of LR involves a multidisciplinary approach that considers the patient's initial pathology, number of locations/resectability of recurrent disease, treatment history, and serum TM. No randomized trials identify superior approaches to these patients and are unlikely to be done secondary to the rarity and heterogeneity of the condition. Numerous cohort studies have investigated responses to therapy in LR patients. In general, the patients fare worse overall than early recurrences and surgical resection plays a larger role in patients with NSGCT. Chemotherapy naïve status suggests an improved response to therapy. Tumor histology at initial presentation and recurrence will have an effect on outcomes. Surgical resection of residual disease is ultimately required in most cases suggesting first line use with resectable disease, in particular with solitary lesions.

### 19.3.6 Chemotherapy

As the cornerstone of initial management of disseminated GCT, chemotherapy was the initial treatment for recurrence in most early studies focusing on LR. Overall, response to chemotherapy alone by patients with LR has been less than satisfactory. In 1988, Borge reported 9 NSGCT patients with relapse >3 years after treatment and no patient fully responded to chemotherapy alone (Borge et al. 1988). Baniel et al. observed a 26% CR rate with patients managed primarily by chemotherapy with durable CR in only 2/65 (3%) cases (Baniel et al. 1995a). Most with CR subsequently relapsed with cancer and surgical resection salvaged 7 of 11 patients. This contrasts to CR with surgery alone in 11 of 16 patients showing surgery is more effective as a solitary therapy albeit in selected patients. Gerl et al. noted durable complete response in chemotherapy in 2/20 (10%) cases and both patients had surgery for residual necrosis (Gerl et al. 1997). In a follow-up to the Baniel study, durable CR to chemotherapy was somewhat improved (5/32 cases) although still low and four of these patients underwent resection of necrosis (George et al. 2003). As a smaller proportion of patients in this report received chemotherapy as first-line treatment for recurrent disease, patient selection is a likely factor. Chemotherapy for non-GCT has not been assessed in larger cohorts. In a small series of 12 patients with non-GCT limited to a single cell type, chemotherapy regimens based on the specific malignant cell was administered (Donadio et al. 2003). Whereas seven patients showed some response, only three patients achieved longer term survival. Most of the responding patients also received surgery. Therefore, a motif through all is that chemotherapy rarely spares patients surgical therapy.

In nonchemotherapy naïve patients, complete and prolonged responses to chemotherapy are rare and residual masses should be removed with surgery. Patients with late relapse of disease in multiple sites or in areas requiring resection of multiple organs or vascular reconstruction may benefit from chemotherapy prior to radical surgery in order to downsize the magnitude of the surgery. While not studied in a randomized fashion, MSKCC has used paclitaxel, ifosfamide, and cisplatin (TIP) with superior results to other salvage chemotherapy regimens in LR patients (Ronnen et al. 2005). In these patients, CR was achieved by TIP in 7 of 14 patients and seemed to work best if other salvage regimens have not been attempted. Three of the seven patients required surgery for CR. Half of the CR patients had residual masses removed. Treating physicians should regularly assess if tumors are demonstrating resistance to chemotherapy by radiographic growth and/or increasing serum TM. TM negative radiographic growth suggests the presence of teratoma or chemoresistant carcinoma/sarcoma. Steadily increasing TM on therapy should prompt change in approach, e.g., desperation surgery.

### 19.3.7 Surgery

As chemotherapy rarely obviates surgery, more consideration is given in its use as an initial therapeutic strategy in the management of LR in NSGCT. Chemotherapy may be part of treatment of LR, but with 60% or more tumors having teratoma and a substantial minority containing chemo-refractory yolk sac tumor, it rarely works in isolation. Any extirpative surgery in testicular cancer requires experience and careful planning. The difficulty of resecting residual masses can be frequently underestimated and surgeons should be prepared for tumors adherent to the great vessels or major branches and bowel. Removal of adjacent organs with or without vascular reconstruction is occasionally necessary. Incomplete resection will almost certainly ensure recurrence that will be more difficult to remove on reoperation. Complete resection of disease should be the primary goal. Baniel et al. reported 11 of 16 patients who became continuously disease free (DF) with surgery alone including three with carcinoma (Baniel et al. 1995a). George investigated a primary surgery cohort of LR patients and 22/49 remained continuously DF (George et al. 2003). As many as four of these patients may have had additional therapies to achieve DF status, but a solid proportion required surgery alone.

The conversion over time from a primary chemotherapy approach to using surgery earlier seems to have had improved outcomes. Cohorts from the 1980s and 1990s had DF rates of 40–60% (Borge et al. 1988; Baniel et al. 1995a; George et al. 2003). A more recent study by Geldart et al. reports an impressive 75% of patients with prolonged NED after treatment of LR in a nonchemotherapy naive group (Geldart et al. 2006). All CR had surgery as part of the LR treatment program with 80% achieving NED with surgery alone. Oldenburg similarly described a 73% cure rate in LR NSGCT patients and 53% avoiding chemotherapy (Oldenburg et al. 2006).

Despite these results, chemotherapy still plays a role in management of LR. Disease in more than one site is rarely (<20%) cured with surgery alone and may suggest chemotherapy to reduce tumor load prior to surgery (George et al. 2003). Chemotherapy naïve patients respond more readily (40% vs. 9%) suggesting a lower threshold for upfront use (George et al. 2003). Some have used positive TMs as an indication for primary chemotherapy in the LR setting (Oldenburg et al. 2006). We do not believe that elevated TMs necessitate primary chemotherapy in the face of radiographically resectable disease.

### 19.3.8 Outcome Based on Pathology and Distribution

All types of GCT have been encountered in pathologic specimens at LR. Fibrosis or necrosis is uncommonly found and denotes CR to chemotherapy. One of six patients with CR to chemotherapy in George et al.'s report had an additional recurrence so follow-up is not obviated (George et al. 2003). Finding teratoma in the LR specimen carries a good prognosis with survival rates of 60–100% on retrospective review (Baniel et al. 1995a; Oldenburg et al. 2006; George et al. 2003; Geldart et al. 2006). These patients may also have further LR and require life-long monitoring. Active GCT at LR carries an intermediate prognosis. Recurrences and death from disease are more common in this group with 40% prolonged NED after treatment (George et al. 2003). Reliable measures for outcomes of transformed teratomatous elements are more difficult to derive due to relatively few reported patients (Michael et al. 2000). Generally, adenocarcinoma and sarcoma may be cured surgically, but frequently recur. Furthermore, localized disease showed better outcome compared to patients with LR at multiple sites: while 55% of patients with relapse affecting only one site remained DF, this rate decreased to only 20% of patients with LR occurring at multiple sites (George et al. 2003).

### 19.3.9 Follow-Up

Risk stratification of GCT patients would assist in developing long-term follow-up protocols as early detection is intuitively felt to confer improved survival. Comprehensive follow-up protocols would be expensive and overly burdensome to the health care system as LR has a relatively low rate of occurrence. There appear to be several risk factors for LR in NSGCT patients. Shahidi et al. analyzed numerous variables in a single-institution series and found that patients with differentiated teratoma in a post chemotherapy resection specimen had an increased predilection for LR (HR 3.9, range 1.9–7.9) (Shahidi et al. 2002). The presence of positive TM on initial diagnosis may also be a risk factor, but clearly not as potent. Also from Shahidi et al.'s study, recurrence after 5 years in patients with initial low stage seminoma or nonseminoma was very rare. Observations from Gerl et al. suggest that patients with an early relapse may have a substantially higher risk of LR (29% at 10 years) (Gerl et al. 1997). Previous LR is another strong indicator of LR as 22 of 91 patients in Michael et al. experienced multiple LR (Michael et al. 2000). These data imply that long-term follow-up protocols might be best directed towards patients with the aforementioned risk factors. Careful patient counseling about the risk of LR and attendant symptoms should be performed. The utility of radiographic imaging in this group of patients has been incompletely defined beyond 5 years. As serum tumor marker elevation may precede radiographic disease, physical examination with biannual TMs from years 2 to 5 post treatment and annual TMs after 5 years would be a reasonable minimum recommendation.

Main points of late relapse in GCT

- LR is defined as recurrence of disease 2 years or more after initial successful treatment leading to tumor remission.
- The course of the disease differs between patients showing relapse from seminoma and nonseminoma, and treatment should be guided by histologic findings.
- Most relapses in patients with seminomas occur before 60 months after initial diagnosis and treatment. As most patients are chemotherapy naïve, polychemotherapy is the cornerstone of treatment and leads to high cure rates.
- LR in patients with NSGCT usually occurs later, can show great histologic variability, and is complex to manage. Chemotherapy resistance is frequently encountered, both in cases showing classical nonseminoma histology, and in the histologic variants "growing teratoma" and non-GCT. Treatment involves a multidisciplinary approach, with surgical resection almost always being the key to cure.
- The biology of LR is poorly understood, but likely involves mechanisms of tumor dormancy and reactivation, and possibly primary chemotherapy resistance of micrometastatic disease. Further research to uncover underlying mechanisms is warranted.

## 19.4 Appendix

See Fig. 19.1.

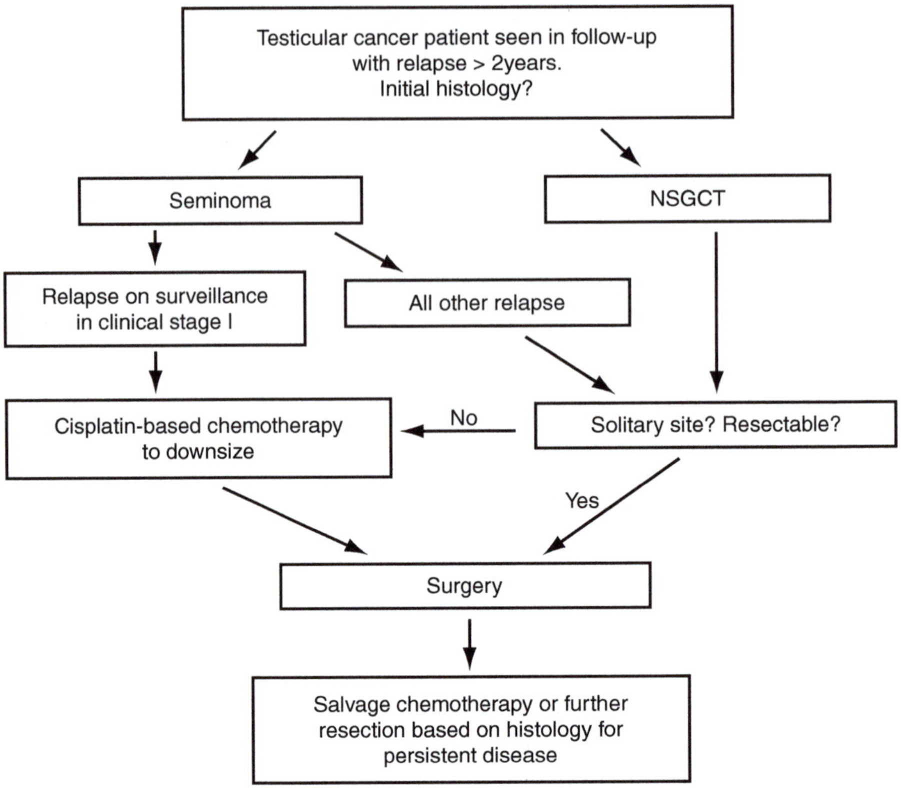


**Fig. 19.1** Treatment algorithm in late testicular cancer relapses

## References


Albers P, Siener R, Kliesch S et al (2003) Risk factors for relapse in clinical stage I nonseminomatous testicular germ cell tumors: results of the German Testicular Cancer Study Group trial. J Clin Oncol 21:1505

Baniel J, Foster RS, Gonin R et al (1995a) Late relapse of testicular cancer. J Clin Oncol 13:1170

Baniel J, Foster RS, Einhorn LH et al (1995b) Late relapse of clinical stage I testicular cancer. J Urol 154:1370

Bauman G, Venkatesan V, Ago C et al (1998) Postoperative radiotherapy for stage I/II seminoma: results for 212 patients. Int J Radiat Oncol Biol Phys 42:313–317

Borge N, Fossa SD, Ous S et al (1988) Late recurrence of testicular cancer. J Clin Oncol 6:1248

Boyer MJ, Cox K, Tattersall MHN et al (1997) Active surveillance after orchiectomy for nonseminomatous testicular germ cell tumors: late relapse may occur. Urology 50:588

Chung PWM, Warde PR (2006) Surveillance in stage I testicular seminoma. Urol Oncol 24:75

Chung PWM, Gospodarowicz MK, Panzarella T et al (2004) Stage II testicular seminoma: patterns of recurrence and outcome of treatment. Eur Urol 45:754

Classen J, Schmidberger H, Meisner C et al (2003) Radiotherapy for stages IIA/B testicular seminoma: final report of a prospective multicenter clinical trial. J Clin Oncol 21:1101

Classen J, Schmidberger H, Meisner C et al (2004) Para-aortic irradiation for stage I testicular seminoma: results of a prospective study in 675 patients. A trial of the German testicular cancer study group (CTCSG). Br J Cancer 90:2305

Dieckmann K-P, Albers P, Classen J et al (2005) Late relapse of testicular germ cell neoplasms: a descriptive analysis of 122 cases. J Urol 173:824

Donadio A, Motzer RJ, Bajorin DF et al (2003) Chemotherapy for teratoma with malignant transformation. J Clin Oncol 21:4285–4291

Donohue JP, Thornhill JA, Foster RS et al (1993) Primary retroperitoneal lymph node dissection in clinical stage A nonseminomatous germ cell testis cancer. Br J Urol 71:236

Geldart TR, Gale J, McKendrick J et al (2006) Late relapse of metastatic testicular nonseminomatous germ cell cancer: surgery is needed for cure. BJU Int 98:353

George DW, Foster RS, Hromas RA et al (2003) Update on late relapse of germ cell tumor: a clinical and molecular analysis. J Clin Oncol 21:113

Gerl A, Clemm C, Schmeller N et al (1997) Late relapse of germ cell tumors after cisplatin-based chemotherapy. Ann Oncol 8:41

Hartmann J, Fossa S, Nichols CR et al (2001) Incidence of metachronous testicular cancer in patients with extragonadal germ cell tumors. J Natl Cancer Inst 93:17

Krege S, Boergermann C, Baschek R et al (2006) Single agent carboplatin for CS IIA/B testicular seminoma. A phase II study of the German testicular cancer study group (GTCSG). Ann Oncol 17:276

Lipphardt M, Albers P (2004) Late relapse of testicular cancer. World J Urol 22:47–54

Michael H, Lucia J, Foster RS et al (2000) The pathology of late recurrence of testicular germ cell tumors. Am J Surg Pathol 24:257

Oldenburg J, Alfsen G, Waehre H et al (2006) Late recurrences of germ cell malignancies: a population-based experience over three decades. Br J Cancer 94:820

Oliver RTD, Mason MD, Mead GM et al (2005) Radiotherapy versus single-dose carboplatin in adjuvant treatment of stage I seminoma: a randomised trial. Lancet 366:293

Read G, Stenning SP, Cullen MH et al (1992) Medical Research Council prospective study of surveillance for stage I testicular teratoma. J Clin Oncol 10:1762

Ronnen EA, Kondagunta GV, Bacik J et al (2005) Incidence of late-relapse germ cell tumor and outcome to salvage chemotherapy. J Clin Oncol 23:6999

Shahidi M, Norman AR, Deamaley DP et al (2002) Late recurrence in 1263 men with testicular germ cell tumors. Cancer 95:520

Sogani P, Perrotti M, Herr HW et al (1998) Clinical stage I testis cancer: long-term outcome of patients on surveillance. J Urol 159:855

Sugimura J, Foster RS, Cummings OW et al (2004) Gene expression profiling of early- and late- relapse nonseminomatous germ cell tumor and primitive neuroectodermal tumor of the testis. Clin Cancer Res 10:2368

Warde PR, Specht L, Horwich A et al (2002) Prognostic factors for relapse in stage I seminoma managed by surveillance: a pooled analysis. J Clin Oncol 20:4448

# Part V

# Late Effects and Follow-Up

# 20 Testicular Cancer: Late Effects of Treatment

Sophie D. Fosså, Lois B. Travis, and Alv A. Dahl

## 20.1 Introduction

The introduction of cisplatin-based chemotherapy into the treatment of testicular cancer (TC) (Einhorn et al. 1989) has changed not only the treatment strategies and improved survival rates (Horwich et al. 2006; Sant et al. 2007), but also the pattern of long-term effects, defined as adverse health problems persisting or occurring one or more years after treatment. This chapter reviews the clinically most significant long-term health problems in testicular cancer survivors (TCSs) treated during the last 30 years. However, many TCSs treated from 1960 onwards are still alive and are at risk to develop clinically significant late effects. Therefore, we also discuss chronic toxicity after older treatment strategies.

## 20.2 General Considerations

It is important to separate treatment-induced chronic morbidity from conditions which are related to the malignancy itself. Posttreatment impaired gonadal function in a TCS may thus be independent from treatment representing a consequence of the prenatally developed "testicular dysgenesis syndrome" (TDS) (Bay et al. 2006). Similarly, the diagnosis of a new TC should be viewed as a consequence of a preexisting carcinogenetic process. Finally, the diagnosis of a second malignancy in a TCS should always lead to the consideration that the multipotent primary germ cell malignancy may have relapsed as an adenocarcinoma, a sarcoma, or even as a hematolgical malignancy (Lutke Holzik et al. 2003).

The understanding of radiotherapy (RT)-related late complications requires insight into radiobiological processes which take place during even many years after discontinuation of treatment (Stone et al. 2003). Irradiated malignant and benign cells either die because of irreversible DNA damages or they survive with or without persisting mutations. In case of cell kill of the malignant cells, the therapeutic aim of cure is achieved. On the other hand, irradiation at high doses may lead to irreversible stem cell death of the normal tissues and is followed during the next 10–30 years by gradually increasing fibrosis and shrinkage of the tissue, paralleled by intima thickening and gradual stenosis of irradiated small vessels. In case of incomplete DNA-repair, a surviving cell may have become more susceptible for subsequent environmental mutagenic influences, and the RT-induced nonlethal genetic changes may thus represent the initial step of cancer development (Allan and Travis 2005).

Many late effects in TCSs (second cancer, gastrointestinal ulcera and stenosis, cardiotoxicity, and cerebral atrophy) are diagnosed 1–3 decades after treatment discontinuation when TCSs no longer are followed-up at their responsible oncological unit. It is therefore difficult to establish true incidence rates of the possible complications although cancer-registries, public statistics on cause-specific death, and large surveys provide some epidemiological insight.

## 20.3 Second Cancer

*Solid tumors*: On the basis of data from national cancer registries, several authors have reported increased incidence and mortality rates due to second cancer in TCSs

S.D. Fosså (✉)
Department of Clinical Cancer Research, Cancer Clinic, Rikshospitalet – Radiumhospitalet Medical Center, Montebello, Oslo, Norway

M.P. Laguna et al. (eds.), *Cancer of the Testis*,
DOI: 10.1007/978-1-84800-370-5_20, © Springer-Verlag London Limited 2010

(van Leeuwen et al. 1993; Gietema et al. 2000; Fossa et al. 2004; Zagars et al. 2004). By international collaboration, Travis et al. (2005) recently quantified solid tumor risk among 40,576 1-year survivors of TC over four decades of follow-up. Second solid cancers developed in 2,285 patients (O/E = 1.41; 95% CI: 1.35–1.47). Similarly, for seminoma and nonseminoma a strong decrease with increasing age at TC diagnosis was observed for both the excess relative risk (ERR) and excess absolute risk (EAR) of solid tumors.

Relative risks of solid cancer were significantly increased for TCSs initially treated with radiation only (RR = 2.0), chemotherapy only (RR = 1.8) ,or radiation and chemotherapy (RR = 2.9). The highest site-specific RRs were observed for cancers of stomach, pancreas, and connective tissue, followed by pleura and bladder (Table 20.1). Among TCSs initially managed with radiation only, RR for sites in standard infradiaphragmatic RT fields (RR = 2.7) clearly exceeded that for remaining sites (RR = 1.6). Cumulative risks for all solid cancers were 36 and 31% for men diagnosed with seminoma and nonseminoma at an age of 35 and after 40 years of follow-up, respectively, compared with 23% for the general population, and compared to 36 and 28% for patients diagnosed at age 35 and 50, respectively (Fig. 20.1).

*Leukemias*: The increased risk of leukemia in TCS has been well-established (Pedersen-Bjergaard et al. 1991; Nichols et al. 1993; Bokemeyer et al. 1995; Travis et al. 2000). On the basis of a review of clinical trials, Smith et al. (1999) showed that the 6-year cumulative risk of secondary leukemia among patients who received 1,500–2,999 mg/m$^2$ of etoposide was small (0.7%). Kollmannsberger et al. (1999), in a recent literature review, reported that the cumulative risk of leukemia for TC patients who received etoposide at cumulative doses of <2,000 and >2,000 mg/m$^2$ was 0.5 and 2%, respectively, at a median of 5 years of follow-up. In an international case–control study of secondary myelodysplastic syndrome or leukemia in 18,567 1-year TCSs, leukemia risk increased with increasing radiation dose to active bone marrow and for TCSs given chest irradiation in addition to abdominal/ pelvic fields irradiation (Travis et al. 2000). Radiation dose to active bone marrow and cumulative amount of cisplatin were predictive of increased risks of leukemia in a statistical model that took into account all treatment variables. It is not known whether combined modality therapy for TC confers a higher risk of leukemia than chemotherapy alone.

*Contralateral TC (CTC)*: In relatively small studies, estimates of the cumulative risk of metachronous CTC 20–25 years after initial diagnosis of TC have ranged from 2.4 to 5.2% (review in Fossa et al. 2005). Fossa et al. (2005) evaluated the risk of CTC among 29,515 U.S. TCSs (1973–2001), 287 of whom developed CTC (O/E = 12.4; 95% CI: 11.0–13.9). The 15-year cumulative risk of CTC was 1.9% (95% CI: 1.7–2.1%). Nonseminomatous histology of the first TC and increasing age were associated with a significantly decreased risk of CTC.

The treatment of extragonadal germ cell tumors (EGCT) is similar to strategies for TC, with the potential for the development of similar long-term sequelae. Survivors experience significant excesses of subsequent TC (Fossa et al. 2003a; Hartmann et al. 2001), likely because of the existence of carcinoma in situ in one or both testicles (Bay et al. 2006). In one large, international survey of 635 patients with EGCT (Hartmann et al, 2001), the cumulative risk of developing a metachronous TC was 10.3% at 10 years.

## 20.4 Nonmalignant Somatic Sequelae

### 20.4.1 Gonadal Toxicity and Fertility Issues

*General:* In agreement with the hypothesis of prenatally developing TDS, morphological alterations in the contralateral testicle are observed in up to 25% of the patients with a newly diagnosed unilateral TC (Hoei-Hansen et al. 2003), in part explaining why sperm cell counts are decreased in up to 50% of unilaterally orchiectomized TC patients before any further treatment (Fossa et al. 1984; Hansen et al. 1989; Carroll et al. 1987). Treatment intensity, the patient's age at diagnosis, and the pretreatment serum level of Follicle Stimulating Hormone are of importance for the speed and degree of posttreatment recovery (Lampe et al. 1997; Petersen et al. 1998; Palmieri et al. 1996; Jacobsen et al. 2001; Aass et al. 1991). Overall, about 70% of TCSs who attempt posttreatment fatherhood are successful (Brydoy et al. 2005) (Fig. 20.2).

*Radiotherapy:* Testicular radiation doses of up to 4 Gy are followed by transient azoospermia with recovery sometimes after several years. Higher doses usually

**Table 20.1** Estimated relative risk of second cancers according to time since testicular cancer (TC) diagnosis for patients diagnosed with TC at age 35 years (minimally modified from (Travis et al. 2005))

| | Time since testicular cancer diagnosis | | | | | | | | Excess number (%)[a] |
|---|---|---|---|---|---|---|---|---|---|
| | All ≥10 years intervals | | 10–19 years | | 20–29 years | | ≥30 years | | All ≥10 years intervals |
| | Obs. | RR (95% CI) | Obs. | RR (95% CI) | Obs. | RR (95% CI) | Obs. | RR (95% CI) | |
| **Cancer site** | | | | | | | | | |
| All solid tumors | 1,694 | 1.9 (1.8–2.1) | 802 | 2.1 (1.9–2.3) | 563 | 2.0 (1.8–2.2) | 329 | 1.7 (1.6–1.9)[b] | 698 (100)[c] |
| Esophagus | 26 | 1.7 (1.0–2.6) | 13 | 2.0 (<1–3.8) | 7 | 0.9 (<1–2.3) | 6 | 2.1 (<1–4.0) | 9 (1.3) |
| Stomach | 129 | 4.0 (3.2–4.8) | 64 | 4.9 (3.7–6.4) | 49 | 4.5 (3.3–5.9) | 16 | 1.9 (1.0–3.2)[d] | 88 (12.6) |
| Colon | 153 | 2.0 (1.7–2.5) | 62 | 1.8 (1.3–2.6) | 52 | 2.1 (1.5–2.8) | 39 | 2.2 (1.6–3.0) | 66 (9.5) |
| Rectum/anus | 101 | 1.8 (1.4–2.3) | 60 | 2.7 (1.9–3.8) | 22 | 1.3 (<1–1.9) | 19 | 1.7 (1.1–2.6) | 39 (5.5) |
| Pancreas | 95 | 3.6 (2.8–4.6) | 44 | 4.1 (2.8–5.9) | 38 | 4.3 (3.0–6.0) | 13 | 2.3 (1.3–3.7) | 63 (9.0) |
| Lung | 256 | 1.5 (1.2–1.7) | 148 | 2.2 (1.7–2.7) | 73 | 1.4 (1.1–1.8) | 35 | 1.0 (<1–1.4)[d] | 65 (9.3) |
| Pleura | 12 | 3.4 (1.7–5.9) | 7 | 6.0 (2.3–12) | 3 | 2.6 (0.5–6.6) | 2 | 1.9 (0.4–6.1) | 8(1.1) |
| Prostate | 249 | 1.4 (1.2–1.6) | 88 | 1.1 (<1–1.6) | 91 | 1.4 (1.1–1.8) | 70 | 1.5 (1.2–1.8) | 52 (7.4) |
| Kidney | 80 | 2.4 (1.8–3.0) | 29 | 1.7 (1.0–2.6) | 30 | 2.5 (1.7–3.6) | 21 | 3.0 (1.9–4.4)[e] | 43 (6.2) |
| Bladder | 211 | 2.7 (2.2–3.1) | 75 | 2.0 (1.4–2.7) | 85 | 3.2 (2.5–4.0) | 51 | 2.6 (2.0–3.5) | 115 (16.4) |
| Malignant melanoma | 70 | 1.8 (1.3–2.3) | 43 | 1.9 (1.3–2.6) | 23 | 2.1 (1.4–3.1) | 4 | 0.8 (0.3–1.7) | 30 (4.2) |
| Thyroid | 16 | 2.3 (1.0–4.4) | 15 | 4.2 (1.8–8.2) | 1 | 1.0 (<1–3.4) | 0 | – | 9 (1.2) |
| Other solid tumors[f] | 277 | 1.6 (1.4–1.9) | 145 | 1.5 (1.2–1.9) | 80 | 1.6 (1.3–2.0) | 52 | 1.9 (1.4–2.4) | 98 (14.1) |

*(continued)*

**Table 20.1** (continued)

| | Time since testicular cancer diagnosis | | | | | | | | Excess number (%)[a] |
|---|---|---|---|---|---|---|---|---|---|
| | All ≥10 years intervals | | 10–19 years | | 20–29 years | | ≥30 years | | All ≥10 years intervals |
| | Obs. | RR (95% CI) | Obs. | RR (95% CI) | Obs. | RR (95% CI) | Obs. | RR (95% CI) | |
| **Radiotherapy only** | | | | | | | | | |
| All solid tumors | 892 | 2.0 (1.9–2.2) | 399 | 2.2 (1.9–2.5) | 300 | 2.0 (1.8–2.3) | 193 | 1.8 (1.6–2.1)[g] | 387 (100)[c] |
| Sites in-field[h] | 445 | 2.7 (2.4–3.0) | 174 | 2.6 (2.1–3.2) | 165 | 2.9 (2.4–3.4) | 106 | 2.5 (2.0–3.0) | 246 (63.7) |
| Other sites | 447 | 1.6 (1.4–1.8) | 225 | 1.9 (1.6–2.3) | 135 | 1.5 (1.3–1.8) | 87 | 1.4 (1.1–1.7)[i] | 141 (36.3) |

The table is restricted to those sites for which significantly increased RR were observed in 10-year survivors of TC. The RR is a decreasing function of age at TC diagnosis; results are presented for age 35 years, which is the mean age of the cohort

*RR* relative risk; *CI* confidence interval; *Obs.* observed number of cases

[a]Percent contribution to the total excess is shown within the parentheses; percentages may not sum to 100 due to rounding

[b]*P* trend (negative) = 0.007

[c]Obtained as sum of site-specific excesses

[d]*P* trend (negative) <0.001

[e]*P* trend (positive) = 0.02

[f]Includes 172 tumors for which site was specified and 105 tumors of unknown or ill-defined primary site (refer to Appendix Table 1 for complete list of solid tumors for all time periods)

[g]P trend (negative) = 0.013

[h]Restricted to those sites which are included in typical infradiaphragmatic radiotherapy fields for TC: stomach, small intestine, colon, rectum, liver, gallbladder and ducts, pancreas, kidney, and bladder

[i]*P* trend (negative) = 0.005

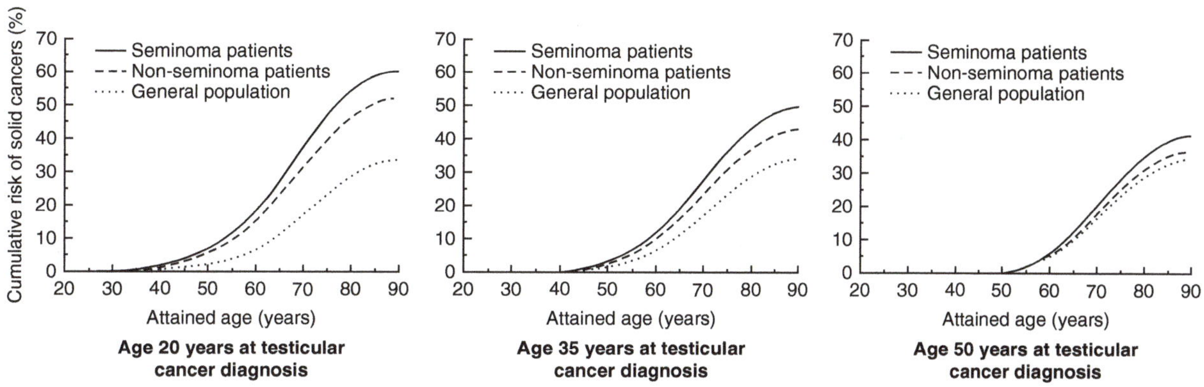


**Fig. 20.1** Cumulative risk (%) of developing a second solid cancer for men with seminomas and nonseminomatous germ cell tumors according to age at testicular cancer (TC) diagnosis and attained age. Risks beyond age 60 years for men diagnosed with TC at age 20 years, or beyond age 75 years for men diagnosed with TC at age 35 years represent extrapolation of estimated trends (with permission from JNCI (Travis et al. 2005))

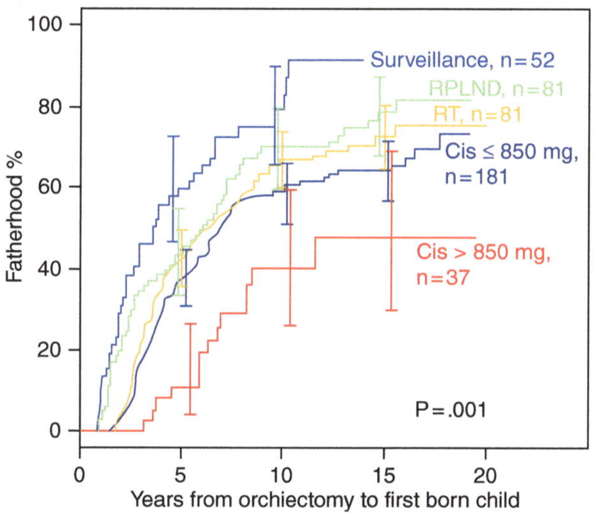


**Fig. 20.2** Actuarial posttreatment paternity rates in each treatment group for patients who attempted conception without the use of cryopreserved semen. $P<0.001$ from two-sided log-rand test. *RPLND* retroperitoneal lymph node dissection; *RT* radiotherapy; *cis* cisplatin. Vertical bars indicate 95% confidence intervals (with permission of JNCI (Brydoy et al. 2005))

lead to permanent depletion of sperm cell production although the exact cumulative testicular doses of 18–20 Gy of sterilizing radiation as applied to patients with carcinoma in situ are followed by the Sertoli cell only syndrome and the risk of insufficient Leydig cell function (Petersen et al. 2002, 2003). With a target dose of 30 Gy to a so-called dog-leg field, the shielded remaining testicle receives a mean dose averaging 50 cGy (Jacobsen et al. 1997). This results in transient postradiation azoospermia in almost all patients, lasting for 6–10 months with gradual recovery during the second year. If the infradiaphragmatic target field is restricted to the para-aortic region, the testicular doses are limited to 20–30 cGy even without any testicular shielding.

*Cytostatics:* The high proliferation rate during spermatogenesis is paralleled by a high sensitivity to cytostatics. Alkylating agents, in particular cyclophosphamide, reduce spermatogenesis in dependency from the cumulative dose. Cisplatin monotherapy and the standard combinations used in the treatment of TC (BEP [bleomycin, etoposide, cisplatin] or VIP [vinblastine, ifosphamide, cisplatin]) have only a modest effect on long-term spermatogenesis, posttreatment paternity can almost be expected in 60–80% of TCSs if pretreatment spermatogenesis is within the normal range (Lampe et al. 1997; Petersen et al. 1998; Reiter et al. 1998; Taksey et al. 2003).

*Surgery:* The fertility in TCSs is threatened not only by reduced spermatogenesis but also by postsurgery "dry ejaculation," resulting from the resection of retroperitoneal sympaticomimetic nerve fibers. Though the introduction of nerve-sparing techniques (Donohue et al. 1990; Jacobsen et al. 1999) and of the surveillance strategy in nonmetastatic patients (Chung and Warde 2006; Segal 2006) have considerably reduced this complication, TCSs with primarily advanced disease or those with recurrent disease still have to face this late adverse effect.

*Clinical consequences:* Semen analysis and the determination of FSH, LH (lutenizing hormone), and testosterone in the serum are the standard tools for monitoring of the gonadal function. Though modern cytotoxic treatment of TC enables recovery of transiently impaired spermatogenesis in the majority of patients, semen cryopreservation, preferably done before orchiectomy (Petersen et al. 1999), should be considered in all patients who do not exclude future paternity. In TC patients, unable to produce an ejaculate, testicular sperm extraction or cryopreservation of testicular tissue should be considered (Rosenlund et al. 1998; Damani et al. 2002). Attempts to reduce the effect of cytotoxic treatment on spermatogenesis by hormones have not been successful, although new trials are encouraged (Meistrich and Shetty 2003). Assisted reproduction techniques (ARTs) with "fresh" or deep-frozen semen are important for TCSs unsuccessful in their attempts to father a child. However, the number of men using their deep-frozen semen is low, given the high rate of "natural" posttreatment fatherhood (Magelssen et al. 2005).

Finally, the risk of clinical or subclinical endocrine hypogonadism should not be overlooked in long-term TCSs (Nord et al. 2003; Huddart et al. 2005). Both RT at doses above 14 Gy and high-dose chemotherapy may permanently reduce Leydig cell function, mirrored by high serum LH and low testosterone. Approximately 16% of TCSs display clinical or subclinical hypogonadism and approximately 5% of all TCSs need androgen substitution after unilateral orchiectomy (Nord et al. 2003).

## 20.4.2 Cardiovascular Long-Term Sequelae

*Radiotherapy:* Even as late as in 1970s, mediastinal RT represented a therapeutic modality in selected TC patients with supra-diaphragmatic lymph node metastases, increasing the risk of long-term cardiac morbidity and mortality by direct injury to the myocardium and/or the coronary arteries (Zagars et al. 2004; Hanks et al. 1992; Van den Belt-Dusebout et al. 2006). Whether infradiaphragmatic high-voltage RT increases the risk of severe cardiac events is still unclear. While the Dutch group did not find increased morbidity risks (Van den Belt-Dusebout et al. 2006) after such RT, Zagars et al. (2004) demonstrated slightly increased mortality rates >20 years after infradiaphragmatic RT at doses of >30 Gy. Also Huddart et al (2003) reported an increased risk of adverse cardiovascular adverse events after infradiaphragmatic RT alone. By such RT, only the most distal parts of the heart are within the target field if at all, but the whole organ receives a mean cardiac dose of 0.7 Gy by leaking and scattered irradiation (Travis et al. 2005). Further, by RT to the paraaortic region, the renal arteries and the medial parts of the kidney are included in the radiation field, with the possibility of premature hypertension due to subclinically reduced renal function (Fosså et al. 2003).

*Chemotherapy:* Anthracyclines at cumulative doses of >500 $mg/m^2$ have a detrimental effect on the myocardium (Floyd et al. 2005; Keefe 2001). During 1970s and early 1980s, Adriamycin was frequently used in the combination chemotherapy of TC patients and was combined with mediastinal RT in metastatic TC patients. Recent publications have described an increased incidence of cardiovascular long-term risk factors (hypercholesterolemia, hypertension, overweight, and metabolic syndrome) and morbidity after cisplatin-based chemotherapy (Sagstuen et al. 2005; Haugnes et al. 2006; Nuver et al. 2005a). It is too early to decide whether the CVB (cisplatin, vinblastine, bleomycin) regimen is more cardiotoxic than today's BEP (Van den Belt-Dusebout et al. 2006). The development of these cardiovascular risk factors is probably related to cisplatin. Cisplatin (Nuver et al. 2005b) and recently also adriamycin (Chow et al. 2006) have been shown to result in endothelial dysfunction during the treatment phase.

## 20.4.3 Neurological Complications

Long-term sequelae in TCSs may affect the motoric, sensoric, and autonomous nerve system.

*Radiotherapy:* Progressive radiation myelopathy is a severe late sequelae in less than 1% of the patients who are irradiated by target doses of ≥50 Gy (Fossa et al. 1989), eventually also at lower doses if applied in combination with chemotherapy. Though the brain usually is regarded to be relatively radio-resistant, experience in survivors after brain tumors and malignant lymphoma indicates a non-neglectable risk (white matter necrosis, hydrocephalus) in TCSs who survive after high-dose cerebral RT, in particular if combined with chemotherapy. (Gavrilovic et al, 2006).

*Chemotherapy:* The late peripheral neurological sequelae after modern chemotherapy are usually less severe but are reported by 20–25% of long-term survivors (Mykletun et al. 2005a; Oldenburg et al. 2006; Fossa et al. 2003b).

Patients receiving cumulative doses of >850 mg cisplatin display sensoric neuropathy more often than those with lower cumulative doses.

Ototoxicity represents a special type of cisplatin-based neurotoxicity. In dependency from both the cumulative dose and serum concentration during treatment, the drug damages the outer hair cells of the inner ear (van Ruijven et al. 2004), clinically expressed as hearing loss and, in particular, tinnitus (Fossa et al. 2003b) in approximately 20% of the patients. The reduction of hearing predominantly usually occurs above the 4,000 Hz threshold, thereby less affecting daily speech. Individual genetic susceptibility explains in part the considerable inter-patient variability: the germline 105Val/105Val polymorphism of GSTP1 protects against cisplatin-induced ototoxicicity, whereas the GST-M1+ polymorphism is associated with increased risk (Oldenburg et al. 2007).

*Surgery:* "Dry ejaculation" is the consequence after retroperitoneal lymph node dissection (RPLND) combined with excessive resection of the sympathicamimetic nerve fibers (Donohue et al. 1990; Jacobsen et al. 1999; Oldenburg et al. 2007). The risk of this complication is reduced by unilateral RPLND or in particular by nerve-sparing RPLND. Disturbed temperature perception and sweating ability are other disturbing consequences of radical RPLND (Oldenburg et al. 2007).

### 20.4.4 Other Long-Term Sequelae

After infradiafragmatic RT, probably 11 of 15 patients record slight changes of their bowel function (tendency for diarrhea, meterorism, and dyspepsia) (Yeoh et al. 1995). Though these symptoms usually do not influence on a patient's daily life, they indirectly indicate minor chronic radiation-induced inflammatory processes in the bowel mucosa and submucosa. In more severe cases, these postradiation processes may after many years end up as gastro-duodenal ulcera (Fossa et al. 1989; Hamilton et al. 1987) and fibrotic changes clinically mimicking malignant tumors (Moul 1992; Stensvold et al. 2004). In general, the development of these severe adverse effects takes many years (10–30 years) and the most severe conditions are diagnosed when the patient no longer has regular follow-up at the oncological clinic.

Infradiafragmatic RT at doses of >20 Gy or standard cisplatin-based chemotherapy is associated with long-term reduction of the renal function (Fosså et al. 2003). However, even after a median observation time of 11 years, the impairment remains subclinical, but a possible impact of these changes on cardiovascular morbidity should not be overseen.

Though cutaneous and pulmonary toxicity is of concern during the acute phase of treatment with bleomycin, long-term pulmonary effects related to this drug have not been observed.

## 20.5 Psychosocial Sequelae (Including Sexuality)

*General:* Psychological distress, health-related quality of life (QoL), as well as sexual dysfunctions and paternity distress have been the focus for several quantitative investigations in TCSs, but because of the lack of randomized designs most of the results are on evidence level III. Further issues associated with reproduction, sexuality, and masculine self-image are usually not covered by validated instruments assessing QoL, leaving the published results open for discussion.

TCSs like men in the general population may have significant pretreatment problems such as unemployment, economical worries, mental disorders, relational problems, and other somatic illnesses. The influence of such pretreatment issues on posttreatment adaptation among TCSs is not well known. Socio-cultural differences in relation to masculinity, sexuality, fertility, and employment should also be kept in mind when findings are compared across studies.

*Partnered relationship:* In most studies, the majority of TCSs (70–90%) were in partnered relationships when TC was diagnosed. The rate of divorce and broken relationships for TCSs is 5–10% in most follow-up studies. Those couples that did separate or divorce saw the cancer as a significant factor in their break-up (Schover and von Eschenbach 1985; Rieker et al. 1985).

Few wives found their husbands less attractive or masculine as TCSs, and in the few studies of wives, the majority found their sexual satisfaction unchanged (Gritz et al. 1989). The main concern of the wives was to become pregnant, particularly if the couple did not have children before the TC was diagnosed. Moynihan (1987) found that 22% of TCSs partners had psychiatric morbidity, mainly anxiety and fertility worries. Tuinman et al. (2007) reported a high correlation between sexual satisfaction in TCSs and their spouses, but the TCSs pairs reported less sexual satisfaction than a reference group.

*Changes in body image:* van Basten et al. (1996) have pointed the devasting effect orchiectomy may have on masculine self-esteem. Indeed, in some studies 15–33% of TCSs have reported permanent decrease in overall attractiveness (Gritz et al. 1989; Rudberg et al. 2002; Arai et al. 1996). On the other hand, no negative impact of orchidectomy was reported in a Scottish (Blackmore 1988) and in an Italian sample (Caffo and Amichetti 1999), however. These differences could reflect different cultural attitudes towards orchidectomy.

*Sexual problems*: Studies of the sexual function in long-term TCSs have been summarized in two systematic reviews (Jonker-Pool et al. 2001; Nazareth et al. 2001). Jonker-Pool et al. (2001) concluded: "it is very difficult to make a clear picture based on the outcome of the existing studies," and Nazareth et al. (2001) stated that "better evidence is needed in studies that control for the impact of the TC, the treatment modality and psychological reactions to both." Jonker-Pool et al. (2001) reviewed 36 studies done between 1975 and 2000, with a mean follow-up time of 6.9 years. Overall, they found that 20% of TCSs had lack of desire, 12% had erectile disorder, 44% ejaculation disorder, and 19% sexual dissatisfaction. Except for ejaculation disorder, these prevalence rates hardly differed from normative American data (Laumann et al. 1999). The review found significant differences in sexual function according to the treatment modalities for TC: surveillance, RPLND, radiation, and chemotherapy. The review concluded that reduced function in the *psychological domains* (drive, satisfaction) was treatment-independent, while changes in *physiological domains* (erection, ejaculation) were associated with extent of disease and treatment modalities.

On the basis of six controlled studies, Nazareth et al. (2001) calculated that the odds ratios for TCSs compared to controls were 1.6 (95% CI 1.1–2.3) for lack of drive, 2.6 (95% CI 1.6–4.1) for erectile dysfunction, and 13.7 (95% CI 7.9–23.9) for ejaculatory dysfunction.

Generally, there seems to be a high correlation between sexual functioning before and after treatment for TC (Aass et al. 1993; Incrocci et al. 2002). Findings must be considered in relation to age (Jonker-Pool et al. 1997), and to the prevalence in the general population. Thirty to fifty percent of TCSs report a decrease in sexual functioning compared to before treatment for TC (Aass et al. 1993; Jonker-Pool et al. 1997; Tinkler et al. 1992). Two-third reported decreased sexual activity, and one-third was dissatisfied with their sexual functioning (van Basten et al. 1999). Ejaculatory dysfunctions showed a high prevalence related to the type of retroperitoneal lympadenectomy. Erectile dysfunction is reported at the same level as in the general population (approximately 10%) (van Basten et al. 1999).

In a national multicenter study from Norway (Dahl et al. 2007), TCSs had significantly worse scores on ejaculatory function compared to age-matched controls from the general population. In the young group (20–39 years), sexual satisfaction was nevertheless significantly better in TCSs compared to NORM. Overall sexual problems were observed in 35% of the young TCSs (NORM 29%) and among 41% of the middle-aged group (40–59 years) (NORM 40%). In multivariate analyses, overall sexual problems in TCSs were significantly associated with increasing age, being without partner, and a higher anxiety score, while ejaculation problems showed significant association with no partner, and a trend for chemotherapy and neurotoxic side effects. Treatment before 1986 had moderate clinical relevance for ejaculation, while for hypogonadism, neurotoxic side effects, having anxiety disorder or chronic fatigue, had at least moderate clinical effect on sexual functioning. This study confirmed a main finding of the two reviews (Jonker-Pool et al. 2001; Nazareth et al. 2001), namely that ejaculation frequently is compromised in TCSs. The results were also in agreement with the statement by Jonker-Pool et al. (2001) that the psychological domains of drive and satisfaction were treatment-independent, but, in contrast to theses authors also, the physiological function of erection was found without relation to treatment.

*Fertility issues:* Biological inability to father a child presents a serious challenge to a man's perception of his masculinity, to his self-esteem, and to his intimate relations. Fertility distress was identified as a source of upset and worry at least 25% of the time during the preceding 6 months. Fertility stress seems to be common (Rieker et al. 1990) in TCSs and represents a major problem among those childless and those with ejaculatory dysfunction. No significant relationship is found between TC-related infertility and marital separation (Schover and von Eschenbach 1985; Moynihan 1987).

*Health-related quality of life (HRQoL):* Post-treatment QoL is not identical to therapy-related psychological, psychosocial, or somatic morbidity, but relates to the patient's overall perception of physical and psychosocial well-being, including family life, leisure activity, and occupational situation. Older studies with less standardized instruments, found that TCSs generally were strong, fit, and satisfied compared to controls (van Basten et al. 1996; Fossa et al. 1988, 1991; Heidenreich and Hoffman 1999; Douchez et al. 1993). Newer studies with validated instruments have confirmed older observations (van Basten et al. 1996; Fossa et al. 1988, 1991; Heidenreich and Hoffman 1999; Douchez et al. 1993) that generally QoL is as good in TCSs as in the general male population (Rudberg et al. 2000; Joly et al. 2002), or with only minimal differences compared to controls from the general male population (Mykletun et al. 2005b). The lack of difference in QoL in long-term TCSs compared to normative data, and between TC treatment groups, might be due to "response shift" (Norman 2003). The influence of treatment modalities on QoL is, however, still unsettled, mostly because of small samples with lack of statistical power. Joly et al. (2002) found no differences, while Rudberg et al. (2000) found that those treated with chemotherapy scored less favorably concerning HRQoL. Fosså et al. (2003b) reported that 2 years after chemotherapy, 36% of TCSs displayed improved and 13% deteriorated HRQoL, compared to baseline. Mykletun et al. (2005b) reported that variation of QoL in TCSs was significantly related to self-reported side-effects and TC-related mental distress stress, but not directly to TC treatment strategies (Fig. 20.3). The association between TC treatment strategies and TC-related mental

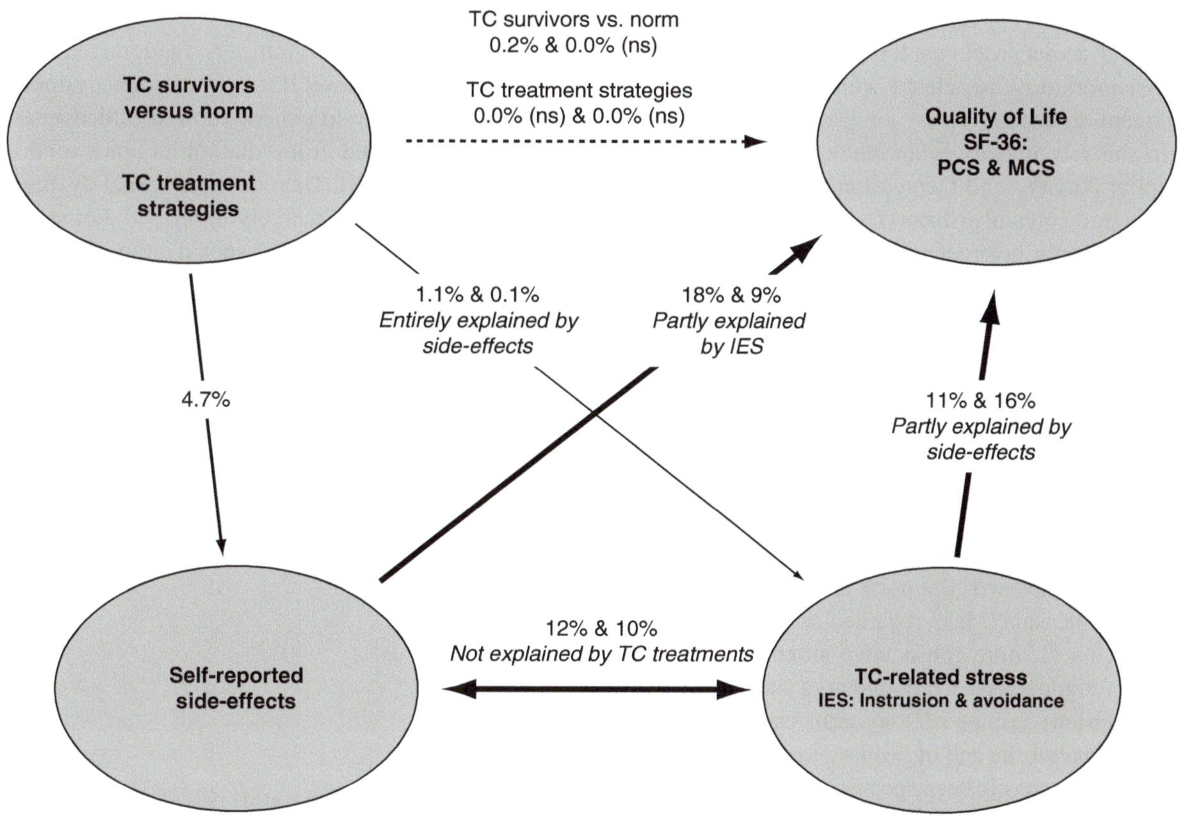


Numbers are explained (p<.05) as also outlined in the tables. Adjustment for TC treatment strategies did not explain any of the associations in the path-analysis. Arrow-styles illustrate effect-sizes in terms of explained variance.

**Fig. 20.3** Path-analysis showing the relation between treatment strategies side effects, TC-related distress, and quality of life in long-term TC survivors (with permission of JCO (Mykletun et al. 2005a))

distress was only marginal. TC-related distress many years after primary treatment is probably more related to psychological characteristics of the patient prior to TC than to treatment itself.

*Mental distress:* Most studies report a higher level of anxiety symptoms and higher prevalence of anxiety disorders among TCSs compared to controls and in the general population (Fossa et al. 1991; Kaasa et al. 1991; Jones and Payne 2000; Fossa and Dahl 2002). There is indication that a considerable proportion of TCSs live with a low feeling of safety (Jones and Payne 2000). This view from questionnaire investigations is in agreement with Moynihan's (1987) study based on diagnostic psychiatric interviews. Among 102 TCSs, she found a 14% prevalence rate of anxiety disorders and 9% of depressions up to 5 years after primary treatment. The presence of these disorders was significantly associated with health worries, fear of relapse, unemployment, and financial difficulties. Nonsignificant associations were observed for treatment strategies, social class, marital status at diagnosis, fertility problems, and sexual problems. It is unclear if there is more mental morbidity associated with the more intensive treatment regimens.

In the recent Norwegian study, the self-reporting Hospital Anxiety and Depression Scale (HADS) was used to study mental distress (Dahl et al. 2005). HADS-defined anxiety disorder was more prevalent in TCSs (19, vs. 14% in the general population). In contrast, the prevalence of HADS-defined depression did not differ between TCSs and controls (10% in both groups). In multivariate analyses of cases, HADS-defined anxiety disorder in TCSs was associated with young age, peripheral neuropathy, economic problems, alcohol problems, sexual problems, relapse anxiety, and having been treated for mental problems.

*Fatigue:* Fatigue is defined as "a feeling or state of tiredness that exceeds the norm and is experienced as clearly unpleasant". It is regarded as chronic when it lasts for six or more consecutive months. Severe and chronic fatigue has been reported in as many as 25–30% across various groups of long-term cancer survivors even years after the end of primary treatment.

Fatigue has rarely been specifically studied in TCSs, but most health-related QoL instruments include scales for the assessment of fatigue, vitality, or energy. Two studies using such instruments found no score differences between TCSs and normal controls (Rudberg et al. 2000; Joly et al. 2002), which is in agreement with Fleer et al.'s (2005) finding 1 year after treatment.

A study from Norway used the Fatigue Questionnaire (FQ) in 791 TCSs treated at the Norwegian Radium Hospital, and found that TCSs reported significantly higher fatigue scores at a mean of 11 years after primary treatment compared to an age-adjusted general population sample and a higher prevalence than among controls (TCSs: 17% vs. controls:10%) (Fossa et al. 2003c). Age, anxiety, and depression, but not treatment modality, were associated with chronic fatigue in that study.

*Living conditions, work and social functioning:* The continuation of planned education and professional life after treatment obviously is of great importance for TCSs, but only few reports have dealt with this issue. Older studies indicate that the vast majority of TCSs continue in work (Schover and von Eschenbach 1985; Moynihan 1987) and experience even greater work satisfaction in general than an age-matched population sample. There appears to be little change in relation to friends and social contacts (Rudberg et al. 2000).

*Psychological interventions:* A randomized controlled trial (evidence level II) of psychological support in relation to primary treatment showed effectiveness which hardly differed from that of nonintervention (Moynihan et al. 1998). Treatment for sexual dysfunctions in TCSs has been scarcely described, but seems to follow general principles for such dysfunctions.

In summary, as a group TCSs have a life-long slightly increased risk of medical and psychosocial long-term sequelae, the type and incidence of which are related to their primary malignancy and its treatment. Combined efforts of epidemiologist and clinicians have to identify high-risk patients who will need life-long regular follow-up by medical specialists, whereas most TCSs probably can be controlled by their family doctors according to evidence-based guidelines.

## References

Aass N, Fossa SD, Theodorsen L et al (1991) Prediction of long-term gonadal toxicity after standard treatment for testicular cancer. Eur J Cancer 27:1087–1091

Aass N, Grünfeld B, Kaalhus O et al (1993) Pre- and posttreatment sexual life in testicular cancer patients: a descriptive investigation. Br J Cancer 67:1113–1117

Allan JM, Travis LB (2005) Mechanisms of therapy-related carcinogenesis. Nat Rev Cancer 5:943–955

Arai Y, Kawakita M, Hida S et al (1996) Psychosocial aspects in long-term survivors of testicular cancer. J Urol 155:574–578
Bay K, Asklund C, Skakkebaek NE, Andersson AM (2006) Testicular dysgenesis syndrome: possible role of endocrine disrupters. Best Pract Res Clin Endocrinol Metab 20:77–90
Blackmore C (1988) The impact of orchiectomy upon the sexuality of the man with testicular cancer. Cancer Nurs 11:33–40
Bokemeyer C, Schmoll HJ, Kuczyk MA et al (1995) Risk of secondary leukemia following high cumulative doses of etoposide during chemotherapy for testicular cancer (letter). J Natl Cancer Inst 87:58–60
Brydoy M et al (2005) Paternity following treatment for testicular cancer. J Natl Cancer Inst 97:1580–1588
Caffo O, Amichetti M (1999) Evaluation of sexual life after orchidectomy followed by radiotherapy for early stage seminoma of the testis. BJU Int 83:462–468
Carroll PR, Whitmore WF Jr, Herr HW et al (1987) Endocrine and exocrine profiles of men with testicular tumours before orchiectomy. J Urol 137:420–423
Chow AY, Chin C, Dahl G, Rosenthal DN (2006) Anthracyclines cause endothelial injury in pediatric cancer patients: a pilot study. J Clin Oncol 24:925–928
Chung P, Warde P (2006) Surveillance in stage I testicular seminoma. Urol Oncol 24:75–79
Dahl AA, Haaland CF, Mykletun A et al (2005) Study of anxiety and depression in long-term survivors of testicular cancer. J Clin Oncol 23:2389–2395
Dahl AA, Bremnes R, Dahl O et al (2007) Is the sexual function compromised in long-term testicular cancer survivors? Eur Urol 52:1438–1447
Damani MN, Master V, Meng MV, Burgess C, Turek P, Oates RD (2002) Postchemotherapy ejaculatory azoospermia: fatherhood with sperm from testis tissue with intracytoplasmic sperm injection. J Clin Oncol 20:930–936
Donohue JP et al (1990) Nervesparing retroperitoneal lymphadenectomy with preservation of ejaculation. J Urol 144: 287–292
Douchez J, Droz JP, Desclaux B et al (1993) Quality of life in long-term survivors of non-seminomatous germ cell testicular tumors. J Urol 149:498–501
Einhorn LH, Williams SD, Loehrer PJ et al (1989) Evaluation of optimal duration of chemotherapy in favorable-prognosis disseminated germ cell tumours: a Southeastern Cancer Study Group protocol. J Clin Oncol 7:387–391
Fleer J, Sleijfer DT, Hoekstra HJ, Tuinman MA, Hoekstra-Weebers JE (2005) Prevalence, changes in and correlates of fatigue in the first year after diagnosis of testicular cancer. Anticancer Res 25:4647–4653
Floyd JD, Nguyen DT, Lobins RL, Bashir Q, Doll DC, Perry MC (2005) Cardiotoxicity of cancer therapy. J Clin Oncol 23:7685–7696
Fossa SD, Dahl AA (2002) Short Form 36 and Hospital Anxiety and Depression Scale. A comparison based on patients with testicular cancer. J Psychosom Res 52:79–87
Fossa SD, Åbyholm T, Aakvaag A (1984) Spermatogenesis and hormonal status after orchiectomy for cancer and before supplementary treatment. Eur Urol 10:173–177
Fossa SD, Aass N, Kaalhus O (1988) Testicular cancer in young Norwegians. J Surg Oncol 39:43–63
Fossa SD, Aass N, Kaalhus O (1989) Long-term morbidity after infradiaphragmatic radiotherapy in young men with testicular cancer. Cancer 64:404–408
Fossa SD, Aass N, Ous S et al (1991) Long-term morbidity and quality of life in testicular cancer patients. Scand J Urol Nephrol Suppl 138:241–246
Fossa SD, Aass N, Heilo A, Daugaard G, E Skakkebaek N, Stenwig AE, Nesland JM, Looijenga LH, Oosterhuis JW (2003a) Testicular carcinoma in situ in patients with extragonadal germ-cell tumours: the clinical role of pretreatment biopsy. Ann Oncol 14:1412–1418
Fossa SD, de Wit R, Roberts T et al (2003b) Quality of life in good prognosis patients with metastatic germ cell cancer: a prospective study of the European Organization for Research and Treatment of Cancer Genitourinary Group/Medical Research Council Testicular Cancer Study Group (30941/TE20). J Clin Oncol 21:1107–1118
Fossa SD, Dahl AA, Loge JH (2003c) Fatigue, anxiety, and depression in long term survivors of testicular cancer. J Clin Oncol 21:1249–1254
Fossa SD, Aass N, Harvei S, Tretli S (2004) Increased mortality rates in young and middle-aged patients with malignant germ cell tumours. Br J Cancer 90:607–612
Fossa SD, Chen J, Schonfeld SJ, McGlynn KA, McMAster ML, Gail MH, Travis LB (2005) Risk of contralaterial testicular cancer: a population-based study of 29,515 U.S. men. J Natl Cancer Inst 97:1056–1066
Fosså SD, Aass N, Winderen M, Börmer OP, Olsen DR (2003) Long-term renal function after treatment for malignant germ cell tumours. Ann Oncol 13:222–228
Gavrilovic IT, Hormigo A, Yahalom J et al (2006) Long-term follow-up of high-dose methotrexate-based therapy with and without whole brain irradiation for newly diagnosed primary CNS Lymphoma. J Clin Oncol 24:4570–4574
Gietema JA, Meinardi MT, Messerschmidt J, Gelevert T, Alt F, Uges DR et al (2000) Circulating plasma platinum more than 10 years after cisplatin treatment for testicular cancer. Lancet 355:1075–1076
Gritz ER, Wellisch DK, Wang H-J et al (1989) Long-term effects of testicular cancer on sexual functioning in married couples. Cancer 64:1560–1567
Hamilton CR, Horwich A, Bliss JM et al (1987) Gastrointestinal morbidity of adjuvant radiotherapy in stage I malignant teratoma of the testis. Radiother Oncol 10:85–90
Hanks GE, Peters T, Owen J (1992) Seminoma of the testis: long-term beneficial and deleterious results of radiation. Int J Rad Oncol Biol Phys 24:913–919
Hansen PV, Trykker H, Andersen J et al (1989) Germ cell function and hormonal status in patients with testicular cancer. Cancer 64:956–961
Hartmann JT, Fossa SD, Nichols CR, Droz JP, Horwich A, Gerl A, Beyer J, Pont J, Fizazi K, Hecker H, Kanz L, Einhorn L, Bokemeyer C (2001) Incidence of metachronous testicular cancer in patients with extragonadal germ cell tumors. J Natl Cancer Inst 93:1733–1738
Haugnes HS, Aass N, Fossa SD, Dahl O, Klepp O, Wist EA, Svartberg J, Wilsgaard T, Bremnes RM (2006) Components of the metabolic syndrome in long-term survivors of testicular cancer. Ann Oncol 18:241–248
Heidenreich A, Hoffman R (1999) Quality-of-life issues in the treatment of testicular cancer. World J Urol 17:230–238
Hoei-Hansen CE, Holm M, Rajpert-De Meyts E, Skakkebaek NE (2003) Histological evidence of testicular dysgenesis in contralateral biopsies from 218 patients with testicular germ cell cancer. J Pathol 200:370–374

Horwich A, Shipley J, Huddart R (2006) Testicular germ-cell cancer. Lancet 367:754–765

Huddart RA, Norman A, Shahidi M, Horwich A, Coward D, Nicholls J et al (2003) Cardiovascular disease as a long-term complication of treatment for testicular cancer. J Clin Oncol 21:1513–1523

Huddart RA, Norman A, Moynihan C, Horwich A, Parker C, Nicholls E, Dearnaley DP (2005) Fertility, gonadal and sexual function in survivors of testicular cancer. Br J Cancer 93:200–207

Incrocci L, Hop WCJ, Wijnmaalen A et al (2002) Treatment outcome, body image, and sexual functioning after orchiectomy and radiotherapy for stage I-II testicular seminoma. Int J Radiat Oncol Biol Phys 53:1165–1173

Jacobsen KD, Olsen DR, Fossa K, Fossa SD (1997) External beam abdominal radiotherapy in patients with seminoma stage I: field type, testicular dose, and spermatogenesis. Int J Radiat Oncol Biol Phys 38:95–102

Jacobsen KD, Ous S, Wæhre H et al (1999) Ejaculation in testicular cancer patients after post-chemotherapy retroperitoneal lymph node dissection. Br J Cancer 80:249–255

Jacobsen KD, Theodorsen L, Fossa SD (2001) Spermatogenesis after unilateral orchiectomy for testicular cancer in patients following surveillance policy.J Urol 165(1):93–96

Joly F, Héron JF, Kalusinski L et al (2002) Quality of life in long-term survivors of testicular cancer: a population-based case-control study. J Clin Oncol 20:73–80

Jones GY, Payne S (2000) Searching for safety signals: the experience of medical surveillance among men with testicular teratomas. Psychooncology 9:385–394

Jonker-Pool G, van Basten JP, Hoekstra HJ et al (1997) Sexual functioning after treatment for testicular cancer. Cancer 80: 454–464

Jonker-Pool G, Van de Wiel HBM, Hoekstra HJ et al (2001) Sexual functioning after treatment for testicular cancer – review and meta-analysis of 36 empirical studies between 1975-2000. Arch Sex Behav 30:55–74

Kaasa S, Aass N, Mastekaasa A et al (1991) Psychosocial well-being in testicular cancer patients. Eur J Cancer 27:1091–1095

Keefe D (2001) Anthracycline induced cardiomyopathy. Semin Oncol 28:2–7

Kollmannsberger C, Hartmann JT, Kanz L et al (1999) Therapy-related malignancies following treatment of germ cell cancer. Int J Cancer 83:860–863

Lampe H, Horwich A, Norman A et al (1997) Fertility after chemotherapy for testicular germ cell cancers. J Clin Oncol 15:239–245

Laumann EO, Paik A, Rosen RC (1999) Sexual dysfunction in the United States. Prevalence and predictors. JAMA 281: 537–544

Lutke Holzik MF, Hoekstra HJ, Mulder NH, Suurmeijer AJ, Sleijfer DT, Gietema JA (2003) Non-germ cell malignancy in residual or recurrent mass after chemotherapy for non-seminomatous testicular germ cell tumor. Ann Surg Oncol 10:131–135

Magelssen H, Haugen TB, von During V, Melve KK, Sandstad B, Fossa SD (2005) Twenty years experience with semen cryopreservation in testicular cancer patients: who needs it? Eur Urol 48:779–785

Meistrich ML, Shetty G (2003) Suppression of testosterone stimulates recovery of spermatogenesis after cancer treatment. Int J Androl 26:141–146

Moul JW (1992) Retroperitoneal fibrosis following radiotherapy for stage I testicular seminoma. J Urol 147:124–126

Moynihan C (1987) Testicular cancer: the psychosocial problems of patients and their relatives. Cancer Surv 6:477–510

Moynihan C, Bliss JM, Davidson J et al (1998) Evaluation of adjuvant psychosocial therapy in patients with testicular cancer: randomised controlled trial. BMJ 316:429–435

Mykletun A, Dahl AA, Haaland CF, Bremnes R, Dahl O, Klepp O, Wist E, Fossa SD (2005a) Side effects and cancer-related stress determine quality of life in long-term survivors of testicular cancer. J Clin Oncol 23:3061–3068

Mykletun A, Dahl AA, Haaland CF et al (2005b) Side effects and cancer-related stress determine quality of life in long-term survivors of testicular cancer. J Clin Oncol 23:3061–3068

Nazareth I, Lewin J, King M (2001) sexual dysfunction after treatment for testicular cancer: a systematic review. J Psychosom Res 51:735–743

Nichols CR, Breeden ES, Loehrer PJ et al (1993) Secondary leukemia associated with a conventional dose of etoposide: review of serial germ cell tumor protocols. J Natl Cancer Inst 85:36–40

Nord C, Bjøro T, Ellingsen D et al (2003) Gonadal hormones in long- term survivors 10 years after treatment for unilateral testicular cancer. Eur Urol 44:322–328

Norman G (2003) Hi! How are you? Response shift, implicit theories and differing epistemologies. Qual Life Res 12: 239–249

Nuver J, Smit AJ, Wolffenbuttel BH, Sluiter WJ, Hoekstra HJ, Sleijfer DT et al (2005a) The metabolic syndrome and disturbances in hormone levels in long-term survivors of disseminated testicular cancer. J Clin Oncol 23:3718–3725

Nuver J, Smit AJ, van der Meer J, van den Berg MP, van der Graaf WT, Meinardi MT et al (2005b) Acute chemotherapy-induced cardiovascular changes in patients with testicular cancer. J Clin Oncol 23:9130–9137

Oldenburg J, Fossa SD, Dahl AA (2006) Scale for chemotherapy-induced long-term neurotoxicity (SCIN): psychometrics, validation, and findings in a large sample of testicular cancer survivors. Qual Life Res 15:791–800

Oldenburg J, Kraggerud SM, Cvancarova M et al (2007) Cisplatin-induced long-term hearing impairment is associated with specific glutathione s-transferase genotypes in testicular cancer survivors. J Clin Oncol 25:708–714

Palmieri G, Lotrecchiano G, Ricci G et al (1996) Gonadal function after multimodality treatment in men with testicular germ cell cancer. Eur J Endocrinol 134:431–436

Pedersen-Bjergaard J, Daugaard G et al (1991) Increased risk of myelodysplasia and leukaemia after etoposide, cisplatin, and bleomycin for germ-cell tumours. Lancet 338:359–363

Petersen PM, Skakkebæk NE, Giwercman A (1998) Gonadal function in men with testicular cancer: biological and clinical aspects. APMIS 106:24–36

Petersen PM, Skakkebæk NE, Rørth M et al (1999) Semen quality and reproductive hormones before and after orchiectomy in men with testicular cancer. J Urol 161:822–826

Petersen PM, Giwercman A, Daugaard G, Rorth M, Petersen JH, Skakkeaek NE, Hansen SW, von der Maase H (2002) Effect of graded testicular doses of radiotherapy in patients treated for carcinoma-in-situ in the testis. J Clin Oncol 20:1537–1543

Petersen PM, Daugaard G, Rorth M, Skakkebaek NE (2003) Endocrine function in patients treated for carcinoma in situ in the testis with irradiation. APMIS 111:93–98

Reiter WJ, Kratzik C, Brodowicz T et al (1998) Sperm analysis and serum follicle-stimulating hormone levels before and after adjuvant single-agent carboplatin therapy for clinical stage I seminoma. Urology 52:117–119

Rieker PP, Edbril SD, Garnick MB (1985) Curative testis cancer therapy: psychosocial sequelae. J Clin Oncol 3:1117–1126

Rieker PP, Fitzgerald EM, Kalish LA (1990) Adaptive behavioral responses to potential infertility among survivors of testis cancer. J Clin Oncol 8:347–355

Rosenlund B, Westlander G, Wood M, Lundin K, Reismer E, Hillensjo T (1998) Sperm retrieval and fertilization in repeated percutaneous epididymal sperm aspiration. Hum Reprod 13:2805–2807

Rudberg L, Nilsson S, Wikblad K (2000) Health-related quality of life in survivors of testicular cancer 3 to 13 years after treatment. J Psychosoc Oncol 18:19–31

Rudberg L, Carlsson M, Nilsson S et al (2002) Self-perceived physical, psychologic, and general symptoms in survivors of testicular cancer 3 to 13 years after treatment. Cancer Nurs 25:187–195

Sagstuen H, Aass N, Fosså SD, Dahl O, Klepp O, Wist E et al (2005) Blood pressure and body mass index in long-term survivors of testicular cancer. J Clin Oncol 23:4980–4990

Sant M, Aareleid T, Artioli ME, et al. Ten-year survival and risk of relapse for testicular cancer: a EUROCARE high resolution study. Eur J Cancer 2007; 43:585-92

Schover LR, von Eschenbach AC (1985) Sexual and marital relationships after treatment for nonseminomatous testicular cancer. Urology 25:251–255

Segal R (2006) Surveillance programs for stage I nonseminomatous germ cell tumors of the testis. Urol Oncol 24:68–74

Smith MA, Rubinstein L, Anderson JR et al (1999) Secondary leukemia or myeloodysplastic syndrome after treatment with epipodophyllotoxins. J Clin Oncol 17:569–577

Stensvold E, Aass N, Gladhaug I, Stenwig AE, Claussen OP, Fossa SD (2004) Erroneous diagnosis of pancreatic cancer after radiotherapy of testicular cancer. Eur J Surg Oncol 30: 352–355

Stone HB, Coleman CN, Anscher MS, McBride WH (2003) Effects of radiation on normal tissue: consequences and mechanisms. Lancet Oncol 4:529–536

Taksey J, Bissada NK, Chaudhary UB (2003) Fertility after chemotherapy for testicular cancer. Arch Androl 49:389–395

Tinkler SD, Howard GCW, Kerr GR (1992) Sexual morbidity following radiotherapy for germ cell tumours of the testis. Radiat Oncol 25:207–212

Travis LB, Andersson M, Gospodarowicz M, van Leeuwen FE, Bergfeldt K, Lynch CF et al (2000) Treatment-associated leukemia following testicular cancer. J Natl Cancer Inst 92: 1165–1171

Travis LB, Fossa SD, Schonfeld SJ, McMaster ML, Lynch CF, Storm H, Hall P, Holowaty E, Andersen A, Pukkala E, Andersson M, Kaijser M, Gospodarowicz M, Joensuu T, Cohen RJ, Boice JD Jr, Dores GM, Gilbert ES (2005) Second cancers among 40, 576 testicular cancer patients: focus on long-term survivors. J Natl Cancer Inst 97:1354–1365

Tuinman MA, Hoekstra HJ, Sleijfer DT et al (2007) Testicular cancer: a longitudinal pilot study on stress response symptoms and quality of life in couples before and after chemotherapy. Support Care Cancer 15:279–286

van Basten JP, Jonker-Pool G, van Driel MF et al (1996) Fantasies and facts of the testes. Br J Urol 78:756–762

van Basten JPA, van Driel HJ, Hoekstra D et al (1999) Objective and subjective effects of treatment for testicular cancer on sexual function. BJU Int 84:671–678

Van den Belt-Dusebout AW, Nuver J, de Wit R, Gietema JA, ten Bokkel Huinink WW, Rodrigus PTR et al (2006) Long-term risk of cardiovascular disease in 5-year survivors of testicular cancer. J Clin Oncol 24:467–475

van Leeuwen FE, Stiggelbout AM, van den Belt-Dusebout AW, Noyon R, Eliel MR, van Kerkhoff EH et al (1993) Second cancer risk following testicular cancer: a follow-up study of 1, 909 patients. J Clin Oncol 11:415–424

van Ruijven MW, de Groot JC, Smoorenburg GF (2004) Time sequence of degeneration pattern in the guinea pig cochlea during cisplatin administration. A quantitative histological study. Hear Res 197:44–54

Yeoh E, Horowitz M, Russo A et al (1995) The effects of abdominal irradiation for seminoma of the testis on gastrointestinal function. J Gastroenter Hepat 10:125–130

Zagars GK, Ballo MT, Lee AK, Strom SS (2004) Mortality after cure of testicular seminoma. J Clin Oncol 22:640–647

# Fertility Issues

# 21

Gedske Daugaard, Fiona McDonald, Elisabeth Carlsen, and Robert Huddart

## 21.1 Background

The high cure rate, coupled with the young age of patients with germ cell tumors, makes the impact of treatment on reproductive function, fertility, and progeny outcome an important issue.

Even before treatment, testicular germ cell tumor patients are known to have lower fertility, lower semen quality, and higher follicle stimulating hormone (FSH) levels than age-matched controls (Petersen et al. 1999a). This suggests that there is a degree of pre-existing impairment of spermatogenesis in the non-tumor testicular tissue prior to any treatment.

The initial management of testicular germ cell tumor patients is usually unilateral orchidectomy. This surgery and subsequent adjuvant treatment can further impair reproductive function and fertility. In particular, the chemotherapy regimens used to treat testicular germ cell tumors frequently lead to azoospermia, but the majority of patients have been shown to recover from this toxicity. Among patients who are normospermic before standard chemotherapy, 80% will recover spermatogenesis by 5 years after completion of treatment (Lampe et al. 1997).

However despite the issues of poor semen quality and impaired reproductive function many still have a chance of paternity. With the development of modern assisted reproductive techniques even men with significant gonadal dysfunction have the potential to father a child (Sakamoto et al. 2007). There are various factors contributing to the abnormal reproductive hormone levels and failure of normal spermatogenesis in testicular germ cell tumor patients. Some of these will be highlighted below together with data on the effects of different treatments on fertility.

## 21.2 Sub-fertility as Risk Factor of Testicular Cancer

Studies have shown that there is an increased risk of testicular cancer among men with reduced fertility that goes beyond the effect of cryptorchidism (Doria-Rose et al. 2005). However, it is not clear whether the sub-fertility is the result of an emerging tumor, or whether both sub-fertility and testicular cancer share a common etiology.

In a case-control study, fertility patterns prior to testicular cancer diagnosis were investigated by comparing previous pregnancies involving 201 men subsequently diagnosed with testicular cancer and those fathered by 204 age and neighborhood matched controls (Baker et al. 2005). Regardless of tumor histology, men diagnosed with testicular cancer were less likely to have ever fathered a live-born infant prior to their diagnosis (OR 0.67, 95% CI 0.42–1.06) and had fewer offspring prior to their diagnosis than control men (means 1.8 and 2.1, respectively). Cases were more likely than controls to report having had an infertility diagnosis (OR 9.47, 95% CI 1.19–75.2) or a low sperm count documented (OR 5.85, 95% CI 1.28–26.7) prior to their cancer diagnosis. No difference in reported pregnancy losses between the two groups was observed. In another study, the incidence ratio of testicular cancer was investigated in over 32,000 men who had previously had semen analysis performed (Jacobsen et al. 2000). Men in couples with documented fertility problems

G. Daugaard (✉)
Department of Oncology 5073, Copenhagen University Hospital, Rigshospitalet, Blegdamsvej 9, Copenhagen, Denmark

M.P. Laguna et al. (eds.), *Cancer of the Testis*,
DOI: 10.1007/978-1-84800-370-5_21, © Springer-Verlag London Limited 2010

were more likely to go on to develop testicular cancer than other men (standardized incidence ratio 1.6, 95% confidence interval 1.3–1.9). This observed risk was relatively constant with increasing time between semen analysis and cancer diagnosis. Low sperm concentration, poor motility of spermatozoa, and high proportion of morphologically abnormal spermatozoa were all associated with an increased risk of testicular cancer. A more recent study has observed decreased fertility among brothers of patients with testicular cancer compared to both controls and sisters of the patients (Richiardi and Akre 2005).

A number of studies have suggested that abnormalities of the contralateral testis contribute to pre-treatment sub-fertility in testicular germ cell tumor patients. A study of biopsy material from the contralateral testis of over 200 patients with unilateral testicular germ cell tumors found significant changes in 24% of cases (Berthelsen and Skakkebaek 1983). These significant findings included carcinoma in situ as well as impairment of spermatogenesis, ranging in severity and including complete lack of sperm production. A similar study found an incidence of carcinoma in situ of 8.7% and of testicular dysgenesis of 25.2% in biopsies of the contra-lateral testis from over 200 patients with unilateral testicular germ cell tumors (Hoei-Hansen et al. 2003). Abnormal or absent spermatogenesis was reported in 48.6% of these patients. A recent study analyzed testicular ultrasound data from 328 men for evidence of microlithiasis including patients previously treated for testicular germ cell tumors, their unaffected male relatives, and healthy male controls (Coffey et al. 2007). Testicular microlithiasis being more frequent in testicular germ cell tumor cases than controls (36.7 vs. 17.8%, age adjusted $P<0.0001$), this study also found that microlithiasis was more common in unaffected male relatives than controls (34.5 vs. 17.8%, age adjusted $P=0.02$). It also observed that testicular germ cell tumor case and matched relative pairs showed greater concordance for testicular microlithiasis than would be expected by chance ($P=0.05$).

These studies together argue in favor of a common etiology between sub-fertility and testicular germ cell tumors. It is possible that a pre-existing defect in germ cells leads to both defective spermatogenesis and testicular cancer with both being part of a testicular dysgenesis syndrome (TDS) (Skakkebaek et al. 2001). The cause of such a defect in the germ cell line remains unclear but may be either genetic or environmental in nature. There are both experimental and epidemiological studies suggesting that TDS is a result of disruption of embryonal programming and gonadal development during fetal life. Impaired gonadal development resulting in the arrest of gonocyte differentiation and retention of its embryonic features, associated with an increasing genomic instability, is the most probable model for pathogenesis of carcinoma in situ, the precursor of testicular cancer (Meyts 2006). Interestingly, it has been observed that patients being treated for extragonadal germ cell tumors with no gonadal involvement also have testicular abnormalities (Carroll et al. 1987). Testicular biopsies from eight such patients revealed a range of abnormalities including fibrosis, edema, and decreased spermatogenesis. Again, a primary germ cell defect may be a common etiological factor accounting for this observation, with defective spermatogenesis in the testes and development of an extragonadal germ cell tumor in incompletely migrated germ cells.

Factors other than a congenital or acquired primary germ cell defect may also influence spermatogenesis in patients with testicular germ cell tumors prior to orchidectomy. Local effects of the tumor itself may contribute to impaired spermatogenesis. Evidence for this is based on the observation that in testicular germ cell tumor orchidectomy specimen spermatogenesis appears to be more defective in the testicular tissue closest to the tumor than further from it (Ho et al. 1992). However, uniform spermatogenesis was observed in testicular tissue from orchidectomy specimens containing benign testicular lesions. Mass effect alone is unlikely therefore to cause this impaired spermatogenesis but it may be a contributory factor, for example in combination with any local paracrine action of secretory substances from the tumor.

Development of a testicular tumor can cause disruption of the blood–testis barrier. One of the functions of this barrier is to prevent auto-antibodies forming against sperm. With disruption of this barrier, anti-sperm antibodies can develop and this autoimmunity may contribute to impaired fertility. A small study on 52 patients with non-seminomatous low-stage testicular germ cell tumors found anti-sperm antibodies using immunofluorescent techniques in 21% of cases (Foster et al. 1991). A similar study revealed anti-sperm antibodies in 73% of patients with testicular germ cell tumors before orchidectomy compared to 8% in healthy controls (Guazzieri et al. 1985). This study also noted that the percentage of patients with antibodies decreased following treatment of the tumor.

Spermatogenesis is a complex process that is well controlled by the hypothalamic–pituitary–gonadal axis.

The various hormones involved not only control the initiation of spermatogenesis but also ensure normal spermatozoa maturation. Any imbalance in this hormonal status could lead to disturbances in this process. A diagnosis of a testicular germ cell tumor may alter the balance of these hormones and thus impair spermatogenesis in one of two ways.

Firstly, the tumor tissue may secrete hormones such as beta-human chorionic gonadotrophin (β-hCG) and alpha-fetoprotein (AFP). Elevated levels of β-hCG have been shown to cause increase in serum testosterone and even greater increase in serum estradiol by conversion of testosterone thereby suppressing LH and FSH levels. A paracrine–endocrine mechanism for impaired spermatogenesis has also been proposed in which intra-testicular β-hCG produced by testicular tumor cells exerts a luteinizing hormone-like effect on the Leydig cells leading to increased production of estradiol and testosterone by the remaining normal testicular tissue and suppression of serum LH levels (Petersen et al. 1999a). Subsequent elevation of intra-testicular levels of estradiol may contribute to impaired spermatogenesis.

Secondly, any malignancy in general can evoke a systemic response in the body. Cytokines such as interleukins and tumor necrosis factor secreted by tumor tissue along with the bodies defence mechanisms mediate this systemic response and may lead to the over- or under-secretion of hormones by endocrine glands. Also stress associated with a cancer diagnosis itself can impair semen quality through disrupted hormone levels (Meirow and Schenker 1995). However, studies of sperm counts in patients with malignancies other than testicular germ cell tumors indicate that sperm counts in these patients were not significantly different from those of healthy controls (Petersen et al. 1998, 1999a). Impairment of spermatogenesis may therefore be limited to patients with a germ cell tumor and not a malignant disease in general.

## 21.3 Reproductive Hormones and Testicular Cancer

### *21.3.1 The Hypothalamic–Pituitary–Gonadal Axis*

The reproductive hormonal axis in men consists of three main components: the hypothalamus, the pituitary gland, and the testis. This axis normally functions in a tightly regulated manner to produce concentrations of circulating steroids required for normal male sexual function and fertility.

The integrating center of the axis is the hypothalamus and is the site of production of the gonadotropin-releasing hormone (GnRH). This is transported to the pituitary gland where it stimulates the synthesis and release of gonadotropic hormones, LH and FSH. Secretion of GnRH is modulated by both the central nervous system and circulating gonadal steroids. GnRH has a very short half-life in the blood (approximately 5 min). The pituitary gland is therefore exposed to high levels of GnRH in hypophyseal-portal blood for brief periods of time. This pulsatile pattern of GnRH release appears to be essential for stimulatory effects on LH and FSH release. The LH and FSH released by the pituitary gland into the systemic blood circulation are carried to the target end organs, the testes.

In the testis, LH stimulates testosterone secretion by the Leydig cells. The secreted testosterone acts on numerous target end organs causing the development of male secondary sexual characteristics and is essential for spermatogenesis. FSH stimulates the Sertoli cells, permitting initiation and maintenance of spermatogenesis. Sertoli cells also produce Inhibin B. Estradiol is produced both from the testis (Sertoli cells and Leydig cells) and from peripheral conversion of androgens.

Negative feedback on the pituitary gland and hypothalamus is primarily by testosterone and Inhibin, controlling LH and FSH, respectively. Although the concentration of estradiol in male serum is relatively low compared with testosterone, it is a much more potent inhibitor of LH and FSH secretion.

## 21.4 Reproductive Hormones and Treatment

### *21.4.1 Orchidectomy Alone*

There are only limited published data on the hormone function of testicular germ cell tumor patients treated with orchidectomy alone and subsequent surveillance follow-up. The largest series is of 179 patients (Huddart et al. 2005). 11% of patients had sub-normal testosterone level, 6% had raised LH level and 42% of patients had raised FSH level after orchidectomy. Of these patients 114 had documented baseline hormones post orchidectomy and a follow-up hormone profile taken a minimum of 5 years post-orchidectomy. In this group the median FSH rose from 7 to 9 iu/l, the median testosterone rose from 13 to 14 nmol/l and the median LH fell from 6 to 5 iu/l between baseline and follow-up. This rise in testosterone over time is unexpected as testosterone levels usually decline with age. An explanation for this may be that the tumor or subsequent orchidectomy causes temporary reduction in testosterone levels at diagnosis that then is able to recover over time. The rise in testosterone may explain the median fall in LH level during the follow-up period. The median rise in FSH over the follow-up period is consistent with data discussed later (Jacobsen et al. 2001) regarding recovery of spermatogenesis over time following unilateral orchidectomy alone. In this study it is interesting to note that elevated serum FSH levels at baseline following orchidectomy was associated with incomplete recovery of spermatogenesis particularly if combined with oligospermia or azoospermia in the immediate post-operative period.

### 21.4.2 Chemotherapy

A number of studies have observed increases in both FSH and LH as a result of chemotherapy following orchidectomy. For example, 22 patients treated with cisplatin-based chemotherapy following orchidectomy were compared to 9 patients treated with orchidectomy alone (Hansen et al. 1990). FSH was elevated in 86% of patients treated with chemotherapy compared to 11% in the reference group and LH was elevated in 59% of patients compared again to 11% in the reference group.

Studies have provided evidence to suggest the level of gonadal dysfunction is greatest immediately after chemotherapy. In one study, involving 232 patients treated with cisplatin-containing chemotherapy, it was shown that there was a higher rate of elevation of FSH and LH in the first year following treatment compared to a median of 8 years after follow-up (LH 32% vs. 3.6%, FSH 89% vs. 64%) (Brennemann et al. 1997). This suggests that there is recovery over time of the detrimental effect the chemotherapy has on gonadal function. Although similar findings are reported in other studies (Huddart et al. 2005) there are also reports on patients treated with chemotherapy where no improvement in LH and FSH levels are observed on longitudinal follow-up (Gerl et al. 2001). Variables in these studies that may account for this observation include differing schedules of chemotherapy, monotherapy, or polychemotherapy, with different agents being used in varying doses. Greater degrees of hormonal dysfunction are seen in patients treated with more intensive chemotherapy (Bokemeyer et al. 1996).

Various studies have observed a decrease in testosterone as a result of chemotherapy following orchidectomy. The largest series of 290 patients treated with platinum-based chemotherapy revealed abnormally low levels of testosterone in 15% on long-term follow-up (Huddart et al. 2005). This, however, was not significantly different to testosterone levels below the normal range in 13% of the 179 patients followed up after orchidectomy alone. The patients who required chemotherapy, however, had lower baseline FSH levels and higher baseline testosterone and LH levels than patients treated with orchidectomy alone. This may be due to disease related factors including interaction between LH and βHCG levels.

Interestingly, this study also included a group of 81 patients treated with both chemotherapy and radiotherapy. 34% of these patients had sub-normal testosterone levels on follow-up, significantly different to the surveillance group, and a further 4% were receiving testosterone replacement.

### 21.4.3 Scattered RT

The main role of radiotherapy in curable testicular germ cell tumor patients is in the adjuvant setting following unilateral orchidectomy in early stage seminoma (stage I and IIA). Until a few years ago irradiation to both the para-aortic lymph nodes and the ipsilateral iliac lymph nodes (dogleg field) was the standard adjuvant field treated in this group of patients provided there was no history of previous inguinoscrotal surgery and subsequent disturbed testicular lymphatics. More recently the standard radiotherapy field treated became confined to the para-aortic lymph nodes only (PA strip) with consequent reduction in the size of the radiation field (Fossa et al. 1999).

There is limited data available on the effect of scattered radiation from subdiaphragmatic radiotherapy on reproductive hormones. In a study discussed in more detail later (Jacobsen et al. 1997) patients treated with dogleg radiotherapy but not those treated with PA strip radiotherapy had a significant rise in their FSH levels after receiving radiotherapy. This was observed in both the patients with sperm counts in the abnormal and normal range prior to radiation. The same study observed the usual rapid post-treatment improvement in spermatogenesis following adjuvant radiotherapy was less likely in those patients who already had a lower than normal sperm count and a raised FSH level before radiotherapy. Using modern radiation techniques and radiation doses of less than 30 Gy, the scatter radiation dose to the contra-lateral testis is low enough for radiation-induced changes in reproductive hormone levels to be unlikely.

### 21.4.4 Testicular RT for CIS

An important study has investigated 48 patients presenting with unilateral testicular germ cell cancer and CIS of the contra-lateral testis (Petersen et al. 2002). The CIS-bearing testis was treated with daily irradiation doses of 2 Gy, 5 days a week, to a cumulative dose of 20 Gy (21 patients), 18 Gy (3 patients), 16 Gy (10 patients), and 14 Gy (14 patients). All patients treated at dose levels 16–20 Gy achieved histologically verified complete remission without signs of recurrence of CIS after an observation period of more than 5 years. One of the14 patients treated at dose level 14 Gy had a relapse of CIS 20 months after irradiation.

Reproductive hormone function was examined before and regularly after radiotherapy in 44 of 48 patients. The level of testosterone was significantly lower after radiotherapy compared to baseline (median 12.2 vs. 11.6 nmol/l). Testosterone continued to fall at a stable rate for more than 5 years after treatment (3.6% per year) without dose dependency. The levels of LH and FSH both significantly increased after radiotherapy (8.5 vs. 12.6 iu/l and 19.2 vs. 33.6 iu/l respectively). The need for androgen replacement therapy was similar at all dose levels. Testicular irradiation was a safe treatment at a dose level of 20 Gy. A lower dose of 14 Gy may lead to risk of relapse of CIS. Impairment of hormone production without clinically significant dose dependency was seen in the dose range 14–20 Gy.

## 21.5 Semen Quality and Testicular Cancer

### 21.5.1 Spermatogenesis

Spermatogenesis is a three-phase process by which spermatogonia develop into mature spermatozoa. The process of sperm formation and maturation occurs in the seminiferous tubules and epididymis in a stepwise fashion. During the first phase the diploid spematogonium within the seminiferous tubules undergoes mitotic division to form a diploid primary spermatocyte. In the second phase, each primary spermatocyte duplicates its DNA and subsequently undergoes the first meiotic division to form two secondary spermatocytes. This is rapidly followed by the second meiotic division which produces four haploid spermatids. The spermatids then elongate. The third phase of spermatogenesis is a maturation phase taking place primarily in the epididymis. During this phase the spermatozoa also acquire motility.

The process of spermatogenesis from spermatogonia to mature spermatozoa is estimated to last approximately 70 days. This fact should be taken into consideration when evaluating the possible effect of any cytotoxic chemotherapy or other factors on spermatogenesis.

### 21.5.2 Evaluation of Semen Quality

Spermatogenesis can be directly evaluated by microscopy of a testicular biopsy. In the normal spermatogenic epithelium all cell types will be represented including late spermatids. Spermatogenesis is however usually evaluated indirectly by analysis of a semen sample as this is non-invasive. A semen sample can be used to give an estimate of fertility potential and most semen samples are analyzed for this reason.

In order to be able to evaluate the quality of a semen sample certain parameters are measured. These semen parameters include semen volume, sperm concentration, sperm morphology, and sperm motility as well as some biochemical markers including pH. Semen sample collection also needs to be optimal including a minimum period of abstinence prior to collection. Standards for collection of samples and normal semen parameters have been established by the World Health Organisation (WHO). Only when all these parameters are within the normal range will the semen quality be reported as normal. The reference ranges given by WHO have changed over the years. In the current guidelines (World Health Organisation 1999) the following references are given: Semen volume ≥2 ml, sperm concentration ≥20 mill/ml, total sperm count ≥40 mill/ml, and percentage of motile spermatozoa ≥40%.

The reference range for proportion of sperm with normal morphological features is still being debated. One study indicates that a percentage of spermatozoa with normal morphologic features as low as 12% may represent a normal semen sample (Guzick et al. 2001). Another study has shown that the concentration of sperm is important for fertility. Optimal pregnancy rates were obtained if the concentration was >40 mill/ml (Bonde et al. 1998). As the percentage of sperm with normal morphologic features appears to be an important semen quality to aid assessment of fertility further studies and guidance are needed.

Another important aspect to remember is that semen quality can vary substantially over time in an individual man. It has been shown in one study that the intra-individual variation in sperm concentration was up to 65% but this variation was somewhat less for sperm motility and sperm morphology (Carlsen et al. 2003). One of the factors affecting sperm concentration in particular is duration of abstinence. Increasing duration of abstinence up to 4–5 days was shown in the same study to increase sperm concentration and thereby total sperm count linearly. Beyond that time there was no advantage observed in increasing the abstinence period since sperm morphology and motility started to deteriorate. Another factor affecting sperm concentration observed in this study was episodes of fever. A febrile episode significantly decreased the number of spermatozoa in the ejaculate by up to 35% for up to 2 months.

These known factors that can affect an individual's sperm quality over time are unable to account for all the observed variations. Therefore it is recommended that an individual has at least two samples analyzed with a period of time in-between to provide a more accurate assessment of semen quality.

## 21.6 Semen Quality and Treatment

### 21.6.1 Orchidectomy Alone

It has been shown that there is significant decrease in sperm concentration and total sperm count after unilateral orchidectomy for testicular cancer (Petersen et al. 1998). Information about the natural course of spermatogenesis in such patients following surgery is provided by a study that observed testicular cancer patients who were followed up after unilateral orchidectomy with surveillance alone (Jacobsen et al. 2001). The analysis of the long-term spermatogenesis of the remaining testicle showed that the reduced spermatogenesis in many cases recovered during the first year following the procedure. Among 60 patients with non-relapsing testicular cancer, at baseline following orchidectomy, 60% of patients were normospermic and this rose to 75% of patients by 1 year. The combination of oligospermia or azoospermia with elevated FSH at baseline following surgery was associated with poor chance of recovery of spermatogenesis (only 2/7 cases revealed any recovery).

### 21.6.2 Chemotherapy

Spermatogenesis is adversely affected by most chemotherapeutic agents. The most susceptible cells are those most actively dividing and consist of spermatogonia and spermatocytes. Non-dividing spermatids and mature spermatozoa are less susceptible as are Leydig cells. Repopulation of the seminiferous tubules occurs as long as some spermatogonial stem cells remain. These cells slowly divide, eventually resulting in a resumption of spermatogenesis.

The specific combination of drugs used for therapy and the dose administered are important factors determining the likely degree of impairment of spermatogenesis. As single drugs, alkylating agents seem to result in the greatest amount of testicular damage. Cisplatin is one of the alkylating agents that interferes with cell division by crosslinking DNA and one of its side effects is impairment of spermatogenesis. Due to its efficacy in germ cell tumors however, cisplatin is at present the main chemotherapeutic agent used in the treatment of these patients (Einhorn and Donohue 1977). Cisplatin is usually given as part of a combination regimen. The most common chemotherapeutic combination in testicular cancer management uses cisplatin with bleomycin and etoposide – BEP chemotherapy (Williams et al. 1987). Other chemotherapeutic agents with efficacy in testicular cancer include: ifosfamide, vinblastine, carboplatin, paclitaxel, gemcitabine, and oxaliplatin. Carboplatin and oxaliplatin are platinum-derived compounds similar to cisplatin with less damaging effect on spermatogenesis, but less efficaciousness in treating germ cell tumors.

Studies have been performed looking at the effect a course of platinum-based chemotherapy has on sperm quality in patients being treated for testicular germ cell tumors. The majority of patients will show temporary or permanent azoospermia (Ohl and Sonksen 1996). In one study, analysis of 170 patients with semen analysis performed pre-chemotherapy and performed again at least 1 year after chemotherapy revealed that of the 89 patients who were normospermic pre-chemotherapy, 64% were normospermic at least 1 year after their treatment (Lampe et al. 1997). This study also showed clear evidence for continued recovery beyond 1 year with the probability of spermatogenesis increasing to 48% by 2 years and 80% by 5 years. It also noted there was a significantly higher probability of recovery of a normal sperm count in the 54 patients treated with carboplatin-rather than cisplatin-based therapy. The effect of the platinum-based chemotherapy on sperm counts appears to be dose related and this study revealed reduced probability of sperm count recovery in patients treated with more than four cycles of platinum-based chemotherapy.

There is further evidence of the importance of the cumulative dose of cisplatin in recovery of a patient's sperm count. Since the introduction of surveillance strategies for patients with a testicular germ cell tumor following unilateral orchidectomy, one study collected data from other previously published studies to compare sperm counts on patients with germ cell tumors treated with and without cisplatin-based chemotherapy treatment to estimate the extent to which the chemotherapy affects long-term fertility. At 2-year follow-up, there was no significant difference in sperm count and rate of azoospermia between the two groups when the cumulative dose of cisplatin was less than or equal to 400 mg/m$^2$. Above this dose irreversible suppression of sperm production was observed (DeSantis et al. 1999). Similar results have been reported by other authors (Fossa et al. 1993; Drasga et al. 1983; Petersen et al. 1994).

While chemotherapy treatment strategies in good-prognosis patients focus on reducing treatment toxicity, aggressive high-dose chemotherapy (HDC) regimens are becoming increasingly used in poor-prognosis patients since the dose-limiting hematological toxicity can be overcome by autologous stem-cell rescue. The long-term effects of such chemotherapy regimens are important and fertility, as one of these effects, has been investigated (Ishikawa et al. 2004). In this small study the HDC given to 27 testicular cancer patients consisted of 1,250 mg/m$^2$ carboplatin, 1,500 mg/m$^2$ etoposide, and 7.5 g/m$^2$ ifosfamide. Information on gonadal function during follow-up was available for ten of the patients. Spermatogenesis recovered after cessation of HDC in five of ten patients. The mean sperm count in the non-azoospermic group of patients was 42.4 mill/mL. Therefore, despite a high chance of long-term infertility following high-dose platinum-based chemotherapy it is also possible that spermatogenesis may recover.

While some recovery of spermatogenesis is demonstrated by means of standard semen analysis in testicular cancer patients after platinum-based chemotherapy, sperm genomic integrity and its implication on the patient's fertility remain poorly understood. A detrimental effect of cancer and cytotoxic treatment on chromatin condenzation and DNA integrity in spermatozoa has been demonstrated (O'Donovan 2005). In this small study DNA integrity and chromatin condenzation in the spermatozoa of 33 men with cancer (testicular cancer, lymphoma, and leukemia) before and after treatment were assessed and compared to 14 control men with proven fertility. It found that in men with cancer, the percentage of spermatozoa with highly condensed DNA was lower and DNA integrity was less than in the controls both before and after cancer treatment. These findings are important because of the potential effects that impaired chromatin condenzation and DNA integrity may have on fertilization and embryo development. Another small study analyzed sperm chromatin packaging pre- and post-chemotherapy in 22 patients treated for testicular germ cell tumors (Spermon et al. 2006). They observed an improvement in DNA condenzation following chemotherapy but an abnormally high percentage of DNA-damaged sperm in these samples compared to controls. It is clear that despite some recovery following platinum-based chemotherapy the sperm quality does not match that of controls and it remains difficult to outline guidance concerning fertility potential of these patients.

### 21.6.3 Scattered RT

As with chemotherapy, spermatogenesis is adversely affected by radiation. The spermatogonia and spermatocytes are the most radiosensitive cells as they are the most rapidly dividing. Following radiation, any surviving spermatogonial stem cells have to be able both to divide to sustain the pool of stem cells, re-populate the seminiferous tubules, and also differentiate and progress through the spermatogenic cycle to produce mature spermatozoa. Leydig cells are relatively radioresistant.

A recent study of 68 patients compared dogleg radiotherapy including testicular shielding to para-aortic radiotherapy without testicular shielding with regard to the gonadal radiation dose and spermatogenesis at 1-year (Jacobsen et al. 1997). The mean testicular dose was significantly lower with PA strip irradiation at 0.09 Gy compared to 0.32 Gy with dogleg irradiation despite the fact testicular shielding was only used with the dogleg field. The dogleg radiation but not the PA strip irradiation led to a significant reduction in sperm count 1 year after treatment in patients with pre-treatment sperm counts within the normal range. In patients with sperm counts below the normal range prior to radiotherapy no significant further reduction in sperm counts was observed after radiotherapy in either group.

Another study compared the toxicity associated with dogleg radiotherapy and PA strip radiotherapy in 478 men using a mid-plane dose of 30 Gy in 2 Gy fractions (Fossa et al. 1999). In patients with sperm counts within the normal range pre-radiotherapy, the median time to the first post-treatment sperm count within the normal range was 13 months for the PA strip patients and 20 months for the DL patients. In patients with sperm counts below the normal range pre-radiotherapy, the median time to the first sperm count within the normal range was 24 months for the PA patients and 37 months for the DL patients. The difference between the two groups declined with longer follow-up. Reduction in field size from dogleg to para-aortic irradiation has a fertility-saving effect by reducing the length of time for recovery from any transient reduction in sperm count caused.

Unfortunately no data are available comparing long-term gonadal function of early stage seminoma patients treated with adjuvant radiotherapy with stage I seminoma patients followed up with surveillance alone after orchidectomy.

### 21.6.4 Testicular RT for CIS

Patients treated with radiotherapy for carinoma-in-situ (CIS) of the contra-lateral testis to doses of between 14 Gy and 20 Gy are rendered sterile. This is consistent with the known effect of such doses of radiation on the male testes (Sandeman 1966).

## 21.7 Protective Strategies

In the past various approaches have been investigated in an attempt to protect gonadal function from the toxic side effects of radiotherapy and chemotherapy. These approaches have attempted to make gonads quiescent during treatment by interrupting the hypothalamo–pituitary–gonadal axis thereby trying to protect against damage during treatment. For example, administration of luteinizing hormone releasing hormone (LHRH) agonists is able to suppress the pituitary–gonadal axis. The protective effects of LHRH agonists during chemotherapy or irradiation have been investigated in 11 pre-clinical and 4 clinical studies (Kreuser et al. 1993). In only 6 out of 11 pre-clinical models could protection be demonstrated. Disappointingly, in the four subsequent clinical trials no significant influence on severity and duration of germ cell impairment could be demonstrated. The protective effects of other agents have also be studied but so far hormonal manipulations designed to protect gonadal function against damage from chemotherapy and radiotherapy have been disappointing.

## 21.8 Cryopreservation of Semen

Testicular cancer is a malignancy with very good prognosis in most cases and usually affects men in the beginning of their reproductive age. Therefore many of these young men may wish to have children after completion of treatment. Men with testicular cancer often have reduced semen quality even before treatment. Reduction in semen quality following orchidectomy, chemotherapy, and radiotherapy leading to temporary or permanent infertility is well documented. As it is difficult to predict the fertility outcome following such treatment for an individual, it is recommended that cryopreservation of semen to all patients with testicular germ cell tumors is offered prior to treatment (Gandini et al. 2006). This should ideally be prior to surgery as there have been a few reported cases with azoospermia following unilateral orchidectomy in men who had sperm production (Petersen et al. 1999b) prior to orchidectomy. Depending on the quality of semen and the amount of time available it is advantageous to deposit at least two ejaculates for isolation and extracorporal storage of semen. The semen is cryopreserved at −186 °C and can be stored for many years. A considerable number of testicular germ cell tumor patients who do have cryopreservation of their semen are able to achieve fatherhood without the need to use their stored sample but for some patients assisted reproductive techniques with their cryopreserved semen offer the only chance for post-treatment paternity. Furthermore, the psychological impact of pre-treatment cryopreservation can be important for all testicular germ cell tumor patients (Magelssen et al. 2005).

## 21.9 Hypogonadism

Hypogonadism is a clinical syndrome complex defined by a low serum testosterone level and low sperm production. Symptoms include loss of energy, fatigue, depression, anxiety, weight gain, loss of libido, erectile dysfunction, and reduction in muscle mass. Long-term low testosterone levels are also associated with osteoporosis, type II diabetes, and cardiovascular disease.

A few studies have looked into the risk of some of these symptoms and adverse events in patients treated for testicular germ cell tumors. In one of the previously mentioned studies (Huddart et al. 2005) sexuality and quality of life were also assessed and patients treated with chemotherapy and radiotherapy were found to be significantly less interested in sex than patients on surveillance. Additional significant findings include an association of radiotherapy treatment and reduced sexual enjoyment and an association of chemotherapy treatment with worries about fathering children. In this study low testosterone levels were significantly associated with lower quality of life scores for physical, social, role functioning, and global quality of life. Also patients with a low testosterone level had significantly higher average systolic and diastolic blood pressure. The same investigators have also reported a significant association between low testosterone levels in patients treated for germ cell tumor and higher body mass index compared to patients with a normal testosterone level following treatment (Huddart and Norman 2003). They have also observed a twofold or greater risk of developing cardiovascular disease (Huddart et al. 2003)after a median of 10.2 years of follow-up after treatment for testicular germ cell tumor. Similar results are reported in other studies (Jonker-Pool et al. 1997; Wiechno et al. 2007) along with the observed association of retroperitoneal lymph node dissection (RPLND) for residual disease following chemotherapy with erectile dysfunction and dry ejaculation.

The frequency of hypogonadism on long-term follow-up of these patients may be as low as 5% in patients treated with orchidectomy alone (Gerl et al. 2001) but as high as 38% in patients treated with orchidectomy, chemotherapy, and radiotherapy (Huddart et al. 2005). These observations suggest that screening for testicular dysfunction should be a routine part of testicular cancer follow-up care. The screening should include both serum testosterone and serum LH, as increased LH level signals decreased Leydig cell function in spite of normal testosterone. However, careful thought will need to be given to the issue of how one manages any detected hypogonadism. Testosterone can be replaced by a number of routes (e.g., patches, gels, implanted pellets), but the most common are still by intramuscular injections, which when commenced are likely to be lifelong. There is no specific testosterone threshold at which symptoms of hypogonadism occur with each patient having an individual testosterone threshold (Lackner et al. 2007). Hormone supplementation is indicated for the symptomatic patient with obvious sexual dysfunctional problems. The correct management approach for the 'asymptomatic' man with reasonable sexual activity is more difficult. It is likely that decisions on this will have to be individualized after careful patient assessment and discussion of issues, but replacement therapy needs to be considered for this patient group.

## 21.10 Conclusion

The majority of studies mentioned assessing the long-term effects of testicular cancer treatment on fertility have used reproductive hormone levels and semen analysis of sperm quality as surrogate markers of fertility. These markers are relatively simple to obtain and analyze in large numbers. However the degree to which deficiencies in these surrogate markers compromise the ability to father a child is not clear. Fertility is defined by the ability of a sexually active, non-contracepting couple to achieve pregnancy within 1 year (Sherins 1995), and attempting paternity is a better measure for fertility than semen quality (Turek et al. 1998). This is important to bear in mind when assessing many of the studies mentioned in this chapter together with the fact that one quarter of the couples in the general population of industrialized countries attempting conception appears to be sub-fertile (Schmidt et al. 1995).

In view of the increased uptake of semen cryopreservation and the use of assisted reproductive techniques to achieve pregnancies with spermatozoa of poor quality in this patient group, larger and more detailed studies are needed to be performed to assess the incidence of congenital anomalies, miscarriage, and stillbirth in pregnancies achieved using assisted reproduction from the cryopreserved semen of men treated for cancer.

The management of testicular germ cell tumors has changed over the years with increasing knowledge about patterns of disease relapse as well as improving imaging, surgical, and radiotherapy techniques and newer chemotherapy schedules. The goal continues to be maintaining and improving on the cure rate for the disease whilst minimizing long-term toxicity. As far as minimizing the effect of treatment on fertility, new approaches are needed to minimize gonadal toxicity possibly with reduction in number of courses of chemotherapy or dose of radiotherapy, or potentially the use of newer less gonadotoxic drugs. Long-term fertility assessments, including paternity achievement, need to continue to be reported as this provides important information for the counseling and management of these men.

## References


Baker JA et al (2005) Fertility patterns prior to testicular cancer diagnosis. Cancer Causes Control 16(3):295–299

Berthelsen JG, Skakkebaek NE (1983) Gonadal function in men with testis cancer. Fertil Steril 39(1):68–75

Bokemeyer C et al (1996) Evaluation of long-term toxicity after chemotherapy for testicular cancer. J Clin Oncol 14(11): 2923–2932

Bonde JP et al (1998) Relation between semen quality and fertility: a population-based study of 430 first-pregnancy planners. Lancet 352(9135):1172–1177

Brennemann W et al (1997) Gonadal function of patients treated with cisplatin based chemotherapy for germ cell cancer. J Urol 158(3 Pt 1):844–850

Carlsen E et al (2003) History of febrile illness and variation in semen quality. Hum Reprod 18(10):2089–2092

Carroll PR et al (1987) Testicular failure in patients with extragonadal germ cell tumors. Cancer 60(1):108–113

Coffey J et al (2007) Testicular microlithiasis as a familial risk factor for testicular germ cell tumour. Br J Cancer 97(12): 1701–1706

DeSantis M et al (1999) Impact of cytotoxic treatment on long-term fertility in patients with germ-cell cancer. Int J Cancer 83(6):864–865

Doria-Rose VP, Biggs ML, Weiss NS (2005) Subfertility and the risk of testicular germ cell tumors (United States). Cancer Causes Control 16(6):651–656

Drasga RE et al (1983) Fertility after chemotherapy for testicular cancer. J Clin Oncol 1(3):179–183

Einhorn LH, Donohue JP (1977) Improved chemotherapy in disseminated testicular cancer. J Urol 117(1):65–69

Fossa SD et al (1993) Semen quality after treatment for testicular cancer. Eur Urol 23(1):172–176

Fossa SD et al (1999) Optimal planning target volume for stage I testicular seminoma: A Medical Research Council randomized trial. Medical Research Council Testicular Tumor Working Group. J Clin Oncol 17(4):1146

Foster RS et al (1991) Detection of antisperm-antibodies in patients with primary testicular cancer. Int J Androl 14(3): 179–185

Gandini L et al (2006) Effect of chemo- or radiotherapy on sperm parameters of testicular cancer patients. Hum Reprod 21(11):2882–2889

Gerl A et al (2001) The impact of chemotherapy on Leydig cell function in long term survivors of germ cell tumors. Cancer 91(7):1297–1303

Guazzieri S et al (1985) Sperm antibodies and infertility in patients with testicular cancer. Urology 26(2):139–142

Guzick DS et al (2001) Sperm morphology, motility, and concentration in fertile and infertile men. N Engl J Med 345(19): 1388–1393

Hansen SW, Berthelsen JG, von der Maase H (1990) Long-term fertility and Leydig cell function in patients treated for germ cell cancer with cisplatin, vinblastine, and bleomycin versus surveillance. J Clin Oncol 8(10):1695–1698
Ho GT et al (1992) Influence of testicular carcinoma on ipsilateral spermatogenesis. J Urol 148(3):821–825
Hoei-Hansen CE et al (2003) Histological evidence of testicular dysgenesis in contralateral biopsies from 218 patients with testicular germ cell cancer. J Pathol 200(3):370–374
Huddart RA, Norman A (2003) Changes in BMI after treatment of testicular cancer are due to age and hormonal function and not chemotherapy. Br J Cancer 89(6):1143–1144; author reply 1145
Huddart RA et al (2003) Cardiovascular disease as a long-term complication of treatment for testicular cancer. J Clin Oncol 21(8):1513–1523
Huddart RA et al (2005) Fertility, gonadal and sexual function in survivors of testicular cancer. Br J Cancer 93(2):200–207
Ishikawa T, Kamidono S, Fujisawa M (2004) Fertility after high-dose chemotherapy for testicular cancer. Urology 63(1): 137–140
Jacobsen KD et al (1997) External beam abdominal radiotherapy in patients with seminoma stage I: field type, testicular dose, and spermatogenesis. Int J Radiat Oncol Biol Phys 38(1):95–102
Jacobsen R et al (2000) Risk of testicular cancer in men with abnormal semen characteristics: cohort study. BMJ 321(7264): 789–792
Jacobsen KD, Theodorsen L, Fossa SD (2001) Spermatogenesis after unilateral orchiectomy for testicular cancer in patients following surveillance policy. J Urol 165(1):93–96
Jonker-Pool G et al (1997) Sexual functioning after treatment for testicular cancer: comparison of treatment modalities. Cancer 80(3):454–464
Kreuser ED, Klingmuller D, Thiel E (1993) The role of LHRH-analogues in protecting gonadal functions during chemotherapy and irradiation. Eur Urol 23(1):157–163; discussion 163–164
Lackner JE et al (2007) Hypogonadism and androgen deficiency symptoms in testicular cancer survivors. Urology 69(4):754–758
Lampe H et al (1997) Fertility after chemotherapy for testicular germ cell cancers. J Clin Oncol 15(1):239–245
Magelssen H et al (2005) Twenty years experience with semen cryopreservation in testicular cancer patients: who needs it? Eur Urol 48(5):779–785
Meirow D, Schenker JG (1995) Cancer and male infertility. Hum Reprod 10(8):2017–2022
Meyts ER (2006) Developmental model for the pathogenesis of testicular carcinoma in situ: genetic and environmental aspects. Hum Reprod Update 12(3):303–323
O'Donovan M (2005) An evaluation of chromatin condensation and DNA integrity in the spermatozoa of men with cancer before and after therapy. Andrologia 37(2–3):83–90
Ohl DA, Sonksen J (1996) What are the chances of infertility and should sperm be banked? Semin Urol Oncol 14(1):36–44
Petersen PM et al (1994) Dose-dependent impairment of testicular function in patients treated with cisplatin-based chemotherapy for germ cell cancer. Ann Oncol 5(4):355–358
Petersen PM et al (1998) Gonadal function in men with testicular cancer. Semin Oncol 25(2):224–233
Petersen PM et al (1999a) Semen quality and reproductive hormones before orchiectomy in men with testicular cancer. J Clin Oncol 17(3):941–947
Petersen PM et al (1999b) Semen quality and reproductive hormones before and after orchiectomy in men with testicular cancer. J Urol 161(3):822–826
Petersen PM et al (2002) Effect of graded testicular doses of radiotherapy in patients treated for carcinoma-in-situ in the testis. J Clin Oncol 20(6):1537–1543
Richiardi L, Akre O (2005) Fertility among brothers of patients with testicular cancer. Cancer Epidemiol Biomarkers Prev 14(11 Pt 1):2557–2562
Sakamoto H et al (2007) Testicular sperm extraction in patients with persistent azoospermia after chemotherapy for testicular germ cell tumor. Int J Urol 14(2):167–170
Sandeman TF (1966) The effects of x irradiation on male human fertility. Br J Radiol 39(468):901–907
Schmidt L, Munster K, Helm P (1995) Infertility and the seeking of infertility treatment in a representative population. Br J Obstet Gynaecol 102(12):978–984
Sherins RJ (1995) Are semen quality and male fertility changing? N Engl J Med 332(5):327–328
Skakkebaek NE, Rajpert-De Meyts E, Main KM (2001) Testicular dysgenesis syndrome: an increasingly common developmental disorder with environmental aspects. Hum Reprod 16(5):972–978
Spermon JR et al (2006) Sperm integrity pre- and post-chemotherapy in men with testicular germ cell cancer. Hum Reprod 21(7):1781–1786
Turek PJ, Lowther DN, Carroll PR (1998) Fertility issues and their management in men with testis cancer. Urol Clin North Am 25(3):517–531
Wiechno P et al (2007) The quality of life and hormonal disturbances in testicular cancer survivors in Cisplatin era. Eur Urol 52(5):1448–1454
Williams SD et al (1987) Treatment of disseminated germ-cell tumors with cisplatin, bleomycin, and either vinblastine or etoposide. N Engl J Med 316(23):1435–1440
World Health Organisation (1999) WHO laboratory manual for the examination of human semen and sperm-cervical mucus interaction, 4th edn. Cambridge University Press, Cambridge

# Follow-Up After Primary Treatment 22

Vassilios Tzortzis, M. Pilar Laguna Pes, and Jerome P. Richie

## 22.1 Introduction

With overall cure rates superior to 95% in early stages and to 80% for metastatic disease, testicular germ cell tumor (TGCT) is unique among urologic malignancies and is considered the model for curable cancer. Factors contributing to this high cure rate are effective diagnoses, accurate staging, effective early treatment based on chemotherapeutic combinations, radiotherapy and surgery when necessary and a strict follow-up.

Creation of well-organized and cost-effective follow-up schedules for patients treated for cancer is important from both medical and socioeconomic perspectives. In spite of the fact that relatively little information exists on the value of follow-up of asymptomatic patients after potentially curative therapy, testis cancer is an excellent model for postorchidectomy or curative therapy surveillance (Edelman et al. 1997).

## 22.2 Rationale for Follow-Up

Early detection and efficient treatment of recurrences are the major reasons for maintaining a follow-up schedule. Relapses may be salvageable with a combination of further chemotherapy and surgery, and studies suggest that around 50% of patients who relapse after primary treatment will be cured, depending on the pattern of relapse and the stage at detection (Fossa et al. 1999a; Huddart and Birtle 2005). It is recognized that most of the recurrences occur in the first 2 years (98.5%) and late relapses (occurring greater than 2 years or later after successful treatment) may have a greater propensity for chemoresistance and confer a worse prognosis (Shahidi et al. 2002a; Ronnen et al. 2005a).

In addition to the early detection of the recurrences, the concern of a follow-up protocol in this particular neoplasm (the highest cure rate among solid tumors) is to detect a metachronous contralateral carcinoma of the testis, second primary cancers, and secondary and late effects of the treatment (cardiovascular toxicity, neuropathy, psychological morbidity related to germ cell cancer or its therapy and infertility).

Today, there is no universally accepted standard follow-up protocol for patients with testicular cancer. Prospective studies to evaluate follow-up policies have not been performed even though a great deal of time and economical resources is spent. To study the efficacy of different follow-up policies, a randomized trial should be performed. However, such a trial would require substantial compliance from both physicians and patients over a long period (5–10 years) while less-intensive strategies may be considered not safe for the patients. The only study with high level of evidence currently available is the RCT of Rustin et al. comparing two different retroperitoneal CT scan schedules (3 vs. 5) during the first 2 years of follow-up in patients with Stage I NSGCT on surveillance (Rustin et al. 2007).

In general, the following considerations may be applied for the selection of an appropriate schedule and testing in the follow-up of testis tumor:

- The results of therapy are dependent on the bulk of disease; thus, an intensive strategy to detect presymptomatic disease may be justifiable.
- Most recurrences after curative therapy will occur in the first 2 years; consequently, surveillance

M.P. Laguna (✉)
Department of Urology, AMC University Hospital, Amsterdam, The Netherlands

M.P. Laguna et al. (eds.), *Cancer of the Testis*,
DOI: 10.1007/978-1-84800-370-5_22, © Springer-Verlag London Limited 2010

should be most frequent and intensive during this time.

- Although less frequent, late relapses can occur beyond 5 years and therefore yearly follow-up for life may be advocated in some stages and histological types.
- After RPLND, relapse in the retroperitoneum is rare and the most likely site of recurrence is the chest.
- The value of chest X-ray (CXR) has been recently questioned in the follow-up of patients with disseminated disease after complete remission.
- CT of the chest has a higher predictive value than CXR; however, the radiation exposure is greater.
- After chemotherapy or radiotherapy, a long-term risk for the development of secondary malignancies and serious comorbidities exists.
- Contemporary follow-up schedules should balance an optimal detection (type of test and timing) while minimizing radiation exposure risk.

## 22.3 Diagnostic Tests in Follow-Up

Diagnostic tests should be performed with a frequency and duration consistent with the nature of the risk and should include only tests with high-positive and -negative predictive values. Diagnostic tests in the follow-up of the patients with testicular cancer include physical examination, serum tumor markers and radiological imaging.

1. *Physical examination* consists of clinical assessment of the neck, supraclavicular fossa, inguinal region, scrotum and contralateral testis. Testis examination seems to be sufficient for detecting contralateral tumors and therefore must be recommended lifelong. The finding of a palpable mass in a nodal region as first sign of relapse is very rare, limiting the importance of physical examination (Khadra and Oakeshott 2002).
2. Measurements of the s*erum tumor markers* β-HCG and AFP are of crucial significance in the follow-up, although they do not obviate the need for clinical and imaging assessment. Beta-HCG and/or AFP are elevated at relapse in about 2/3 of NSGCT and approximately 1/3 of seminomas (Bosl and Motzer 1997). Trigo et al. found HCG and AFP elevated as first indicators in 40% of NSGCTs and 25% of seminoma patients (Trigo et al. 2000). Recent findings (Venkitaraman et al. 2007) suggest that although LDH is vital in the prognosis of metastatic disease and thus should be routinely included, its use in detecting relapses is questionable because of the increased false-positive finding. However, it was suggested that the s-LD-1 isoform might be more specific for TGCT and be a more precise tumor marker (von Eyben et al. 2001). Nonmalignant causes of persistently elevated levels of both AFP and β-HCG may be considered and false-positive causes of tumor marker elevation should be excluded before subjecting patients to adjuvant therapy. Liver impairment secondary to drugs (chemotherapy, anesthetics or antiepileptics), hepatitis and alcohol abuse may all lead to an elevated AFP level. Furthermore, persistent HCG elevations may be caused by hypogonadism and marijuana use.
3. *Radiological tests*. The available literature on the value of CXR in the follow-up of patients with testicular cancer is controversial. Several series based on their observations, that an abnormal chest radiograph is rarely the only indicator of recurrent disease, have proposed that routine chest radiographs are unnecessary (Gels et al. 1995; Sharir et al. 1999). Buchholz et al. reported the lack of value of CXR during posttreatment surveillance after radiation therapy for low-stage seminoma (Buchholz et al. 1998). Similar findings have been reported in patients with advanced stage NSTC who achieved a complete response after chemotherapy and surgical resection of a residual mass (Gietemsa et al. 2002). On the contrary, Colls et al. found that among 248 patients under surveillance, approximately 5% of recurrences were detected by chest radiograph alone (Colls et al. 1999a). Furthermore, Harvey et al. found that all pulmonary relapses were easily visible on CXR, and patients with intrathoracic disease had at least one other indicator of relapse (elevated serum marker/other disease site) and there is no evidence to suggest that relapses would have been detected at an earlier stage with the addition of chest CT to the surveillance protocol (Harvey et al. 2002).

For the evaluation of the mediastinum and lungs, CT is more sensitive than plain X-ray, although, nodules of <1 cm may present as false-positive finding. Thoracic relapses in NSCCT are usually marker-positive, and the great majority of GCTs that relapse will have significant disease burden outside the chest (Oldenburg et al. 2006). Chest CT may pick up small marker-negative lesions not visible on CXR, but it is uncertain if the detection of such small lesions is likely to have prognostic significance (Martin et al. 2007).

Abdominal CT with oral and intravenous contrast media is mandatory, although false-negative findings can occur because of the inability of this modality to detect foci of disease in normal-sized nodes or to differentiate benign and malignant enlargement. It has been shown that, by using 10–15 mm as the upper limit of normal, up to 44% of scans were false-negative (Richie et al. 1982; Rowland et al. 1982). For practical purposes then, a cutoff of 10 mm is used. Nodes measuring between 8 and 10 mm are considered suspicious (Dalal et al. 2006).

While pelvic CT forms an integral part of initial staging, routinely scanning of the pelvis as part of the follow-up is controversial. Although there is no firm evidence, there is an assumed increased risk of pelvic lymph node disease following scrotal violation, and, for this reason, a pelvic CT may be included in the follow-up protocol on those scarce cases of primary scrotal violation (White et al. 1997). The removal of routine pelvic CT scanning from surveillance programs significantly reduces patient radiation exposure and has led to a substantial resource saving.

Pelvic CT scan alone is also recommended in those patients with Stage I seminoma treated with radiation therapy limited to the para-aortic (PA) and interaortocaval field.

Several retrospective studies have suggested improved diagnostic accuracy of FDG-PET scan compared with CT imaging in a range of settings (de Wit et al. 2005; Hoh et al. 1998). In a Danish study, 70% of patients with normal-sized nodes who subsequently developed relapse could be identified at presentation by the use of PET. The negative predictive value of PET was 92% (Lassen et al. 2003). Huddart et al. found a higher than expected relapse rate on surveillance in FDG-PET negative patients and suggest that $^{18}$FDG-PET scanning is not sufficiently sensitive to identify patients at low risk of relapse in this setting (Huddart et al. 2007). Some authors reported that the use of PET in the evaluation of retroperitoneal lymph nodes and radiographic abnormalities after chemotherapy presents no apparent advantage over CT, mainly because neither PET nor CT have the ability to detect microscopic nodal disease. The cause of most false-negative findings has to be seen in the insufficient differentiation between adult teratoma and tumor necrosis in patients with nonseminomatous testicular cancer (Cremerius et al. 1999; Ganjoo et al. 1999).

$^{18}$FDG-PET scanning, however, is recommended in the case of seminoma postchemotherapy retroperitoneal mass of ≥3 cm (De Santis et al. 2004).

MRI does not provide any additional information and must be offered in patients to whom intravenous contrast media cannot be given. The only advantage is the avoidance of radiation in young patients (Hogeboom et al. 1993). The value of MRI may be further enhanced in the future by the use of ultramagnetic small paramagnetic iron oxide (USPIO) contrast agents (Bellin et al. 1998).

## 22.4 Follow-Up Schedules

In testis cancer, follow-up schedules are tailored to tumor type and treatment policy. This consideration is of capital importance in Stage I and in low-bulk Stage II disease for both seminoma and NSGCT. In those stages, different postorchidectomy treatment policies may be chosen not only depending on the presence or absence of risk factors (for Stage I) but also driven by the centers or country preferences.

Although the different treatment policies result in similar cure rates in low stages and in general most of the recurrences present during the first 2 years after curative treatment, the sites of recurrence may vary depending on whether a local or systemic approach were taken. Consequently, for a proper understanding of follow-up schedules data on recurrence risk is mandatory.

Frequency and type of examinations depend on the estimated risk of relapse and treatment strategy. Currently, no unanimous guidelines exist and there is a lack of clear consensus on how to follow-up patients after the first treatment approach. While most of the guidelines agree on the type of examination to be performed, important variation exists in the frequency of the examinations not only for the different treatment policies, which is logical and related to the risk and timing of recurrence, but also for the same treatment policy among the different guidelines.

For the purposes of the present chapter, a review of the literature and online guidelines on follow-up has been performed. The eight more detailed and broadly available guidelines or recommendations were selected for analysis and listed in addendum I (Albers et al. 2008a; van As et al. 2008; Huddart and Kataja 2008a, b; Motzer et al. 2008; www ocsyd se; wwwtcrc acor org; www bccancer bc ca; Segal et al. 2001). The Cancer Care Ontario described only follow-up for early stage NSGCT in surveillance (Segal et al. 2001) and the Princess Margaret Hospital guidelines were already included in the TCRC guidelines. Although all the guidelines state the minimum times a given test is recommended during follow-up, a wide variation in schedules exists. As the evidence in the subject is low, no schedule can be chosen over another except for the frequency of abdominopelvic CT scan in Stage I NSGCT in surveillance (Rustin et al. 2007). For this reason, frequency of the tests to be performed will be expressed in a range per year.

## 22.4.1 Seminoma

### 22.4.1.1 Stage I Seminoma

It is estimated that 70–80% of seminomas present with clinical Stage I disease at diagnosis. In 15–20% of the cases, there is nodal involvement (radiological confirmation) at the level of the retroperitoneum and only 5% of patients present with distant metastasis (Groll et al. 2007). Approximately 30% present with elevation of β-hCG at diagnosis or in the course of the disease. Consequently, in most cases, measurement of blood markers will not be a reliable test for follow-up (McCaffrey et al. 1998). Postorchidectomy treatment options in Stage I seminoma are retroperitoneal radiotherapy, surveillance and a neoadjuvant single cycle of carboplatin chemotherapy.

#### Recurrence After Postorchidectomy Adjuvant Radiotherapy

Low doses of radiotherapy (20–24 Gy) limited to the retroperitoneal or the hockey stick field achieve an overall survival rate of approximately 99% at 5–10 years (Fossa et al. 1999b; Melchior et al. 2001). Relapse rates range from 3 to 4% and recurrence typically occurs outside the irradiated area. The commonest site of recurrence is at the supradiaphragmatic lymph nodes, mediastinum, lungs or bones. In a small proportion of cases, the tumor will relapse in the inguinal or external iliac nodes (Livsey et al. 2001). Most common time of recurrences presentation is within 18 months after treatment, although late relapses have also been described. Owing to the extremely low risk of relapse after 5 years (approaching 0%), follow-up beyond 5 years may be unnecessary after radiotherapy (Shahidi et al. 2002b).

#### Recurrence After Postorchidectomy Adjuvant Chemotherapy

One or two courses of carboplatin is an effective alternative treatment in Stage I seminoma. The relapse rate is less than 2%, but the number of patients treated in a prospective setting is still low and the length of follow-up is also limited in most studies. In general, this treatment is well tolerated, with only mild, acute and intermediate-term toxicity (Oliver et al. 2005). A disadvantage of adjuvant chemotherapy is that unlike following radiotherapy, continued surveillance of the retroperitoneum is mandatory.

#### Recurrence During Postorchidectomy Surveillance

At least 80% of patients with seminoma Stage I will be overtreated if an active treatment is given prophylactically. The risk of relapse at 5 years after surveillance ranges between 15 and 20% (Chung et al. 2002). Nevertheless, there is no increased risk of death. The median time to relapse ranges from 12 to 18 months, but up to 29% of relapses can develop later. The sites of relapse are the PA lymph nodes in up to 82% of cases; pelvic lymph nodes, inguinal nodes and lungs can also be affected (Warde and Jewett 1998). Owing to the high and often late rate of relapse, close and active follow-up is mandatory for at least 5 years. Some authors recommend a 10-year follow-up (van As et al. 2008).

#### Follow-Up Schedules for Seminoma Stage I

Very recently, the European Consensus Conference on Diagnosis and Treatment of Germ Cell Cancer (EGCCCG), based on the study of Martin et al. (Martin

**Table 22.1** Variations in the number of times a test is performed during follow-up in the different schedules for seminoma Stage I in postorchidectomy surveillance and postorchidectomy adjuvant chemotherapy or radiotherapy

| | Year 1 | Year 2 | Year 3 | Year 4 | Year 5 | Year 6–10 |
|---|---|---|---|---|---|---|
| Physical examination | 3–5 | 2–4 | 1–4 | 1–2 | 1–2 | 0–1 |
| Tumor markers | 3–6 | 2–6 | 1–4 | 1–2 | 1–2 | 0–1 |
| Chest X-ray | 2–6 | 1–6 | 1–2 | 1–2 | 1–2 | 0–1 |
| Abdominopelvic CT scan | 1–4 | 1–4 | 0–4 | 0–2 | 0–2 | 0–1[a] |

Frequency is expressed in times per year. Sources: EAU, ESMO, NCCN, RMH, SWENOTECA, TCRC and BCCA guidelines
[a]See remarks in Table 22.2 against NCCN on CT years 4–7

et al. 2007), created recommendations for the frequency of follow-up visits and the diagnostic imaging procedures based on the treatment chosen and the resulting pattern of relapse for seminoma Stage I. Surveillance is the only strategy that has an annual hazard rate of relapse >5%; consequently, follow-up visits every 4 months for the first 2 years is recommended. For the third and fourth year, the annual hazard is between 1 and 5% and the visits can be set every 6 months. In the period from 5 to 10 years, the annual hazard is between 0.3 and 1% and the follow-up appointments can be reduced to once per year. Relapses more than 10 years on surveillance are extremely rare and the follow-up can be ended. After radiotherapy, the annual hazard rate of relapse is between 1 and 5% and six monthly visits are recommended for the first to third year. For the fourth to sixth year, the hazard rate is 0.3–1% and the visits can be reduced to once per year. After 6 years the annual hazard rate of relapse is below 0.3% and the follow-up can be ended. There is a limited experience with the use of carboplatin and recommendation can be made only for the first 3 years. The annual hazard rate for this period is 1–5% and the follow-up visits must be set every 6 months. There is little evidence to provide guidance for the investigations required. Clinically assessable regions such as the neck, supraclavicular fossa, inguinal region, scrotum and contralateral testis should be examined at every visit. If the relapse risk for failure is >1%, CT of the pelvis and/or abdomen must be performed. To detect chest relapses, a CXR rather than chest CT it is recommended, given the lower radiation dose and lack of evidence of a significant impact on prognosis of discovering metastases at an earlier stage. For surveillance and adjuvant carboplatin strategies, a CXR at alternating visits initially, and then annually when the hazard rate is <1%, would reflect the lower risk of relapse at this site. Given the low frequency of an isolated pelvic relapse on surveillance, a similar intermittent approach with pelvic CT imaging would also be reasonable. This may also be the case with adjuvant carboplatin, although details are lacking in published results to date to allow this recommendation to be evidence-based (Krege et al. 2008).

Variations in the minimal number of each test performed per year according to the different guidelines consulted are displayed in Table 22.1. Frequency of the testis is, in general, in the lower range after postorchidectomy radiotherapy and in the higher range in the surveillance policy. Specific remarks for the different policies are described in Table 22.2. Of note some guidelines with broad diffusion recommend the same follow-up schedule and test frequency irrespective of the policy after orchidectomy.

#### 22.4.1.2 Seminoma Stage IIa/b

##### Treatment and Recurrence

There is considerable variability in the treatment of the Stage IIa/b seminoma. In Stage IIa, radiotherapy remains the preferred treatment option over chemotherapy. In Stage IIb, chemotherapy with three cycles of standard-dose bleomycin, etoposide and cisplatin (BEP), or four cycles of etoposide (EP), represents a treatment alternative to radiotherapy, particularly in patients with larger multinodal retroperitoneal disease, although there may be a higher risk of acute toxicity (Patterson et al. 2001). With modern radiation techniques, relapse-free survival at 6 years for Stage IIa is 95%. In fact, patients with Stage II (N1) disease have

**Table 22.2** Remarks on follow-up of seminoma Stage I according to EAU, RMH, NCCN, ESMO, SWENOTECA, TCRC and BCCA guidelines

| Guidelines | Remarks |
|---|---|
| EAU | A single follow-up schedule is recommended for the three treatment options |
| RMH | In the surveillance policy, Pelvic CT only if scrotal violation or previous pelvic surgery. Follow-up recommended until 10 yearsIn adjuvant radiotherapy CT abdomen only on clinical indication. Pelvic CT not recommended on third and fourth year. Follow-up not recommended after fifth year<br>In adjuvant chemotherapy (single agent carboplatin), physical examination and tumor markers recommended in the first year at months: 1,3,6,9 and 12. Pelvic CT scan only if scrotal violation or previous pelvic surgery. CT scan abdomen is not recommended on third and fourth year. Follow-up recommended until year tenth |
| NCCN | In adjuvant radiotherapy, only pelvic CT scan recommended during the first 3 years. Follow-up recommended until fifth year Owing to low morbidity of radiation, surveillance is often not recommended in Stage I seminoma, except for patients at high risk (horseshoe or pelvic kidney, inflammatory bowel disease or prior radiotherapy)<br>In surveillance of adjuvant chemotherapy, follow-up is recommended up to 10 years with chest X-ray (CXR) in alternative visits<br>In both policies, controls every 6 months from year 4 to 7 with CT scan every visit<br>An intense imaging and markers follow-up is recommended during the first 3 years |
| ESMO | A unique schedule is recommended irrespective of the treatment policy Physical examination and markers are performed the first year at month 1 and then every 3 months<br>Pelvic CT is recommended in patients treated with adjuvant radiotherapy and abdominal CT in patients treated with adjuvant Carboplatin<br>CT scan (pelvic or abdominal) not performed on third and fourth year |
| SWENOTECA | Two different follow-up schedules, one for surveillance or adjuvant Carboplatin or metastatic seminoma and another one for postorchidectomy radiotherapy in Stage I. In the follow-up for metastatic seminoma retroperitoneum is followed four times in case of residual tumor<br>Follow-up schedule lasts for 6 years in postorchidectomy radiotherapy.<br>After radiotherapy if PA, pelvic examination once per year and abdominal at 24 months; if hockey stick abdominal and pelvic at month 24 |
| TCRC | A very detailed follow-guideline depending on type of treatment including Princess Margaret Hospital guidelines Princess Margaret Hospital guidelines for seminoma Stage I in surveillance recommend CXR every 8 months during years 1–3. Years 4–7 no tumor markers are recommended and CXR once a year. Physical examination and abdominal CT scan is recommended twice a year during years 4–7. Regarding follow-up years 8–10, no tumor markers are performed and CXR, physical examination and abdominal CT scan once a year<br>Princess Margaret Hospital guidelines for seminoma Stage I after radiotherapy includes the same schedule as for surveillance but CT scan is not recommended from years 4 to 10 |
| BCCA | Abdominopelvic CT scan is recommended every 24 months during years 7–10 If high-risk seminoma Stage I in surveillance protocol, CXR and abdominopelvic CT scan are recommended three times a year during the first 2 years<br>The follow-up schedule is less stringent after radiotherapy with only tumor markers and CXR twice a year during the first 2 years. Abdominal CT scan is performed once a year |

enjoyed survival rates above 90%, which statistically do not differ from those of patients with Stage I disease (Arranz Arija et al. 2001).

Table 22.3 describes the variations in the follow-up schedules among guidelines (Albers et al. 2008a; van As et al. 2008; Huddart and Kataja 2008a, b; Motzer et al. 2008; www ocsyd se) for Stage IIa–b seminoma treated by postorchidectomy radiotherapy. Owing to the scarcity of this group of patients, no clear follow-up guidelines can be formulated but a similar strategy to the one recommended for Stage I after radiotherapy seems reasonable. Specific remarks on the different guidelines can be found in Table 22.4. Variations in follow-up schedules of seminoma Stage IIa–b treated

**Table 22.3** Variations in the number of times a test is performed during follow-up in the different schedules for seminoma Stage IIa–b radiotherapy (in times per year)

| | Year 1 | Year 2 | Years 3–4 | Year 5 | Years 5–10 |
|---|---|---|---|---|---|
| Physical examination | 3–4 | 3–4 | 2–4* | 1–2 | 1* |
| Tumor markers | 3–6 | 3–4 | 2–4* | 1–2 | 1* |
| Chest X-ray | 2[a]–6 | 1–4 | 0–4* | 1 | 0 or 1* |
| Abdominal CT scan | 2[a]–4 | 0–2 | 0 or 1 | 0 or 1 | 0 or 1* |

Sources: EAU, RMH, NCCN, ESMO, SWENOTECA and TCRC

[a]At third and twelfth months

*Per year

**Table 22.4** Remarks on follow-up seminoma Stage II a–b radiotherapy according to EAU, RMH, NCCN, ESMO, SWENOTECA and TCRC guidelines

| Guidelines | Remarks |
|---|---|
| EAU | EAU recommends a simplified follow-up schedule for Stages II and advanced seminoma, irrespective of adjuvant treatment modality<br>If postchemotherapy evaluation shows any mass >3 cm, CT scan abdomen should be repeated 2–4 months later to ensure mass regression. FDG-PET scan must be performed if available<br>A chest CT is indicated if abnormality is detected on CXR and after pulmonary resection<br>In patients with headaches, focal neurological findings or any central nervous system, brain CT has to be performed |
| RMH | Pelvic CT only in scrotum violation or previous pelvic surgery in adjuvant radiation |
| NCCN | Abdominopelvic CT scan at month fourth of first year only, when no residual mass and normal tumor markers<br>If residual mass and normal tumor markers PET scan is preferable as results may alter the management<br>A strict follow-up with physical examination, tumor markers and CXR three or four times on third year. On fourth year only twice<br>No follow-up mentioned after year 5 |
| ESMO | Only one schedule for seminoma Stages II a–c and III. No follow-up mentioned after year 5<br>If normal posttreatment CT scan, abdomino pelvic CT is recommend once a year on year 1, 2 and 5<br>If abnormal posttreatment CT scan, it should be repeated every 6 months until normal or abnormalities stabilized. A PET scan may help to identify patients who have residual cancer active cancer. Consider biopsy or resection for large residual or growing masses |
| SWENOTECA | Swenoteca has a single follow-up schedule for seminoma in surveillance , adjuvant carboplatinum or metastatic seminoma. This schedule prolongs until 10 years<br>The only variation includes four times retroperitoneal scanning instead of three in case of residual tumor |
| TCRC | Two follow-up schedules are recommended. In one of them ( Nichols) tumor markers and CXR are performed 12 times the first year, six times the second year, two times years 3–5 and afterwards once a year. CT scan is not mentioned<br>In the Princess Margaret Hospital schedule, no tumor markers are recommended years 4–7 but CXR is performed twice during these years. Years 8–10 no tumor markers but CXR recommended once a year. CT scan is not mentioned |

by chemotherapy will be included with more advanced seminoma (Stage IIc–IV) as it has been proposed by the Royal Marsden Hospital, the NCCN, ESMO, SWENOTECA, TCRC and EAU (Albers et al. 2008a; van As et al. 2008; Huddart and Kataja 2008a; Motzer et al. 2008; www ocsyd se; wwwtcrc acor org) (Tables 22.5 and 22.6).

#### 22.4.1.3 Seminoma Stage IIc and III

##### Treatment and Recurrence

For patients with Stage IIc disease treated by radiation therapy alone, approximately half of patients develop metastatic disease outside the treated fields.

**Table 22.5** Variations in the follow-up of seminoma Stage IIa–b and IIC to IV after chemotherapy. Frequency expressed in number of times per year

| | Year 1 | Year 2 | Years 3–4 | Year 5 |
|---|---|---|---|---|
| Physical examination | 3–6 | 3–4 | 2–3[a] | 1–2[a] |
| Tumor markers | 6 | 3 or 4 | 2–3[a] | 1 or 2[a] |
| Chest X-ray | 3–6 | 1–4 | 0–3 | 1 |
| Abdominopelvic CT scan[b] | 0–3 | 0–3 | 0–2 | 0 or 1 |

Sources: EAU, RMH, NCCN, ESMO, SWENOTECA and TCRC guidelines

[a]Per year

[b]Until CR with or without surgery

**Table 22.6** Remarks on follow-up seminoma after chemotherapy (Stages II a–b and IIc–IV). According to EAU, RMH, NCCN, ESMO, SWENOTECA and TCRC guidelines

| Guidelines | Remarks |
|---|---|
| EAU | Abdominopelvic CT scan once a year after fifth year<br>A unique follow-up schema for advanced seminoma and nonseminoma<br>A chest CT is indicated if abnormality is detected on CXR and after pulmonary resection<br>In patients with headaches, focal neurological findings or any central nervous system, brain CT has to be performed |
| RMH | Pelvic CT only in scrotum violation or previous pelvic surgery<br>In Stage IIa–IV, after chemotherapy a more intensive physical examination, TM and CXR during the first year (six times)<br>CT scan until CR with or without surgery. Frequency of CT scan determine by MDT<br>Late effects (clinical examination, blood pressure, height and weight assessed at 2, 5 and 10 years<br>Discharge after 5 years |
| NCCN | The most stringent schedule with physical examination, tumor markers and CXR three times on the third year and twice on fourth year<br>Abdominopelvic CT scan to be performed at fourth month of year 1 status postsurgery. Otherwise abdominal pelvic CT scan every 3 months until stable |
| ESMO | Physical examination and CXR are performed the first month and then every 3 months during the first year<br>If abnormal posttreatment CT scan, repeat CT scan every 6 months until normal or abnormalities stabilized. A PET scan may help to identify patients who have residual active cancer<br>Consider biopsy or resection for large, residual or growing masses |
| SWENOTECA | The same follow-up schedule for surveillance, adjuvant carboplatin or metastatic seminoma, with physical examination only three times the first year and four times retroperitoneal exploration if residual tumor during the first year. Also follow-up is prolonged up to 10 years |
| TCRC | Only follow schedules for seminoma Stage I and III treated by chemotherapy<br>No frequency of abdominal CT scan mentioned |

Cisplatin-based chemotherapy has been found to be highly effective against disseminated testicular seminoma. More than 90% of patients who present with Stage III disease achieve a complete response to chemotherapy alone, and approximately 90% of the responders remain disease-free during follow-up evaluation up to 4 years (de Wit et al. 2001). With large volume seminoma, a residual mass may be found following chemotherapy. In most cases, this represents fibrotic scar tissue which can be resolved in time, but if it is larger than 3 cm, the probability of an active malignancy is higher (Puc et al. 1996). Data suggests that 80% of patients with active disease can be identified on PET scan and this test should be performed in case of masses ≥3 cm, 4–6 weeks after chemotherapy (De Santis et al. 2004). Van As et al. suggest that following

PET a CT scans must be performed at regular intervals (6 monthly to annually) until complete response or stabilization of the mass. When this is achieved, the low rate of relapse makes further scanning unnecessary (van As et al. 2008).

Current guidelines for follow-up of patients with metastatic seminoma are based on observational and case studies and differ among the different centers and societies. Although, this fact precludes a high level of evidence-based guidelines, this is the best available evidence to date. Variations in follow-up schedules are reported in Tables 22.5 and 22.6.

## 22.4.2 Nonseminomatous Germ Cell Testis Cancer (NSGCT)

### 22.4.2.1 NSGCT Stage I

The majority of patients presenting with NSGCT will have no evidence of disease beyond the testis (Stage I disease). Up to 20–30% of the pathologically defined low-risk patients and 35–50% of high-risk patients (mainly vascular and lymphatic invasion) will experience relapse. Relapses occur in the retroperitoneum (54–78%) and in the lung (13–31%), and very rarely in more than one visceral organ (Klepp et al. 1990). A risk-depended treatment is applied and three major strategies have evolved to deal with recurrence risk: surveillance and treatment at relapse, adjuvant retroperitoneal lymph node dissection (RPLND) with or without adjuvant chemotherapy in case of pathological positive nodes and adjuvant chemotherapy. If treatment is performed correctly, the cure rate should be 99% regardless of the management chosen.

#### Recurrence During Postorchidectomy Surveillance

The main rationale for surveillance is that salvage therapy is highly successful and chemotherapy can be spared to a considerable number of patients. The results of a surveillance policy depend upon a careful preoperative staging procedure (define risks factors), and intensive follow-up management in highly motivated patients. NSGCTs are suitable for a surveillance policy because most of them produce serological tumor markers and the time within which relapse occurs can be predicted. In particular, 80% of the relapses will occur in the first 12 months after orchidectomy and approximately 12% during the second year (Read et al. 1992). The median time to relapse is 6 months (range 1–62 months), but relapses after 3–5 years, and even later, may still occur, with an annual rate of 4% (Oliver et al. 2004). Approximately 20% of metastases will occur in the retroperitoneum and 10% in the mediastinum and lungs (Colls et al. 1999b). Historically, an intensive follow-up protocol with a serial abdominopelvic CT scan was performed with the intention to diagnose better prognosis disease at relapse.

An analysis on the follow-up intervals in Stage I NSGCT in surveillance has been performed by Segal et al. (Segal et al. 2006). Relapse rate varied in the 18 studies included between 23 and 36% at a median follow-up of 74 months. Pooled median relapse time was 6 months. In almost all the studies, clinical examination and tumor markers were performed monthly during the first year while abdominopelvic CT scan intervals varied between 2 and 3 months. In the second year of follow-up, there were more differences in the frequency of visits, serological and radiological investigations with some schedules skiping abdominopelvic CT scans. There was little variation in the measured outcomes associated with the frequency of CT scans during the first year of surveillance. Although the frequency of CT scans did not seem to influence outcome beyond 2 years of follow-up, there was still a 3% risk of abdominal recurrences after 2 years and the available data showed a small but significantly worse outcome by discontinuing abdominal imaging after 2 years. On the basis of this data, on the fact that 15% of the recurrences presented with negative tumor markers and that the prognosis was significantly improved when the recurrent abdominal masses were nonpalpable, they propose that an aggressive follow-up schedule including abdominopelvic CTs can every 3 or 4 months during the first year and every 4 months during the second year. Two CT scans were recommended in the third year and once a year in the fourth and fifth year.

More recently, the unique randomized MRC TE08 trial supports a lack of benefit of frequent CT scans during the first years and recommends a CT at 3 and 12 months only. In addition, they support that the omission of chest CTs may be safe. From their data, it is also clear that relapse after 5 years is so infrequent that the follow-up may be discontinued at this point (Rustin et al. 2007). In a pool analysis of Groll et al., late relapses were 2%; today, most clinicians discharge patients from surveillance after 5 years (Groll et al. 2007).

Variations in the follow-up schedules and specific recommendations are shown in Tables 22.7 and 22.8.

## Recurrence After Postorchidectomy and Nerve-Sparing RLND

Retroperitoneal lymph node dissection allows more accurate staging as around 30% of all patients with

**Table 22.7** Variations in the follow-up of NSGCT Stage I in postorchidectomy surveillance expressed in the number of times a test is performed per year

| | Year 1 | Year 2 | Year 3 | Year 4 | Year 5 |
|---|---|---|---|---|---|
| Physical examination | 4–12 | 2–6 | 2–4 | 2 or 3 | 1 or 2 |
| Tumor markers | 4–12 | 4–6 | 2–4 | 2 or 3 | 1 or 2 |
| Chest X-ray | 2–12 | 2–6 | 0–4 | 0–3 | 0–2 |
| Retroperitoneal CT scan | 2[a]–6 | 1–4 | 0–3 | 0–2 | 0 or 1 |

Sources: EAU, RMH, NCCN, SWENOTECA, ESMO, BCCA, TCRC and CCO guidelines

[a]At months 3 and 12

**Table 22.8** Remarks on the follow-up of NSGCT Stage I on postorchidectomy surveillance according to EAU, RMH, NCCN, SWENOTECA, ESMO, BCCA, TCRC

| Guidelines | Remarks |
|---|---|
| EAU | Abdominopelvic CT scan twice only the first year, at months 3 and 12. Thereafter, only if indicated<br>CXR to be performed only during the first 2 years<br>Follow-up recommended up to 10 years by physical examination and tumor markers once a year |
| RMH | Very strict follow-up during the first year with physical examination and CXR seven times (at months 1, 3, 5, 7, 9, 11 and 12); Tumor markers monthly during first year<br>Abdominal CT scan at months 3 and 12 the first year and once during second year. Pelvic CT scan to be performed in case of pelvis at high risk |
| NCCN | Very strict follow-up during first year with Physical examination, tumor markers and CXR every 1 or 2 months<br>Abdominal CT scan every 2–3 months during first year. Pelvic CT scan only if pelvis at high risk<br>Abdominal CT scan every 3–4 months during second year<br>Follow-up recommended more than 6 years (with annual CT scan) |
| ESMO | Physical examination, tumor markers and CXR monthly during first year and every two months during second year<br>Abdominal CT scan only, unless pelvis at risk |
| SWENOTECA | Only one follow-up schedule for nonseminoma Stage I irrespective of the treatment policy; however, if two cycles BEP have been administered serum markers are determined only four times (instead of 7) in the first year and retroperitoneal scanning only two times (instead of 4)<br>Follow-up until year 10 with Physical examination, serum markers and CXR once a year |
| TCRC | No retroperitoneal CT scan after 5 years<br>Specific mention of rationale for long-term follow-up |
| BCCA | For low-risk tumors in surveillance, retroperitoneal CT scan is recommended twice a year, at 3 and 12 months. Second year only one CT scan at month 24. Thereafter, only one more at fifth year (month 56)<br>For high-risk tumors, three retroperitoneal CT scans recommended during the first year, at months 3, 6 and 12. During second year, two CT scans at months 18 and 24 and thereafter once a year until fifth year<br>Follow-up recommended up to tenth year |

No specific remarks in CCO guidelines

Stage I and 50% of those with risk factors in the primary tumors will be understaged by conventional radiological and marker evaluation (Huddart and Kataja 2008b; Krege et al. 2008; Mead et al. 1992; Sohaib and Husband 2007). Ten to thirteen percent of patients without evidence of nodal metastases demonstrates pulmonary relapse within the first year (Albers et al. 2008b). RPLND properly performed should eliminate the retroperitoneal nodes as a site of relapse, and thus the need for repeated abdominal CT scans; however, *in-field* or outside template retroperitoneal recurrences have been described (Albers et al. 2008b) and a postoperative baseline CT might be recommended. Variations in the follow-up and specific remarks are displayed in Tables 22.9 and 22.10.

**Table 22.9** Variations in the follow-up (times a test is performed per year) of NSGCT Stage I postorchidectomy adjuvant chemotherapy after complete response or pathological Stage I after RPLND

| | Year 1 | Year 2 | Year 3 | Year 4 | Year 5 |
|---|---|---|---|---|---|
| Physical examination | 4–12 | 3–6 | 2 | 2 | 1 or 2 |
| Tumor markers | 4–12 | 3–6 | 2 | 2 | 1 or 2 |
| Chest X-ray | 2–12 | 1–6 | 0–2 | 0–2 | 0 or 1 |
| Abdominopelvic CT scan | 0–2 | 0–2 | 0 or 1 | 0 or 1 | 0 or1 |

Source: EAU, RMH, NCCN, ESMO. SWENOTECA, TCRC, BCCA

**Table 22.10** Remarks on the follow-up of NSGCT Stage I of postorchidectomy adjuvant chemotherapy or pathological Stage I after RPLND according to EAU, RMH, NCCN, ESMO, SWENOTECA, TCRC and BCCA guidelines

| Guidelines | Remarks |
|---|---|
| EAU | Recommends follow-up up to 10 years. From year 6 to 10, by means of physical examination and tumor markers once a year<br>Abdominopelvic CT scan , once a year during the first 2 years, timing not specified |
| RMH | Follow-up over 5 years not mentioned<br>Physical examination and tumor markers five times during first year (at months 1, 3, 6, 9 and 12)<br>Adominal CT scan only at sixth month |
| NCCN | Follow-up recommended beyond year 6 with physical examination, markers and CXR once a year and CT scan every one or 2 years<br>The same follow-up is recommended for Stages I and more advanced after chemotherapy or RPLND and complete response |
| ESMO | No specific recommendations for follow-up of Stage I chemotherapy<br>Recommended follow-up after chemotherapy in general includes clinical examination, CXR and tumor markers bimonthly the first year. Every 3 months the second years and every 6 months from third to fifth year. Thereafter annually. CT scans only as clinically indicated |
| SWENOTECA | A unique follow-up schedule for any Stage I nonseminoma. Only during the first year, the intensity of the serum markers determination (four times) and of retroperitoneal scanning (two times) is lower than in a surveillance policy<br>Follow-up until year 10 with physical examination, serum markers and CXR once a year |
| TCRC | Guidelines on follow-up are detailed in Stage I according to treatment, but no follow-up is mentioned for chemotherapy<br>Adjuvant chemotherapy is not mentioned as an option in the TCRC guidelines<br>In the case of RPLND and pathological Stage I, no retroperitoneal CT scan mentioned although it might be used depending on the type of RPLND performed<br>In the case of RPLND and pathological Stage II and adjuvant chemotherapy, no specific schedule for retroperitoneal CT scan mentioned. It can be used occasionally |
| BCCA | After chemotherapy treatment, only one CXR per year until fifth year |

#### Recurrence After Postorchidectomy Adjuvant Chemotherapy

Patients within the high-risk group may receive chemotherapy. Proponents of adjuvant chemotherapy point out that, although two cycles of adjuvant chemotherapy represent overtreatment for some patients, low relapse rates and less-intensive follow-up are the clear benefits (Cullen et al. 1996). Furthermore, adjuvant chemotherapy prevents relapses that would require a higher total dose of chemotherapy (Studer et al. 2000). The need for repeated and long-term assessment of the retroperitoneum after adjuvant chemotherapy is still not clear.

Variations in the proposed follow-up of different guidelines are presented in Tables 22.9 and 22.10.

### 22.4.2.2 NSGCT Stages II–IV

Cure rates of 90, 75–80 and 50% in advanced disease with "good," "intermediate" and "poor" prognostic criteria (IGCCCG classification), respectively, have been reported (Mead et al. 1992). Roughly one-third of patients will have residual PA masses after treatment. Necrotic or fibrotic tissue, teratoma, pure embryonal carcinoma or mixed tumors can be found. Patients with primary pure embryonal carcinoma should undergo primary chemotherapy immediately or after a period of surveillance. In patients with primary teratoma or mixed tumors, two options can be considered: retroperitoneal lymph node dissection (RPLND) or surveillance. The 2-year disease-free survival rate for such patients is 60–80%. Recurrence, usually in the lungs, will occur within the first year, although relapses that occur >2 years posttreatment is reported (Ronnen et al. 2005b). In this case, three or four cycles of combination chemotherapy may provide a high cure rate. Standard observation is initiated after patients are rendered disease-free. Radiological assessment continues until residual disease has either been surgically resected or completely resolved, with a CT scan performed at this point as a baseline for follow-up. The use of PET scan in this situation is under evaluation. Variations in the follow-up protocols for patients with advanced NSGCT are shown in Tables 22.11 and 22.12.

## 22.5 Secondary Effects of Follow-Up

The upcoming data on the late effects after treatment and surveillance protocols are beginning to shape strategies with a trend to minimize treatment interventions and intensity of follow-up schedules. The potential benefit of repeated imaging studies during follow-up must be weighed against the consequent financial and health costs. Prolonged follow-up with excessively frequent imaging may expose patients to the risk of radiation exposure. A typical chest CT has an associated radiation dose equivalent to 400 CXRs (8 vs. 0.02 mSv) (Sohaib and Husband 2007). Current recommendations are to limit occupational doses to 100 mSv over 5 years (ICRP 1991). A whole trunk CT produces dose of 10–30 mSv, equivalent to 1,000 chest radiographs, and is associated with a 1:1,000 risk of second cancer/leukemia in a 25-year-old patient over the subsequent 40 years. It could be postulated that five whole-body CTs could induce one second cancer every 200 patients (Rehani and Berry 2000).

**Table 22.11** Variations in the Follow-up of NSGCT Stage II–IV after complete response to chemotherapy and or RPLND in the number of times a test is performed per year

| | Year 1 | Year 2 | Year 3 | Year 4 | Year 5 | Years 6–10 |
|---|---|---|---|---|---|---|
| Physical examination | 4–6 | 3–6 | 1–3 | 2 or 3 | 2 or 3 | 1[a] |
| Tumor markers | 4–7 | 3–6 | 1–4 | 2 or 3 | 2 | 1[a] |
| Chest X-ray | 3–6 | 3–6 | 1–3 | 2 or 3 | 2 | 1[a] |
| Abdominopelvic CT scan | 0–2 | 0–2 | 0 or 1 | 0 or 1 | 0 or 1 | 0 or 1 |

Sources: EAU, RMH, NCCN, ESMO, SWENOTECA, TCRC and BCCA guidelines

[a]Once a year

**Table 22.12** Remarks in the follow-up of NSGCT Stage II–IV according to EAU, RMH, NCCN, ESMO, SWENOTECA, TCRC and BCCA guidelines

| Guidelines | Remarks |
|---|---|
| EAU | Unique follow-up schedule for advanced NSGCT and seminoma<br>Abdominal CT scan to be performed at least annually if teratoma is found in the retroperitoneum<br>A chest CT scan to be performed if abnormality on CXR and after pulmonary resection<br>A brain CT scan to be performed in patients with headaches, focal neurological findings or any central nervous system symptoms |
| RMH | Follow-up recommended beyond 10 years with physical examination and tumor markers every 2 years. CXR stops at 10 years<br>Abdominopelvic CT only once, at 5 years |
| NCCN | Abdominopelvic CT scan twice the first year, once or twice the second year and once thereafter. From year 6 onwards, every 12 or 24 months years 6 and subsequent<br>The same schedule is recommended after RPLND<br>No recommendations are given for Stage IIIC or more ( Poor Risk) |
| ESMO | No recommendations for Stage IV<br>Abdominal CT scan only if clinical indicated<br>Follow-up after 5 years with physical examination, tumor markers and CXR once a year |
| SWENOTECA | The frequency of the retroperitoneal scanning is higher than in other schedules with four times during first year and two in years 3, 4 and 5<br>From years 6 to 10, retroperitoneal scanning is performed once a year only if mature teratoma is found in RPLND; otherwise; a retroperitoneal CT is performed at year 7 and 10 |
| TCRC | In pathological Stage II with RPLND and 2BEP, occasional CT scan could be discussed<br>Abdominal CT scan every 2 years for patients with large-volume teratoma<br>Distinguish schedules for good and poor risk<br>In poor risk, follow-up is more intensive during the first year, with tumor markers and CXR recommended every months (12 times) |
| BCCA | For Stages II–IV, tumor type or treatment, follow-up schedule is based on prognostic group<br>The frequency of CXR and abdominal CT scan is higher during the three first years for Intermediate and poor prognostic groups<br>CXR is performed more frequently if intrathoracic disease<br>If supradiafragmatic disease CXR is replaced by CT, thorax in all prognostic groups |

Ultrasound and magnetic resonance imaging have been suggested in surveillance programs in order to reduce this radiation exposure. However, ultrasound is not as reliable as CT in the assessment of retroperitoneal nodes and limited data suggest that MRI may be used instead of CT for abdominal disease (Sohaib et al. 2005). Promising approaches may include new developments in functional and magnetic resonance imaging, and dissection of the molecular determinants of tumor development, especially metastasis.

## 22.6 Follow-Up of the Secondary Effects After Treatment

Testicular cancer survivors require more intensive surveillance than their age-matched counterparts because of an elevated risk of serious comorbidities and early mortality. Fossa et al. report that more than 40% of deaths in patients who survive at least a year from their initial diagnosis are from nonmalignant causes (Fossa et al. 2007). Causes include gastrointestinal disorders (intestinal vascular lesions, hepatobiliary disease, and ulcers), cardiovascular disease, infections, respiratory illnesses, infertility and anxiety (Fossa et al. 2004; Dahl et al. 2005). Other authors reported that acute nephrotoxicity, ototoxicity, Raynaud's phenomenon and neuropathy can persist in 20–40% of these patients (Petersen and Hansen 1999). Authors found that the increased incidence of hypercholesterolemia and overweight in such patients, especially in the younger ones, represent significant risk factors for cardiovascular disease (Gietema et al. 1992; Nuver et al. 2005) and Vaughn et al. report that survivors of TGCTs are at increased risk of hypogonadism and metabolic syndrome (Vaughn et al. 2002). Metabolic syndrome (abdominal obesity, hypertriglyceridemia, low high-density lipoprotein, hypertension or insulin resistance) may occur in 25–40% of testicular cancer survivors, compared with only 3–4% of the general population (Haugnes et al. 2007).

Although data are lacking and no evidence-based guidelines exist, the Royal Marsden group include in their follow-up protocol a long-term cardiovascular status assessment of these patients (van As et al. 2008). They report that blood pressure, glucose, fasting cholesterol, LH and testosterone must be evaluated at 2, 5 and 10 years. In addition, patients should be encouraged to make appropriate lifestyle modifications including adoption of a healthful diet, smoking cessation, and exercising regularly.

Feldman et al. recommend annual evaluation of blood pressure, glucose, renal function, body mass index and evaluation of lipid profiles at least every 5 years (more frequently if another risk factor is present) with referral to the appropriate specialist if abnormalities are detected. Early treatment of these conditions, including patients with borderline values who in other settings are suitable for an observational approach, must be advised (Feldman et al. 2008).

While infradiafragmatic radiotherapy and chemotherapy increase the risk of major complications (including second malignancies and cardiovascular risk) 1.8- and 1.9-fold, smoking may also play an important role with a 1.7-fold increased risk of major complication in long-term testis cancer survivors when comparing with those patients treated also by surgery, suggesting counseling about smoking should be given to those patients treated by chemotherapy or radiation (Van den Belt-Dusebout et al. 2007).

## 22.7 Follow-Up for Second Primary Cancers

The risk of contralateral second primary tumor depends on the patient's age and exposure to chemotherapy. In a review of the literature, Herr et al. reported that the risk of contralateral metachronous tumor formation in men treated for testis cancer ranges from 1.5 to 3.2% in the United States, and up to 5.2% in Europe (Herr and Sheinfeld 1997). Patients aged <30 years with seminoma display the highest risk, whereas older men with nonseminoma disease have the lowest risk. In the case of biopsy-proven untreated testicular intraepithelial neoplasia (TIN) in the contralateral testis, the cumulative probability for development of testicular cancer ranges between 30 and 70% after 7–15 years. Lifelong self-examination of the remaining testis must be encouraged in all patients and some authors have recommended the inclusion of a routine testicular ultrasonography in the follow-up of patients with GCTs. Significant controversy exists as to whether the contralateral testis should be biopsied. In patients with a testicular volume of <12 mL, the role of biopsy (at least 2 years after chemotherapy) is discussed in order to detect carcinoma in situ (Dieckmann and Loy 1996).

Concern about increased risk of second primary cancers, other than testicular, has been raised in the last years. Long-term survivors of testis cancer treated by chemotherapy of radiotherapy have and elevated risk to develop malignant mesothelioma of the pleura, esophagus, lung, colon, bladder, pancreas and stomach cancer. Patterns of development are similar for seminoma and nonseminoma, with slightly lower risk for those nonseminoma patients treated after 1975. Relative and excess absolute risk decrease with increasing age at testis cancer diagnosis, while young patients may experience higher levels of risk as they reach older ages (Travis et al. 2005). In fact, recent data confirms that even at 20 years after treatment the risk for second malignant neoplasms was 2.6-fold increased after subdiafragmantic radiotherapy and 2.1-fold increased after chemotherapy when compared with surgery only. Subdiafragmatic radiotherapy strongly increases the risk for second malignancies but not for cardiovascular risk whereas chemotherapy increases both secondary malignancies and cardiovascular risk (Van den Belt-Dusebout et al. 2007).

Owing to the increased risk of these patients to develop melanomas, regular skin examinations for pigmented lesions must be included in the long-term evaluation (Travis et al. 2005).

Although no specific follow-up protocol exist for the early detection of secondary malignancies of others organs, a high level of suspicious should be maintained in the long-term survivors after treatment.

## 22.8 Costs and Follow-Up

The cost-effectiveness of the follow-up protocols of testicular cancer patients has been less frequently argued than that of other solid cancers. This is because a delay in detecting relapses often results in advanced disease with worst prognosis because of the extraordinarily short doubling time of testicular cancer cells. On the other hand, since the vast majorities of men are relatively young and show an excellent response to treatment, routine follow-up consumes considerable time and money. Thus, cost-effective follow-up in TGCT is critical more than any other urologic malignancy.

The frequency of follow-up visits and the diagnostic imaging procedures are based on the treatment chosen and the resulting pattern of relapse. Although comparative studies on costs have inherent difficulties, especially in different health care systems, and thus may never be carried out in a reliable manner, calculation must take in to consideration the cost of physician's visits (hospital outpatient care setting or physician office), tumor marker evaluation and imaging procedures (Sokoloff et al. 2007).

The majority of follow-up protocols include routine examination of serum HCG, AFP and LDH. For seminomas, the cost-efficacy of these tests was questionable (Ackers and Rustin 2006). In patients with NSGCT, elevation of tumor markers at recurrences are most common in Stage II and consequently more cost effective than in Stage I (Koch 1998).

Regarding imaging procedures, Sharir et al. reported that the removal of routine CXR would not have changed progression detection in their patients during follow-up of Stage I NSGCT (Sharir et al. 1996). Sharda et al. found that surveillance was more expensive (39% excess cost) than adjuvant radiotherapy with the large majority of the cost (91%) attributed to the follow-up. CT scans constitutes 70% of the total cost in the surveillance group (Sharda et al. 1996). Francis et al. found that the cost per patient of a 10-year follow-up schedule was 4,900£ and 4,612£ for seminoma and NSGCT Stage I, respectively. In the same study, a 10-year follow-up cost comparison after surveillance, nerve-sparing RPLND, adjuvant chemotherapy and radiotherapy for Stage I GCT revealed that there are no significant differences in costs among these treatment modalities (Francis et al. 2000). Edelman et al. report that the cost of their 5-year follow-up schedule was 13 million $ (2.5 million $/1,000 patients). This cost was calculated based on the utilization of CXR as the method for lung metastases. If a thoracic CT was used instead of X-ray, the cost would increase to $34 million (Edelman et al. 1997). Similar findings were reported from Kakehi et al. According to their 5-year surveillance protocol for NSGCT Stage I, the cost was related to the imaging modality for the evaluation of chest relapses (CT or X-ray) (Kakehi et al. 2002).

Wright et al., examining the CT imaging of 167 patients with testicular germ-cell cancer, found that pelvic CT scanning is no longer considered mandatory in all patients on surveillance with Stage I testicular NSGCT. Following an initial staging CT scan of the chest, abdomen and pelvis, subsequent pelvic CT scanning is only required in the follow-up of patients with an identifiable risk factor for pelvic recurrence. The removal of routine pelvic CT scanning from surveillance schedules significantly reduces patient radiation exposure and has led to a substantial resource saving (Wright and White 1999).

## 22.9 Considerations

There is a paucity of high-evidence data regarding the most effective follow-up regimens after primary treatment of testis cancer to identify relapses. Optimal use of imaging, frequency of physician visits and serum marker level measurements need to be further addressed. However, on the basis of data published in the literature, a very frequent follow-up would only be necessary for Stage I NSGCT on surveillance and during the first 2 years after orchidectomy. Up to now, there is only high evidence for omitting frequent abdominopelvic CT scans in the first 2 years of follow-up. Most likely routine follow-up after 5 years is not required for patients with seminoma at any stage and patients with Stage I NSGCTs. For patients with Stage II–III NSGCTs at presentation, there is a continuing low risk of recurrence and lifelong follow-up should be considered. Patients and physicians have to be aware of the existence of an increased risk for second malignancies and cardiovascular effect on those patients treated by radiotherapy and chemotherapy and in smokers. Appropriate counseling has to be given especially to those in whom testis cancer was diagnosed before 35 years of age.

## 22.10 Addendum I: Guidelines Consulted and Abbreviations

- European Association of Urology (EAU). www.uroweb.org
- European Society for Medical Oncology (ESMO). www.esmo.org
- National Comprehensive Cancer Network (NCCN). www.nccn.org
- Royal Marsdem Hospital (RMH). www.icr.ac.uk
- Swedish and Norwegian Testicular Cancer Project (SWENOTECA). www.ocsyd.se
- The Testicular Cancer Resource Center (TCRC). www.tcrc.acor.org
- British Columbia Cancer Agency (BCCA). www.bccancer.bc.ca
- Cancer Care Ontario (CCO). www.cancercare.on.ca

## References


Ackers C, Rustin G (2006) The use of lactate dehydrogenase (LDH) as a marker for relapse in patients on surveillance for stage I germ cell tumours. Br J Cancer 94:1231–1232

Albers P, Albrecht W, Algaba F et al (2008) EAU Guidelines on testicular cancer. www.uroweb.org

Albers P, Siener R, Krege S et al (2008b) Randomized phase III trial comparing retroperitoneal lymph node dissection with one course of bleomycin and etoposide plus cisplatin chemotherapy in the adjuvant treatment of clinical stage I Nonseminomatous testicular germ cell tumors: AUO trial AH 01/94 by the german Testicular Cancer Study Group. J Clin Oncol 26:2966–2972

Arranz Arija JA, Garcia del Muro X, Guma J et al (2001) E400P in advanced seminoma of good prognosis according to the International Germ Cell Cancer Collaborative Group (IGCCCG) classification: the Spanish Germ Cell Cancer Group experience. Ann Oncol 12:487–491

Bellin M, Roy C, Kinkel K et al (1998) Lymph node metastases: safety and effectiveness of MR imaging with ultrasmall superparamagnetic iron oxide particles: initial clinical experience. Radiology 207:799–808

Bosl GJ, Motzer RJ (1997) Testicular germ-cell cancer. N Engl J Med 337:242–253

Buchholz TA, Walden TL, Prestidge BR (1998) Cost-effectiveness of post-treatment surveillance after radiation therapy for early stage seminoma. Cancer 82:1126–1133

British Columbia Cancer Agency. www.bccancer.bc.ca

Chung P, Parker C, Panzarella T et al (2002) Surveillance in stage I testicular seminoma-risk of late relapse. Can J Urol 9:1637–1640

Colls MB, Harvey VJ, Skelton L et al (1999a) Late results of surveillance of clinical stage I nonseminoma germ cell testicular tumours: 17 years' experience in a national study in New Zealand. BJU Int 83:76–82

Colls BM, Harvey VJ, Skelton L et al (1999b) Late results of surveillance of clinical stage I nonseminoma germ cell testicular tumours: 17 years' experience in a national study in New Zealand. Br J Urol Int 83:76–82

Cremerius U, Wildberger JE, Borchers H et al (1999) Does positron emission tomography using 18-fluoro-2-deoxyglucose improve clinical staging of testicular cancer? Results of a study in 50 patients. Urology 54:900–904

Cullen MH, Stenning SP, Parkinson MC et al (1996) Short-course adjuvant chemotherapy in high-risk stage I nonseminomatous germ cell tumors of the testis: a Medical Research Council report. J Clin Oncol 14:1106–1113

Dahl AA, Haaland CF, Mykletun A et al (2005) Study of anxiety disorder and depression in long-term survivors of testicular cancer. J Clin Oncol 23:2389–2395

Dalal PU, Sohaib SA, Huddart R (2006) Imaging of testicular germ cell tumours. Cancer Imaging 6:124–134

De Santis M, Becherer A, Bokemeyer C et al (2004) 2-18fluoro-deoxy- D-glucose positron emission tomography is a reliable predictor for viable tumor in postchemotherapy seminoma: an update of the prospective multicentric EMPET trial. J Clin Oncol 22:1034–1039

Dieckmann KP, Loy V (1996) Prevalence of contralateral testicular intraepithelial neoplasia in patients with testicular germ cell neoplasms. J Clin Oncol 14:3126–3132

Edelman MJ, Meyers FJ, Siegel D (1997) The utility of follow-up testing after curative cancer therapy: A critical review and economic analysis. J Gen Intern Med 12:318–331

Feldman DR, Bosl GJ, Sheinfeld J et al (2008) Medical treatment of advanced testicular cancer. JAMA 299:672–684

Fossa SD, Stenning SP, Gerl A et al (1999a) Prognostic factors in patients progressing after cisplatin-based chemotherapy for malignant non-seminomatous germ cell tumours. Br J Cancer 80:1392–1399

Fossa SD, Horwich A, Russell JM et al (1999b) Optimal planning target volume for stage I testicular seminoma: a Medical Research Council randomized trial. J Clin Oncol 17:1146

Fossa SD, Aass N, Harvei S, Tretli S (2004) Increased mortality rates in young and middle-aged patients with malignant germ cell tumours. Br J Cancer 90:607–612

Fossa SD, Gilbert E, Dores GM et al (2007) Noncancer causes of death in survivors of testicular cancer. J Natl Cancer Inst 99:533–544

Francis R, Bower M, Brunstrom G et al (2000) Surveillance for stage I testicular germ cell tumours: results and cost benefit analysis of management options. Eur J Cancer 36:1925–1932

Ganjoo KN, Chan RJ, Sharma M, Einhorn LH (1999) Positron emission tomography scans in the evaluation of postchemotherapy residual masses in patients with seminoma. J Clin Oncol 17:3457–3460

Gels ME, Hoekstra HJ, Sleijfer DT et al (1995) Detection of recurrence in patients with clinical stage I nonseminomatous testicular germ-cell tumors and consequences for further follow-up: a single-center 10-year experience. J Clin Oncol 13:1188–1194

Gietema JA, Sleijfer DT, Willemse PH et al (1992) Longterm follow-up of cardiovascular risk factors in patients given chemotherapy for disseminated nonseminomatous testicular cancer. Ann Intern Med 116:709–715

Gietemsa JA, Meinardi MT, Sleifer DT et al (2002) Routine chest X-rays have no additional value in the detection of relapse during routine follow-up of patients treated with chemotherapy for disseminated non-seminomatous testicular cancer. Ann Oncol 13:1616–1620

Groll RJ, Warde P, Jewett MA (2007) A comprehensive systematic review of testicular germ cell tumor surveillance. Crit Rev Oncol Hematol 64:182–197

Harvey ML, Geldart TR, Duell R et al (2002) Routine computerised tomographic scans of the thorax in surveillance of stage I testicular non-seminomatous germ-cell cancer – a necessary risk? Ann Oncol 13:237–242

Haugnes HS, Aass N, Fossa SD et al (2007) Components of the metabolic syndrome in long-term survivors of testicular cancer. Ann Oncol 18:241–248

Herr HW, Sheinfeld J (1997) Is biopsy of the contralateral testis necessary in patients with germ cell tumors? J Urol 158: 1331–1334

Hogeboom WR, Hoekstra HJ, Mooyart EL et al (1993) Magnetic resonance imaging of retroperitoneal lymph node metastases of non-seminomatous germ cell tumors of the testis. Eur J Surg Oncol 19:429–437

Hoh CK, Seltzer MA, Franklin J et al (1998) Positron emissions tomography in urological oncology. J Urol 159:347–356

Huddart R, Kataja V (2008) Testicular seminoma: ESMO clinical recommendations for diagnosis, treatment and follow-up. Ann Oncol 19(suppl 2):ii49–ii51

Huddart R, Kataja V (2008) Mixed or on-seminomatous germ-cell tumors: ESMO clinical recommendations for diagnosis, treatment and follow-up. Ann Oncol 19(suppl 2):ii52–ii54

Huddart RA, Birtle AJ (2005) Recent advances in the treatment of testicular cancer. Expert Rev Anticancer Ther 5:123–138

Huddart RA, O'Doherty MJ, Padhani A et al (2007) $^{18}$Fluorodeoxyglucose positron emission tomography in the prediction of relapse in patients with high-risk, clinical stage I nonseminomatous germ cell tumors: preliminary report of MRC Trial TE22 – the NCRI Testis Tumour Clinical Study Group. J Clin Oncol 25:3090–3095

ICRP: International Commission on Radiological Protection (1991) ICRP: Recommendations of the International Commission on Radiological Protection, ICRP publication 60. Pergamon Press, Oxford, UK

Kakehi Y, Kamoto T, Kawakita M et al (2002) Follow-up of clinical stage I testicular cancer patients: cost and risk benefit considerations. Int J Urol 9:154–161

Khadra A, Oakeshott P (2002) Pilot study of testicular cancer awareness and testicular self-examination in men attending two South London general practices. Fam Pract 19:294–6

Klepp O, Olsson AM, Henrikson H et al (1990) Prognostic factors in clinical stage I nonseminomatous germ cell tumours of the testis: multivariate analysis of a prospective multicenter study. J Clin Oncol 8:509–518

Koch MO (1998) Cost-effective strategies for the follow-up of patients with germ cell tumors. Urol Clin North Am 25: 495–502

Krege S, Beyer J, Souchon R et al (2008) European Consensus Conference on Diagnosis and Treatment of Germ Cell Cancer: A Report of the Second Meeting of the European Germ Cell Cancer Consensus Group (EGCCCG): Part II. Eur Urol 53:497–513

Lassen U, Daugaard G, Eigtved A et al (2003) Whole-body FDG-PET in patients with stage I nonseminomatous germ cell tumours. Eur J Nucl Med Mol Imaging 30:396–402

Livsey JE, Taylor B, Mobarek N et al (2001) Patterns of relapse following radiotherapy for stage I seminoma of the testis: implications for follow-up. Clin Oncol (R Coll Radiol) 13:296–300

Martin JM, Panzarella T, Zwahlen DR et al (2007) Evidence-based guidelines for following stage 1 seminoma. Cancer 109:2248–2256

McCaffrey JA, Bajorin DF, Motzer RJ (1998) Risk assessment for metastatic testis cancer. Urol Clin North Am 25: 389–395

Mead GM, Stenning SP, Parkinson MC et al (1992) The Second Medical Research Council study of prognostic factors in nonseminomatous germ cell tumors. Medical Research Council Testicular Tumour Working Party. J Clin Oncol 10:85–94

Melchior D, Hammer P, Fimmers R et al (2001) Long term results and morbidity of paraaortic compared with paraaortic and iliac adjuvant radiation in clinical stage I seminoma. Anticancer Res 21:2989–2993

Motzer RJ, Bolger GB, Boston B et al (2008) NCCN Practice guidelines in oncology. Testicular cancer. V.2.2008. www.nccn.org

Nuver J, Smit AJ, Sleijfer DT et al (2005) Left ventricular and cardiac autonomic function in survivors of testicular cancer. Eur J Clin Invest 35:99–103

Oldenburg J, Alfsen GC, Waehre H et al (2006) Late recurrences of germ cell malignancies: a population- based experience over three decades. Br J Cancer 94:820–27

Oliver RT, Ong J, Shamash J et al; Anglian Germ Cell Cancer Group (2004) Long-term follow-up of Anglian Germ Cell Cancer Group surveillance versus patients with Stage 1 nonseminoma treated with adjuvant chemotherapy. Urology 63:556–561

Oliver RT, Mason MD, Mead GM et al (2005) Radiotherapy versus single-dose carboplatin in adjuvant treatment of stage I seminoma: a randomised trial. Lancet 366(9482):293–300

Patterson H, Norman AR, Mitra SS et al (2001) Combination carboplatin and radiotherapy in the management of stage II testicular seminoma: comparison with radiotherapy treatment alone. Radiother Oncol 59:5–11

Petersen PM, Hansen SW (1999) The course of longterm toxicity in patients treated with cisplatin-based chemotherapy for non-seminomatous germ-cell cancer. Ann Oncol 10: 1475–1483

Puc HS, Heelan R, Mazumdar M et al (1996) Management of residual mass in advanced seminoma: results and recommendations from the Memorial Sloan–Kettering Cancer Center. J Clin Oncol 14:454–460

Read G, Stenning SP, Cullen MH et al (1992) Medical Research Council prospective study of surveillance for stage I testicular teratoma. Medical Research Council Testicular Tumors Working Party. J Clin Oncol 10:1762–1768

Rehani MM, Berry M (2000) Radiation doses in computed tomography: the increasing doses of radiation need to be controlled. BMJ 320:593–594

Richie JP, Garnick MB, Finberg H (1982) Computerized tomography: how accurate for abdominal staging of testis tumors? J Urol 127:715–717

Ronnen EA, Kondagupta GV, Bacik J et al (2005a) Incidence of late-relapse germ cell tumor and outcome to salvage chemotherapy. J Clin Oncol 23:6999–7004
Ronnen EA, Kondagunta GV, Bacik J et al (2005b) Incidence of late-relapse germ cell tumor and outcome to salvage chemotherapy. J Clin Oncol 23:6999–7004
Rowland RG, Weisman D, Williams SD et al (1982) Accuracy of preoperative staging in stages A and B nonseminomatous germ cell testis tumors. J Urol 127:718–720
Rustin GJS, Mead GM, Stenning SP et al (2007) A randomised trial of 2 versus 5 CT scans in the surveillance of patients with stage 1 nonseminomatous germ cell tumours of the testis: Medical Research Council Trial TE08. J Clin Oncol 25: 1310–1315
Segal R, Lukka H, Klotz L, Eady A, Bestic N, Johnston M and the Genitourinary Cancer Disease Site Group (2001) Surveillance programs for early stage non seminomatous testicular cancer. Practice guideline report no 3-5. www.cancercare.on.ca
Segal R et al (2006) Surveillance in Stage I NSGCT of the testis. Urol Oncol 24:68–74
Shahidi M, Norman AR, Dearnaley DP et al (2002a) Late recurrence in 1263 men with testicular germ cell tumors. Multivariate analysis of risk factors and implications for management. Cancer 95:520–530
Shahidi M, Norman AR, Dearnaley DP, Nicholls J, Horwich A, Huddart RA (2002b) Late recurrence in 1263 men with testicular germ cell tumors. Multivariate analysis of risk factors and implications for management. Cancer 95:520–530
Sharda NN, Kinsella TJ, Ritter MA (1996) Adjuvant radiation versus observation: A cost analysis of alternative management schemes in early-stage testicular seminoma. J Clin Oncol 14:2933–2939
Sharir S, Foster R, Donahue J et al (1996) What is appropriate follow-up after treatment? Semin Urol Oncol 14:45–53
Sharir S, Jewett MA, Sturgeon JF et al (1999) Progression detection of stage I nonseminomatous testis cancer on surveillance: implications for the follow-up protocol. J Urol 161:472–476
Sohaib SA, Husband J (2007) Surveillance in testicular cancer: who, when, what and how? Cancer Imaging 7:145–147
Sohaib SA, Huddart R, Dearnaley DP, Horwich A (2005) Sensitivity of MRI in the diagnosis of retroperitoneal disease in testicular germ cell tumours. AJR Am J Roentgenol 184(suppl):63
Sokoloff MH, Joyce GF, Wise M et al (2007) Testis cancer. J Urol 177:2030–2041
Studer UE, Burkhard FC, Sonntag RWJ (2000) Risk adapted management with adjuvant chemotherapy in patients with high risk clinical stage I nonseminomatous germ cell tumor. Urology 163:1785–1787
Swedish and Norwegian Testicular Cancer Project. www.ocsyd.se
The testicular Cancer Resource Center. wwwtcrc.acor.org
Travis LB, Fossa SD, Schonfeld SJ et al (2005) Second cancers among 40, 576 testicular cancer patients: focus on long-term survivors. J Natl Cancer Inst 97:1354–1365
Trigo JM, Tabernero JM, Paz-Ares L et al (2000) Tumor markers at the time of recurrence in patients with germ cell tumors. Cancer 88:162–168
van As NJ, Gilbert DC, Money-Kyrle J et al (2008) Evidence-based pragmatic guidelines for the follow-up of testicular cancer: optimising the detection of relapse. Br J Cancer 98:1894–1902
Van den Belt-Dusebout AW, de Wit R, Gietema JA, Horenblas S, Lowuman MW, Ribot JG, Hoekstra HJ, Ouwen GM, Aleman BM, Leeuwen FE (2007) Treatment-specific risks of second malignancies and cardiovascular disease in 5 years survivors of testicular cancer. J Clin Oncol 25:4370–4378
Vaughn DJ, Gignak GA, Meadows AT (2002) Long-term medical care of testicular cancer survivors. Ann Intern Med 136: 463–470
Venkitaraman R, Johnson B, Huddart RA et al (2007) The utility of lactate dehydrogenase in the follow-up of testicular germ cell tumours. BJU Int 100:30–32
von Eyben FE, Madsen EL, Blaabjerg O et al (2001) Serum lactate dehydrogenase isoenzyme 1 and relapse in patients with nonseminomatous testicular germ cell tumors clinical stage I. Acta Oncol 40:536–540
Warde P, Jewett MAS (1998) Surveillance for stage I testicular seminoma. Is it a good option? Urol Clin North Am 25: 425–433
White PM, Howard GC, Best JJ et al (1997) The role of computed tomographic examination of the pelvis in the management of testicular germ cell tumours. Clin Radiol 52:124–129
de Wit R, Roberts JT, Wilkinson PM et al (2001) Equivalence of three or four cycles of bleomycin, etoposide, and cisplatin chemotherapy and of a 3- or 5-day schedule in good-prognosis germ cell cancer: a randomized study of the European Organization for Research and Treatment of Cancer Genitourinary Tract Cancer Cooperative Group and the Medical Research Council. J Clin Oncol 19:1629–1640
de Wit M, Hartmann M, Kotzerke J et al; German Multicenter PET Study Group (2005) 18F-FDG-PET in clinical stage I and II non-seminomatous germ cell tumors: first results of the German multicenter trial. J Clin Oncol 23(suppl):4504Wright AR, White PM (1999) Testicular cancer–who needs surveillance pelvic CT? Clin Radiol 54:78

# Part VI

# Testicular Cancer in Childhood and Non-Germ Cell Tumors

# Testicular Cancer in Childhood

# 23

Jonathan H. Ross

## 23.1 Introduction

The age distribution of testicular cancer is bimodal with a large peak in young adulthood and a smaller peak in early childhood. Tumors occurring in adolescence have a similar histological pattern and natural history to those occurring in older adults. However, prepubertal testis tumors occur with distinct histologic patterns and a natural history that differs from that of adult tumors (Table 23.1). Not surprisingly, the management of prepubertal tumors differs as well. The incidence of testis tumors in children is 0.5–2.0 per 100,000 children accounting for 1–2% of all pediatric tumors (Coppes et al. 1994). Yolk sac tumors account for the overwhelming majority of malignant prepubertal testis tumors. The appropriate management of prepubertal yolk sac tumors has been clarified by recent multicenter trials (Haas et al. 1999; Rogers et al. 2004; Cushing et al. 2004; Mann et al. 2000; Lo Curto et al. 2003; Schlatter et al. 2003). Much rarer malignancies in children include some stromal tumors and dysgerminomas occurring in association with gonadoblastoma in dysgenetic gonads. However, unlike in adults, the majority of tumors in children are actually benign, with teratomas being the most common (Pohl et al. 2004). This has important implications for the initial management of testis tumors in children.

J.H. Ross, MD
Chief Division of Pediatric Urology,
Rainbow Babies and Children's Hospital,
Associate Professor, University Hospitals Case Western
Reserve College of Medicine, USA

## 23.2 Presentation and Evaluation

Testis tumors most commonly present as a testicular mass. A minority of patients will have a hydrocele at presentation, which may be secondary to the tumor or coincidental. The presence of a hydrocele may delay the diagnosis of a testis tumor, and an ultrasonogram should be considered for any boy with a hydrocele in whom the testis cannot be palpated. Occasionally, patients will present with pain due to an acute bleed into the tumor. Physical examination will usually reveal a hard mass in the testicular parenchyma. These masses must be distinguished from benign extratesticular lesions such as epididymal cysts. As part of the physical examination, signs of androgenization or feminization should be sought. Metastatic disease is uncommon, and the primary sites – the retroperitoneum and lungs – are unlikely to result in symptoms or physical findings. In rare cases, metastases to the bone or central nervous system may occur. Symptoms or signs of involvement at these locations are important in guiding the radiographic evaluation.

The initial radiographic evaluation of children with a suspected testis tumor is limited. Because most prepubertal testis tumors are benign, any metastatic evaluation is usually deferred until tissue confirmation of the tumor's histology is obtained. However, when a malignancy is suspected (for example, in children with an elevated alpha-fetoprotein (AFP) level and in adolescents) a computerized tomography scan (CT) of the abdomen may be obtained preoperatively. Imaging of the primary tumor is sometimes helpful. Ultrasonography is most often employed. It is able to distinguish testicular tumors from benign extratesticular lesions. The extent of testicular involvement can also be determined, which is helpful if testis-sparing

M.P. Laguna et al. (eds.), *Cancer of the Testis*,
DOI: 10.1007/978-1-84800-370-5_23, © Springer-Verlag London Limited 2010

**Table 23.1** Comparison of behavior of different testis tumors in adults and in prepubertal children

| Tumor | Adult | Prepubertal |
|---|---|---|
| Seminoma | Common malignant tumor in older men. Also occurs in dysgenetic testes or as dysgerminoma in dysgenetic gonads of young adult patients with Y chromatin | May present in childhood in dysgenetic gonads/testes |
| Nonseminomatous mixed germ cell tumor | Common malignant tumor in young men | Vanishingly rare |
| Pure yolk sac | Very rare malignant tumor | Most common malignant tumor |
| Teratoma | Sometimes malignant | Most common benign tumor |
| Sertoli cell | Approximately 10% are malignant | May rarely be malignant in older children |
| Leydig cell | Approximately 10% are malignant | Benign |
| Granulosa cell | Very rare – sometimes malignant | Juvenile granulosa cell tumors occur mostly in infants and are benign |

surgery is being considered. However, testis-sparing may be feasible even when there seems little normal testicle present on ultrasound (Patel et al. 2007). The ultrasonographic appearance of specific testis tumors has been described, but the ultrasound findings are too inconsistent to allow a definitive diagnosis on the basis of ultrasound alone.

Tumor markers play an important role in the evaluation and follow-up of childhood testis tumors. AFP is the most important tumor marker. Levels are elevated in 80–90% of children with a yolk sac tumor, and AFP has a biological half-life of approximately 5 days (Uehling and Phillips 1994). Elevated levels of AFP preoperatively should preclude consideration of a testis-sparing approach. An important caveat is that AFP levels are normally quite high in infancy. An "elevated" level in a boy less than 1 year of age does not rule out the possibility of a benign tumor, such as teratoma (Grady et al. 1997). The beta subunit of human chorionic gonadotropin (HCG) is an important marker in adolescent testis tumors, but it is rarely elevated in children because the histologic types that lead to elevated HCG levels are rarely encountered in prepubertal testis tumors.

## 23.3 Surgical Approach

The standard approach to a testis tumor is an inguinal orchiectomy as described in Chap. 6.2. However, increasing consideration has been given to performing testis-sparing surgery for benign testicular tumors (Ross et al. 2002). This is particularly attractive in prepubertal patients because many, if not most, tumors are benign in this population. The preoperative evaluation plays a significant role in patient selection for testis-sparing surgery. An elevated AFP level in a child over 1 year of age virtually always reflects the presence of a yolk sac tumor and precludes a testis-sparing approach. However, in infants, and older children with a normal AFP, the likelihood of a benign tumor is considerable. This is also true in boys presenting with androgenization. For these patients, an inguinal exploration should be considered so that testis-sparing surgery may be performed if a benign histology is confirmed. The initial approach is the same as for an inguinal orchiectomy. Once the testis is delivered into the inguinal incision, the spermatic cord is occluded with a noncrushing clamp. The field is draped off with towels and the tunica vaginalis is opened. The tumor is excised with a margin of normal parenchyma or enucleated and sent for frozen section. If a benign histology is confirmed, then the testicular defect is closed with absorbable suture and the testis is returned to the scrotum. If a malignancy is detected, or the frozen section is nondiagnostic, then an orchiectomy is performed. Reports from small series suggest that this approach is safe and is effective in preserving testicular tissue (Valla 2001).

Once the primary tumor is excised, the type of adjunctive management selected will depend on the tumor's histology and the results of radiographic and biochemical studies. The intensity of follow-up also depends on the malignant potential of the primary tumor.

## 23.4 Germ Cell Tumors

Yolk sac tumor accounts for nearly all malignant prepubertal testis tumors. Yolk sac tumors have been referred to by a number of other names including endodermal sinus tumor, orchioblastoma, juvenile embryonal carcinoma, mesoblastoma vitellinum, clear cell adenocarcinoma, extraembryonal mesoblastoma, and archenteronoma (Coppes et al. 1994). The majority of patients present under 2 years of age.

Metastatic evaluation of yolk sac tumors includes a CT scan of the abdomen and pelvis to rule out retroperitoneal lymph node or other intra-abdominal metastases and a chest X-ray or chest CT scan to rule out pulmonary metastases. Bone scans and head CT scans are obtained only when there is clinical suspicion of metastases at these sites. Serum AFP level is also measured postoperatively. Its half-life is approximately 5 days, and a persistent elevation of AFP after orchiectomy suggests the presence of metastatic disease. However, AFP levels as high as 50,000 ng/mL can occur in normal infants, and levels greater than 50 ng/mL can occur in children up to 6 months of age (Brewer and Tank 1993). Therefore, serial measurements are particularly important in small children.

A tumor-node-metastasis (TNM) staging system exists for testis tumors, but its applicability to pediatric tumors is limited owing to the infrequent employment of retroperitoneal lymph node dissection (RPLND) in these patients. Several other systems have been proposed. The staging system used in the Intergroup Pediatric Oncology Group/Children's Study Group (now the Children's Oncology Group) studies is shown in Table 23.2. While the details of various staging systems vary, they are all based on the local extent of the tumor, the normalization or persistence of elevated tumor markers, and the radiographic evidence of regional lymphatic or distant metastases. Approximately 80% of children with yolk sac tumors have stage I disease.

**Table 23.2** Pediatric oncology group/Children's cancer group staging system for testicular germ cell tumors (Rogers et al. 2004)

| Stage | |
|---|---|
| I | Limited to the testis and normalization of tumor markers after tumor excision |
| II | Microscopic residual disease in the scrotum, significant extension into the spermatic cord, transcrotal orchiectomy, limited retroperitoneal disease (<2 cm), or persistent elevation of tumor markers after tumor excision |
| III | Retroperitoneal lymph node involvement (>2 cm) |
| IV | Distant metastases |

Historically, RPLND was the most common form of adjunctive therapy for the treatment of yolk sac tumors. However, with the widespread use of AFP to detect occult metastases and improvements in multiagent chemotherapy, the reliance on RPLND to diagnose and treat metastatic disease in prepubertal patients has waned. Although some series suggested improved survival with RPLND, the studies were uncontrolled and the majority of patients who "benefited" had no histopathological evidence of disease in the resected nodes (Green 1983). In theory, RPLND is less beneficial for children than for adults because yolk sac tumors in children have a predilection for hematogenous spread, with only a minority of metastases being limited to the retroperitoneum. A review of the Prepubertal Testis Tumor Registry of the Urology section of the American Academy of Pediatrics found that metastases were limited to the retroperitoneum in only 32% of patients with metastatic disease, whereas metastatic disease in 46% of these patients occurred at hematogenous sites *without* retroperitoneal involvement (Grady et al. 1994). The operative morbidity of RPLND in children is significant, including wound complications, bowel obstruction, chylous ascites, and anejaculation as adults due to injury to the sympathetic nerves (Green 1983). Currently, retroperitoneal surgery is limited to excisional biopsy of retroperitoneal masses in patients with a normal AFP and excisional biopsy of residual masses following chemotherapy – both rare events.

Chemotherapy is very effective in treating metastatic yolk sac tumor. The most commonly used regimens include cisplatin or carboplatin in combination with other agents such as etoposide and bleomycin. Because children with metastatic disease often have multiple sites of spread, chemotherapy is particularly appropriate for these patients.

Radiation is not a standard form of treatment for metastatic yolk sac tumor. Whereas yolk sac tumor is radiosensitive, the doses required when radiation is used as a primary therapy are prohibitively toxic (Connolly and Gearhart 1993). Lower doses of radiation may play a role in combination with surgery and chemotherapy for high-risk patients.

As with adult germ cell tumors, the selection of adjuvant therapy for yolk sac tumor depends on the stage of the tumor. The trend in managing stage I tumors is toward observation. Most series reported during the 1990s have found no survival advantage to adjuvant therapy in this group (Table 23.3) (Rogers et al. 2004; Mann et al. 2000; Schlatter et al. 2003; Fernandes et al. 1989; Leonard et al. 1991). Approximately 80% of patients have stage I disease and the recurrence rate for these patients managed by observation is approximately 15%. Virtually all of the stage I patients suffering a recurrence can be salvaged with chemotherapy. Patients with stage I tumor are therefore generally observed closely without adjuvant therapy. Patients are evaluated 1 month after orchiectomy with a CT scan of the abdomen and pelvis, a chest X-ray, and a serum AFP. Serum AFP is then measured monthly for 6 months, then every 3 months from 6 months to 2 years. A chest X-ray and abdominal/pelvic CT scan are obtained every 3 months for the first year, and every 6 months during the second year. Recurrent disease is usually treated with chemotherapy, even if it appears to be limited to the retroperitoneum. If the patient remains free of disease for 2 years, then he is almost certainly cured, though annual follow-up is continued.

Patients with a negative metastatic evaluation, but a failure of the AFP to normalize, are generally treated with 3–4 cycles of chemotherapy. The potential toxicities of the chemotherapy regimens employed include myelosuppression, ototoxicity and renal toxicity from platinum-based agents, and pulmonary toxicity from bleomycin. High-grade ototoxicity was rare in the United Kingdom study which utilized carboplatinum rather than cis-platinum (Mann et al. 2000). However, carboplatin is more myelotoxic. In determining the need for chemotherapy, it must be remembered that a "normal" AFP in infants may be quite high. Patients with positive lymph nodes on CT scan are also treated with chemotherapy, although consideration may be given to performing a modified RPLND in the presence of minimal retroperitoneal disease and a normal AFP. An RPLND should also be considered when retroperitoneal disease is not responding to chemotherapy or for a persistent mass after chemotherapy when the AFP level has normalized. Some of these residual masses will contain only necrotic tumor and calcifications (Uehling and Phillips 1994).

Chemotherapy is the mainstay of treatment for patients with hematogenous metastases. Chemotherapy with second-line agents should be used for patients failing to respond to standard agents. Surgical excision and radiation should also be considered for those with limited sites of metastatic disease who fail to respond to chemotherapy.

The typical germ cell tumors seen in adults, such as embryonal or mixed germ cell tumors, occur almost exclusively after puberty. There is little data regarding the behavior of these germ cell tumors in adolescents, though they appear to exhibit behavior similar to that seen in adults. Until further studies on adolescent germ cell tumors are performed, most patients will be managed as adults with observation, retroperitoneal lymph node dissection, and/or chemotherapy depending on the specific histology and stage of the disease. The details of these various approaches are discussed elsewhere in this text. While teratomas are virtually always benign in

**Table 23.3** Results of large multicenter studies of prepuberatal malignant germ cell tumors of the testis

| | Number of patients | Recurrence rate of stage 1 tumors on observation (%) | Survival for stage 1 tumors (%) | Survival for those with stage II–IV disease (%) |
|---|---|---|---|---|
| United Kingdom's Children's Cancer Study Group (Mann et al. 2000) | 62 | 5 | 100 | 100 |
| German Cooperative Studies (Haas et al. 1999) | 110 | 15 | 100 | 80 |
| U.S. Pediatric Intergroup Study (Rogers et al. 2004; Cushing et al. 2004; Schlatter et al. 2003) | 94 | 17 | 100 | 100 |
| Italian Cooperative Study[a] (Lo Curto et al. 2003) | 36 | 19 | 100 | 100 |
| Total | 302 | 14 | 100 | 98 |

[a]Includes 6 patients over 10 years of age

prepubertal patients and testis-sparing surgery is a reasonable consideration in that population, teratomas in adolescents may behave in a malignant fashion (Ulbright 2004). Therefore, postpubertal teratomas should be evaluated and followed on the same protocol as other malignant germ cell tumors occurring in adolescents.

## 23.5 Stromal Tumors

Stromal testis tumors are rare in children, and there are no large series to guide their management. However, anecdotal reports and small series in the literature offer some experience on which to base therapy (Thomas et al. 2001). Leydig cell and juvenile granulosa cell tumors are universally benign in children (Coppes et al. 1994; Thomas et al. 2001). Sertoli cell tumors account for only 2% of primary prepubertal testis tumors. A review of 60 cases of Sertoli cell tumors reported only 4 cases in patients under 20 years of age – the youngest being 15 years old (Young et al. 1998). Approximately 10% of adult Sertoli cell tumors are malignant. These malignant tumors are usually characterized by large tumor size, areas of necrosis, vascular invasion, cellular atypia, and increased mitotic activity. In contrast to general series dominated by adult patients, the median age of patients in the Prepubertal Testis Tumor Registry was 6 months, with a range of 4 months to 10 years. There were no reports of metastatic disease. Sertoli cell tumors are usually hormonally inactive in children, although they may occasionally cause gynecomastia or isosexual precocious puberty (Kratzer et al. 1997). Whereas all reported cases to date have been benign in children under 5 years of age, there have been a few cases of malignant Sertoli cell tumors in older children (Cortez and Kaplan 1993; Kolon and Hochman 1997). Orchiectomy is sufficient treatment in infants, although a metastatic evaluation could be considered in infants with worrisome histologic findings. Older children should undergo an abdominal CT scan and chest X-ray to rule out metastases. When metastatic disease is present, aggressive combination treatment including RPLND, chemotherapy, and radiation therapy should be considered.

The large cell calcifying Sertoli cell tumor is a clinically and histologically distinct entity with a higher incidence of multifocality and hormonal activity (Coppes et al. 1994; Washecka et al. 2002). These tumors are composed of large cells with abundant cytoplasm and varying degrees of calcification ranging from minimal amounts to massive deposits. Approximately one-third of patients with large cell calcifying Sertoli cell tumor have an associated genetic syndrome and/or endocrine abnormality. The two syndromes most commonly associated with large cell calcifying Sertoli cell tumor are Peutz–Jeghers syndrome and Carney's syndrome. Peutz–Jeghers syndrome is an autosomal dominant disorder consisting of mucocutaneous pigmentation and hamartomatous intestinal polyposis. Features of Carney's syndrome include myxomas of the skin, soft tissue, and heart, myxoid lesions of the breast, lentigines of the face and lips, cutaneous blue nevi, Cushing's syndrome, pituitary adenoma, and schwannoma. Awareness of this familial syndrome is important because patients and their first-degree relatives are at risk for the potentially lethal associated entities. Whereas they are occasionally malignant in adults, large cell calcifying Sertoli cell tumors have been universally benign in patients under 25 years of age. Orchiectomy is sufficient treatment for children.

Histologically, "mixed" or "undifferentiated" stromal tumors consist of areas of gonadal stromal neoplasia and undifferentiated regions of spindle cells that may exhibit a high mitotic rate. Although some of these tumors have histologic characteristics commonly associated with malignancy, most are benign. There are inadequate data in the literature to formulate rigid guidelines for managing these tumors. While histologic features may not correlate with invasive or metastatic potential, a high index of suspicion is appropriate when there are a large number of mitotic figures, the tumor is poorly differentiated or when local invasion is present in the primary tumor (Thomas et al. 2001). Whereas aggressive behavior has not occurred in young infants, there are reports of such behavior in older children. Because orchiectomy cures most of these patients, RPLND and adjuvant therapy are probably not appropriate in the absence of radiographic evidence of metastatic disease. However, given the uncertainty, postoperative evaluation and follow-up for the development of metastatic disease seem prudent.

## 23.6 Gonadoblastoma

Gonadoblastomas contain both germ cells and stromal cells. Usually, three distinct elements are present: large germ cells resembling seminoma, sex cord nongerminal elements such as Sertoli or granulosa cells, and stromal elements such as Leydig cells (Rutgers and Scully 1987). Gonadoblastomas occur more frequently in postpubertal patients, but they may be seen in childhood. Gonadoblastoma occurs almost exclusively in dysgenetic gonads, usually in association with a disorder of sexual development. Gonadoblastoma is more likely to occur in dysgenetic gonads occurring in patients with a Y chromosome or evidence of some Y chromatin. Gonadoblastomas occur in 3% of patients with true hermaphroditism, and 10–30% of patients with mixed gonadal dysgenesis or pure gonadal dysgenesis and an XY karyotype (Savage and Lowe 1990; Ramani et al. 1993). They also occur commonly in the dysgenetic testis syndrome.

Gonadoblastomas are usually asymptomatic – often detected incidentally when dysgenetic gonads are removed. However, virilization has been associated with some of these tumors. Forty percent of gonadoblastomas are bilateral (Savage and Lowe 1990). Whereas gonadoblastomas are benign, overgrowth of the germinal components leading to a dysgerminoma (or seminoma) occurs in as many as 50% of cases (Ramani et al. 1993). Approximately 10% of patients develop overtly malignant tumors. Whereas most invasive tumors associated with disorders of sexual development occur in young adulthood, there are several reports in children as well (Ramani et al. 1993). Intraepithelial germ cell neoplasia may be identified in many of these gonads and is associated with germ cell tumors.

Gonadoblastomas are treated by orchiectomy. Indeed, any dysgenetic gonad in a child with a Y chromosome should be removed prophylactically in infancy or early childhood. Tumors are much less likely in patients who lack a Y chromosome such as those with Turner's syndrome or XX patients with pure gonadal dysgenesis. When malignant degeneration is present, a metastatic evaluation and appropriate follow-up are indicated. Fortunately, these tumors are radiosensitive and have a favorable prognosis. However, if unfavorable elements such as choriocarcinoma or embryonal carcinoma are present, the outlook is poor.

## References


Brewer J, Tank E (1993) Yolk sac tumors and alpha-fetoprotein in first year of life. Urology 42:79

Connolly JA, Gearhart JP (1993) Management of yolk sac tumors in children. Urol Clin North Am 20:7

Coppes MJ, Rackley R, Kay R (1994) Primary testicular and paratesticular tumors of childhood. Med Pediatr Oncol 22:329

Cortez JC, Kaplan GW (1993) Gonadal stromal tumors, gonadoblastomas, epidermoid cysts, and secondary tumors of the testis in children. Urol Clin North Am 20:15

Cushing B, Giller R, Cullen JW et al (2004) Randomized comparison of combination chemotherapy with etoposide, bleomycin, and either high-dose or standard-dose cisplatin in children and adolescents with high-risk malignant germ cell tumors: a pediatric intergroup study–Pediatric Oncology Group 9049 and Children's Cancer Group 888. J Clin Oncol 22:2691

Fernandes E, Etcubanas E, Rao B et al (1989) Two decades of experience with testicular tumors in children at St. Jude Children's Research Hospital. J Pediatr Surg 24:677

Grady R, Ross JH, Kay R (1994) Patterns of metastatic spread in prepubertal yolk sac tumor of the testis. J Urol 153:1259

Grady R, Ross JH, Kay R (1997) Epidemiologic features of teratomas of the testis in a prepubertal population. J Urol 158:1191

Green DM (1983) The diagnosis and treatment of yolk sac tumors in infants and children. Cancer Treat Rev 10:265

Haas RJ, Schmidt P, Gobel U, Harms D (1999) Testicular germ cell tumors an update – results of the German Cooperative Studies 1982-1997. Klinische Padiatrie 211:300

Kolon TF, Hochman HI (1997) Malignant Sertoli cell tumor in a prepubescent boy. J Urol 158:608

Kratzer SS, Ulbright TM, Talerman A et al (1997) Large cell calcifying Sertoli cell tumor of the testis. Am J Surg Pathol 21:171

Leonard M, Jeffs R, Leventhal B et al (1991) Pediatric testicular tumors: the Johns Hopkins experience. Urology 37:253

Lo Curto M, Lumia F, Alaggio R et al (2003) Malignant germ cell tumors in childhood: results of the first Italian cooperative study "TCG 91". Med Pediatr Oncol 41:417

Mann JR, Raafat F, Robinson K et al (2000) The United Kingdom Children's Cancer Study Group's second germ cell tumor study: carboplatin, etoposide, and bleomycin are effective treatment for children with malignant extracranial germ cell tumors, with acceptable toxicity. J Clin Oncol 18:3809

Patel AS, Coley BD, Jayanthi VR (2007) Ultrasonography underestimates the volume of normal parenchyma in benign testicular masses. J Urol 178:1730–1732

Pohl HG, Shukla AR, Metcalf PD et al (2004) Prepubertal testis tumors: actual prevalence rate of histological types. J Urol 172:2370

Ramani P, Yeung CK, Habeebu SSM (1993) Testicular intratubular germ cell neoplasia in children and adolescents with intersex. Am J Surg Pathol 17:1124

Rogers PC, Olson TA, Cullen JW et al (2004) Treatment of children and adolescents with stage II testicular and stages I and II ovarian malignant germ cell tumors: a Pediatric Intergroup Study–Pediatric Oncology Group 9048 and Children's Cancer Group 8891. J Clin Oncol 22:3563

Ross JH, Rybicki L, Kay R (2002) Clinical behavior and a contemporary management algorithm for prepubertal testis tumors: a summary of the Prepubertal Testis Tumor Registry. J Urol 168:1675

Rutgers JL, Scully RE (1987) Pathology of the testis in intersex syndromes. Semin Diagn Pathol 4:275

Savage MO, Lowe DG (1990) Gonadal neoplasia and abnormal sexual differentiation. Clin Endocrinol 32:519

Schlatter M, Rescorla F, Giller R et al (2003) Excellent outcome in patients with stage I germ cell tumors of the testes: a study of the Children's Cancer Group/Pediatric Oncology Group. J Pediatr Surg 38:319

Thomas JC, Ross JH, Kay R (2001) Stromal testis tumors in children: a report from the prepubertal testis tumor registry. J Urol 166:2338

Uehling DT, Phillips E (1994) Residual retroperitoneal mass following chemotherapy for infantile yolk sac tumor. J Urol 152:185

Ulbright TM (2004) Gonadal teratomas: a review and speculation. Adv Anat Pathol 11:10–23

Valla JS (2001) Testis-sparing surgery for benign testicular tumors in children. J Urol 165:2280

Washecka R, Dresner MI, Honda SA (2002) Testicular tumors in Carney's complex. J Urol 167:1299

Young RH, Koelliker DD, Scully RE (1998) Sertoli cell tumors of the testis, not otherwise specified: a clinicopathologic analysis of 60 cases. Am J Surg Pathol 22:709

# 24 Primary Non-Germ Cell Tumors of the Testis

Walter Albrecht and John P. Stein

## 24.1 Background

Testicular stromal tumors in adults are rare and account for only 2–4% of testicular tumors. The Testicular Cancer Working Group of the European Association of Urology (EAU) has included these tumors into the EAU Germ Cell Tumour Guidelines (Albers et al. 2006). This paper presents the to-date management of testicular stromal tumors.

Only about 800 cases are published, the majority are Leydig cell and Sertoli cell tumors. Because of their metastatic ability and associated hormonal disorders, these two are of clinical relevance.

Stromal tumors arise in the supportive and hormone-producing tissues of the testicles.

Leydig cell tumors develop from normal hormone-producing interstitial cells of the testicle. Sertoli cell tumors develop from Sertoli cells, which support and nourish the sperm-producing germ cells.

## 24.2 Methods

A Medline search for Leydig cell tumors (synonym: interstitial cell tumor) and Sertoli cell tumors (synonym: androblastoma) was performed. Pure laboratory work without clinical data, female and pediatric tumors and animal cases, double publications, and papers with unclear histology or missing data on clinical course were excluded. The majority of the remaining publications are case reports, with only a few papers reporting series of more than 10 cases, most of them published in the pathology literature. The true incidence of stromal tumors remains therefore uncertain and the proportion of metastatic tumors can only be given approximately.

The individual publications have been rated according to evidence-based medicine (EBM) categories.

Nevertheless, the symptoms for preoperative suspicion of testicular stromal tumors and the characteristics of tumors at high risk for metastases are sufficiently well established (EBM IIA and EBM IIB) to enable recommendations to be made regarding diagnosis and surgical approach.

## 24.3 Pathology and Classification

The non-germ cell tumors of the testicle include the sex cord/gonadal stromal tumors and the miscellaneous nonspecific stromal tumors.

The different histological subtypes of testicular tumors are defined according to the WHO classification 2004 (adapted) (WHO 2004).

Sex cord/gonadal stromal tumors

- Leydig cell tumor
- Malignant Leydig cell tumor
- Sertoli cell tumor
  - NOS – general
  - Sclerosing
  - Large cell calcifying
- Malignant Sertoli cell tumor
- Granulosa cell tumor
  - Adult type
  - Juvenile type

W. Albrecht
Urology Department, Landesklinikum
Weinviertel Mistelbach, Austria

M.P. Laguna et al. (eds.), *Cancer of the Testis*,
DOI: 10.1007/978-1-84800-370-5_24, 

- Thecoma/fibroma group of tumors
- Other sex cord/gonadal stromal tumors
  - Incompletely differentiated
  - Mixed
- Tumors containing germ cell and sex cord/gonadal stromal (gonadoblastoma)

Miscellaneous nonspecific stromal tumors

- Ovarian epithelial tumors
- Tumors of the collecting ducts and rete testis
- Tumors (benign and malignant) of nonspecific stroma

## 24.4 Leydig Cell Tumors

### 24.4.1 Clinical Data

The literature research on Leydig cell tumors resulted in 515 tumors in adults, including three publications (Cheville et al. 1998; Kim et al. 1985; Matveev and Gurarii 1997) reporting larger series on a total of 90 patients. Follow-up data of more than 2 years are available for about 95 patients.

### 24.4.2 Epidemiology

Leydig cell tumors constitute about 1–3% of adult testicular tumors (Kim et al. 1985; Ulbright et al. 1999) and 3% of testicular tumors in infants and children (Ulbright et al. 1999). The tumor is most common in the third to sixth decade in adults with a similar incidence observed in every decade. Another peak incidence is seen in children between 3 and 9 years. Three percent of Leydig cell tumors are bilateral (Kim et al. 1985). Occasionally, they occur in patients with Klinefelter's syndrome (Ulbright et al. 1999).

### 24.4.3 Pathology of Leydig Cell Tumors

Leydig cell tumors are the most common type of sex cord/gonadal stromal tumors. Histopathologically, they are well outlined and usually up to 5 cm in diameter. They are also solid, colored yellow to tan, with hemorrhage and/or necrosis present in 30% of cases. Microscopically, the cells are polygonal, with eosinophilic cytoplasm with occasional Reinke crystals, regular nucleus, solid arrangement, and capillary stroma. The cells express vimentin, inhibin, protein S100, steroid hormones, calretinin, and cytokeratin (focally) (WHO 2004).

About 10% of Leydig cell tumors are malignant tumors, generally in older patients without endocrine symptoms (Kim et al. 1985), which present with the following parameters:

- Large size (>5 cm)
- Cytologic atypia
- Increased mitotic activity (>3 per 10 high-power field [HPF])
- Increased MIB-1 expression (18.6 vs. 1.2% in benign) (Cheville et al. 1998)
- Necrosis
- Vascular invasion (Cheville et al. 1998)
- Infiltrative margins
- Extension beyond the testicular parenchyma
- p53 overexpression (McCluggage et al. 1998)
- DNA aneuploidy (Cheville et al. 1998; McCluggage et al. 1998)
- Older patients

### 24.4.4 Diagnosis

Either patients present with a painless enlarged testis or the tumor is an incidental ultrasound finding. In up to 80%, hormonal disorders with high estrogen and estradiol levels and low testosterone, as well as increased levels of luteinising hormone (LH) and follicle-stimulating hormone (FSH) are reported (Mineur et al. 1987; Reznik et al. 1993), while negative results are always obtained for the testicular germ cell tumor markers, alpha-fetoprotein (AFP), β-human chorionic gonadotrophin (β-HCG), lactate dehydrogenase (LDH), and placental alkaline phosphatase (PLAP). Sperm abnormalities are not infrequent (Haddad et al. 2005). Approximately 30% of patients present with gynaecomastia (Bercovici et al. 1984; Haas et al. 1989) and 3% of tumors are bilateral (Kim et al. 1985).

Leydig cell tumors must be distinguished from the multinodular tumor-like and often bilaterally occurring lesions of the androgenital syndrome (Ruthgers et al. 1988). Diagnostic work-up must include markers, hormones (at least testosterone, LH, and FSH; if not conclusive, additionally estrogen, oestradiol, progesterone, and cortisol), ultrasound of both testes, and CT scan of chest and abdomen.

On ultrasound, it may be possible to observe well-defined, small, hypoechoic lesions with hypervascularization, but the appearance is variable and is indistinguishable from germ cell tumors (Maizlin et al. 2004; Ponce de Leon Roca et al. 2000).

The proportion of metastatic tumors in all published case reports is only 10%. Within three larger series with longer follow-up, 18 metastatic tumors were found in a total of 83 cases (21.7%) (Cheville et al. 1998; Kim et al. 1985; Matveev and Gurarii 1997). Histopathological signs of malignancy have been listed above (Cheville et al. 1998; McCluggage et al. 1998). In addition, patients of older age have a greater risk of harboring a tumor of malignant potential.

## 24.5 Sertoli Cell Tumor

### *24.5.1 Clinical Data*

The literature research for clinical data on Sertoli cell tumors resulted in 265 tumors in adults, including three publications (from the same group) (Young et al. 1998; Proppe and Scully 1980; Zukerberg et al. 1991) reporting on a total of 80 patients. Follow-up data of more than 2 years are available in less than 40 patients.

### *24.5.2 Epidemiology*

Sertoli cell tumors account for less than 1% of testicular tumors; the mean age at diagnosis is around 45 years with rare cases under the age of 20 (Young et al. 1998; Giglio et al. 2003). On rare occasions, these tumors may develop in patients with the androgen insensitivity syndrome and Peutz–Jeghers syndrome.

### *24.5.3 Pathology of Sertoli Cell Tumors*

The tumor is well circumscribed, yellow, tan, or white, with an average diameter of 3.5 cm (Young et al. 1998). Microscopically, the cells are eosinophilic to pale with vacuolated cytoplasm due to lipids that in some cases acquire a lipoid-rich aspect. The nuclei are regular with grooves and there may be inclusions. The arrangement of the cells is tubular or solid; a cord-like or retiform pattern is possible. The stroma is fine and capillary, but in some cases a sclerosing aspect predominates. The cells express vimentin, cytokeratins, inhibin (40%), and protein S-100 (30%) (Young et al. 1998).

The Large cell calcifying Sertoli cell tumor can be sporadic (unilateral and unifocal) or associated with dysplastic syndromes as Peutz–Jeghers syndrome (bilateral and multifical) (Proppe and Scully 1980; Plata et al. 1995). Its characteristic microscopic aspect is a hyalinized stroma with broad areas of calcification. The tumoral cells are eosinophilic with prominent nucleoli with rare mitosis.

The sclerosing Sertoli cell tumor is very infrequent with small tubules of bland cells and entrapped non-neoplastic tubules (Zukerberg et al. 1991; Anderson 1995).

The rate of malignant tumors ranges between 10 and 22% and less than 50 cases are reported (Jacobsen 1993; Kratzer et al. 1997; Henley et al. 2002).

Signs of a malignant Sertoli tumor are as follows:

- Large size (>5 cm)
- Pleomorphic nuclei with nucleoli
- Increased mitotic activity (>5 per 10 HPF)
- Necrosis
- Vascular invasion

### *24.5.4 Diagnosis*

Either patients present with an enlarged testis or the tumor is an incidental ultrasound finding (Grabrilove et al. 1980). Most classic Sertoli tumors are unilateral and unifocal. Hormonal disorders are infrequent, although gynaecomastia is sometimes seen (Young et al. 1998). The testicular tumor-markers, AFP, β-HCG, LDH, and PLAP are always negative.

Diagnostic work-up has to include tumor markers, hormones (at least testosterone, LH, and FSH; if not conclusive, additionally estrogen, oestradiol, progesterone, and cortisol), ultrasound of both testes, and CT scan of chest and abdomen.

Sertoli cell tumors are generally hypoechoic on ultrasound but they can be of variant appearance and therefore cannot be safely distinguished from germ cell tumors (Giglio et al. 2003). Only the large cell calcifying form has a characteristic image with brightly echogenic foci due to calcification (Gierke et al. 1994; Chang et al. 1998).

The large cell calcifying form is diagnosed in younger men and is associated with genetic syndromes (Carney's complex (Washecka et al. 2002) and Peutz–Jeghers syndrome (Young et al. 1995)) or, in about 40% of cases, endocrine disorders. Forty-four percent are bilateral, either synchronous or metachronous, and 28% show multifocality (Kratzer et al. 1997).

The characteristics of metastatic tumors have been depicted above (Jacobsen 1993; Kratzer et al. 1997; Henley et al. 2002). However, among patients whose tumors have been histopathologically classified as "malignant" using these or similar characteristics (i.e., 18.8% of tumors in all reported cases), only 7% showed metastatic disease during follow-up. In the largest series with the longest follow-up, tumors of 7.5% of patients had been classified as "malignant" at primary diagnosis and 11.7% showed metastatic disease long-term (Young et al. 1998). In general, affected patients are of higher age, and tumors are nearly always palpable and show more than one sign of malignancy (Young et al. 1998).

Up to 20% of the large cell calcifying form tumors are malignant. There are some hints that discrimination between an early and late onset type may define a different risk for metastatic disease (5.5% compared with 23%) (Giglio et al. 2003). Metastases in the infrequent sclerosing subtype are rare.

## 24.6 Granulosa Cell Tumor

This is a rare tumor, with two variants – juvenile and adult.

The juvenile type is benign. It is the most frequent congenital testicle tumor and represents 6.6% of all prepuberal testicular neoplasms. The cystic appearance is characteristic of this tumor type (Kaplan et al. 1986).

With the adult type, the average age at presentation is 44 years. The typical morphology is of a homogeneous, yellow–gray tumor with elongated cells, and with grooves in micro-follicular and Call–Exner bodies' arrangement.

Malignant tumors represent around 20% of cases. They are usually >7 cm diameter.

Vascular invasion and necrosis are features suggestive of malignant biology (Al-Bozom et al. 2000).

## 24.7 Thecoma/Fibroma Group of Tumors

These tumors are very rare and benign (WHO 2004).

## 24.8 Other Sex Cord/Gonadal Stromal Tumors

Sex cord/gonadal stromal tumors may be incompletely differentiated or mixed forms.

There is limited experience with incompletely differentiated sex cord/gonadal stromal tumors and there are no cases of reported metastasis (WHO 2004). In mixed tumor forms, all the histological components should be reported.

However, the clinical behavior is most likely to reflect the predominant pattern or the most aggressive component of the tumor (Perito et al. 1992).

## 24.9 Tumors Containing Germ Cell and Sex Cord/Gonadal Stromal (Gonadoblastoma)

If the arrangement of the germ cells are in nested pattern and the rest of the tumor is composed of sex cord/gonadal stroma, the term gonadoblastoma is used. It is most frequent in gonadal dysgenesis with ambiguous genitalia. Bilateral tumors are present in 40% of cases. The prognosis is correlated with the invasive growth of the germinal component (Scully 1970).

In case of a diffuse arrangement of the different components, there are some doubts about the neoplastic nature of the germinal cells and some authors consider them to be entrapped rather than neoplastic (Ulbright et al. 2000).

## 24.10 Miscellaneous Tumors of the Testis

### 24.10.1 Tumors of Ovarian Epithelial Types

These tumors resemble the epithelial tumors of the ovary. Cystic appearance with occasional mucinous material can be observed. Microscopically, the aspect is identical to their ovarian counterparts and their evolution is similar to the different epithelial ovarian subtypes. Some Brenner types can be malignant (WHO 2004).

### 24.10.2 Tumors of the Collecting Ducts and Rete Testis

These tumors are very rare. Benign (adenoma) and malignant (adenocarcinoma) tumors have been reported, with malignant tumors showing local growth with a mortality rate of more than 50%.

### 24.10.3 Tumors (Benign and Malignant) of Nonspecific Stroma

These are very uncommon and have similar criteria, prognosis, and treatment as the soft tissue sarcomas.

## 24.11 Treatment

Testicular tumors of small volume, otherwise asymptomatic, are often misinterpreted as germ cell tumors and inguinal orchie ctomy is performed. It is highly recommended to perform an organ-sparing procedure in every small intraparenchymal lesion to gain the histological diagnosis. Especially in patients with symptoms of gynaecomastia, hormonal disorders, or typical imaging on ultrasound (calcifications, small circumscribed tumors), a nongerm-cell tumor should be considered and immediate orchiectomy should be avoided (Wegner et al. 1997). In cases of germ cell tumor in either frozen section or paraffin histology, orchiectomy is recommended as long as a contralateral normal testicle is present. Secondary orchiectomy can be performed, if final pathology reveals a nonstromal (e.g., germ cell) tumor. Organ-sparing surgical approaches in a center with experience are justified as long as the remaining testicular parenchyma is sufficient for endocrine (and in stromal tumors also exocrine) function (Heidenreich et al. 1997).

In tumors with histological signs of malignancy, especially in patients of older age, orchiectomy and retroperitoneal lymphadenectomy are recommended to prevent metastases (Mosharafa et al. 2003). Tumors metastasizing to lymph nodes, lung, or bone respond poorly to chemotherapy or radiation and survival is poor.

## 24.12 Follow-Up

Recommendations for appropriate follow-up cannot be given in general because of the lack of follow-up data in most reported cases and the lethal outcome of metastatic tumors, irrespective of the therapy chosen. In the absence of signs of malignancy, an individualized surveillance strategy after orchiectomy is recommended (CT scans may be most appropriate as specific tumor-markers are not available). In cases with preoperative hormonal disorders, the affected tests should be monitored during follow-up for possible signs of recurrence (Maeda et al. 2002).

## References

Albers P, Albrecht W, Algaba F, Bokemeyer C, Cohn-Cedemark G, Fizazi K, Horwich A, Laguna MP and the Testicular Tumor Working Group of the EAU. Guidelines on testicular tumors (2010). European Association of Urology Guidelines; ISBN 978-90-79754-70-0

Al-Bozom IA, El-Faqih SR, Hassan SH, El-Tiraifi AE, Talic RF (2000) Granulosa cell tumour of the adult type. A case report and review of the literature of a very rare testicular tumour. Arch Pathol Lab Med 124:1525–1528. EBM III

Anderson GA (1995) Sclerosing Sertoli cell tumour of the testis: a distinct histological subtype. J Urol 154:1756–1758, review. EBM III

Bercovici JP, Nahoul K, Tater D, Charles JF, Scholler R (1984) Hormonal profile of Leydig cell tumours with gynecomastia. J Clin Endocrinol Metab 59:625–630. EBM III

Chang B, Borer JG, Tan PE, Diamond DA (1998) Large-cell calcifying Sertoli cell tumour of the testis: case report and review of the literature. Urology 52:520–522. EBM III

Cheville JC, Sebo TJ, Lager DJ, Bostwick DG, Farrow GM (1998) Leydig cell tumour of the testis: a clinicopathologic, DNA content, and MIB-1 comparison of nonmetastasizing and metastasizing tumours. Am J Surg Pathol 22:1361–1367. EBM IIA

Gierke CL, King BF, Bostwick DG, Choyke PL, Hattery RR (1994) Large-cell calcifying Sertoli cell tumour of the testis: appearance at sonography. AJR Am J Roentgenol 163:373–375. EBM III

Giglio M, Medica M, De Rose AF, Germinale F, Ravetti JL, Carmignani G (2003) Testicular Sertoli cell tumours and relative sub-types. Analysis of clinical and prognostic features. Urol Int 70:205–210, review. EBM III

Grabrilove JL, Freiberg EK, Leiter E, Nicolis GL (1980) Feminizing and non-feminizing Sertoli cell tumour. J Urol 124:757–767

Haas GP, Pittaluga S, Gomella L, Travis WD, Sherins RJ, Doppman JL, Linehan WL, Robertson C (1989) Clinical occult Leydig cell tumour presenting with gynecomastia. J Urol 142:1325–1327. EBM III

Haddad O, Leroy X, Lemaitre L, Biserte J, Rigot JM (2005) [Infertility and testicular tumour based on a series of 25 patients]. Prog Urol 15:1096–1100 (French). PMID: 16429659

Heidenreich A, Holtl W, Albrecht W, Pont J, Engelmann UH (1997) Testis preserving surgery in bilateral testicular germ cell tumors. Br J Urol 79:253–257. EBM IIb

Henley JD, Young RH, Ulbright TM (2002) Malignant Sertoli cell tumours of the testis: a study of 13 examples of a neoplasm frequently misinterpreted as seminoma. Am J Surg Pathol 26:541–550. EBM III

Jacobsen GK (1993) Malignant Sertoli cell tumours of the testis. J Urol Pathol 1:233–255. EBM III

Kaplan GW, Cromie WJ, Kelalis PP, Silber I, Tank ES Jr (1986) Gonadal stromal tumours: a report of the prepuberal testicular tumours registry. J Urol 136:300–302. EBM III

Kim I, Young RH, Scully RE (1985) Leydig cell tumours of the testis. A clinicopathological analysis of 40 cases and review of the literature. Am J Surg Pathol 9:177–192. EBM III

Kratzer SS, Ulbright TM, Talerman A, Srigley JR, Roth LM, Wahle GR, Moussa M, Stephens JK, Millos A, Young RH (1997) Large cell calcifying Sertoli cell tumour of the testis: contrasting features of six malignant and six benign tumours and a review of the literature. Am J Surg Pathol 21:1271–1280. EBM III

Maeda T, Itoh N, Kobayashi K, Takahashi A, Masumori N, Tsukamoto T (2002) Elevated serum estradiol suggesting recurrence of Leydig cell tumor nine years after radical orchiectomy. Int J Urol 9:659–661. EBM III

Maizlin ZV, Belenky A, Kunichezky M, Sandbank J, Strauss S (2004) Leydig cell tumours of the testis: gray scale and color Doppler sonographic appearance. J Ultrasound Med 23:959–964. EBM III

Matveev BP, Gurarii LL (1997) [Leydig-cell tumours of the testis]. Urol Nefrol (Mosk) (4)34–36. (Russian) EBM III

McCluggage WG, Shanks JH, Arthur K, Banerjee SS (1998) Cellular proliferation and nuclear ploidy assessments augment established prognostic factors in predicting malignancy in testicular Leydig cell tumours. Histopathology 33:361–368. EBM III

Mineur P, de Cooman S, Hustin J, Verhoeven G, de Hertogh E (1987) Feminizing testicular Leydig cell tumour: hormonal profile before and after unilateral orchidectomy. J Clin Endocrinol Metab 64:686–691. EBM IIB

Mosharafa AA, Foster RS, Bihrle R, Koch MO, Ulbright TM, Einhorn LH, Donohue JP (2003) Does retroperitoneal lymph node dissection have a curative role for patients with sex cord-stromal testicular tumours? Cancer 98:753–757. EBM III

Perito PE, Ciancio G, Civantos F, Politano VA (1992) Sertoli-Leydig cell testicular tumour. case report and review of sex cord/gonadal stromal tumour histogenesis. J Urol 148:883–885. EBM III

Plata C, Algaba F, Andujar M, Nistal M, Stocks P, Martinez JL, Nogales FF (1995) Large cell calcifying Sertoli cell tumour of the testis. Histopathology 26:255–259. EBM III

Ponce de Leon Roca J, Algaba Arrea F, Bassas Arnau L, Villavicencio Mavrich H (2000) [Leydig-cell tumours of the testis]. Arch Esp Urol 53:453–458. (Spanish) EBM III

Proppe KH, Scully RE (1980) Large-cell calcifying Sertoli cell tumour of the testis. Am J Clin Pathol 74:607–619. EMB III

Reznik Y, Rieu M, Kuhn JM, Mandard JC, Bottet P, Lemonnier D, Bekka S, Mahoudeau J (1993) Luteinizing hormone regulation by sex steroids in men with germinal and Leydig cell tumours. Clin Endocrinol (Oxf) 38:487–493. EBM IIB

Ruthgers JL, Young RH, Scully RE (1988) The testicular "tumour" of the adrenogenital syndrome. A report of six cases and review of the literature on testicular masses in patients with adrenocortical disorders. Am J Surg Pathol 12:503–513. EBM III

Scully RE (1970) Gonadoblastoma. A review of 74 cases. Cancer 25:1340–1356. EBM III

Ulbright TM, Amin MB, Young RH (1999) Tumours of the testis, adnexia, spermatic cord and scrotum. AFIP 1999. EBM III

Ulbright TM, Srigley JR, Reuter VE, Wojno K, Roth LM, Young RH (2000) Sex-cord-stromal tumours of the testis with entrapped germ cells: a lesion mimicking unclassified mixed germ cell sex cord-stromal tumours. Am J Surg Pathol 24:535–542. EBM III

Washecka R, Dresner MI, Honda SA (2002) Testicular tumours in Carney's complex. J Urol 167:1299–1302. EBM III

Wegner HE, Dieckmann KP, Herbst H, Andresen R, Miller K (1997) Leydig cell tumour – comparison of results of radical and testis sparing surgery in a single center. Urol Int 59:170–173. EBM IIB

WHO (2004) WHO histological classification of testis tumours. In: Eble JN, Sauter G, Epstein JI, Sesterhenn IA (eds) Pathology & genetics. Tumours of the urinary system and male genital organs. IARC Press, Lyon, p 218, 250–262. EBM III

Young S, Gooneratne S, Straus FH, Zeller WP, Bulun SE, Rosenthal IM (1995) Feminizing Sertoloi cell tumours in boys with Peutz–Jeghers syndrome. Am J Surg Pathol 19:50–58. EBM III

Young RH, Koelliker DD, Scully RE (1998) Sertoli cell tumours of the testis, not otherwise specified: a clinicopathologic analysis of 60 cases. Am J Surg Pathol 22:709–721. EMB III

Zukerberg LR, Young RH, Scully RE (1991) Sclerosing Sertoli cell tumour of the testis. A report of 10 cases. Am J Surg Pathol 15:829–834. EMB III

# Index

**D**

MIX
Papier aus verantwortungsvollen Quellen
Paper from responsible sources
FSC® C105338

If you have any concerns about our products,
you can contact us on
**ProductSafety@springernature.com**

In case Publisher is established outside the EU,
the EU authorized representative is:
**Springer Nature Customer Service Center GmbH**
**Europaplatz 3, 69115 Heidelberg, Germany**

Printed by Libri Plureos GmbH
in Hamburg, Germany